Coding for Pediatrics 2021

A MANUAL FOR PEDIATRIC DOCUMENTATION AND PAYMENT

For Use With AMA *CPT* 2021

26th EDITION

Author
Committee on Coding and Nomenclature (COCN)
American Academy of Pediatrics
Linda D. Parsi, MD, MBA, CPEDC, FAAP, Editor
Cindy Hughes, CPC, CFPC, Consulting Editor
Becky Dolan, MPH, CPC, CPEDC, Staff Editor

American Academy of Pediatrics
DEDICATED TO THE HEALTH OF ALL CHILDREN®

American Academy of Pediatrics Publishing Staff

Mary Lou White, *Chief Product and Services Officer/SVP, Membership, Marketing, and Publishing*

Mark Grimes, *Vice President, Publishing*

Mary Kelly, *Senior Editor, Professional/Clinical Publishing*

Laura Underhile, *Editor, Professional/Clinical Publishing*

Meghan Corey, *Editorial Assistant*

Jason Crase, *Senior Manager, Production and Editorial Services*

Leesa Levin-Doroba, *Production Manager, Practice Management*

Peg Mulcahy, *Manager, Art Direction and Production*

Maryjo Reynolds, *Marketing Manager, Practice Publications*

Published by the American Academy of Pediatrics
345 Park Blvd
Itasca, IL 60143
Telephone: 630/626-6000
Facsimile: 847/434-8000
www.aap.org

The American Academy of Pediatrics is an organization of 67,000 primary care pediatricians, pediatric medical subspecialists, and pediatric surgical specialists dedicated to the health, safety, and well-being of infants, children, adolescents, and young adults.

While every effort has been made to ensure the accuracy of this publication, the American Academy of Pediatrics (AAP) does not guarantee that it is accurate, complete, or without error.

The recommendations in this publication do not indicate an exclusive course of treatment or serve as a standard of medical care. Variations, taking into account individual circumstances, may be appropriate. Vignettes are provided to illustrate correct coding applications and are not intended to offer advice on the practice of medicine.

Any websites, brand names, products, or manufacturers are mentioned for informational and identification purposes only and do not imply an endorsement by the American Academy of Pediatrics (AAP). The AAP is not responsible for the content of external resources. Information was current at the time of publication.

This publication has been developed by the American Academy of Pediatrics. The contributors are expert authorities in the field of pediatrics. No commercial involvement of any kind has been solicited or accepted in development of the content of this publication. Disclosures: Ms Arnold disclosed a consulting relationship with Thermo Fisher Scientific. Dr Lago disclosed an employee relationship with Cotiviti, Inc. Dr Parsi disclosed an ownership and consulting relationship with The PEDS MD Company.

Please visit www.aap.org/cfp for an up-to-date list of any applicable errata for this publication.

Special discounts are available for bulk purchases of this publication. Email Special Sales at aapsales@aap.org for more information.

Printed in the United States of America

CPT copyright 2020 American Medical Association (AMA). All rights reserved.

Fee schedules, relative value units, conversion factors, and/or related components are not assigned by the AMA, are not part of *CPT*, and the AMA is not recommending their use. The AMA does not directly or indirectly practice medicine or dispense medical services. The AMA assumes no liability for data contained or not contained herein.

CPT is a registered trademark of the AMA.

This publication has prior approval of the American Academy of Professional Coders (AAPC) for 4.0 continuing education units. Granting of this approval in no way constitutes endorsement by AAPC of the publication content or publication sponsor.

11-35Q   1 2 3 4 5 6 7 8 9 10

MA0988
ISBN: 978-1-61002-446-4
eBook: 978-1-61002-447-1
ISSN: 1537-324X

Disclaimer

Every effort has been made to include the new and revised 2021 *Current Procedural Terminology* (CPT®); *International Classification of Diseases, 10th Revision, Clinical Modification (ICD-10-CM)*; and Healthcare Common Procedure Coding System (HCPCS) codes, their respective guidelines, and other revisions that might have been made. Due to our publishing deadlines and the publication date of the American Medical Association *CPT,* additional revisions and/or additional codes may have been published subsequent to the date of this printing. It is the responsibility of the reader to use this manual as a companion to the *CPT, ICD-10-CM,* and HCPCS publications. Vignettes are provided throughout this publication to illustrate correct coding applications. They are not intended to offer medical advice on the practice of medicine. Further, it is the reader's responsibility to access the American Academy of Pediatrics website (www.aap.org/cfp) routinely to find any corrections due to errata in the published version. At the time of publication, *CPT* and the Centers for Medicare & Medicaid Services were in conflict with regard to when prolonged services (**99417**) begin. We have presented the timing from *CPT* as part of this publication. For more information or to check for a resolution, please visit www.aap.org/coding.

Copyright Acknowledgment

Current Procedural Terminology (CPT®) is a listing of descriptive terms and 5-digit numeric identifying codes and modifiers for reporting medical services and procedures performed by physicians. This presentation includes only the *CPT* descriptive terms, numeric identifying codes, and modifiers for reporting medical services and procedures that were selected by the American Academy of Pediatrics (AAP) for inclusion in this publication. The inclusion of a *CPT* service or procedure description and its code number in this publication does not restrict its use to a particular specialty group. Any procedure or service in this publication may be used to report the services provided by any qualified physician or, when appropriate, other qualified health care professional.

The American Medical Association (AMA) and the AAP assume no responsibility for the consequences attributable to or related to any use or interpretation of any information or views contained in or not contained in this publication.

Any 5-digit numeric *CPT* code, service descriptions, instructions, and/or guidelines are copyright 2020 (or such other date of publication of *CPT* as defined in the federal copyright laws) AMA. All rights reserved.

The most current *CPT* is available from the AMA.

No fee schedules, basic unit values, relative value guides, conversion factors or scales, or components thereof are included in *CPT.*

Contents

This publication has prior approval of the American Academy of Professional Coders (AAPC) for 4.0 continuing education units (CEUs). Granting of this approval in no way constitutes endorsement by the AAPC of the publication, content, or publication sponsor. To earn your CEUs, complete the 40-question quiz online (www.aap.org/cfp). Click on "2021 Coding for Pediatrics Quiz." A passcode will be required; enter AAPCFP26.

The following online-exclusive content can be accessed at www.aap.org/cfp, access code AAPCFP26:
- AAP Position on Medicare Consultation Policy
- Care Plan Oversight Billing Worksheet Template
- Chronic Care Management Tracking Worksheet
- Commonly Administered Pediatric Vaccine Updates
- Evaluation and Management Key Components
- Example Worksheet for Tracking CCM Service Times
- FAQ: Immunization Administration
- General Documentation Checklist
- Medicare Requirements for Incident-to Services by Nonphysician Professionals and Clinical Staff
- Medicare Telemedicine Codes
- Primary Care Exception Rule Guidelines
- Responding to Retrospective Audit and Carrier Take-back
- RUC Survey Times for Hospital Care and Critical Care Services
- Sample Audit Log
- Shared Savings
- Skin Graft Code Descriptors
- Template Letter to Payers That Deny Code 99211 for Evaluation of a TB Skin Test

Foreword

The American Academy of Pediatrics (AAP) is pleased to publish the 26th edition of *Coding for Pediatrics*—an instructional manual and reference tool for use by primary care pediatricians, pediatric subspecialists, and others involved in the provision of care to children. This manual supports the delivery of quality care to children by providing the pediatric practitioner with the knowledge to best support appropriate business practices. This edition includes the 2021 *Current Procedural Terminology (CPT®)* and *International Classification of Diseases, 10th Revision, Clinical Modification (ICD-10-CM)* code changes with guidelines for their application.

Most significantly, this manual provides pediatric-specific guidance to coding for all evaluation and management (E/M) services by providing guidance and examples of documentation and code selection using the 1995 and 1997 E/M documentation guidelines and the new and distinctly different guidelines for office and other outpatient E/M services.

With a focus on creating ease of reference, *Coding for Pediatrics 2021* is divided into the following parts:

- **Part 1: Coding Basics and Business Essentials** includes information on code sets, compliance, and business topics such as billing and payment methodologies.
- **Part 2: Primarily for the Office and Other Outpatient Settings** includes information on coding and billing of services such as office visits, outpatient consultations, and preventive services.
- **Part 3: Primarily for Hospital Settings** includes information on coding for inpatient and observation services, including newborn care and surgical procedures.
- **Part 4: Digital Medicine Services** includes discussion of the evolving codes for reporting telemedicine services, remote monitoring and interpretation, and other services provided via digital technology.
- Quick references to *CPT* and *ICD-10-CM* code changes applicable to pediatrics are provided in Appendixes I and II. A table of pediatric vaccine product codes can be found in Appendix III, and direct supervision and reporting guidelines can be found in Appendix IV.
- A **continuing education quiz** to earn 4.0 continuing education units from the American Academy of Professional Coders is available online at www.aap.org/cfp.
- Supplemental material can be found on the *Coding for Pediatrics* website (www.aap.org/cfp) for a wealth of information, including a documentation checklist and tracking worksheets for care management and care plan oversight services.

Each chapter includes "Test Your Knowledge!" questions (answers can be located in **Appendix V**). Additionally, resources for more information on each chapter's contents can be located at the end of chapter.

As in previous years, the AAP is also pleased to also offer *Coding for Pediatrics 2021* as an eBook.

Coding for Pediatrics 2021 does not replace *CPT, ICD-10-CM,* or the Healthcare Common Procedure Coding System; rather, it supplements those manuals. Every effort has been made to include the 2021 codes and their respective guidelines; however, revised codes and/or guidelines may have been published subsequent to the date of this printing. Errata to this manual will be posted as appropriate on the *Coding for Pediatrics* website (www.aap.org/cfp).

The AAP actively works with the American Medical Association (AMA) *CPT* Editorial Panel and the AMA/Specialty Society Relative Value Scale Update Committee (RUC) to develop pediatric specialty codes and assign them appropriate relative value units. Since 1995, the AAP has contributed to the process that evaluates and reviews changes to the Medicare Resource-Based Relative Value Scale (RBRVS). Pediatricians have been actively involved in the AMA RUC Practice Expense Review Committee to review direct practice expenses for all existing codes. As importantly, the AAP is represented on the AMA *CPT* Editorial Advisory Panel and on the *ICD-10-CM* Editorial Advisory Board. The AAP continues to be involved in all areas of payment. The AAP Committee on Coding and Nomenclature oversees all areas of coding as they relate to pediatrics, including *CPT* procedure coding, *ICD-10-CM* diagnosis coding, and the valuation of *CPT* services through the Medicare RBRVS.

The AAP will continue to request new code changes and attempt to expeditiously notify membership of changes through various means. *AAP Pediatric Coding Newsletter™*—a monthly newsletter available in print and online—provides up-to-date coding and payment information. The newsletter and other online resources can be accessed through the AAP newsletter website (https://coding.aap.org). Other resources include coding seminars presented at the AAP National Conference & Exhibition; webinars sponsored by the AAP (www.aap.org/webinars/coding); instructional materials in *AAP News,* including the Coding Corner; *Pediatric ICD-10-CM: A Manual for Provider-Based Coding; Pediatric Office-Based Evaluation and Management Coding: 2021 Revisions; Pediatric Coding Basics: An Introduction to Medical Coding;* and various quick reference cards. The use of these resources should provide pediatricians with the skills needed to report their services appropriately. The AAP Health Care Financing Strategy staff stands ready to assist with coding problems and questions not covered in this manual. The AAP Coding Hotline can be contacted at https://form.jotform.com/Subspecialty/aapcodinghotline.

During development of this book, multiple new codes and new coding guidelines have been added to *CPT* and *ICD-10-CM* for use in reporting care during the 2019 coronavirus public health emergency. Due to ongoing nature of these changes, the AAP has maintained an up-to-date document detailing the changes at https://downloads.aap.org/AAP/PDF/COVID%202020.pdf.

Acknowledgments

Coding for Pediatrics 2021, 26th Edition, is the product of the efforts of many dedicated individuals.

Our mission is to make coding easier to understand so that pediatric providers can continue to serve children well. We have sought to make this book easier to understand by categorizing care areas and by using many examples (vignettes) of different coding situations. This knowledge is key to helping all pediatric providers stay in compliance and correctly code with confidence. We hope you enjoy reading this book, and we will continue to strive to always serve you with excellence.

This work has been made immeasurably easier and the final edition dramatically improved by the dedicated work of many collaborators. First and foremost, I must thank Cindy Hughes, CPC, CFPC, consulting editor, for her professional input. Additionally, I must thank the Committee on Coding and Nomenclature (COCN) support staff at the American Academy of Pediatrics (AAP), particularly Becky Dolan, MPH, CPC, CPEDC, staff editor, for her many excellent suggestions as well as for reviewing major portions of the project. Thank you also to Teri Salus, MPA, CPC, CPEDC, for her review of new *Current Procedural Terminology* (*CPT*®) codes and suggestions for changes to content. I would also like to thank the members of COCN and the AAP Coding Publications Editorial Advisory Board. The members of these committees have each contributed extensive time in reviewing and updating content of the manual. We want to especially thank the following reviewers:

Margie C. Andreae, MD, FAAP
Cheryl Arnold, MHSA, FACMPE
Greg Barabell, MD, CPC, FAAP
Vita Boyar, MD, FAAP
David M. Kanter, MD, MBA, CPC, FAAP
S. Kalyan Katakam, MD, MPH, FAAP
Steven E. Krug, MD, FAAP
Jamie C. Lago, MD, CPC, FAAP
Edward A. Liechty, MD, FAAP
Jeanne Marconi, MD, FAAP
Richard A. Molteni, MD, FAAP
Renee F. Slade, MD, FAAP
Sanjeev Y. Tuli, MD, FAAP

None of this work is possible without the support of the COCN members who work tirelessly to develop and value codes and fight for pediatrics "at the table." The committee strives to keep pediatrics at the forefront of coding and valuation. The excellent teams listed as follows are truly experts in these areas and are devoted to representing the AAP and its members:

CPT Team
Joel F. Bradley, MD, FAAP (*CPT* Advisor)
Renee F. Slade, MD, FAAP (*CPT* Alternate Advisor)
Teri Salus, MPA, CPC, CPEDC (AAP Staff to *CPT*)

American Medical Association/Specialty Society Relative Value Scale Update Committee (RUC) Team
Steven E. Krug, MD, FAAP (RUC Advisor)
Margie C. Andreae, MD, FAAP (RUC Representative)
Eileen D. Brewer, MD, FAAP (RUC Alternate Representative)
Linda Walsh, MAB (AAP Staff to RUC)

International Classification of Diseases (ICD) Team
Jeffrey F. Linzer Sr, MD, FAAP (AAP Representative to *ICD*)
Edward A. Liechty, MD, FAAP (AAP Alternate Representative to *ICD*)
Becky Dolan, MPH, CPC, CPEDC (AAP Staff to *ICD*)

I am most grateful to the invaluable input of the following AAP committees and individuals: the Committee on Medical Liability and Risk Management, specifically Richard L. Oken, MD, FAAP, and AAP staff Julie Ake, senior health policy analyst; the Private Payer Advocacy Advisory Committee, specifically Sue Kressly, MD, FAAP; Greg Barabell, MD, CPC, FAAP; and AAP staff Lou Terranova, senior health policy analyst; and the Section on Neonatal-Perinatal Medicine coding trainers. In addition, we reached out to other AAP members for their expertise on specific content areas.

This project would not have been completed were it not for the outstanding work of AAP staff. In Membership, Marketing, and Publishing, Mary Kelly, senior editor, professional/clinical publishing; Laura Underhile, editor, professional/clinical publishing; Jason Crase, senior manager, production and editorial services; Peg Mulcahy, manager, art direction and production; Leesa Levin-Doroba, production manager, practice management; and Maryjo Reynolds, marketing manager, practice publications, deserve special recognition for their outstanding skill and dedication to this project. At the AAP, I am especially appreciative of the support and professional expertise of Linda Walsh, MAB, senior manager, healthy policy and coding, and AAP staff support to the AAP COCN, dedicated advocates for all of us who provide medical care to children. A special thank-you to our AAP Board of Directors reviewer, Richard Tuck, MD, FAAP. Dr Tuck is a former COCN member and is an expert on this topic. We are so grateful to have his leadership and review for this manual!

Finally, we all would like to give a big thank-you to all our readers, billers, coders, medical team, and dedicated pediatric providers who work tirelessly around the clock to provide the best care to all children. Your work inspires us to work very hard behind the scenes to provide you the latest and most accurate coding information. By all of us working together, we can accomplish the highest standards of care and be a voice for our children and their future.

Respectfully,
Linda D. Parsi, MD, MBA, CPEDC, FAAP
Editor

How to Use This Manual

Step 1. Use either the Table of Contents or Index to locate information on specific services, codes, or broader subjects.	**Contents** An Introduction to the Official Code Sets 5 Telling the Encounter Story 5
Step 2. Use chapter content to review code descriptors and instructions for reporting. Before reporting, verify current codes and complete selection and reporting instructions in the appropriate code set manual or application.	**99464** Attendance at delivery (when requested by the delivering physician or other qualified health care professional) and initial stabilization of newborn Code **99464** is not reported when hospital-mandated attendance is the only underlying basis for providing the service.
Step 3. Examples are used as guidance on meeting the criteria specified by codes and reporting instructions. However, note that codes must be assigned based on the service provided and supporting documentation.	➤ **The pediatrician administers 3 injections of allergen extract for a patient with allergic rhinitis due to pollen.** The extract was prepared and supplied by an allergist. The pediatrician will report code **95117** with *ICD-10-CM* code **J30.1**.
Step 4. Note key points of information highlighted in each chapter.	If the physician performs the venipuncture as a convenience or because staff is not trained in the procedure, code **36415** is reported because the physician's skill was not required.
Step 5. Resources for additional information are listed at the end of each chapter as well as online at www.aap.org/cfp.	CHAPTER 7. OFFICE AND OTHER OUTPATIENT EVALUATION AND MANAGEMENT SERVICES |||||| 177 **Resources** **Documentation** American Academy of Pediatrics Initial History Questionnaire Documentation Form for office or outpatient visits (available for purchase at http://shop.aap.org) **Examples of Office E/M Code Levels** "Office E/M 2021: Level 2 Visits" (August 2020 *AAP Pediatric Coding Newsletter*) (https://coding.solutions.aap.org/article.aspx?articleid=2765198; subscription required) "Office E/M 2021: Level 3 Visits" (September 2020 *AAP Pediatric Coding Newsletter*) (https://coding.solutions.aap.org/article.aspx?articleid=2765216; subscription required) "Office E/M 2021: Level 4 Visits" (October 2020 *AAP Pediatric Coding Newsletter*) (https://coding.aap.org; subscription required) "Office E/M 2021: Requirements, Examples, and Use of the Prolonged Service Code" (November 2020 *AAP Pediatric Coding Newsletter*) (https://coding.aap.org; subscription required) **Medical Decision-making** "Office E/M 2021: An Overview of Medical Decision-making" (February 2020 *AAP Pediatric Coding Newsletter*) (https://coding.solutions.aap.org/article.aspx?articleid=2759684; subscription required) "Office E/M 2021: Determining the Number and Complexity of Problems Addressed" (April 2020 *AAP Pediatric Coding Newsletter*) (https://coding.solutions.aap.org/article.aspx?articleid=2763373; subscription required) "Office E/M 2021: Determining Levels of Amount and/or Complexity of Data" (May 2020 *AAP Pediatric Coding Newsletter*)
Step 6. While every effort is made to provide accurate and up-to-date coding guidance, changes do happen. Any corrections and code or instruction changes published subsequent to the date of this printing are posted online at www.aap.org/cfp.	

Part 1
Coding Basics and Business Essentials

Part 1: Coding Basics and Business Essentials

The Basics of Coding

Contents

An Introduction to the Official Code Sets

In the United States, the Health Insurance Portability and Accountability Act of 1996 (HIPAA) requires the use of 5 specific code sets for purposes of health care transactions. The 4 code sets primarily used by physicians are listed in **Table 1-1**. The fifth designated code set, *Code on Dental Procedures and Nomenclature* (*CDT*), is primarily used to report dental procedures to dental insurance plans.

Table 1-1. Code Sets Required by Health Insurance Portability and Accountability Act of 1996		
Code Set	**Used to Report**	**Examples**
International Classification of Diseases, 10th Revision, Clinical Modification (ICD-10-CM)	Diagnoses and other reasons for encounters	**Z00.110** Health examination for newborn under 8 days old **Z00.111** Health examination for newborn 8 to 28 days old
Current Procedural Terminology (CPT®)[a]	Most professional services, vaccine and immune globulin products, and tracking performance measurement	**99291** Critical care, evaluation and management of the critically ill or critically injured patient; first 30-74 minutes **90686** Influenza virus vaccine, quadrivalent (IIV4), split virus, preservative free, 0.5 mL dosage, for intramuscular use
Healthcare Common Procedure Coding System (HCPCS)[b]	Supplies, medications, and services (when a *CPT* code does not describe the service as covered by health plan benefits)	**S0630** Removal of sutures; by a physician other than the physician who originally closed the wound **J0171** Injection, Adrenalin, epinephrine, 0.1 mg
National Drug Code (NDC)	Specific prescription drug, vaccine, and insulin products and dosages	**00006-4047-41** RotaTeq 2-mL single-dose tube, package of 10 **60574-4114-01** Synagis 0.5-mL in 1 vial, single dose

[a] Also known as Level I of the HCPCS code set.
[b] Refers to Level II HCPCS codes assigned by the Centers for Medicare & Medicaid Services.

The national standards for code sets created by HIPAA restricts the creation of codes by local or regional payers that previously complicated reporting methodologies. Each code set, other than *CDT*, is used to facilitate communication of standardized health information for purposes such as prior authorization of medical care and submission of health care claims in pediatric practice. Understanding the purpose and constructs of the 4 code sets used by physicians is important to successful interactions with health plans and supports accurate health care statistics.

New codes are listed in quick references in **Appendix I** and **II**.
- Quick Reference to 2021 *ICD-10-CM* Pediatric Code Changes (effective with services provided on or after October 1, 2020)
- Quick Reference to 2021 *CPT®* Pediatric Code Changes (effective with services provided on or after January 1, 2021)

Telling the Encounter Story

Because physicians do not submit full documentation, various code sets and other supportive information tell payers what happened and what should be paid (**Figure 1-1**). Learning to appropriately select codes for diagnoses, services, supplies, and medications is important to support appropriate payment by health plans. In the end, the codes submitted on a claim tell the story of what happened during a patient encounter.

However, documentation of an encounter must support the codes assigned for each diagnosis and service and may be requested by a payer to support the accuracy of code assignment. The following 7 general principles of documentation apply to all services:
1. The medical record should be complete and legible.
2. The documentation of each patient encounter should include
   - Reason for the encounter and relevant history, physical examination findings, and prior diagnostic test results
   - Assessment, clinical impression, or diagnosis
   - Plan for care
   - Date and legible identity of the observer
3. If not documented, the rationale for ordering diagnostic and other ancillary services should be easily inferred.
4. Past and present diagnoses should be accessible to the treating and/or consulting physician.

●=New code   ▲=Revised code   #=Re-sequenced code   +=Add-on code

5. Appropriate health risk factors should be identified.
6. The patient's progress, response to and changes in treatment, and revision of diagnosis should be documented.
7. The *Current Procedural Terminology* (*CPT*®) and *International Classification of Diseases, 10th Revision, Clinical Modification* (*ICD-10-CM*) codes reported on the health insurance claim form or billing statement should be supported by the documentation in the medical record.

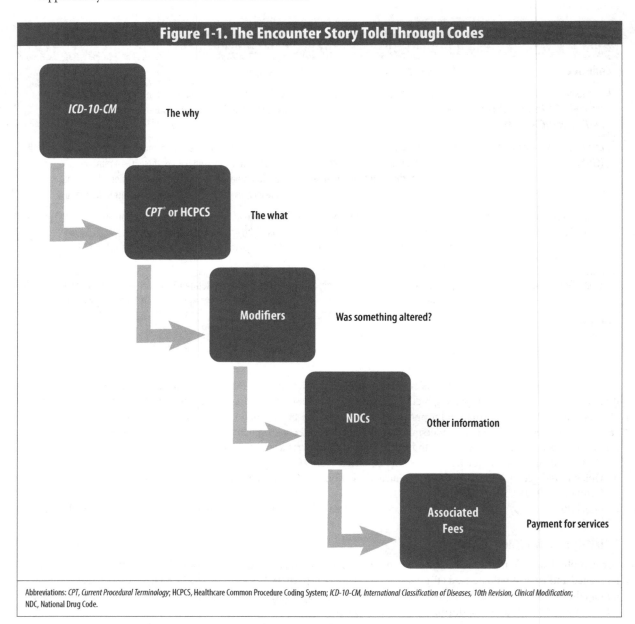

Figure 1-1. The Encounter Story Told Through Codes

ICD-10-CM — The why

CPT® or HCPCS — The what

Modifiers — Was something altered?

NDCs — Other information

Associated Fees — Payment for services

Abbreviations: *CPT, Current Procedural Terminology; HCPCS, Healthcare Common Procedure Coding System; ICD-10-CM, International Classification of Diseases, 10th Revision, Clinical Modification; NDC, National Drug Code.*

International Classification of Diseases, 10th Revision, Clinical Modification (ICD-10-CM)

The United States uses a clinical modification of the World Health Organization *International Classification of Diseases, 10th Revision* (*ICD-10*), called *ICD-10-CM*, as the official system for reporting morbidity and mortality associated with health care data.

- Physicians assign diagnoses and other reasons for encounters to which *ICD-10-CM* codes are assigned.
- Although the values assigned to procedure codes are the basis for amounts paid for services, payers are increasingly using *ICD-10-CM* codes when determining the appropriateness of services submitted on a claim (eg, level of evaluation and management [E/M] service).

Updates to *ICD-10-CM* are implemented each October 1 following publication in early to midsummer. Interim code updates may occur in April when there is a significant indication for a code to identify a new health condition.

Oversight and resolution of coding questions related to *ICD-10-CM* is performed by the American Hospital Association (AHA) Editorial Advisory Board for *Coding Clinic for ICD-10-CM and ICD-10-PCS* and the public-private "cooperating parties": the Centers for Medicare & Medicaid Services (CMS), National Center for Health Statistics, AHA, and American Health Information Management Association. The increased granularity and specificity in *ICD-10-CM* are also at the specific request of certain medical societies. No clinical diagnosis codes are added for payment purposes.

The American Academy of Pediatrics (AAP) holds a seat on the editorial advisory board. Findings are published quarterly by the AHA in *Coding Clinic. ICD-10-CM* codes and accompanying guidelines and findings by the editorial advisory board are part of the standard transaction code sets under HIPAA and must be recognized by all payers. For *ICD-10-CM*, the hierarchy of official coding guidelines and instructions is as follows:

1. *ICD-10-CM* alphabetic index and tabular list
2. *Official Guidelines for Coding and Reporting*
3. AHA *Coding Clinic* advice

Pediatricians with suggestions for changes to existing or new *ICD-10-CM* codes related to pediatric care are encouraged to forward their suggestions to coding staff at the AAP headquarters. The AAP staff and advisor who are involved in the process can be of great assistance. To contact the AAP Coding Staff, complete the form at https://form.jotform.com/Subspecialty/aapcodinghotline.

ICD-10-CM Code Structure

In *ICD-10-CM*, a code is a complete set of alphanumeric characters for which there are no further subdivisions, 3 to 7 characters long, describing a condition or reason for an encounter or related factors, such as external causes.

The first character of each code is a letter. The second through seventh characters may be letters or numbers. For codes that extend beyond 3 characters, the first 3 characters are found to the left of a decimal with the remaining characters to the right.

Pattern: XXX.XXXX

Although typically illustrated in capital letters, the alphabetic characters are not case sensitive.

Examples of complete codes are illustrated in **Table 1-2** along with explanatory notes for each type of code.

Table 1-2. Examples of *International Classification of Diseases, 10th Revision, Clinical Modification* Codes	
Code	**Explanatory Notes**
R05 Cough	Describes the symptom of cough when no further diagnosis is documented at the end of the encounter.
J06.9 Acute upper respiratory infection	Considered a definitive diagnosis; therefore, **R05** would not be reported in addition when cough is an integral symptom of the upper respiratory infection.
J11.83 Influenza due to unidentified influenza virus with otitis media	Combination code representing an etiology or underlying condition of influenza and a manifestation or secondary infection of otitis media. When a combination code does not exist, report multiple codes, as necessary, to describe the documented conditions.
Z00.129 Encounter for routine child health examination without abnormal findings	Describes a routine child health examination without abnormal findings. Code **Z00.121** is reported when a routine child health examination includes abnormal findings (eg, new condition, exacerbation of a chronic illness).
W07.XXXA Fall from chair, initial encounter	Note the letter **X** is used as a placeholder in code **W07.XXXA**. The placeholder must be used to complete the code so the seventh character is in the appropriate position. External cause codes are never primary.

Assignment of the seventh character is based on whether the patient is undergoing active treatment (services to establish a pattern of healing) and not whether the provider is seeing the patient for the first time over the course of treatment for an injury.

See examples of the seventh characters that apply to most injuries, **A**, **D**, and **S**, in **Table 1-3**. Categories for traumatic fractures have additional seventh character values (eg, **C**, initial encounter for open fracture type IIIA, IIIB, or IIIC).

Table 1-3. Examples of Seventh Characters A, D, and S *When selecting a seventh character to indicate the type of encounter, a helpful mnemonic for the seventh character is **A** as active treatment/management, **D** as during healing, and **S** as scars and other sequela.*		
A Initial Encounter (Active Care)	**D Subsequent Encounter (Routine Healing Phase)**	**S Sequela (Late Effect)**
A physician repairs a laceration to the face (active treatment).	A pediatrician removes facial sutures placed by an emergency department physician.	A pediatrician evaluates a complaint of scar contracture that resulted from repair of a facial laceration.
S01.81XA Laceration without foreign body of other part of head, initial encounter	**S01.81XD** Laceration without foreign body of other part of head, subsequent encounter	**L90.5** Scar conditions and fibrosis of skin **S01.81XS** Laceration without foreign body of other part of head, subsequent encounter. NOTE: Sequela (eg, scar) must always be reported first.

ICD-10-CM Guidelines

The official conventions found in the *ICD-10-CM Official Guidelines for Coding and Reporting* are outlined in sections that include descriptions of symbols, abbreviations, and other instructional notes. The guidelines are organized into 4 sections. Only sections I and IV pertain to reporting physician services. Sections II and III relate to hospital or facility technical services and are not discussed here. *ICD-10-CM* guidelines can be found in *ICD-10-CM* manuals or at www.cdc.gov/nchs/icd/icd10cm.htm.

The following excerpts from the *ICD-10-CM* guidelines provide an overview of the information pertinent to pediatric care as provided in each section of the guidelines:

Section I—Conventions, General Coding Guidelines, and Chapter-Specific Guidelines

A. Conventions

The conventions of *ICD-10-CM* include punctuation, notes, and terminology used throughout the code set.

[ ] Brackets
- Identify manifestation codes in the Alphabetic Index (eg, otitis externa due to impetigo **L01.00** [**H62.40**])
- Enclose synonyms, alternative wording, or explanatory phrases in the tabular list (eg, **S04.811** Injury of olfactory [1st] nerve, right side).

( ) Parentheses—Enclose supplementary words (ie, nonessential modifiers) that may be included in the medical record but do not affect code selection; for example, bronchiolitis (acute) (infective) (subacute) **J21.9**. If a nonessential modifier is mutually exclusive to a sub-term of the main term, the sub-term is given priority.

- Dash—Indicates that additional characters are required for code completion (eg, **R10.-**). A dash is also used throughout this publication to indicate incomplete codes.

Notes
- **Includes:** Further defines or gives examples of the content of a category.
- **Excludes1:** Not coded here—used to indicate codes for conditions that would not occur in conjunction with the code category where the note is found. An exception to the *Excludes1* definition is the circumstance when the 2 conditions are unrelated to each other. If it is not clear whether the 2 conditions involving an *Excludes1* note are related, coders are instructed to query the provider.
- **Excludes2:** Not included here—used to indicate codes for conditions not included in the code category where the note is found but that may be additionally reported when both conditions are present.
- **Code first:** A sequencing rule in the tabular list to report first a code for an underlying cause or origin of a disease (etiology), if known.
- **Code also:** An instruction that another code may be necessary to fully describe a condition. The sequence of the codes depends on the circumstances of the encounter.
- **See:** In the alphabetic index, this instructs that another term should be referenced to find the appropriate code.
- **See also:** In the alphabetic index, this instructs that another term may provide additional entries that may be useful.
- **Use an additional code:** A sequencing rule often found at the listing of an etiology code, this instruction directs to also report a code for the manifestation.

Terminology

- **And:** Means and/or when appearing in a title in *ICD-10-CM;* for example, **Q16.1**, congenital absence, atresia and stricture of auditory canal (external) includes absence, atresia, or stricture.
- **Combination code:** A single code that represents multiple conditions or a single condition with an associated secondary process or complication.
- **First-listed diagnosis:** For reporting of professional services, the diagnosis, condition, problem, or other reason for the encounter or visit shown in the medical record to be chiefly responsible for the services provided is listed first and followed by other conditions that affected management or treatment.
- **NEC:** Not elsewhere classifiable. Indicates a code for other specified conditions that is reported when the medical record provides detail that is not captured in a specific code.
- **NOS:** Not otherwise specified. Indicates a code for an unspecified condition that is reported when the medical record does not provide sufficient detail for assignment of a more specific code.
- **Sequela:** A late effect of an illness or injury that is no longer in the acute phase. There is no time limit on when a sequela code can be used. The residual may be apparent early, such as in cerebral infarction, or it may occur months or years later, such as that due to a previous injury.
- **With and In:** The classification presumes a causal relationship between the 2 conditions linked by the terms *with* or *in*. These conditions should be coded as related even in the absence of provider documentation explicitly linking them, unless the documentation clearly states that the conditions are unrelated or when another guideline exists that specifically requires a documented linkage between 2 conditions (eg, sepsis guideline for "acute organ dysfunction that is not clearly associated with the sepsis").

    For conditions not specifically linked by these relational terms in the classification or when a guideline requires that a linkage between 2 conditions be explicitly documented, provider documentation must link the conditions to code them as related.

B. General Coding Guidelines

- Assign a code for signs and symptoms when no definitive diagnosis has been reached at an encounter.
- Do not report additional codes for conditions that are integral or routinely associated with a disease process (eg, wheezing in asthma).
- When the same condition is documented as acute and chronic, codes for both conditions are reported if the alphabetic index lists the conditions at the same indentation level. The acute condition is sequenced first.
- When a combination code describes 2 diagnoses, or a diagnosis and its associated manifestation or complication, report only the combination code. If a manifestation or complication is not identified in a combination code, it should be separately reported.
- When reporting a sequela (late effect) of an injury or illness, report first the current condition and then the sequela code.
- If both sides are affected by a condition and the code category does not include a code for the bilateral condition, assign codes for right and left. When a patient has a bilateral condition and each side is treated during separate encounters, assign the bilateral code for each encounter where the condition exists on both sides. Do not assign a bilateral code if the condition no longer exists bilaterally.
- Coders generally may not assume a complication of care without documentation of the cause-and-effect relationship (eg, infection in a patient with a central venous line).
- Unspecified codes are appropriately selected when information to support a more specific code was not available at the time of the encounter (eg, type of pneumonia is not known).

C. Chapter-Specific Guidelines

See guidelines for specific diagnoses and/or conditions found in each chapter of *ICD-10-CM*. Chapter guidelines are important to coding for pediatric care and need to be followed for appropriate code selection.

When selecting electronic coding applications, look for inclusion of chapter-specific guidelines when using the code search functionality. *Pediatric ICD-10-CM: A Manual for Provider-Based Coding*, a manual published by the AAP, adds chapter-specific guidance to each chapter for easy reference.

Section IV—Diagnostic Coding and Reporting Guidelines for Outpatient Services

Selecting a Code

- The coding conventions and guidelines of Section I take precedence over these outpatient guidelines.
- Never assign a code for a condition that is unconfirmed (eg, probable or rule out obstruction). Instead, assign codes for signs and symptoms (eg, vomiting, abdominal distension).
- Use codes in categories **Z00–Z99** when circumstances other than a disease or an injury are recorded as the reason for encounter.

Sequencing of Diagnosis Codes

- Physicians and other providers of professional services should list first the condition, symptom, or other reason for encounter that is chiefly responsible for the services provided. List also any coexisting conditions. However, always defer to the manual to determine if sequencing is outlined in the guidelines.

> Diagnosis codes must be appropriately linked to services on a claim to support the medical necessity of that service. See the Reporting Codes for Payment section later in this chapter for more information.

Reporting Previously Treated Conditions

- Do not code conditions that have been previously treated but no longer exist. Personal history codes **Z85–Z87** may be used to identify a patient's historical conditions. Codes for family history that affects current care are also reported (**Z80–Z84**).
- Report codes for chronic or recurring conditions as many times as the patient receives care for each condition.

Reporting Diagnoses for Diagnostic Examinations

- The condition, symptoms, or other reason for a diagnostic examination or test should be linked to the service. For laboratory or radiology testing in the absence of related conditions, signs, or symptoms, report code **Z01.89**, encounter for other specified special examinations.
- When diagnostic tests have been interpreted by a physician and the final report is available at the time of coding, code any confirmed or definitive diagnosis(es) documented in the interpretation. Do not code related signs and symptoms as additional diagnoses.

Reporting Preoperative Evaluations

- When the reason for an encounter is a preoperative evaluation, a code from subcategory **Z01.81-**, encounter for pre-procedural examinations, is reported first, followed by codes for the condition that is the reason for surgery and codes for any findings of the preoperative evaluation.
- Please see **Chapter 9** for discussion of reporting health examinations (preventive care).

The Pathway to *ICD-10-CM* Code Selection

To correctly select codes in *ICD-10-CM*, it is important to know how the alphabetic index and tabular list are used to locate the most specific code for documented diagnoses.

It is important to recognize and follow instructions found in the alphabetic index and tabular list. These are the prevailing instructions for reporting that are supplemented by the guidelines and guidance published in AHA *Coding Clinic for ICD-10-CM*. Refer to the AAP manuals *Pediatric Coding Basics* and *Pediatric ICD-10-CM* for more information.

Tabular List

The tabular list is the end point for code selection. It is an alphanumeric list of *ICD-10-CM* codes structured as an indented list of 22 chapters with further divisions, including blocks, categories, subcategories, and codes. Chapters are based on condition, body system, consequences of external causes, external causes, and other factors influencing health status or contact with health services. Examples of notes found at each level of the tabular list (eg, chapter, block) follow.

> Look for instructional notes at each division within the tabular list (ie, chapter, block, category, or code), as these give important guidance to correct code selection.

Diagnosis Coding Tips

- Specificity in coding is important to demonstrating the reason for a service or encounter, including the nature or severity of conditions managed. See further discussion of this important topic in the Appropriate Use of Unspecified Codes section later in this chapter.
- Physicians and other practitioners should become familiar with the documentation elements that are captured in *ICD-10-CM* code categories for conditions commonly seen in their practice. For example, when documenting care for otitis media, key documentation elements include whether the condition
  - Affects the right, the left, or both ears
  - Is acute, acute recurrent, or chronic
  - Is suppurative or nonsuppurative
  - Is with or without spontaneous rupture of the tympanic membrane
    Exposure to or use of tobacco is also reported in conjunction with otitis media.
- Pay close attention to the terminology for nonspecific diagnoses. For example, the diagnosis "reactive airways disease" is to be coded as asthma per the guidelines.
    In children treated for an asthma-like condition who have not been diagnosed with asthma, it may be more appropriate to report the signs or symptoms as the primary diagnosis.
- When testing is performed to rule out or confirm a suspected diagnosis or condition on a patient with a sign(s) or symptom(s), it is considered a diagnostic examination and is not screening. Therefore, the code that explains the reason for the test (ie, sign or symptom) should be reported.

Examples

➤ **A chest radiograph is ordered due to positive purified protein derivative testing.** Code **R76.11** (nonspecific reaction to tuberculin skin test without active tuberculosis) is assigned on the order to indicate the reason for testing.

➤ **A tuberculin purified protein derivative test is performed to screen for tuberculosis in a patient with no symptoms and no known exposure.** Code **Z11.1** (encounter for screening for respiratory tuberculosis) is assigned as the reason for the test.

- If, after evaluation and study of a suspected condition, there is no diagnosis or there are no signs or symptoms that are appropriate, report the codes for observation and evaluation for suspected conditions not found.
    Codes for observation and evaluation for suspected conditions not found in a neonate (*ICD-10-CM* codes **Z05.0–Z05.9**) are distinct from those for reporting suspected conditions not found in older children and adults (*ICD-10-CM* code **Z03.89**).
- Use aftercare codes (**Z42–Z49**, **Z51**) for patients who are receiving care to consolidate treatment or managing residual conditions.
- Conditions that were previously treated and no longer exist cannot be reported. Therefore, it is correct coding to report care following completed treatment with *ICD-10-CM* code **Z09**, encounter for follow-up examination after completed treatment for conditions other than malignant neoplasm.
  - Personal history codes (**Z86.-**, **Z87.-**) may be used to provide additional information on follow-up care.
  - If a payer does not accept follow-up care codes as primary and requires that the service be reported with the diagnosis code that reflects the condition that had been treated, report the follow-up care codes as secondary. However, get the payer's policy in writing and inquire why it is not following coding guidelines.
- Do not select a diagnosis code that is "close to" the diagnosis or condition documented in the medical record. For example, do not report unspecified joint pain (**M25.50**) if the diagnosis is right knee pain (**M25.561**). Modify code selection methods to support correct code assignment.
- Pay attention to age factors within certain code descriptors. For example, report *ICD-10-CM* code **R10.83** for infantile colic and *ICD-10-CM* code **R10.84** for colic in a child older than 12 months.
- There is no limit to the number of diagnosis codes that can be documented.
  - Space is only allotted for up to 12 codes on the CMS-1500 paper claim form and each service line may be connected to 1 to 4 of the included codes. You may submit as many claim forms as necessary to report the diagnoses.
  - Electronic claims in HIPAA version 5010 may also include up to 12 diagnosis codes.
- "Recurrent" is not defined by *ICD-10*. Therefore, to use a recurrent code, the documentation should reflect that a practitioner believes it to be a recurrence.

- "Confirmed" influenza or other conditions do not require a positive laboratory test result or other test. What is required is that the practitioner, through training and experience, believes the patient has the condition based on clinical assessment and documents the condition in the chart.
- Do not report "suspected" or "rule out" diagnoses for physician services. Code to the nearest clinical certainty, which may be signs or symptoms.

Appropriate Use of Unspecified Codes

Unspecified codes are valid *ICD-10-CM* codes used to report conditions for which a more specific diagnosis has not yet been determined and/or testing to determine a more specific diagnosis would not be medically necessary. However, misuse of unspecified codes may result in claim denials and unnecessary delays in receiving prior authorizations for testing or procedures.

Do not report the default code (first code listed in the alphabetic index) when more detail about the patient's condition(s) should be documented to support another, more specific code. For example, do not report **J45.909** for unspecified asthma, uncomplicated, for reevaluation of asthma, which includes clinical classification of intermittent, mild-persistent, moderate-persistent, or severe-persistent asthma. The diagnosis code reported should reflect what is known at the end of the current encounter. Unspecified codes are not appropriate when information to support a more specific code would generally be known (eg, laterality, type of attention-deficit/hyperactivity disorder).

Examples of unspecified codes that may be acceptable are as follows:
- Viral intestinal infection, unspecified (**A08.4**)
- Infectious gastroenteritis and colitis, unspecified (**A09**)
- Acute pharyngitis, unspecified (**J02.9**)
- Pneumonia, unspecified organism (**J18.9**)
- Sprain of unspecified site of right knee (**S83.91X-**)

The following examples of unspecified codes indicate inappropriate coding due to failure to document information (eg, location) that would typically be known at the time of the encounter and/or inappropriate code selection:
- Acute suppurative otitis media without spontaneous rupture of eardrum, unspecified ear (**H66.009**)
- Otitis media, unspecified, unspecified ear (**H66.90**)
- Cutaneous abscess of limb, unspecified (**L02.419**)
- Extremely low birth weight newborn, unspecified weight (**P07.00**)

In short, unspecified codes are necessary and should be reported when appropriate. Physicians must document in enough detail to capture what is known at the time of the encounter, and codes selected must reflect the documented diagnosis(es). If, at the time of code selection, documentation does not appear to include information that would be known at the time of the encounter, it is appropriate for coders to query the physician for more information and/or request an addendum to the documentation to more fully describe the conditions addressed at the encounter.

More About *ICD-10-CM*

The AAP *Pediatric ICD-10-CM: A Manual for Provider-Based Coding* (available through https://shop.aap.org) is a condensed version of the entire *ICD-10-CM* manual and provides only the guidelines and codes that are applicable and of importance to pediatric practitioners. The manual was designed for use in conjunction with the complete *ICD-10-CM* code set. The *ICD-10-CM* codes are found at www.cdc.gov/nchs/icd/icd10cm.htm.

AAP Pediatric Coding Newsletter™ provides timely articles on diagnosis coding for pediatric conditions. Subscriptions are available through https://shop.aap.org.

Healthcare Common Procedure Coding System (HCPCS)

The Healthcare Common Procedure Coding System (HCPCS) includes Level I codes (*CPT*) and Level II codes (CMS national codes). HCPCS Level II codes are the standardized coding system for describing and identifying health care services, equipment, and supplies that are not identified by HCPCS Level I (*CPT*) codes. To differentiate discussion of *CPT* and HCPCS Level II codes, the term HCPCS typically is used in reference to Level II codes unless otherwise stated.

HCPCS codes begin with a single letter (**A–V**) followed by 4 numeric digits (eg, **Q4011**, cast supplies, short arm cast, pediatric [0–10 years], plaster). Commonly used categories of HCPCS include
- **A** codes for medical and surgical supplies
- **H** codes for services such as alcohol/drug and behavioral services
- **J** codes for drugs administered by other than oral method and chemotherapy drugs

- **Q** codes that represent temporary codes (although many codes have been used for years) for certain tests and procedures and supplies such as cast supplies
- **S** codes for screenings and examinations in alignment with certain payer policies (often BlueCross BlueShield plans)
- **T** codes, used mainly by Medicaid agencies to describe specific services such as nursing and certain behavioral health services

HCPCS codes may be reported when the narrative differs from the *CPT* code for the service. Payer policies, particularly Medicaid plan policies, often drive the decision between reporting with *CPT* versus HCPCS. For instance, *CPT* does not include a code for removal of sutures by a physician other than the physician who repaired the wound and instructs to report an E/M service for encounters for suture removal. HCPCS includes code **S0630** (removal of sutures by a physician other than the physician who originally closed the wound). When allowed or required by a payer, code **S0630** may be reported in lieu of an E/M service for suture removal.

HCPCS **J** codes (eg, **J0696**, injection, ceftriaxone sodium, per 250 mg) represent medications only and not the administration of the medication.

- The term *injection* is included in the descriptor to specify that the medication code is reported for the medication when provided via injection or infusion and not oral or topical applications.
- Separate procedure codes, typically *CPT* codes, are used to report medication administration by injection or infusion.
- HCPCS codes for drugs specify the unit of measure for each unit reported on the claim (eg, 250 mg of ceftriaxone sodium is reported with 1 unit on the claim line reporting provision of the medication). (See the National Drug Code [NDC] section later in this chapter for information on reporting units of service in conjunction with NDC reporting.)

> **Do not report the number of milligrams (mg) as the unit of service on a claim. Reporting 900 mg of ceftriaxone sodium with 900 units would be incorrect; 900 mg of ceftriaxone sodium is reported with 4 units (rounding up is allowed by Medicare; other payers may require 3.6 units).**

Modifiers are also included in the HCPCS code set. Modifiers indicate that a service or procedure has been altered by some specific circumstance but not changed in its basic code definition.

> **Modifiers are further discussed in Chapter 2 and illustrated throughout this manual.**

- HCPCS modifiers are more comprehensive than the modifiers included in *CPT,* offering modifiers that designate anatomical sites, provider types, and services payable under specific benefits or policies.
- HCPCS modifiers may be appended to any procedure code (*CPT* or HCPCS) as appropriate.

Examples

F4	Left hand, fifth digit
EP	Service provided as part of Medicaid Early and Periodic Screening, Diagnostic, and Treatment (EPSDT) program
AJ	Clinical social worker

New permanent HCPCS codes are released by the CMS each November for implementation on January 1 of each year. However, temporary HCPCS codes may be implemented on a quarterly basis. Temporary codes are added to address the need for a reporting mechanism prior to the annual update (eg, to meet the requirements of a legislative mandate or to add a new product).

Current Procedural Terminology (CPT)

CPT is published annually by the American Medical Association (AMA). *CPT* codes are Level I codes of HCPCS but are commonly treated as a separate code set. This is the primary procedural coding system for professional services by physicians and other qualified health care professionals (QHPs). *CPT* codes are commonly included in electronic health record (EHR) systems, but instructions for reporting may not be included. *CPT* manuals and code applications or software provide important instructions for appropriate code selection.

CPT includes 3 categories of codes. Category I codes represent procedures or services that have been determined consistent with current medical practice and are performed by many practitioners in clinical practice in multiple locations. Category I codes are 5-digit numeric codes, with exception of codes for proprietary laboratory analyses, which include 4 numeric digits followed by the letter **U**.

- Evaluation and management (**99202–99499**)
- Anesthesia (**01000–01999, 99100–99140**)
- Surgery (**10004–69990**)
- Radiology (**70010–79999**)
- Pathology and laboratory (**80047–89398, 0001U–0017U**)
- Medicine (**90281–99199, 99500–99607**)

Each section of codes is preceded by guidelines specific to code selection and reporting of services included in that section.

- Category I *CPT* codes are updated annually with release of new codes each fall to allow physicians and payers to prepare for implementation on January 1 of each year.
  - Exceptions include the vaccine product codes, which are updated twice annually (January and July) and may be released earlier when specific criteria for rapid release are met. Newly released vaccine codes are posted to www.ama-assn.org/practice-management/cpt/category-i-vaccine-codes.
  - New vaccine codes released July 1 are implemented on January 1, and vice versa.
- Category II *CPT* codes are a set of supplemental tracking codes that can be used for performance measurement. They are 5-digit alphanumeric codes that include 4 numbers followed by the letter **F**. Category II codes are released online 3 times a year, with an effective date of 3 months after release, at www.ama-assn.org/practice-management/cpt/category-ii-codes.

> **See Chapter 3 for more discussion and illustration of Category II codes.**

- Category III *CPT* codes are a set of temporary codes for emerging technology, services, procedures, and service paradigms. Category III codes allow data collection to substantiate the usage of new services and procedures.
  - Assignment of a Category III code to a service is not a statement of support, or lack thereof, for the efficacy of, use of, or payment for the service.
  - Category III codes are 5-character alphanumeric codes with 4 numbers followed by the letter **T**.
  - Category III codes are not assigned relative value units (RVUs), and payment for these services is based strictly on payer policies. If you are performing any procedure or service identified with a Category III *CPT* code, work with your payers to determine their coverage and payment policies.
  - Category III codes are released biannually with an implementation date 6 months following the release date. For instance, a code released on January 1, 2021, is implemented on July 1, 2021, and published in *CPT 2022*. The most recent Category III code listing is found at www.ama-assn.org/practice-management/cpt/category-iii-codes.
  - In general, Category III codes must be replaced for reporting by Category I codes or approved for continued Category III status within 5 years following the Category III code assignment. Category III codes that are not renewed for continued utilization are archived and the codes are not reused.

The AMA hosts a website devoted to *CPT,* www.ama-assn.org/practice-management/cpt, with information on code development and maintenance, summaries of recent *CPT* Editorial Panel actions, and newly released codes.

CPT Conventions and Guidelines

CPT includes an index of procedures used to find codes and code ranges to help guide the user to the correct section(s) of codes.

- Codes should not be selected from the index without verification in the main text of the manual.
- Terms in the index include procedures and services, organs and anatomic sites, conditions, synonyms, eponyms, and abbreviations (eg, EEG).

Appendixes in *CPT* provide clinical examples of E/M services; quick references to modifiers; a summary of new, revised, and deleted codes; add-on and modifier-exempt codes; and other procedure code references. Based on changes to the coding manual, the appendixes may vary from year to year.

CPT is structured to save space in the listing of codes by use of indentations to identify variations of services that have a common base descriptor. For example

99381	Initial comprehensive preventive medicine evaluation and management of an individual including an age and gender appropriate history, examination, counseling/anticipatory guidance/risk factor reduction interventions, and the ordering of laboratory/diagnostic procedures, new patient; infant (age younger than 1 year)
99382	early childhood (age 1 through 4 years)
99383	late childhood (age 5 through 11 years)

●=New code   ▲=Revised code   #=Re-sequenced code   +=Add-on code

99384	adolescent (age 12 through 17 years)
99385	18–39 years

The portion of the code descriptor for **99381** before the semicolon also applies to codes **99382–99385**. Increased indentation of codes that share a portion of the first code's descriptor helps to identify which codes share a common base procedure.

As shown in **Table 1-4**, symbols are used throughout *CPT* to code characteristics such as new or revised codes, new instructions, and other important characteristics of a code (eg, a code placed out of numeric sequence).

CPT includes specific guidelines that are located at the beginning of each section and additional prefatory instructions for categories of codes throughout the *CPT* manual.

● Code-specific instructions often follow a code in parentheses (referred to as *parenthetical instructions*).

Table 1-4. *Current Procedural Terminology* Symbols	
Symbols	**Description**
●	A bullet at the beginning of a code indicates a new code for the current year.
▲	A triangle means the code descriptor has been revised.
+	A plus sign means the code is an add-on code.
Ø	A null sign means the code is a "modifier **51** exempt" code and, therefore, does not require modifier **51** (multiple procedures) even when reported with other procedures.
⚡	The lightning bolt identifies codes for vaccines that are pending US Food and Drug Administration approval.
#	The pound symbol is used to identify re-sequenced codes that are out of numerical sequence. Related codes are placed in an appropriate location, making it easier to locate a procedure or service.
★	A star means the service represented by the code is included in Appendix P of the *CPT* manual as a code to which modifier **95** (synchronous telemedicine service) may be appended to indicate the service was rendered via real-time telemedicine services.

● While code selection is often incorporated in EHRs, knowledge of and access to *CPT* guidelines is important to correct coding. Correct coding is important to obtaining correct claims payment. Always read the applicable guidelines and instructions before selecting a code.

Additional guidance can be found in *CPT Assistant,* a monthly newsletter published by the AMA that provides additional information about the intended use of codes, the related guidelines, and parenthetical instructions. Although widely considered authoritative, *CPT* instruction and *CPT Assistant* are not part of the HIPAA standard transaction code sets. All payers must accept *CPT* codes but are not required to adhere to the published guidelines and instructions. Where payer policy differs from *CPT,* payer contracts typically require adherence to payer policy.

Example

➤ **A health plan policy does not allow separate payment for vision screening in conjunction with a routine child health examination even though *CPT* instructs that the screening is separately reported.** Although the health plan may deny charges associated with a vision screening, the plan must not reject the claim due to inclusion of a vision screening code (eg, **99173**, screening test of visual acuity, quantitative, bilateral).

Some key instructions are
● In the *CPT* code set, the term *procedure* is used to describe services, including diagnostic tests. The section of the book in which a code is placed is not indicative of whether the service is a surgery or not a surgery for insurance or other purposes.
● Select the code for the procedure or service that accurately identifies the service performed.
   — Do not select a code that merely approximates the service provided.
   — If no specific code exists, report the service using the appropriate unlisted procedure code. Unlisted procedure codes are provided in each section of *CPT* (eg, **99429**, unlisted preventive medicine service). When reporting an unlisted procedure code, medical records will need to be submitted to the health plan to identify the service rendered (attach to the claim to avoid delay caused by a health plan request for the records).
   — In some cases, a modifier may be used to indicate a reduced, discontinued, or increased procedural service.

- Many diagnostic services require a technical and professional component.
  - It is important to understand that the technical component (eg, obtaining an electrocardiogram) leads to results or findings.
  - The interpretation and creation of a report of the results or findings is a professional service. Some services specifically require a professional's interpretation and report.
  - Other services include only a technical component and require only documentation of the results or findings (eg, scoring of a developmental screening instrument).
  - Codes and modifiers exist to report the technical or professional component when the complete service is not provided by the same individual or provider (eg, facility provides technical component and physician provides professional component).

> **Never report a code for a global service without a modifier when only the technical or professional component was provided. See Chapter 2 for discussion of appropriate modifiers (eg, 26, TC).**

- Add-on codes (marked with a + before the code) are always performed in addition to a primary procedure and are never reported as stand-alone services. Add-on codes describe additional intraservice work and are not valued to include preservice and post-service work like most other codes.

Example

99291   Critical care, evaluation and management of the critically ill or critically injured patient; first 30–74 minutes
+99292   each additional 30 minutes (List separately in addition to code for primary service)

Code **99292** is never reported in the absence of code **99291** on the same date of service.

Provider Terminology

Physicians may incorporate other health care professionals (eg, medical nutrition therapist, psychologist, behavioral health care manager) into their medical practice, allowing patients to receive more care in their medical home.

Of particular importance to correct reporting of services that include clinical staff and other nonphysician providers (NPPs) is identifying the providers included when terms such as *physician or other QHP* and *qualified, nonphysician health care professional* are used in *CPT* and/or payer instruction.

CPT provides definitions of providers as follows:

- **Physician or other QHP:** an individual who is qualified by education, training, licensure/regulation (when applicable), and facility privileging (when applicable) who performs a professional service within his or her scope of practice and independently reports that professional service
- **Clinical staff member:** a person who works under the supervision of a physician or other QHP and who is allowed by law, regulation, and facility policy to perform or assist in the performance of a specific professional service but does not individually report that professional service

Throughout the *CPT* code set, the use of terms such as *physician, QHP,* or *individual* is not intended to indicate that other entities may not report the service. In selected instances, specific instructions may define a service as limited to professionals or to other entities (eg, hospital, home health agency).

Note: CPT does not include any requirements for licensure but, rather, advises physicians to follow state regulations and the related scopes of practice defined by regulations (eg, regulations defining services that require a nursing license).

> **Coding for services by clinical staff and qualified nonphysician health care professionals is discussed in Chapter 13.**

Use of Time in Procedure Coding

> **New in 2021   The time used in selecting codes for office and other outpatient evaluation and management (E/M) services (99202–99205, 99212–99215) is the physician's or other qualified health care professional's *total time* on the date of the encounter. See Chapter 7 for more information on use of time in selecting codes for office and other outpatient E/M services.**

Most procedures and services in *CPT* are described by specific components of physician work (eg, **94011**, measurement of spirometric forced expiratory flows in an infant or child through 2 years of age). However, time (especially intraservice time) is also used as a proxy for physician work. Many services are reported based solely on time of service or, as in the case of many E/M services, may be reported based on key components of work (ie, history, examination, and medical decision-making) *or* time (see discussion of each type of E/M service for time specifications).

CPT provides general and category-/code-specific instructions for reporting services based on time. An understanding of these instructions is key to selecting codes that most accurately capture the services provided. This chapter will review the general guidelines for reporting time. Service-specific instructions and examples are also provided throughout this manual to help illustrate time-based coding.

Different categories of services use time differently. It is important to review the instructions for each category.

Time-Based Coding Examples

➤ **Moderate (conscious) sedation services are reported based on 15-minute time increments of intraservice time, beginning with administration of a sedating agent(s) and ending after the procedure is completed and the physician or QHP providing the sedation is no longer in personal continuous face-to-face contact with the patient.**

➤ **Intra-arterial and intravenous infusions are reported based on time and whether the infusion is the initial infusion service or a subsequent infusion service.**

➤ **Care plan oversight services for ventilator management of a patient in a home or domiciliary setting are reported for 30 minutes or more per month.**

The Value of Documenting Time

Failure to document time of service may be costly even when it is possible to report a service without documenting time.

Example

➤ **A physician documents an expanded-problem focused history and examination with moderate complexity medical decision-making at a subsequent hospital visit.** The physician also documents that more than 50% of a total of 35 minutes was spent on the floor reviewing laboratory and radiology reports, discussing the patient's care with another physician, and counseling the patient's parents on the child's diagnosis and plan of care.

    Teaching Point: If time were not documented, the documented key components would support code **99232** (level 2 subsequent hospital care). However, documentation of more than 50% of 35 minutes spent in counseling and/or coordination of care on the patient's unit/floor would support code **99233**.

    Code **99232** has 2.04 total RVUs, while code **99233** is assigned 2.94 total RVUs. Persistent failure to document the time of E/M services may result in significant loss of otherwise earned revenue. For example, a payer contract allows $40 per RVU, so a practice is paid $81.60 ($40 × 2.04) for code **99232** and $117.60 ($40 × 2.94) for code **99233**. Therefore, $36 of potential revenue is lost due to lack of documentation; if **99232** is reported 10 times when **99233** is supported, $360 of potential revenue is lost.

Failure to document time also eliminates the possibility of reporting prolonged services and may negatively affect the level of service reported when multiple episodes of care occur on the same date (eg, multiple hospital care services). Routinely noting the time spent face-to-face (outpatient) or on a patient's unit or floor (observation and inpatient) and those instances when more than 50% of that time is spent in counseling and/or coordination of care allows for recognition of occasions where reporting based on time is most advantageous.

General Guidelines

CPT provides overall instructions for time-based reporting in the "Instructions for Use of the CPT Codebook" found in the Introduction of the coding manual. These instructions are followed for reporting time-based services when there are no section guidelines, prefatory instructions, parenthetical instructions, or specified time requirements in code descriptors (see examples in **Table 1-5**).

Section and prefatory instructions, code descriptors, and parenthetical instructions override the general instruction for time-based reporting.

    ●=New code   ▲=Revised code   #=Re-sequenced code   +=Add-on code

Table 1-5. *Current Procedural Terminology* Time Rules	
Time Rules	**Examples**
Midpoint rule: A unit of time is attained when the midpoint is passed (eg, a code described as 60 minutes may be reported when 31 minutes have elapsed). The midpoint rule is not applied when *Current Procedural Terminology* includes category- or code-specific instructions to the contrary. When codes are ranked in sequential typical times and the actual time is between 2 typical times, the code with the typical time closest to the actual time is used. If the actual time of service falls exactly between the typical times of 2 codes, report the code with the lower typical time (ie, the midpoint must be passed to report the greater service).	At least 8 minutes of preventive medicine counseling are required to support code **99401** (midpoint of 7½ minutes is passed). **99401** Preventive medicine counseling and/or risk factor reduction intervention(s) provided to an individual (separate procedure); approximately 15 minutes
Code descriptor describes required time.	**99238** Hospital discharge day management; 30 minutes or less **99239** more than 30 minutes
Prefatory instruction overrides midpoint rule.	Code **99291** is reported once for the first 30–74 minutes of critical care on a given date even if the time spent is not continuous on that date. *Critical care of <30 minutes' total duration on a given date is reported with an evaluation and management code other than* **99291**.

- If your EHR or other coding reference does not include the prefatory and parenthetical instructions provided in *CPT*, code verification by a second party prior to billing may be necessary. Alternatively, it may be possible to insert instructions in the form of notes or alerts in an EHR.
- Some payers may require that the typical time assigned to a service be met or exceeded rather than approximated as allowed for some services by *CPT*.
- It is important to note that a code that is reported "per day" or for services "on the same date" is not reported for all services in a 24-hour period but, rather, all services on a single calendar date.

Examples

99463   Initial hospital or birthing center care, per day, for E/M of normal newborn infant admitted and discharged on the same date

99468   Initial inpatient neonatal critical care, per day, for the E/M of a critically ill neonate, 28 days of age or younger

- Time is the physician's or other reporting provider's time, unless otherwise stated. Time spent by clinical staff is reported only when specified in *CPT* or allowed under incident-to policy established by a payer.

See Chapter 13 for information on reporting services incident to a physician's service.

Documentation of Time

- Documentation of time spent providing services should be evident in the medical record for each service reported based on time (ie, total minutes of service or start and stop times).
- Documentation of time may be automated in an EHR, but physicians should be able to demonstrate that the EHR functionality captures the correct time for code selection as specified by *CPT*. For instance, only intraservice time is used to select codes for moderate sedation. Documentation should clearly reflect the start and stop times for this service.
- When multiple services are provided on the same date, the time spent in time-based services must be clearly distinguished from time spent providing other services.
- In addition to documentation of total time or start and stop times of service, documentation should clearly support the service reported. For example, documentation of psychotherapy should include factors such as modalities and frequency, functional status, mental status examination, diagnosis, treatment plan, prognosis, and progress.
- All documentation must be signed or electronically authenticated with the name and credentials of the physician or other provider of care and date of service.

Key Takeaways for Reporting Time

Examples of time-based reporting are included throughout this manual to further the understanding of time-based reporting. The examples emphasize some key tips for reporting based on time.

- Time must be documented to support coding of time-based services. Failure to document time may lead to lost revenue.
- Time is met when the midpoint is passed unless otherwise specified in *CPT* instruction or code descriptors.
- Time is that of the physician or other individual reporting the service unless otherwise specified (eg, code descriptor specifies clinical staff time).
- Documentation should include the context of time spent in counseling and/or coordination of care, when applicable. (Time of counseling and/or coordination of care is not a factor in code selection for some E/M services, such as office or other outpatient E/M services.)
- Some payers require the specific amount of time (eg, 43 minutes, with 30 minutes spent in counseling and/or coordination of care), while other payers allow less specific documentation (eg, >40 minutes spent face-to-face with >50% spent in counseling and/or coordination of care).

National Drug Code (NDC)

NDCs are universal product identifiers for prescription drugs including vaccines and insulin products. Codes are 10-digit, 3-segment numbers that identify the product, labeler, and trade package size. Medicare, Medicaid, and other government payers (eg, Tricare), as well as some private payers, require the use of NDCs when reporting medication and vaccine product codes.

- The HIPAA standards for reporting NDCs do not align with the 10-digit format; they require an 11-digit code.
  - Conversion to an 11-digit code in 5-4-2 format is required.
  - Leading zeros are added to the appropriate segment to accomplish the 5-4-2 format, as illustrated in **Table 1-6**.

  It is important to verify each payer's requirements for NDC reporting. A payer may require either of the following:
- The NDC that is provided on the outer packaging when a vaccine or other drug is supplied in bulk packages
- The NDC from the vial that was administered

  When reporting NDCs
- A qualifier (N4) precedes the NDC number on the claim form (eg, N400006404720).
- The correct number of NDC units must also be included on claims.
  - The NDC units are often different from HCPCS or *CPT* units.
  - For most payers, NDC units are reported as grams (GR), milligrams (ME), milliliters (ML), or units (UN).
  - The qualifiers GR, ME, ML, and UN are reported before the number of NDC units on a claim to indicate the measure.

Table 1-6. National Drug Code Format Examples		
Product	**10-digit NDC Formats**	**11-digit NDC Formats (Added 0 [zero] is <u>underscored.</u>)**
RotaTeq 2-mL single-dose tube, package of 20	0006-4047-20 (4-4-2)	<u>0</u>0006-4047-20 (5-4-2)
Fluzone Quadrivalent 0.25-mL prefilled single-dose syringe, package of 10	49281-517-25 (5-3-2)	49281-<u>0</u>517-25 (5-4-2)
Synagis 0.5-mL in 1 vial, single dose	60574-4114-1 (5-4-1)	60574-4114-<u>0</u>1 (5-4-2)
Abbreviation: NDC, National Drug Code.		

Example

➤ A claim for supply of 0.5-mL, single-dose, prefilled syringe of pneumococcal 13-valent conjugate vaccine would include 1 unit of service on the claim line with *CPT* code **90670** and ML05 units on the NDC line for this service (example NDC claim line: N400005197105 ML05).

●=New code   ▲=Revised code   #=Re-sequenced code   +=Add-on code

If you are not currently reporting vaccines with NDCs, be sure to coordinate the requirements with your billing software company. For more information on NDCs, visit www.fda.gov/drugs/informationondrugs/ucm142438.htm or visit www.aap.org/cfp (access code AAPCFP26) for updates.

Beyond Code Sets

Who Assigns the Codes?

- Diagnoses should be assigned by the clinician (ie, pediatrician, pediatric nurse practitioner, or physician assistant) indicating a principal (primary) diagnosis that best explains the reason with the highest risk of morbidity or mortality for the patient encounter.
- All contributing (secondary) diagnoses that help explain the medical necessity for the episode of care should also be listed. However, only those conditions that specifically affect the patient's encounter should be listed.
- Code assignment may take place in conjunction with documentation or later, depending on the workflow processes of the practice.

> Documentation of diagnoses, signs and symptoms, or other reasons for a service is not accomplished through code assignment. Per official guidance from *Coding Clinic*, selection of a code cannot replace a written diagnostic statement. Multiple clinical conditions may be represented by a single diagnosis code, and more than 1 code may be required to fully describe a condition. Codes should be assigned to the documented diagnostic statement.

- When codes are selected by physicians at the time of EHR documentation, it is advisable to have trained administrative staff verify that the codes are selected in compliance with *ICD-10-CM* guidelines and conventions. Electronic health records often fail to show complete code descriptors and/or *ICD-10-CM* instructions (eg, exclusion notes).
- Assignment of the specific diagnosis code by clinical or administrative staff should be done under the physician's or reporting provider's supervision.
- The first-listed code on the claim should be the principal diagnosis unless the tabular instructions direct to "code first" a specific condition (eg, code first cystic fibrosis [**E84.-**] in a patient with secondary diabetes [**E08.-**] due to cystic fibrosis).
- Verification of the levels of service, need for modifiers, and compliance with *CPT* and payer policies is advised prior to billing.
- For those practices using a printed encounter form, including 50 to 100 of the most commonly used diagnoses *and* their respective codes on the outpatient encounter form allows the physician or other QHP to mark the appropriate code(s), indicating which is primary.
  - If a specific diagnosis code is not included on the form, write it in.
  - Do not select a diagnosis code that is "closest to" the diagnosis.
  - The AAP has developed a *Pediatric Office Superbill* (an encounter form including *ICD-10-CM* codes). For a copy, go to www.aap.org/cfp (access code AAPCFP26).

Reporting Codes for Payment

In addition to establishing standard code sets, HIPAA also established electronic transaction standards for patient benefit inquiries and submission of health claims and related reports.

- Claims for professional services are typically submitted electronically in a format referred to as 837P (professional claim) as currently configured in version 5010A1.
- Paper claim form submissions using the National Uniform Claim Committee 1500 claim form, version 02/12 (1500 form), are allowed for providers who meet an exception to the HIPAA requirements for electronic claim submission (eg, provider with <10 full-time employees).
  - Paper claims submission increases the length of time between submission and payment and increases the chance of error in either completion of the form or claims processing. Because of this, few physicians routinely submit paper claims and it is advisable to submit electronic claims whenever possible.
  - The 1500 form contains the same information as an electronic claim and is valuable for demonstrating how codes and other information necessary for claims processing must be relayed to payers. An example of a completed 1500 form is found in **Figure 1-2**.

Figure 1-2. Example of a Completed 1500 Form

Example 1500 Claim Form

HEALTH INSURANCE CLAIM FORM

APPROVED BY NATIONAL UNIFORM CLAIM COMMITTEE (NUCC) 02/12

ABC Health Plan
123 Money St.
Anywhere, AK 00000

CARRIER

PICA | PICA

1. MEDICARE (Medicare#) ☐ | MEDICAID (Medicaid#) ☒ | TRICARE (ID#/DoD#) ☐ | CHAMPVA (Member ID#) ☐ | GROUP HEALTH PLAN (ID#) ☐ | FECA BLK LUNG (ID#) ☐ | OTHER (ID#) ☐ | 1a. INSURED'S I.D. NUMBER (For Program in Item 1): 123456789

2. PATIENT'S NAME (Last Name, First Name, Middle Initial): Smith, Boy
3. PATIENT'S BIRTH DATE: MM 11 DD 22 YY 2020 — SEX M ☒ F
4. INSURED'S NAME (Last Name, First Name, Middle Initial): Smith, Momma

5. PATIENT'S ADDRESS (No., Street): 123 Main St.
6. PATIENT RELATIONSHIP TO INSURED: Self ☒ Spouse ☐ Child ☐ Other ☐
7. INSURED'S ADDRESS (No., Street)

CITY: Anywhere | STATE: KS
8. RESERVED FOR NUCC USE
CITY | STATE

ZIP CODE: 12345 | TELEPHONE (Include Area Code): (555) 5555555
ZIP CODE | TELEPHONE (Include Area Code): ( )

9. OTHER INSURED'S NAME (Last Name, First Name, Middle Initial): Smith, Poppa
10. IS PATIENT'S CONDITION RELATED TO:
11. INSURED'S POLICY GROUP OR FECA NUMBER: 98765432102

a. OTHER INSURED'S POLICY OR GROUP NUMBER: 45612378900
a. EMPLOYMENT? (Current or Previous): YES ☐ NO ☒
a. INSURED'S DATE OF BIRTH: MM 01 DD 01 YY 1992 — SEX M ☐ F ☒

b. RESERVED FOR NUCC USE
b. AUTO ACCIDENT? YES ☐ NO ☒ PLACE (State)
b. OTHER CLAIM ID (Designated by NUCC)

c. RESERVED FOR NUCC USE
c. OTHER ACCIDENT? YES ☐ NO ☒
c. INSURANCE PLAN NAME OR PROGRAM NAME: Good Health Plan

d. INSURANCE PLAN NAME OR PROGRAM NAME: Another Good Plan
10d. CLAIM CODES (Designated by NUCC)
d. IS THERE ANOTHER HEALTH BENEFIT PLAN? YES ☒ NO ☐ If yes, complete items 9, 9a, and 9d.

READ BACK OF FORM BEFORE COMPLETING & SIGNING THIS FORM.
12. PATIENT'S OR AUTHORIZED PERSON'S SIGNATURE I authorize the release of any medical or other information necessary to process this claim. I also request payment of government benefits either to myself or to the party who accepts assignment below.
SIGNED: Signature on file DATE: 02/22/2021

13. INSURED'S OR AUTHORIZED PERSON'S SIGNATURE I authorize payment of medical benefits to the undersigned physician or supplier for services described below.
SIGNED: Signature on file

14. DATE OF CURRENT ILLNESS, INJURY, or PREGNANCY (LMP): MM DD YY QUAL.
15. OTHER DATE: QUAL. MM DD YY
16. DATES PATIENT UNABLE TO WORK IN CURRENT OCCUPATION: FROM MM DD YY TO MM DD YY

17. NAME OF REFERRING PROVIDER OR OTHER SOURCE: 17a. | 17b. NPI
18. HOSPITALIZATION DATES RELATED TO CURRENT SERVICES: FROM MM DD YY TO MM DD YY

19. ADDITIONAL CLAIM INFORMATION (Designated by NUCC)
20. OUTSIDE LAB? YES ☐ NO ☐ $ CHARGES

21. DIAGNOSIS OR NATURE OF ILLNESS OR INJURY Relate A-L to service line below (24E) ICD Ind. 0
A. Z00.129 | B. Z23 | C. | D.
E. | F. | G. | H.
I. | J. | K. | L.

22. RESUBMISSION CODE | ORIGINAL REF. NO.
23. PRIOR AUTHORIZATION NUMBER

24. A. DATE(S) OF SERVICE From MM DD YY	To MM DD YY	B. PLACE OF SERVICE	C. EMG	D. PROCEDURES, SERVICES, OR SUPPLIES CPT/HCPCS	MODIFIER	E. DIAGNOSIS POINTER	F. $ CHARGES	G. DAYS OR UNITS	H. EPSDT Family Plan	I. ID QUAL	J. RENDERING PROVIDER ID. #
1	02 22 21		11		99391	25	A	111 00	1		NPI	1234567890
N44928105105 ML05												
2	02 22 21		11		90698		AB	200 00	1		NPI	1234567890
N400006404741 ML2												
3	02 22 21		11		90680		AB	200 00	1		NPI	1234567890
N400005197105 ML05												
4	02 22 21		11		90670		AB	200 00	1		NPI	1234567890
5	02 22 21		11		90460		AB	150 00	3		NPI	1234567890
6	02 22 21		11		90461		AB	100 00	4		NPI	1234567890

25. FEDERAL TAX I.D. NUMBER: 12-4567897 SSN ☐ EIN ☒
26. PATIENT'S ACCOUNT NO.: 11111
27. ACCEPT ASSIGNMENT? (For govt. claims, see back) YES ☒ NO ☐
28. TOTAL CHARGE $ 961 00
29. AMOUNT PAID $
30. Rsvd for NUCC Use

31. SIGNATURE OF PHYSICIAN OR SUPPLIER INCLUDING DEGREES OR CREDENTIALS (I certify that the statements on the reverse apply to this bill and are made a part thereof.): Signature on file SIGNED 02232021 DATE
32. SERVICE FACILITY LOCATION INFORMATION: Pediatric Practice, 111 Some Street, Anywhere, US 99999 a. NPI b.
33. BILLING PROVIDER INFO & PH # (555) 5555555: Pediatric Practice, 111 Some Street, Anywhere, US 99999 a. 01233456789 b.

NUCC Instruction Manual available at: www.nucc.org   PLEASE PRINT OR TYPE   APPROVED OMB-0938-1197 FORM 1500 (02-12)

PATIENT AND INSURED INFORMATION

PHYSICIAN OR SUPPLIER INFORMATION

Chapter 1. The Basics of Coding

Linking the Diagnosis to the Service

- Every claim line for a physician service must be linked to the appropriate *ICD-10-CM* code that represents the reason for the service.
  - Each *ICD-10-CM* code is placed in a diagnosis field labeled 21A–L.
  - A diagnosis pointer in field 24E indicates which diagnosis code relates to each service line by indicating the letter of the related diagnosis field. More than 1 diagnosis field may be linked to a service.
- When using an EHR, physicians should list the primary diagnosis in the EHR first and make certain the software knows that it should be reported as the first listed. In addition, the EHR should be able to link diagnosis codes to the appropriate services.
- The diagnosis code may be the same for each service performed.

Example

➤ **If a child is diagnosed with a urinary tract infection, the code for urinary tract infection (*ICD-10-CM* code N39.0) should be linked to the E/M service (eg, 99213) and a dipstick urinalysis without microscopy (81002) performed.**

Other Coding and Billing Information

Correct code assignment and claim completion are important steps in compliant and effective practice management. However, many other processes and policies are required. Please see **Chapter 4** for additional guidance on coding and billing procedures.

Resources

AAP Coding Assistance and Education

AAP Coding Hotline (https://form.jotform.com/Subspecialty/aapcodinghotline)

AAP *Coding for Pediatrics* Online

www.aap.org/cfp (access code AAPCFP26)
AAP Initial History Questionnaire (https://shop.aap.org/initial-history-questionnaire-documentation-form)

AAP *Pediatric Coding Newsletter*™

ICD-10-CM Collection (https://coding.solutions.aap.org/icd10.aspx; subscription required)

Current Procedural Terminology (CPT)

American Medical Association *CPT* general information (www.ama-assn.org/practice-management/cpt-current-procedural-terminology)
Category II code changes (*CPT* Category II codes alphabetical clinical topics listing: www.ama-assn.org/practice-management/cpt/category-ii-codes)

Category III code list (www.ama-assn.org/practice-management/cpt/category-iii-codes)

Newly released vaccine codes (www.ama-assn.org/practice-management/cpt/category-i-vaccine-codes)

ICD-10-CM Code Files and Guidelines

National Center for Health Statistics *ICD-10-CM* (www.cdc.gov/nchs/icd/icd10cm.htm)

American Academy of Pediatrics *Pediatric ICD-10-CM: A Manual for Provider-Based Coding* (available for purchase at https://shop.aap.org)

National Drug Codes

US Food and Drug Administration National Drug Code Directory (www.fda.gov/drugs/informationondrugs/ucm142438.htm)

Test Your Knowledge!

1. **Which of the following is a general principle of documentation?**
   a. Physicians must always submit full documentation of services with each claim.
   b. Physicians should assign as many codes as possible for each service.
   c. Physicians should copy and paste notes whenever possible.
   d. The medical record should be complete and legible.

2. **Which of the following best describes a first-listed diagnosis?**
   a. The code assigned for the condition a patient self-diagnosed prior to the visit
   b. The codes assigned for the patient's presenting signs and symptoms
   c. The code assigned for the condition chiefly responsible for the services provided
   d. The code assigned to the patient's condition that has the highest risk regardless of the reasons for the services provided

3. **Which of the following is a guideline in *ICD-10-CM*?**
   a. Always assign a code for a condition that is unconfirmed.
   b. Do not report codes for conditions that have been previously treated but no longer exist.
   c. Report additional codes for conditions that are integral to a disease process.
   d. Always assign a code for signs and symptoms.

4. **Which of the following indicates failure to document information that would typically be known at the time of the encounter and/or inappropriate code selection?**
   a. Viral intestinal infection, unspecified (**A08.4**)
   b. Acute pharyngitis, unspecified (**J02.9**)
   c. Sprain of unspecified site of right knee (**S83.91X-**)
   d. Extremely low birth weight newborn, unspecified weight (**P07.00**)

5. **Which of the following is true of the *CPT* code set?**
   a. Three categories of codes are included in the code set.
   b. All codes are updated on January 1 of each year.
   c. *CPT* codes are Level II codes of HCPCS.
   d. *CPT* codes should be selected from an index of procedures.

●=New code ▲=Revised code #=Re-sequenced code +=Add-on code

Modifiers and Coding Edits

Contents

Chapter 2. Modifiers and Coding Edits

Current Procedural Terminology® Modifiers

Current Procedural Terminology (*CPT*®) defines a *modifier* as an indicator that a service or procedure has been altered by some specific circumstance but not changed in its basic code definition. Because a modifier is used to report a service or procedure that was altered, medical record documentation must always support the use of the modifier.

In addition to *CPT* modifiers, the Centers for Medicare & Medicaid Services (CMS) maintains a list of modifiers for use with Healthcare Common Procedure Coding System (HCPCS) and *CPT* codes. Most state Medicaid programs and many commercial payers follow CMS guidelines and may recognize HCPCS modifiers as well.

When are modifiers needed? In brief, a modifier or combination of modifiers is appended to a procedure code when it is necessary to add context of how or when the service was provided. Context often affects payment, such as when a bilateral procedure is reported with a code that does not indicate unilateral or bilateral. By appending modifier **50** (bilateral procedure), the claim for services provides context allowing claims adjudication systems to process for payment at a higher rate (typically 150% of the allowable amount for the unilateral service). Examples of information provided by modifiers include

- A service provided on the same date or within the global period of a previous service is unrelated, more extensive, performed on a different body area, or performed at separate encounters.
- A face-to-face service was provided via telemedicine using real-time, interactive communication technology.
- The same service was repeated on the same date.
- An evaluation and management (E/M) service that might otherwise be considered part of another service is significantly beyond the typical preservice and/or post-service components of the other service.
- The units of services provided were medically necessary but exceed the payer's unit of service edits.
- A service that may be provided for diagnostic or preventive purposes was provided for preventive purposes.

Some modifiers are used exclusively with E/M services, and others are reported only with surgical or other procedures. Refer to **Table 2-1** to review modifiers used with E/M service codes and those used only for other services. Multiple modifiers can be appended to a single *CPT* or HCPCS code.

Payers use coding edits (ie, paired codes and/or unit of service limitations) to aid in automated claims adjudication. Modifiers play an important role in this process.

- When a modifier is appropriately applied to 1 code in a pair of codes reported by a physician on 1 date of service or to a code for services that exceed the units of service typically allowed by payer edits, the payer may allow charges that would otherwise be denied as bundled or non-covered.
- Further illustration of the use of modifiers in relation to payer edits is discussed in the Coding Edits section later in this chapter.

The Health Insurance Portability and Accountability Act of 1996 requires recognition of all *CPT* modifiers, but payers may have their own payment and billing policies for the use of modifiers that can vary from *CPT* guidelines.

- Know and understand their policies. This is important to capturing all payments allowed under your contract.
- If payment is denied inappropriately because of nonrecognition or the incorrect application of a modifier, you should appeal the denied services.
- For additional assistance, contact the American Academy of Pediatrics (AAP) Coding Hotline (https://form.jotform.com/Subspecialty/aapcodinghotline).

Table 2-1. Modifiers and Evaluation and Management Services	
24, 25, 57	E/M-only modifiers
22, 26, 47, 50, 51, 52, 53, 54, 55, 56, 58, 59, 62, 63, 66, 76, 77, 78, 79, 80, 81, 82, 91	Procedure-only (non-E/M service) modifiers (Do not append to E/M services.)
32, 33, 92, 95, 96, 97, 99	Either E/M or procedures
Abbreviation: E/M, evaluation and management.	

22—Increased Procedural Services

- Modifier **22** is used to report procedures when the work required to provide a service is substantially greater than typically required.
- Modifier **22** is only appended to anesthesia, surgery, radiology, laboratory, pathology, and medicine codes.

●=New code   ▲=Revised code   #=Re-sequenced code   +=Add-on code

- Documentation must clearly reflect the substantial additional work and the reason for the additional work (eg, increased intensity, time, technical difficulty of procedure, severity of patient's condition, physical and mental effort required).
  - It is important that the documentation is specific. For instance, documentation that a procedure took longer than 1 hour is less supportive than documentation that the procedure took a total of 85 minutes or lasted from 9:15 to 10:40 am.
  - Reporting of additional diagnosis codes to support the increased work is also important.
- Most payers will require that a copy of the medical record documentation be sent with the claim when modifier **22** is reported.
- For an electronic claim, indicate "additional documentation available on request" in the claim level loop (2300 NTE) or in the line level loop (2400 NTE) segment. If the payer allows electronic claim attachments, follow the payer's instructions to submit the procedure note and, if necessary, a physician statement about the increased difficulty of the procedure.

Examples—Modifier 22

➤ **The physician required 45 minutes to perform a simple repair of a 1-cm laceration on a 2-year-old because the child was combative and several stops and starts were necessary.**
  12011 22 (simple repair superficial wound of face; ≤2.5 cm)

➤ **An appendectomy is performed on a morbidly obese 12-year-old.** The surgery is complicated and requires additional time because of the obesity.
  44950 22 (appendectomy)

24—Unrelated E/M Service by the Same Physician or Other Qualified Health Care Professional During a Postoperative Period

For more information on global surgery guidelines, see chapters 10 and 19.

- Modifier **24** is appended to an E/M code when the physician or other qualified health care professional (QHP) who performed a procedure provides an unrelated E/M service during the postoperative period.
- The CMS has its own system for definition of global periods, and some payers will follow those guidelines or assign a specific number of follow-up days for surgical procedures.

  Link the appropriate *International Classification of Diseases, 10th Revision, Clinical Modification* (*ICD-10-CM*) code to the E/M visit to support that the service was unrelated to the surgical procedure. Do not report the surgical diagnosis code if it was not the reason for the encounter.

Example—Modifier 24

➤ **A physician sees a 6-year-old established patient for swimmer's ear (right ear) and performs a level-2 established patient office or other outpatient E/M service.** Eight days prior to this visit, the physician had performed a removal of a subcutaneous foreign body (by incision) not involving the fascia from the patient's foot. The CMS has assigned a 10-day global postoperative period to code **10120** (removal foreign body subcutaneous tissues, simple), indicating that payment for all follow-up visits within that period related to that surgical service are included under the code. Many payers will follow the CMS global period.

ICD-10-CM	CPT
H60.331 (acute swimmer's ear, right ear)	**99212 24** (established office/outpatient E/M)

25—Significant, Separately Identifiable E/M Service by the Same Physician or Other Qualified Health Care Professional on the Same Day of the Procedure or Other Service

- Modifier **25** is appended only to an E/M service, and only when *all of the following are true:*
  - A separate service identified by a separate procedure code is performed by the same physician or other QHP, or by a physician or other QHP of the same specialty and group.
  - The patient's condition requires a significant E/M service (**99202–99499**) above and beyond the other service provided or beyond the usual preoperative and postoperative care associated with the procedure that was performed.
  - The service is separately identifiable in the documentation of the encounter(s).
- Different diagnoses are not required for reporting of the E/M service on the same date.
- The performed and documented E/M components must support the level of service reported and be separately identifiable from the procedure or other service documentation whether documented in 1 combined note or separate notes.
- *CPT* procedure codes include evaluative elements routinely performed prior to the procedure and the routine postoperative care. An assessment of the problem with an explanation of the procedure to be performed is considered inherent to the procedure and should not be reported separately with an E/M service code.
- When appropriate, modifier **25** may be reported on more than 1 E/M service for a single encounter. An example would be reporting a preventive medicine service (eg, **99393 25**) along with a problem-oriented service (eg, **99212 25**) in addition to giving the patient vaccines with counseling (eg, **90460**).
- **DO *NOT* USE MODIFIER 25 WHEN**
  - **The medical record does not support both services.**
  - **A problem encountered during a preventive medicine visit is insignificant or incidental (eg, minor diaper rash, renewal of prescription medications without reevaluation) or did not require additional work to perform the key components (ie, history, physical examination, and, importantly, medical decision-making [MDM], or time) of the E/M service.**
  - **The E/M service is a routine part of the usual preoperative and postoperative care.**
  - **Modifier 57 (decision for surgery) is more appropriate. The ultimate decision on whether to use modifier 25 or 57 requires knowledge of payer policies. (See modifier 57 later in this chapter.)**

Examples—Modifier 25

➤ **An E/M service is performed on a 6-year-old established patient.** He is given 600,000 units of Bicillin (penicillin G benzathine) by intramuscular injection for strep throat.

ICD-10-CM	CPT
J02.0 (streptococcal pharyngitis)	**99212–99215 25** (established patient E/M visit, office) **J0561** × 6 units (injection penicillin G benzathine, 100,000 units) **96372** (administration therapeutic injection)

    Teaching Point: *CPT* requires that modifier **25** be appended to a significant and separately identifiable E/M service when also reporting the administration of a therapeutic injection.

➤ **A 12-year-old established patient is seen for his preventive medicine visit.** The patient complains of an increasingly severe itchy rash on his hands, arms, and legs for 3 days. He is diagnosed and treated for a moderately severe case of poison ivy, requiring a prescription for a topical steroid. Medical decision-making is straightforward, supporting code **99212**. He has not yet received his tetanus, diphtheria, and acellular pertussis (Tdap) or meningococcal (MenACWY-D) intramuscular vaccines. The physician counsels the parents on the risks and protection from each of the diseases. The Centers for Disease Control and Prevention (CDC) Vaccine Information Statements are given to the parents and the nurse administers the vaccines.

     ●=New code   ▲=Revised code   #=Re-sequenced code   +=Add-on code

ICD-10-CM	CPT
Z00.121 (well-child check with abnormal findings) **Z23** (encounter for immunization)	**99394 25** (preventive medicine visit, established patient, age 12 through 17 years) **90715** (Tdap, 7 years or older, intramuscular) **90734** (MenACWY-D) **90460** × 2 units **90461** × 2 units
L23.7 (allergic contact dermatitis due to plants, except food)	**99212 25** (office/outpatient E/M, established patient)

Teaching Point: Medical record documentation supports that a significant, separately identifiable E/M service was provided and is reported in addition to the preventive medicine service. Modifier **25** is appended to code **99212** to signify that it is significant and separately identifiable from the preventive medicine service. Modifier **25** is also appended to code **99394** to signify it is significant and separately identifiable from immunization administration (required by payers that have adopted Medicare and Medicaid bundling edits).

See Chapter 9 for additional examples and guidelines for reporting a preventive medicine visit and a problem-oriented visit on the same day of service.

➤ **A patient is scheduled for an office encounter for excision of an ingrown toenail.** The physician takes a problem-focused history from the patient, who has no other complaints; examines the affected nail; and agrees with excision, explaining the procedure, risks, and benefits. The ingrown nail is corrected by wedge excision of the nail fold.

ICD-10-CM	CPT
L60.0 (ingrowing nail)	**11765** (wedge excision of skin of nail fold)

Teaching Point: An E/M service with modifier **25** is *not* reported. A separate charge for an E/M service is reported only when the E/M service is significant and separately identifiable from the preservice work of a procedure reported on the same date.

See chapters 10 and 19 for more information on reporting an evaluation and management service on the date of a procedure.

26—Professional Component

Professional, Technical, or Global Services

Certain procedures (eg, cardiac tests, radiographs, surgical diagnostic tests, laboratory tests) are broken down into professional and technical components. *CPT* has a modifier for the professional component (**26**) but does not have a modifier for reporting only the technical component. That falls under the HCPCS modifier set (modifier **TC**).

- Professional component only: The physician who does not own the equipment but performs the written interpretation and report should report the service with modifier **26** appended to the appropriate *CPT* code.
  - Modifier **26** is used to indicate that only the physician or other QHP component (supervision and interpretation) is being reported on a procedure that includes technical and professional (physician) components.
  - The professional component includes the physician work (eg, interpretation of the test, written report).
- Technical component only: Most payers recognize modifier **TC** (technical component only). The facility or provider who owns the equipment and is responsible for the overhead and associated costs would report the same procedure code with modifier **TC** appended.
- Technical and professional components (global): If a service includes a professional and technical component and the physician owns the equipment, employs the staff to perform the service, and interprets the test, the procedure is reported *without a modifier*.

Reporting Modifier 26

- When reporting the professional component of diagnostic tests, interpretation should be documented in a report similar to that which is typical for the physicians who predominantly provide the service. This report should include *all of the following:*
  — Indication(s) for testing
  — Description of test
  — Findings
  — Limitations (when applicable)
  — Impression or conclusion
- If the report of a physician's interpretation is included in the documentation of another service (eg, office visit), it is important that the report is distinct and complete.
- The professional component is not reported when a physician reviews a test and notes agreement with the interpreting physician or when only a quick read without formal interpretation is provided.
- Some codes were developed to distinguish between technical and professional components (eg, routine electrocardiogram [ECG] codes **93000–93010**). Modifier **26** is not appropriate when reporting codes that distinguish professional and technical components and may result in a denial of the charge.

Examples—Modifier 26

➤ **A pediatrician interprets and creates a report of the findings from a radiograph of the foot that was produced by an outpatient radiology practice and transmitted electronically to the pediatrician. The pediatrician's order was for imaging without interpretation and report, so there is no other interpretation and report (ie, a radiologist will not also interpret and report).**

    73620 26 (x-ray foot, 2 views)

    The physician reports modifier **26**, indicating professional component only, because the hospital provided the technical component.

➤ **A pediatrician electronically accesses the image of a foot radiograph that was taken at the outpatient department of the hospital and will be interpreted by a radiologist at that facility. The pediatrician notes findings in the patient's records.**

    The pediatrician's review of the radiograph is not separately reported when a radiologist will provide a final interpretation and report. The physician did not perform the interpretation and report that constitutes the professional component of the foot radiograph. However, the physician's review of the image increases the level of MDM in a related E/M service.

➤ **A cardiologist performs transthoracic echocardiography with spectral and color-flow Doppler on a patient in the hospital.**

    The surgeon would report code **93306 26** (echocardiography, transthoracic, real-time with image documentation [2D], includes M-mode recording, when performed, complete, with spectral Doppler echocardiography, and with color-flow Doppler echocardiography), and the hospital would report code **93306 TC**.

32—Mandated Services

- Modifier **32** is appended to services (eg, second opinion) that are mandated by a third-party payer or governmental, legislative, or regulatory requirements.
- The modifier may be reported with codes for E/M services (eg, for second opinion required by a payer).
- Modifier **32** would be used when, for example, radiological services are requested from a worker's compensation carrier, laboratory testing (eg, drug tests) is requested by a court system, or a physical therapy assessment is requested by an insurer.

Chapter 2. Modifiers and Coding Edits

Example—Modifier 32

➤ **A developmental pediatrician is asked by a managed care organization to provide a second opinion on a family physician's patient for selected treatment services for autism spectrum disorder (ASD).** A comprehensive history and physical examination with high MDM are performed and documented and a report with recommendations is sent back to the managed care organization.

ICD-10-CM	CPT	
F84.0 (autistic disorder)	**99245 32** (office/outpatient consultation)	

33—Preventive Services

CPT modifier **33** is used to communicate to payers that a preventive medicine service (defined by the Patient Protection and Affordable Care Act [PPACA] provisions; the 4 categories are listed as follows) was performed on a patient enrolled in a health care plan subject to the preventive service coverage requirements of the PPACA and, therefore, should not be subject to cost sharing.

- The appropriate use of modifier **33** will reduce claim adjustments related to preventive services and facilitate correct payments to members.
- Modifier **33** should only be appended to codes represented in 1 or more of the following 4 categories:
  — Services rated A or B by the US Preventive Services Task Force
  — Immunizations for routine use in children, adolescents, and adults as recommended by the Advisory Committee on Immunization Practices of the CDC
  — Preventive care and screenings for children as recommended by Bright Futures (AAP) and newborn testing (American College of Medical Genetics and Genomics)
  — Preventive care and screenings provided for women supported by the Health Resources and Services Administration
- **DO *NOT* USE MODIFIER 33**
  — **When the *CPT* code(s) is identified as inherently preventive (eg, preventive medicine counseling)**
  — **When the service(s) is not indicated in the categories noted previously**
  — **With an insurance plan that continues to implement the cost-sharing policy on preventive medicine services**
- Check with your payers before reporting modifier **33** to verify any variations in reporting requirements.

Example—Modifier 33

➤ **A 17-year-old established patient is seen for an office visit on Monday for a missed period and suspected pregnancy.** The physician provides an E/M service with straightforward MDM. The physician determines the patient is not pregnant and does not want to become pregnant but has been sexually active with multiple partners. The physician then spends approximately 10 minutes discussing contraception and risks of sexually transmitted infection (STI) with the patient. Point-of-care HIV-1 and HIV-2 testing is conducted with negative results. Specimen is collected for chlamydia and gonorrhea screening by an outside laboratory. The patient chooses to adopt barrier contraception methods and acknowledges understanding of risks and benefits of this contraception method.

ICD-10-CM	CPT
Z32.02 (encounter for pregnancy test, result negative)	Problem-oriented **99212 25** (office visit) **81025** (urine pregnancy test)
Z30.09 (encounter for other general counseling and advice on contraception) **Z11.4** (encounter for screening for HIV) **Z11.3** (encounter for screening for STI)	Preventive **99401** (preventive counseling, approximately 15 minutes) **86703 33 92** (antibody; HIV-1 and HIV-2; single assay)

Teaching Point: Append modifier **33** to code **86703** to indicate the test was performed as a preventive service because, although recommended as a preventive service, the test is also used for diagnostic purposes. Modifier **92** is reported to indicate use of the HIV test kit (not all payers recognize modifier **92**). Code **99401** is reported for 8 to 23 minutes of service based on the midpoint rule for billing based on time (ie, time is met when the midpoint is passed). Typically, health plans cover services related to contraception (eg, **99401**) without cost to the patient.

For more information on reporting moderate sedation, see chapters 10 and 19.

47—Anesthesia by Surgeon

- Modifier **47** is used only when a physician performing a procedure *also personally performs* the regional and/or general anesthesia. The physician performing the procedure may not report codes **00100–01999** for anesthesia services. Instead, modifier **47** is appended to the code for the procedure performed.
- When performed, a code for regional anesthesia (nerve block) may be reported to indicate the site of the block.
- Modifier **47** is considered informational by many payers and does not affect payment.
  - Medicaid considers all anesthesia (other than moderate conscious sedation) provided by the same physician performing a procedure to be included in the procedure.
  - Other payers may restrict use of modifier **47** to specific procedure codes and provide specific reporting instructions. Be sure to verify payer policy prior to reporting.
- **DO *NOT* USE MODIFIER 47 WHEN**
  - **Administering local anesthesia because it is considered inherent to the procedure**
  - **Performing moderate (conscious) sedation**

Example—Modifier 47

➤ **The surgeon performs a nerve block on the brachial plexus (64415) and removal of a ganglion cyst on the wrist (25111).**
  25111 47 and **64415**
  The regional anesthesia is separate from the procedure.

50—Bilateral Procedure

- Modifier **50** is used to identify bilateral procedures that are performed at the same session.
- It is used only when the services and/or procedures are performed on identical anatomical sites, aspects, or organs.
- Modifier **50** is not appended to any code with a descriptor that indicates the procedure includes bilateral, "one or both," or "unilateral or bilateral."
- The Medicare Physician Fee Schedule Relative Value Files (www.cms.gov/Medicare/Medicare-Fee-for-Service-Payment/PhysicianFeeSched/PFS-Relative-Value-Files.html) include a column (Column Z, BILAT SURG) that identifies codes that may be reported with modifier **50**. Procedures with a 1 indicator can be reported with modifier **50**.

Many private payers also publish lists of codes that may be reported as bilateral procedures.

- When the *CPT* code descriptor indicates a bilateral procedure and only a unilateral procedure is performed, modifier **52** (reduced services) should be appended to the procedure code.
- For Medicaid claims that require use of modifier **50**, only report 1 unit of service on the line item for the bilateral procedure.

Examples—Modifier 50

➤ **A physician removes foreign bodies from both ears.**
  69200 50 (removal foreign body external auditory canal; without general anesthesia)

➤ **A physician performs bilateral computerized corneal topography.**

Modifier **50** would not be appended to code **92025** (computerized corneal topography, unilateral or bilateral, with interpretation and report) because the code descriptor indicates a unilateral or bilateral procedure. (Modifier **52** is also not required for reporting a unilateral service when the code descriptor includes unilateral or bilateral.)

Coding Conundrum: Modifier 50

Nearly all payers now follow *Current Procedural Terminology* guidelines and Medicaid National Correct Coding Initiative (NCCI) instruction for bilateral surgical procedures. The NCCI edits require that bilateral surgical procedures (for which there is no code specifying a bilateral procedure) be reported with modifier **50** and 1 unit of service.

Example: Report removal of foreign bodies from both ears with code **69200 50** with 1 unit.

Bilateral diagnostic procedures may be reported with 2 units of service on 1 claim line, 1 unit of service and modifier **50** on one claim line, or 1 unit of service and modifier **RT** on 1 claim line plus 1 unit of service and modifier **LT** on a second claim line.

Example: Report bilateral x-rays of clavicles with one of the following methods:
73000 (radiologic examination; clavicle, complete) × 2 units
73000 50 x 1 unit
73000 RT x 1 unit and **73000 LT** x 1 unit

51—Multiple Procedures

- Some payers, including some Medicare administrative contractors, have advised against reporting this modifier because their systems automatically assign multiple service reductions to the appropriate services. In these cases, the system ignores modifier **51**. Follow payer guidance for reporting modifier **51**.
- When required, modifier **51** is appended to additional procedures(s) or service(s) when multiple procedures are performed at the same session by the same individual or individuals in the same group practice. The primary procedure or service is reported first without a modifier.
- When multiple procedures or services are reported, payers usually reduce the payment for the second and each additional code by 50% because there is some resource cost duplication when multiple procedures are done at the same visit or session. Medicare and some state Medicaid programs follow this policy.
- Most payers identify procedures that are eligible for modifier **51** and, therefore, are subject to multiple procedure or service payment reductions. Although many claims adjudication systems now automatically identify the primary procedure, it is advisable that the first-reported service is that with the highest relative value, followed by additional services appended with modifier **51**, when applicable.

For information on multiple surgery indicators and adjustments, see Chapter 12, Section 40.6, of the *Medicare Claims Processing Manual* at www.cms.gov/Regulations-and-Guidance/Guidance/Manuals/Downloads/clm104c12.pdf.
- **DO *NOT* USE MODIFIER 51 WHEN**
  — **Reporting add-on procedures (codes identified with the + symbol are exempt from the need to report this modifier because the services are performed in addition to a primary procedure or service).**
  — **Reporting *CPT* codes identified with the symbol Ø (exempt from modifier 51) because they have no associated pre- or post-service valuation and are already reduced (see Appendix E in *CPT* for a list of these codes).**
  — **Different providers perform the procedures.**
  — **Two or more physicians perform different and unrelated procedures (eg, multiple trauma) on the same patient on the same day (unless one of the physicians performs multiple procedures).**
  — **Reporting E/M services, physical medicine and rehabilitation services, or provision of supplies (eg, vaccines).**

Example—Modifier 51

➤ **A child undergoes adenoidectomy and bilateral myringotomy with tube placement at the same surgical session. The surgeon reports**

69436 50   **Tympanostomy (requiring insertion of ventilating tube), general anesthesia**
42830 51   **Adenoidectomy, primary; younger than age 12**

Teaching Point: Code **69436** is reported first because it carries the highest relative value when reported with modifier **50** (6.72 non-facility total relative value units [4.48 times 150%] vs 5.95 for code **42830**). Modifier **51** is appended to code **42830**. If the myringotomy was a unilateral procedure, code **42830** would be listed first and modifier **51** appended to code **69436** (with no modifier **50**).

52—Reduced Services

- Modifier **52** is used when a service or procedure is partially reduced or eliminated (ie, procedure started but discontinued) at the discretion of the physician or other QHP.
- Modifier **52** is not used when a procedure is canceled prior to the induction of anesthesia and/or surgical preparation in the operating room.
- The diagnosis code linked to the procedure reported with modifier **52** should reflect why the procedure was reduced.
- When reporting a reduced service or a procedure code with modifier **52**, do not reduce your normal fee. Let the payer reduce the payment based on its policy.

Examples—Modifier 52

➤ **A peripherally inserted central venous catheter (PICC) without a subcutaneous port is inserted with imaging guidance, but tip location is not confirmed by imaging.**

ICD-10-CM	CPT
J13 (pneumonia due to *Streptococcus pneumoniae*)	**36572 52** (PICC insertion without subcutaneous port, with imaging guidance; younger than 5 years of age)

   Teaching Point: Code **36572** includes confirmation of the tip location. Therefore, modifier **52** would be appended when performed without confirmation of catheter tip location.

➤ **Polysomnography with sleep staging and 4 or more additional parameters of sleep, with attendance by a sleep technologist, is performed on a 7-year-old patient. The study is discontinued after 4 hours of recording due to the patient's inability to sleep.**

ICD-10-CM	CPT
R06.83 (snoring)	**95810 52** (polysomnography; age 6 or older, sleep staging with 4 or more additional parameters of sleep, attended by a technologist)

   Teaching Point: Instructions for reporting polysomnography include appending of modifier **52** when there is less than 6 hours of recording for code **95800**, **95801**, **95806**, **95807**, **95810**, or **95811**.

53—Discontinued Procedure

- Modifier **53** signifies that a procedure was terminated (ie, started but discontinued) due to extenuating circumstances or circumstances in which the well-being of the patient was threatened (eg, patient is at risk or has unexpected, serious complications, such as excessive bleeding or hypotension) during a procedure.
- It is not used to report the elective cancellation of a procedure prior to the patient's anesthesia induction and/or surgical preparation in the operating suite.
- The diagnosis code should reflect the reason for the termination of the procedure.
- Most payers will require that operative or procedure reports be submitted with the claim.

Examples—Modifier 53

➤ **An unsuccessful attempt is made to place a central line in the right subclavian vein.** The line is successfully placed in the left subclavian vein.
   36555 53 RT (insertion non-tunneled centrally inserted central venous catheter; younger than 5 years)
   36555 LT
   Note: Some payers do not recognize modifiers **RT** and **LT**. See the descriptions and use of these modifiers in the Healthcare Common Procedure Coding System Modifiers section later in this chapter.

Chapter 2. Modifiers and Coding Edits

➤ **During catheterization of the right side of the heart, the child experiences ventricular arrhythmia and the procedure is discontinued.**

93451 53 (right heart catheterization)

Coding Conundrum: Modifier 52 or 53?

The main distinction between modifiers **52** (reduced services—service was started but the physician elected to reduce the scope or even eliminate the procedure or service) and **53** (discontinued procedure—reason for terminating the procedure is due to extenuating circumstances or because complications arise that place the patient at risk) is the basis for the decision to alter the procedure. Modifier **52** is often used when the physician plans to reduce the scope or extent of the procedure as noted, whereas modifier **53** is used for situations such as unexpected events that occur in the course of the procedure (eg, cardiac arrest, profuse bleeding, arrhythmia). The following examples demonstrate the appropriate application of these modifiers when a physician performs a routine circumcision:

52: A physician begins a circumcision (**54150**) on a 3-day-old boy. The physician elects to perform the circumcision without a dorsal penile or ring block. In this circumstance, modifier **52** would be reported with code **54150** to indicate the service was reduced from its full descriptor based on the physician's discretion.

53: A physician begins a circumcision (**54150**) on a 3-day-old boy. During the procedure, the physician notices the neonate is showing signs of respiratory distress. The physician determines that the procedure needs to be discontinued to assess the neonate. Due to the severity of the situation, the physician decides not to continue with the procedure. In this circumstance, the physician would append modifier **53** to code **54150**, linking it to *International Classification of Diseases, 10th Revision, Clinical Modification* codes **Z41.2** (encounter for routine and ritual male circumcision) and **P22.9** (respiratory distress, newborn) to indicate why the procedure was discontinued. When reporting a procedure with modifier **53**, it is important to indicate why the procedure was discontinued.

54—Surgical Care Only

Modifier **54** is appended to the surgery procedure code when the physician does the procedure but another physician or other QHP (not of the same group practice) accepts a transfer of care and provides preoperative and/or postoperative management.

55—Postoperative Management Only

Modifier **55** is appended to the surgical code to report that only postoperative care is performed because another physician or other QHP of another group practice has performed the surgical procedure and transferred the patient for postoperative care.

56—Preoperative Management Only

Modifier **56** is appended to the surgical code when only the preoperative care and evaluation are performed because another physician or other QHP of another group practice has performed the surgical procedure.

Coding Conundrum: Modifiers 54, 55, and 56

Modifiers **54**, **55**, and **56** typically are used to report surgical procedures that have a global period of 10 to 90 days. They are not reported with procedures that have 0-day global periods. It is important to learn which guidelines are followed by your major payers. When reporting these modifiers, coordination and communication between the physicians and their billing staff is imperative.

For more information on global surgery guidelines, see **chapters 10** and **19**.

Examples—Modifiers 54, 55, and 56

➤ **An infant undergoes a repair of tetralogy of Fallot.** The patient's pediatric cardiologist provides the postoperative management.

The surgeon reports code **33692** (complete repair tetralogy of Fallot without pulmonary atresia) with modifier **54** appended, and the cardiologist reports code **33692 55** for postoperative care services.

These split care arrangements will usually require a manual review by payers, with some variable amount of the global fee being carved out for the 2 physicians. Check with your payers for their payment policy if this is typical for your practice.

➤ **A child is admitted to the hospital by the pediatrician for intravenous antibiotics for a deep abscess on the right leg.** On the second day of the hospital stay, a surgeon is called in and performs an incision and drainage of the abscess (includes follow-up care within 90 days following the procedure). The child is discharged on day 3 and seen in follow-up by the pediatrician.

Surgeon reports

ICD-10-CM	CPT
L02.415 (cutaneous abscess of right lower limb)	**27603 54** (incision and drainage with surgical care only)

Pediatrician reports

ICD-10-CM	CPT
L02.415	**27603 55** (incision and drainage with postoperative management only)

57—Decision for Surgery

- Modifier **57** is appended to an E/M service that resulted in the initial decision to perform the surgery or procedure.
- Appending modifier **57** to the E/M service indicates to the payer that the E/M service is not part of the global period. The global period for surgical procedures is assigned by the CMS, private payers, or state Medicaid and not by the American Medical Association.
- Many payers will follow the CMS Medicare payment policy that allows reporting of modifier **57** only when the visit on the day before or day of surgery results in a decision to perform a surgical procedure that has a 90-day global period (major procedure).
- Know commercial and state Medicaid policies, maintain a written copy of the policy, and adhere to the policy.

Examples—Modifier 57

➤ **A 10-year-old is seen by the pediatrician for the evaluation of pain in her foot.** Radiograph reveals a metatarsal fracture, and the decision is made to treat the closed fracture.

Code **28470** (closed treatment, metatarsal fracture; without manipulation) has an assigned global surgery period of 90 days. The appropriate E/M code (**99202–99215 57**), based on the medical necessity and performance and documentation of the required key components, would be reported in addition to code **28470**. An E/M code with modifier **57** is reported only by the physician or a physician of the same specialty and group practice of the physician who performs the procedure. Other physicians providing E/M services on the day before or day of a procedure would not append modifier **57**.

➤ **A circumcision is performed on the day of discharge on a 2-day-old born in the hospital, delivered vaginally.**

ICD-10-CM	CPT
Z38.00 (single liveborn infant, delivered vaginally) **Z41.2** (encounter for routine male circumcision)	**99238 25** (hospital discharge management) **54150** (circumcision using clamp/device with dorsal penile or ring block)

Teaching Point: The procedure has a 0-day global period. Per CMS guidelines, modifier **25** would be appended to the E/M service instead of modifier **57**.

●=New code   ▲=Revised code   #=Re-sequenced code   +=Add-on code

58—Staged or Related Procedure or Service by the Same Physician or Other Qualified Health Care Professional During the Postoperative Period

- Modifier **58** is used to indicate that a procedure or service performed during the postoperative period was planned or anticipated (ie, staged), was more extensive than the original procedure, or was for therapy following a surgical procedure.
- Modifier **58** is a recognized modifier under the National Correct Coding Initiative (NCCI). (See the Appropriate NCCI Modifiers section later in the chapter for more on NCCI edits.) Refer to the Medicaid NCCI website, www.medicaid.gov/medicaid/program-integrity/ncci/index.html, for more details on the proper use of modifier **58** to override an edit.
- Typically, payers recognize modifier **58** only when there is a global surgical period associated with the procedure code.
- **DO *NOT* REPORT MODIFIER 58 WHEN**
  - **Treatment of a problem requires a return to the operating/procedure room (eg, unanticipated clinical condition) (see modifier 78).**
  - **Reporting procedures that include as part of their *CPT* descriptor "one or more visits" or "one or more sessions."**

Examples—Modifier 58

➤ **An excision of a malignant lesion (1 cm) on the leg is performed.** The pathology report indicates that the margins were not adequate, and a re-excision is performed 1 week later. The excised diameter is less than 2 cm.
11602 58 (excision, malignant lesion including margins, leg; excised diameter 1.1–2.0 cm) for the second excision
Note: The first excision would be reported using code **11601** (margin diameter 0.6–1.0 cm).

➤ **Closure of a perineal urethrostomy, 5 weeks post-hypospadias repair, is performed as planned.**
53520 58 (closure of urethrostomy)

59—Distinct Procedural Service

> Never use modifier **59** in place of modifier **25** or on an evaluation and management service.

- Modifier **59** is never appended to the code for an E/M service.
- Report modifier **59** only when no other modifier better describes the reason for separately reporting a service that might otherwise be bundled with another procedural service on the same date.
- Never append modifier **59** to bypass payer edits without clinical justification.
- See HCPCS modifiers **XE, XP, XS,** and **XU** for potential alternatives to modifier **59**.
- Per *CPT,* modifier **59** represents one of the following conditions of a procedure:
  - The procedure was provided at a different session from another procedure.
  - The procedure was a different procedure or surgery.
  - The procedure involved a different site or organ system.
  - The procedure required a separate incision or excision.
  - The procedure was performed on a separate lesion or injury (or area of injury in extensive injuries).

Example—Modifier 59

➤ **Influenza A and B tests (87804) were performed. In this case, the rapid influenza test provides the physician with 2 distinct results.**
87804 (infectious agent antigen detection by immunoassay with direct optical observation; influenza)
87804 59
Modifier **59** would be appended to the second test to reflect that 2 distinct tests were performed.

Chapter 2. Modifiers and Coding Edits

Coding Conundrum: Modifier 51 (Multiple Procedures) or 59 (Distinct Procedural Service)?

Modifier **51** is most often used on surgical procedures that are performed during the same session and through the same incision. This modifier identifies potentially overlapping or duplicative relative value units related to the global surgical package or the technical component of certain services (eg, radiology services). Not all payers recognize or require modifier **51**.

Modifier **59** is used to identify distinct and independent procedures that are not normally reported together but are appropriate to the clinical circumstances. They are typically unrelated procedures or services performed on the same patient by the same provider on the same day on different anatomical sites or at different encounters. This is a modifier of last resort. When another modifier, such as **51**, is more appropriate, it should be reported in lieu of modifier **59**.

62—Two Surgeons

- Modifier **62** is used when 2 surgeons work together as primary surgeons performing a distinct part(s) of a procedure. Do not use modifier **62** when 1 surgeon assists another.
- Each surgeon should report his or her distinct operative work by adding modifier **62** to the procedure code and any associated add-on code(s) for that procedure as long as both surgeons continue to work together as primary surgeons.
- Each surgeon should report the co-surgery once using the same procedure code.
- If an additional procedure(s) (including an add-on procedure[s]) is performed during the same surgical session, a separate code(s) may also be reported without modifier **62** added.
- Column AB (CO SURG) of the Medicare Physician Fee Schedule (Resource-Based Relative Value Scale [RBRVS]) identifies procedures that may or may not be performed by co-surgeons. Indicator 1 is assigned to those procedures for which co-surgery is allowed under the Medicare program. See www.cms.gov/Medicare/Medicare-Fee-for-Service-Payment/PhysicianFeeSched/PFS-Relative-Value-Files.html.

Example—Modifier 62

➤ **A neurosurgeon and general surgeon work together to place a ventriculoperitoneal shunt.**

Both physicians would report code **62223 62** with the same diagnosis code. The operative note must include the name of each surgeon, specific role of each surgeon, and necessity for 2 surgeons. Each surgeon should dictate his or her own operative report.

Most payers will require authorization prior to the procedure.

63—Procedure Performed on Infants Less Than 4 kg

- Modifier **63** is used to report procedures performed on neonates and infants up to a *present body weight of 4 kg* that involve significantly increased complexity and physician work commonly associated with these patients.
- Unless otherwise designated, this modifier may only be appended to procedures or services listed in the **20100–69999** code series and codes **92920, 92928, 92953, 92960, 92986, 92987, 92990, 92997, 92998, 93312–93318, 93452, 93463, 93505, 93530–93533, 93561–93564, 93568, 93580, 93582, 93590–93592, 93615,** and **93616.**
- Use of modifier **63** may require submission of an operative note with the claim. The operative note should include the patient's weight. It is also beneficial to report the patient's weight on the claim.
- **DO *NOT* REPORT MODIFIER 63**
  - **When the code descriptor indicates the procedure is performed on young infants or neonates because the relative value for those procedures reflects the additional work (eg, code 49491 for repair initial inguinal hernia on preterm infant)**
  - **With any *CPT* code listed in Appendix F of the *CPT* manual**

Examples—Modifier 63

➤ **A surgeon performed a right heart and retrograde left heart catheterization on a 4-week-old who weighed 3.1 kg with positive findings of congenital anomalies.**

93530 26 63 (combined right heart catheterization and retrograde left heart catheterization, for congenital cardiac anomalies)

●=New code   ▲=Revised code   #=Re-sequenced code   +=Add-on code

Chapter 2. Modifiers and Coding Edits

➤ **A repair of patent ductus arteriosus by ligation is performed on an infant weighing less than 4 kg.**
   33820 63 (repair of patent ductus arteriosus; by ligation)

66—Surgical Team

- Modifier **66** is appended to the basic procedure code when highly complex procedures (requiring the concomitant services of several physicians or other QHPs, often of different specialties, plus other highly skilled, specially trained personnel and various types of complex equipment) are carried out under the surgical team concept.
- Each surgeon reports modifier **66**.
- Each surgeon should dictate his or her own operative report and it should reflect the medical necessity for team surgery.
- Column AC (TEAM SURG) of the Medicare Physician Fee Schedule (RBRVS) identifies procedures that may or may not be performed by a team of surgeons. Indicator 1 is assigned to those procedures for which team surgery is allowed under the Medicare program.
- The operative notes are usually required by the payer.
- If a surgeon is assisting another surgeon, modifier **80**, **81**, or **82** would be more applicable.

Example—Modifier 66

➤ **Multiple surgeons perform different portions of an organ transplant.**
   Each physician would report his or her services with modifier **66** appended to the procedure code.

76—Repeat Procedure or Service by Same Physician or Other Qualified Health Care Professional

- Modifier **76** is used when a procedure or service is repeated by the same physician or other QHP subsequent to the original procedure or service. Use of this modifier may prevent denial as a duplicate service line.
- The repeat procedure may be performed on different days. (Payer guidance may vary.)
- This modifier is appended to non-E/M procedure codes only and is not reported when the code definition indicates a repeat procedure.
- The use of this modifier advises the payer that this is not a duplicate service. (See modifier **91** for repeat clinical diagnostic laboratory test.)
- The CMS only recognizes this modifier on ECGs and radiographs or when a procedure is performed in an operating room or other location equipped to perform procedures. State Medicaid programs or other commercial payers may follow this guideline. Check with payers to determine their policy on use of the modifier.

Examples—Modifier 76

➤ **You see a patient in your office with severe asthma and give 3 nebulized albuterol treatments and steroids over the course of the visit.**
   Report **94640** 3 times with modifier **76** appended to the second and third codes. Only report **94640 76** with 3 units if directed to do so by payer policy because most payers will deny based on the lack of an initial service (ie, code reported without modifier **76**).
   The Medicare and Medicaid NCCI manuals contradict *CPT* instruction for code **94640**, stating that *CPT* code **94640** should only be reported once during a single patient encounter regardless of the number of separate inhalation treatments that are administered. Follow individual payer guidance.

➤ **A physician performs incision and drainage of a cutaneous abscess of the right thigh (10060).** Within the 10-day global period of the procedure, the physician performs a repeat incision and drainage (**10060**) of the right thigh.
   First date of service: **10060**
   Second date of service: **10060 76**

77—Repeat Procedure or Service by Another Physician or Other Qualified Health Care Professional

- Modifier **77** is used when a procedure or service is repeated by another physician or health care professional subsequent to the original procedure or service. Be sure that the same code(s) is reported by each physician to avoid denials when reporting modifier **77**.
- Payers may require documentation to support the medical necessity of performing the same service or procedure on the same day or during the global surgical period (if applicable).

Example—Modifier 77

➤ **A simple repair of a 3-cm laceration of the knee is performed by the pediatrician.** Later that day, the child falls on the knee and opens the wound. A physician at the urgent care center performs another simple repair.

The second physician should report the service with code **12002 77**.

Remember that the diagnosis code selected must provide the medical necessity for the duplicate procedure. Payers may require a copy of the medical record.

78—Unplanned Return to the Operating/Procedure Room by the Same Physician or Other Qualified Health Care Professional Following Initial Procedure for a Related Procedure During the Postoperative Period

- Modifier **78** is used when another procedure is unplanned and related to the initial procedure, requires a return to the operating or procedure room, and is performed during the postoperative period of the initial procedure by the same physician.
- The related procedure might be performed on the same day or any time during the postoperative period. (For repeat procedures, see modifier **76**.)
- Link the appropriate diagnosis code(s) that best explains the reason for the unplanned procedure.

Examples—Modifier 78

➤ **A pediatric surgeon returns to the operating room to stop bleeding from an abdominal procedure performed earlier in the day.**

35840 78 (exploration for postoperative hemorrhage, thrombosis, or infection; abdomen)

The second procedure will usually be paid only for the intraoperative service, not the preoperative or postoperative care already paid in the original procedure.

➤ **An incision and drainage of a deep abscess in the pelvis area 6 days following excision of a lipoma is performed.**

26990 78 (incision and drainage, pelvis area; deep abscess)

79—Unrelated Procedure or Service by the Same Physician or Other Qualified Health Care Professional During the Postoperative Period

- The physician may need to indicate that the performance of a procedure or service during the postoperative period was unrelated to the original procedure. This circumstance may be reported by using modifier **79**.
- The diagnosis must identify the reason for the new procedure within the global period. (For repeat procedures by the same physician on the same day, see modifier **76**.)

Example—Modifier 79

➤ **A patient had closed treatment of a shoulder dislocation with manipulation; 2 months later, the patient requires open treatment of a humeral shaft fracture.**

24515 79 (open treatment of humeral shaft fracture with plate/screws, with or without cerclage)

●=New code   ▲=Revised code   #=Re-sequenced code   +=Add-on code

80—Assistant Surgeon

- Modifier **80** is used when the assistant surgeon assists the surgeon during the entire operation. Note: Modifier **62**, not **80**, is used when 2 surgeons work together as primary surgeons performing a distinct part(s) of a procedure.
- The primary surgeon reports the appropriate *CPT* code for the procedure and the assistant surgeon reports the same code with modifier **80** appended.
- Payers vary on payment rules. The CMS establishes guidelines for payment of assistant surgery for each procedure code. Most payers, including the CMS, will not pay for nonphysician surgery technicians in this role.
- Many payers require documentation to support the necessity of an assistant surgeon.

81—Minimum Assistant Surgeon

- Modifier **81** is used when an assistant surgeon is required for a short time and minimal assistance is provided.
- The assistant surgeon reports the same procedure code as the surgeon with modifier **81** appended.
- Many payers require documentation to support the use of an assistant surgeon for only a portion of a procedure.

82—Assistant Surgeon (When Qualified Resident Surgeon Not Available)

- Modifier **82** is used in teaching hospitals when a resident surgeon is not available to assist the primary surgeon.
- The unavailability of a qualified resident surgeon is a prerequisite for the use of modifier **82** appended to the usual procedure code number(s).

Modifiers 80, 81, and 82

The Medicare Physician Fee Schedule includes in column AA (ASST SURG) indicators identifying procedures that may or may not be billed by an assistant surgeon. Indicator 1 is assigned to those procedures for which an assistant surgeon is allowed to bill under the Medicare program.

Note that a payer may require use of Healthcare Common Procedure Coding System modifier AS (physician assistant, nurse practitioner, or clinical nurse specialist services for assistant-at-surgery) for surgical assistance performed by a qualified health care professional.

91—Repeat Clinical Diagnostic Laboratory Test

- Modifier **91** is used to indicate it is necessary to repeat the same laboratory test on the same day to obtain subsequent test results.
- Modifier **91** is only reported when the laboratory test is performed more than once on the same patient on the same day.
- Modifier **91** cannot be reported when repeat tests are performed to confirm initial results, because of testing problems with the specimen or equipment, or for any reason when a normal one-time, reportable result is all that is required.

Example—Modifier 91

➤ **In the course of treatment for hyperkalemia, a patient had 3 serum potassium determinations (84132) done on the same day in the same office.** The patient had severe diarrhea and dehydration and initial potassium was borderline high. An ECG demonstrated peaked T waves indicating need to recheck potassium values. The second potassium test came back as 6.0, and 10% calcium gluconate (10–15 mL/kg) was given to bring down potassium. A third potassium test was performed to see results.

   84132 91 × 3 units of service

92—Alternative Laboratory Platform Testing

- Modifier **92** is used to indicate that laboratory testing was performed using a kit or transportable instrument that wholly or in part consists of a single-use, disposable analytic chamber.
- This modifier is not required or acknowledged by all payers.
- *CPT* instructs to report this modifier with HIV test codes **86701–86703** and **87389**.

95—Synchronous Telemedicine Service Rendered via a Real-time Interactive Audio and Video Telecommunications System

Modifier **95** is used to indicate a service was rendered via real-time (synchronous) interactive audio and video telecommunications system. This modifier is not applied if the communication is not real-time interactive audio and video.

Codes to which modifier **95** may be applied are found in Appendix P of *CPT 2021* and are preceded by a star symbol in the *CPT* manual.

Appendix P codes that may be of particular interest to pediatricians include

- New and established patient office or other outpatient E/M services (**99202–99205**, **99212–99215**)
- Subsequent hospital care (**99231–99233**)
- Inpatient and outpatient consultations (**99241–99245**, **99251–99255**)
- Subsequent nursing facility care (**99307–99310**)
- Prolonged services in the outpatient setting (**99354**, **99355**)
- Individual behavior change interventions (**99406–99409**)
- Transitional care management services (**99495**, **99496**)

> **For more information on reporting synchronous telemedicine services, see Chapter 20.**

Appendix P also includes codes for services such as psychotherapy, health and behavior assessment and intervention, medical nutrition therapy, and education and training for patient self-management, allowing for telemedicine services provided by certain qualified nonphysician health care professionals in addition to subspecialty physicians.

For a full listing of codes that may be reported for telemedicine services, see Appendix P in your *CPT* reference.

96—Habilitative Services

When a health plan is subject to the PPACA provision for equal and separate benefits for habilitative and rehabilitative services, it may be necessary to append a modifier to identify those services that are habilitative (ie, intended to help the patient learn and retain new skills and functioning).

- Use of modifiers to distinguish services may allow for appropriate claims processing and support the patient's access to the full benefits for each type of service for habilitative and rehabilitative services.
- Not all health plans are subject to the PPACA provision for habilitative and rehabilitative benefits, and covered services may vary. Be sure to verify benefits under each individual patient's plan prior to provision of services.
- When necessary, append modifier **96** (habilitative services) to the procedure code to indicate that the procedure provided was a habilitative service (eg, speech therapy for a child who is a late talker) versus rehabilitative (eg, speech therapy to assist a child with regaining speech following illness or injury).
- See modifier **97** for reporting rehabilitative services.
- When both habilitative and rehabilitative services are rendered on the same date, append the appropriate modifier to the code for each service.

Example—Modifier 96

➤ **A speech pathologist works with a toddler and his mom on speech development due to a profound speech delay.** The patient's health plan requires a modifier to distinguish this habilitative service from rehabilitative services.
92507 96 (adaptive behavior treatment with protocol modification administered by physician or other qualified health care professional, which may include simultaneous direction of technician, face-to-face with one patient, each 15 minutes)

97—Rehabilitative Services

Modifier **97** is appended when it is necessary to designate that a service was rehabilitative in nature (ie, to help restore or improve a patient's skill or function that was lost due to injury or disease). See discussion of modifier **96** for differentiation of habilitative and rehabilitative services.

- Use of modifier **97** to distinguish rehabilitative services may allow for appropriate claims processing and support the patient's access to the full benefits.

Chapter 2. Modifiers and Coding Edits

●=New code ▲=Revised code #=Re-sequenced code +=Add-on code

● Not all health plans are subject to the PPACA provision for habilitative and rehabilitative benefits. Be sure to verify benefits under each patient's plan prior to provision of services.

Example—Modifier 97

➤ **A physician provides 15 minutes of adaptive behavior treatment with protocol modification for a child with ASD.**
   #97155 97

99—Multiple Modifiers

CPT instructs that modifier **99** is reported under certain circumstances when 2 or more modifiers are required to completely describe a service. However, current paper and electronic claims allow listing of up to 4 modifiers per claim line, and payers often instruct to report modifier **99** only when more than 4 modifiers are required on a single code.

Follow individual payer instructions regarding use of modifier **99** and placement of additional modifiers on the claim (eg, in narrative field 19 of the paper claim form).

> For more information on reporting modifiers, see "When Are Modifiers Necessary?" in the November 2016 *AAP Pediatric Coding Newsletter*™ at https://coding.solutions.aap.org/article.aspx?articleid=2571212 (subscription required).

Healthcare Common Procedure Coding System Modifiers

The HCPCS modifiers are used to report specific information not conveyed in code descriptors or by *CPT* modifiers, such as

E1	Upper left eyelid
QW	Performance of tests waived by Clinical Laboratory Improvement Amendments (CLIA)
RT	Right side
SL	State-supplied vaccine
TC	Technical component only
XE	Procedural services performed at separate encounters on the same date

Medicaid programs often use a variety of HCPCS modifiers for state-defined purposes. See your state Medicaid provider manual for information on HCPCS modifiers and definitions assigned in your state (eg, modifier **SY** [persons who are in close contact with member of high-risk population] may be used with codes for certain immunizations). Be sure to review the list of HCPCS modifiers in your 2021 HCPCS reference.

Anatomical Modifiers

An anatomical modifier may be reported to identify specific sites, such as right foot, fifth digit (**T9**).
● The anatomical-specific modifiers are designated as appropriate modifiers under NCCI edits and are listed in the Appropriate NCCI Modifiers section later in this chapter.
● The Medicaid NCCI manual indicates that procedures performed on fingers should be reported with modifiers **FA** and **F1–F9**, and procedures performed on toes should be reported with modifiers **TA** and **T1–T9**. See also modifiers for eyelids (**E1–E4**) and coronary arteries (**LC, LD, LM, RC, RI**).

Medically Unlikely Edit (MUE) values for many finger and toe procedures are 1 (one) based on use of these modifiers for clinical scenarios in which the same procedure is performed on more than 1 finger or toe. (See the Medically Unlikely Edits section later in this chapter for more information.)

Example—Anatomical Modifiers

➤ **A physician must amputate the fourth and fifth phalanges of the left foot.**
   28820 T3 (amputation, toe; metatarsophalangeal joint)
   28820 T4 (amputation, toe; metatarsophalangeal joint)
   Note: Some payers may require that modifier **59** (distinct procedural service) or **XS** (separate structure) be reported. Verify coding edits and payer policy before reporting.

X {E, P, S, U} Modifiers

Modifiers **XE**, **XP**, **XS**, and **XU** more specifically identify reasons for separate reporting of procedures or services that otherwise may be identified by *CPT* modifier **59**.

XE   Separate encounter (different operative session)
XP   Separate practitioner
XS   Separate structure (site/organ)
XU   Unusual nonoverlapping service

- As payer adoption and guidance on use of these modifiers may vary, it is important to verify individual payer policy before reporting.
- As the **XE**, **XP**, **XS**, and **XU** modifiers are more specific, payers may require reporting in lieu of modifier **59**.
- Modifiers **XE**, **XP**, **XS**, and **XU** should not be appended to an E/M code.
- Do not append modifier **59** and the **XE**, **XP**, **XS**, and **XU** modifiers to the same service line of a claim (ie, single code).
- While accepted by most payers, few resources are available to describe appropriate reporting of these modifiers.
- National Correct Coding Initiative edits are not yet updated to require modifiers **XE**, **XP**, **XS**, and **XU** in lieu of modifier **59** for specific code pairs.

EP—Service Provided as Part of Medicaid Early and Periodic Screening, Diagnostic, and Treatment (EPSDT) Program

Some Medicaid and private payers require the use of modifier **EP** to denote services that are provided to covered patients as part of the Early and Periodic Screening, Diagnostic, and Treatment (EPSDT) program services required in the state.

Modifier **EP** can be appended to the preventive medicine service (eg, **99392**) or screening services, such as developmental screening (**96110**).

Example—Modifier EP

➤ **A 9-month-old established patient presents for her routine preventive medicine service.** As part of her state EPSDT services, she receives an age-appropriate history and physical examination, preventive counseling, and anticipatory guidance. A standardized developmental screening, which is required of EPSDT services, is also completed and scored.

    99391 EP (preventive medicine service, established patient <1 year)
    96110 EP (developmental screening)

GA—Waiver of Liability Statement Issued as Required by Payer Policy, Individual Case

GU—Waiver of Liability Statement Issued as Required by Payer Policy, Routine Notice

GX—Notice of Liability Issued, Voluntary Under Payer Policy

Modifiers **GA**, **GU**, and **GX** may or may not be recognized by Medicaid and private payers when reporting services that are not covered under the patient's benefit plan. Follow individual payer policies regarding provision and reporting of advance notice of noncoverage to patients/responsible parties.

GC—This Service Has Been Performed in Part by a Resident Under the Direction of a Teaching Physician

- Modifier **GC** indicates a teaching physician is certifying that the service was rendered in compliance with the CMS requirements for services reported by teaching physicians.
- Requirements for reporting modifier **GC** may vary among commercial health plans. This modifier is typically informational, meaning it does not affect the amount paid for a service.
- If the service was provided solely by the teaching physician, the claim should not be billed with the **GC** modifier.

●=New code   ▲=Revised code   #=Re-sequenced code   +=Add-on code

Chapter 2. Modifiers and Coding Edits

JW—Drug Amount Discarded/Not Administered to Any Patient

- Practice administrators may use as a tool to internally track wasted drugs and vaccines.
- This modifier is reported on claims only when allowed or required by certain payers.
- Medicare requires use of modifier **JW** on codes for the unused portion of a drug or biological from a single-dose vial or package. Medicaid plans may also require reporting of modifier **JW**.
  - Report only when the full amount of a single-dose vial is not used due to patient indications (eg, patient requires lower dose) and required by a payer.
  - Report only when the amount of drug wasted is equal to at least 1 billing unit (ie, do not report wastage when 7 mg of a 10-mg vial is administered and the billing unit is 10 mg, as the remaining 3 mg is already accounted for in the billing unit).
  - Never report for discarded amounts from a multidose vial.
  - Never report modifier **JW** for overfill wastage (ie, an excess amount placed in the single-dose vial by the manufacturer to ensure that an adequate amount can be drawn into the syringe for use).
- Modifier **JW** is not applicable for reporting the following circumstances. However, some practices use the modifier for internal tracking of drug waste.
  - A parent decides to forego an immunization after the vaccine had been drawn up. Report on a claim only when specifically allowed by payer policy. Practices should keep a log of all wasted vaccines.
  - The vial is dropped, and the medication must be discarded.
  - A vaccine is discarded due to temperature out of range during storage.

QW—Clinical Laboratory Improvement Amendments–Waived Tests

- The CLIA-waived tests are those commonly done in a laboratory or an office that are considered simple and low risk.
- One common test in the *CPT* **80000** series that is CLIA waived is the rapid strep test (**87880**).
- Laboratories and physician offices performing waived tests may need to append modifier **QW** to the *CPT* code for CLIA-waived procedures. The use of modifier **QW** is payer specific.
- Some of the CLIA-waived tests are exempt from the use of modifier **QW** (eg, **81002**, **82272**). To review the list of CLIA-waived procedures, go to www.cms.gov/clia.

RT, LT—Right and Left Side

- Modifiers **RT** and **LT** are used for information only and do not affect payment of a procedure unless otherwise specified by a payer.
- Used to identify procedures performed on the left or right side of the body.
- Some plans allow modifiers **RT** and **LT** in place of modifier **50**, but be sure of payer policy for reporting bilateral diagnostic procedures.

  Some payers may require that modifier **59** (distinct procedural service) be reported in addition to or in lieu of the laterality modifiers.

Example—Modifiers RT and LT

➤ **The physician removes a subcutaneous foreign body that extended into the fascia from the left elbow and a subfascial foreign body from the right elbow.**
  24200 LT (removal of a subcutaneous foreign body from the elbow)
  24201 RT (removal of a deep foreign body from the elbow)

X1–X5 Patient Relationship Modifiers

- Modifiers **X1–X5** were introduced for voluntary identification of the reporting physician or practitioner's relationship to a patient during an episode of care.

X1	Continuous/broad services
X2	Continuous/focused services
X3	Episodic/broad services
X4	Episodic/focused services
X5	Only as ordered by another clinician

- At this time, there is no requirement to report modifiers **X1–X5**, and there is no effect on payment whether these modifiers are used or not used.
- In the future, the patient relationship modifiers are intended for use in value-based payment methodologies where the cost of care and outcomes may be attributed to specific physicians and other providers of care.

> **For more information on value-based payment methodologies, see Chapter 3.**

Coding Edits

National Correct Coding Initiative (NCCI) Edits

The NCCI edits were developed for use by the CMS in adjudicating Medicare claims, but they are also used by virtually all private payers, and all Medicaid programs use a Medicaid-specific version of the NCCI edits. The NCCI edits frequently form the basis for proprietary claims editors.

The NCCI edits

- Have been developed based on *CPT* code descriptors and instructions, coding guidelines developed by national medical societies (eg, AAP), Medicare billing history, local and national Medicare carrier policies and edits, and analysis of standard medical and surgical practice.
- Are used by payers in the claims processing system for physician services as well as to promote correct coding.
- Include 2 types of edits: procedure-to-procedure edits and MUEs.
- Physicians should not inconvenience patients or increase risks to patients by performing services on different dates of service to avoid MUE or NCCI procedure-to-procedure edits.
  - This instruction comes from the Medicaid NCCI manual and prohibits practice policies that focus on achieving maximum payment.
  - Delaying patient care to avoid code edits could be seen as an abusive billing practice; policies or practices that might be perceived in this way should be avoided.

Procedure-to-Procedure Edits

- Identify code pairs that normally should not be billed by the same physician or physicians of the same group practice and same specialty (*provider* is used in NCCI manuals) for the same patient on the same date of service.
- Include edits based on services that are mutually exclusive based on code descriptor or anatomical considerations (**Table 2-2**), services that are considered to be inherent to each other, and edits based on coding instructions.
  - If 2 codes of an edit are billed by the same provider for the same patient for the same date of service without an appropriate modifier, only the column 1 code is paid.
  - If clinical circumstances justify appending the appropriate modifier to the column 2 code, payment of both codes may be allowed.

> **The Centers for Medicare & Medicaid Services allows physicians to append modifiers 59, XE, XP, XS, and XU to either the column 1 or column 2 code when reporting 2 codes paired by the Medicare National Correct Coding Initiative (NCCI) edits. Other payers may adopt this policy or require the modifier be appended to the code in column 2 of the NCCI edit file.**

Appropriate NCCI Modifiers

Modifier indicators are assigned to every code pair identified in the NCCI. They dictate whether modifiers are needed or will be accepted to override the edit. These indicators are

0   Under no circumstance may a modifier be used to override the edit.
1   An appropriate modifier may be used to override the edit.
9   This edit was deleted prior to its effective date or there is, essentially, no edit.
     Refer to **Table 2-2** for examples.

●=New code   ▲=Revised code   #=Re-sequenced code   +=Add-on code

Table 2-2. Examples of Medicaid National Correct Coding Initiative Edits			
Column 1 Comprehensive Code	**Column 2 Component Code**	**Modifier Indicator**	**Effective Date**
99460 Initial hospital or birthing center care, per day, for evaluation and management of normal newborn infant	**99462** Subsequent hospital care, per day, for evaluation and management of normal newborn	0	10/1/2010
The NCCI edits preclude any payment for the component code because they are mutually exclusive. Each code represents all normal newborn care on a single date of service by 1 physician or physicians of the same specialty and group practice.			
94640 Pressurized/non-pressurized inhalation treatment	**94664** Demonstration and/or evaluation patient use of nebulizer	1	10/1/2010
*The component code (**94664**) would be denied unless a modifier indicating a distinct procedural service (eg, **59**) is appended to **94664**. Medicaid payment policy allows both services only if the nebulizer treatment and demonstration utilize different devices (eg, treatment with small volume nebulizer and demonstration of handheld inhaler with spacer) or occurred at separate encounters. Please refer to the Medicaid NCCI edit site for more information (www.medicaid.gov/medicaid/program-integrity/ncci/index.html).*			
94060 Bronchodilation responsiveness, spirometry as in **94010**, pre- and post-bronchodilator administration	**94010** Spirometry	0	10/1/2010
*The NCCI edits preclude any payment for the component code (ie, column 2 code **94010**).*			
90460 Immunization administration through 18 years of age, first or only component, with counseling by physician	**99392** Preventive medicine service, established patient age 1–4	1	1/1/2013
*The component code (**99392**) would be denied if modifier **25** (significant, separately identifiable E/M service) were not appended to it. Be aware that the higher valued service may be the component code and would be denied without the application of the correct modifier. Medicaid NCCI edits place routine child health examination codes (eg, **99392**) as component codes to immunization administration codes, although the counseling included in the routine child health examination is distinct from immunization counseling.*			
Abbreviations: E/M, evaluation and management; NCCI, National Correct Coding Initiative.			

- Only certain modifiers can be used to override edits when the service or procedure is clinically justified, and they may be used only on the code pairs that are assigned the 1 indicator. See **Table 2-3** for a list of modifiers that override NCCI edits.
- The CMS now allows modifiers **59**, **XE**, **XS**, **XP**, or **XU** on column 1 and 2 codes.
- For overrides of other mutually exclusive edits or correct coding edits, the appropriate modifier is always appended to the code that appears in column 2 because that is considered the bundled or exclusive procedure.
- To append the appropriate modifier and override an edit, it is imperative that the conditions of that modifier are met.

Medically Unlikely Edits

The *National Correct Coding Initiative Policy Manual for Medicaid Services* describes MUEs as unit of service edits that were established by the CMS to prevent payment for an inappropriate number or quantity of the same service (eg, accidental reporting of 100 rather than 10 units). An MUE for a HCPCS or *CPT* code is the maximum number of units of service, under most circumstances, allowable by the same provider for the same beneficiary on the same date of service.

Medicaid MUEs

- Are applied separately to each line of a claim. If the unit of service on a line exceeds the MUE value, the entire line is denied.
- Are coding edits rather than medical necessity edits.
- May be established based on claims data.
- May limit units of service based on anatomical structures.
- May limit the number of units of service based on *CPT* code descriptors or *CPT* coding instructions.
- Are published on the CMS Medicaid NCCI website at www.medicaid.gov/medicaid/program-integrity/ncci/index.html.

Table 2-3. Modifiers That Can Be Used to Override National Correct Coding Initiative Edits

24 Unrelated E/M service by the same physician or other qualified health care professional during a postoperative period	**F5** Right hand, thumb
	F6 Right hand, second digit
25 Significant, separately identifiable E/M service by the same physician or other qualified health care professional on the same day of the procedure or other service	**F7** Right hand, third digit
	F8 Right hand, fourth digit
	F9 Right hand, fifth digit
57 Decision for surgery	**LC** Left circumflex, coronary artery
58 Staged or related procedure or service by the same physician or other qualified health care professional during the postoperative period	**LD** Left anterior descending coronary artery
	LM Left main coronary artery
	LT Left side
59 Distinct procedural service	**RC** Right coronary artery
78 Unplanned return to the operating/procedure room by the same physician or other qualified health care professional following initial procedure for a related procedure during the postoperative period	**RI** Ramus intermedius coronary artery
	RT Right side
	TA Left foot, great toe
	T1 Left foot, second digit
79 Unrelated procedure or service by the same physician or other qualified health care professional during the postoperative period	**T2** Left foot, third digit
	T3 Left foot, fourth digit
91 Repeat clinical diagnostic laboratory test	**T4** Left foot, fifth digit
E1 Upper left, eyelid	**T5** Right foot, great toe
E2 Lower left, eyelid	**T6** Right foot, second digit
E3 Upper right, eyelid	**T7** Right foot, third digit
E4 Lower right, eyelid	**T8** Right foot, fourth digit
FA Left hand, thumb	**T9** Right foot, fifth digit
F1 Left hand, second digit	**XE** Separate encounter (different operative session)
F2 Left hand, third digit	**XP** Separate practitioner
F3 Left hand, fourth digit	**XS** Separate structure (site/organ)
F4 Left hand, fifth digit	**XU** Unusual nonoverlapping service

Abbreviation: E/M, evaluation and management.

- Are published with an "Edit Rationale" for each HCPCS and *CPT* code.
  - The MUE value assigned for code **96110** (developmental screening, per instrument) is 3 based on CMS NCCI policy. (No further explanation of this rationale is provided in the current Medicaid or Medicare NCCI manuals but may be based on historical claims data.)
  - The MUE value assigned to code **96127** (brief emotional/behavior assessment, per instrument) is 2 based on the nature of the service or procedure (typically determined by the amount of time required to perform a procedure/service or clinical application of a procedure/service).
- Are applied separately to each claim line for a service when modifiers (eg, **59**, **76**, **77**, anatomical) cause the same HCPCS or *CPT* code to appear on separate lines of a claim.

It is important to recognize that the use of modifiers to override the MUE must be justified based on correct selection of the procedure code, correct application of the number of units reported, medical necessity and reasonableness of the number of services, and, if applicable, reason the physician's practice pattern differs from national patterns.

Keeping Up to Date With the NCCI

Medicaid and Medicare NCCI edits are updated quarterly. Each Medicare NCCI version ends with .0 (point zero), .1, .2, or .3 indicating its effective dates.

- Versions ending in .0 (point zero) are effective from January 1 through March 31 of that year.
- Versions ending in .1 are effective from April 1 through June 30 of that year.
- Versions ending in .2 are effective from July 1 through September 30 of that year.
- Versions ending in .3 are effective from October 1 through December 31 of that year.

The CMS releases the Medicare NCCI edits free of charge on its website (www.cms.gov/NationalCorrectCodInitEd/NCCIEP/list.asp). Medicaid NCCI files are published separately free of charge at www.medicaid.gov/medicaid/program-integrity/ncci/edit-files/index.html.

- Although many of the Medicaid edits mirror Medicare edits, this is not always the case. The CMS has instructed that use of the appropriate NCCI file is important to correct coding.
- Online NCCI edits are posted in spreadsheet form, which allows users to sort by procedure code and effective date.
- There is a "Find" tool that allows users to look for a specific code. The edit files are indexed by procedure code ranges for simplified navigation.
- Policy manuals that explain the rationale for edits and correct use of NCCI-associated modifiers are published to the web pages listed previously (see "Reference Documents" link on the Medicaid NCCI page).
  — Updated manuals for the year ahead are published annually in late fall.
  — Changes in the manual are shown in red font for easy identification.
  — Be sure to update your NCCI edit files quarterly and review changes to the NCCI manual each year.

Practice management and electronic health record software may also contain tools for identifying codes affected by NCCI edits.

Reviewing and Using These Edits

1. Be aware of all coding edits that are applicable to your specialty; as each update replaces the former edits, it is important to review them quarterly. Always look for new or deleted edits. Updated files can be found at www.aap.org/coding under the "Coding Resources, National Correct Coding Initiative (NCCI) Edits" tab.
2. Pay close attention to the modifier indicator because it may have changed from the last quarterly update. For example, a code set that initially would not allow override with a modifier may now subsequently allow one, or vice versa.
3. Pay attention to the effective date and deletion date of each code set. The edits are applicable only if they are effective. The effective date is based on the date of service, not the date the claim was submitted. Sometimes a pair is retroactively terminated. If so, you may resubmit claims for payment if the date of service is within the filing time frame of the payer.
4. Use modifiers as appropriate.
   a) Modifiers should be used only when applicable based on coding standards, when medically justified or necessary, and when supported by medical record documentation (progress notes, operative notes, procedure notes, diagrams, or pictures), or, as previously mentioned, when dictated by payers.
   b) Refer to the CMS written guidelines (because they are very explicit about billing surgical procedures) or to your payer's provider manual.
5. When billing surgical procedures, you may need to look at several different codes for possible edits. Be sure to always use the code that is reflective of the total service performed.
6. Appeal denied payment for services for which there is no edit and the policy manual and/or payment policies do not preclude reporting, for which a reported modifier should have allowed payment, and/or for which the edit is inconsistent with *CPT* guidelines. Having knowledge of how this system works is to your benefit when appealing the denial.
7. Some payers have developed or adopted coding edit programs that are different from and often more comprehensive than the NCCI.
   a) If a payer policy differs from the CMS NCCI policy and is not clearly defined in its provider manual, refer to the payer's website.
   b) Make sure you get policies in writing for the services you commonly perform. Your contracts with health plans should be explicit regarding how you will receive initial and updated policies.
8. Report the services provided correctly based on *CPT* code guidelines (unless a payer has clearly stated otherwise).

Resources

AAP Coding Hotline

American Academy of Pediatrics Coding Hotline (https://form.jotform.com/Subspecialty/aapcodinghotline)

Assistant Surgeon Procedure Identification

Medicare Physician Fee Schedule Relative Value Files (www.cms.gov/Medicare/Medicare-Fee-for-Service-Payment/PhysicianFeeSched/PFS-Relative-Value-Files.html; see Column AA [ASST SURG] in the file applicable to the date of service).

Bilateral Procedure Identification

Medicare Physician Fee Schedule Relative Value Files (www.cms.gov/Medicare/Medicare-Fee-for-Service-Payment/PhysicianFeeSched/PFS-Relative-Value-Files.html; see Column Z [BILAT SURG] in file applicable to date of service).

CLIA-Waived Tests

Medicare list of CLIA-waived tests (www.cms.gov/clia)

Co-surgery and Team Surgery Procedure Identification

Medicare Physician Fee Schedule Relative Value Files (www.cms.gov/Medicare/Medicare-Fee-for-Service-Payment/PhysicianFeeSched/PFS-Relative-Value-Files.html; see Column AB [CO SURG] or Column AC [TEAM SURG] in the file applicable to the date of service).

Global Period of Procedures

"The Surgical Package and Related Services," May 2018 *AAP Pediatric Coding Newsletter* (https://coding.solutions.aap.org/article.aspx?articleid=2679119; subscription required)

Modifier Use

"When Are Modifiers Necessary?" November 2016 *AAP Pediatric Coding Newsletter* (https://coding.solutions.aap.org/article.aspx?articleid=2571212; subscription required)

Multiple Surgery Indicators and Adjustments

Medicare Claims Processing Manual, Chapter 12, Section 40.6 (www.cms.gov/Regulations-and-Guidance/Guidance/Manuals/Downloads/clm104c12.pdf)

National Correct Coding Initiative Edits

Medicaid NCCI website (www.medicaid.gov/medicaid/program-integrity/ncci/index.html)
Medicare NCCI website (www.cms.gov/NationalCorrectCodInitEd/NCCIEP/list.asp)
NCCI file links from AAP (www.aap.org/coding; see the "Coding Resources, National Correct Coding Initiative (NCCI) Edits" tab)

Test Your Knowledge!

1. **Which of the following describes an appropriate reason for applying a modifier?**
   a. To add context to how or when the service was provided
   b. To override an edit that would appropriately reduce payment
   c. To indicate that you disagree with a payer's edits
   d. All of the above

2. **Which of the following is described by modifier 24?**
   a. An evaluation and management (E/M) service included the decision for surgery.
   b. Service is separately identifiable in the medical record.
   c. Service is significant and distinct from a procedural service on the same date.
   d. An unrelated E/M service was provided during the postoperative period of a procedure.

3. **Which of the following is a potential substitution for modifier 59?**
   a. **25**, significant, separately identifiable E/M service by the same physician or other qualified health care professional (QHP) on the same day of the procedure or other service
   b. **XS**, separate structure (site/organ)
   c. **51**, multiple procedures
   d. **77**, repeat procedure or service by another physician or QHP

4. **Which modifier indicates a procedure required the concomitant services of several physicians or other QHPs, often of different specialties?**
   a. **66**
   b. **63**
   c. **80**
   d. **22**

5. **Which of the following is an indication of a procedure-to-procedure edit?**
   a. A code pair identifies services that should not normally be billed by the same physician for the same patient on the same date of service.
   b. The code pair represents services that are never covered by health plans.
   c. Units of service would not likely be exceeded by the same physician on the same date.
   d. Two procedures in a code pair are not reported when performed on different dates.

Chapter 2. Modifiers and Coding Edits

Coding to Demonstrate Quality and Value

Contents

Quality and performance measurement are important aspects of the pediatric medical home and the movement from payment by fee for service alone to value-based payment. Physicians who have successfully participated in quality measurement may see incentive payments, such as per-member/per-month payments, annual incentives, or a percentage of savings.

> For more information on value-based payment and other emerging payment models, see Chapter 4.

Physicians, payers, and accreditation organizations may use codes or claims data as a first line of quality measurement. When diagnosis or procedure codes provide necessary information for reviewing quality performance data, more time-consuming and costly medical record review may be avoided.

In January 2017, the American Academy of Pediatrics (AAP) published a policy statement, "A New Era in Quality Measurement: The Development and Application of Quality Measures" (http://pediatrics.aappublications.org/content/139/1/e20163442). This policy statement includes the following recommendation to national policy makers:

> "Quality measures, as much as possible, should be reportable by either *International Classification of Diseases, 10th Revision, Clinical Modification,* or *Current Procedural Terminology*® category II codes to reduce burden on pediatric health care providers. However, the inclusion of measures that also capture patient-centered perspectives on care is essential."

Clinical registries and other electronic data may also be used in quality measurement. This chapter discusses 3 ways that correct coding may support performance measurement.
- Hierarchical condition categories (HCCs)
- Codes that may support Healthcare Effectiveness Data and Information Set (HEDIS) quality measurement
- *Current Procedural Terminology* (CPT) Category II codes

Hierarchical Condition Categories

Hierarchical condition categories are categories of conditions that are assigned weight values and used along with certain demographic and prescription drug claim data in calculating a patient's risk of increased health care use or risk adjustment. **Figure 3-1** shows other components of risk adjustment.

- Health plans offered to individuals under the Patient Protection and Affordable Care Act are subject to revenue adjustment based on the average risk of insured members based in part on HCCs.
- Hierarchical condition categories are also used in shared savings agreements with accountable care organizations (ACOs) and value-based payment to hospitals.
- Even if a pediatrician is not part of an ACO or alternative payment model, health plans and hospitals rely on physicians to document conditions that affect HCC assignment.

International Classification of Diseases, 10th Revision, Clinical Modification (ICD-10-CM) codes are collected from the claims submitted to health plans and used to identify HCCs. Only a small percentage of *ICD-10-CM* codes are assigned to HCCs. Examples of values assigned for certain HCCs can be found in **Table 3-1**.

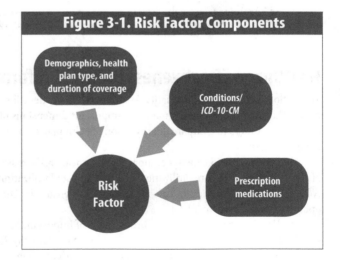

Figure 3-1. Risk Factor Components

Demographics, health plan type, and duration of coverage

Conditions/ ICD-10-CM

Prescription medications

Risk Factor

Most pediatricians do not need to know the weights assigned to various conditions or how those weights are used to calculate risk adjustment factors. What pediatricians need to know is how their documentation affects risk adjustment and how risk adjustment may affect pediatricians and their patients. In addition, choosing a less-specific code than a code supported in the documentation could affect that weight.
- Payment to pediatricians may increasingly be based on quality and cost of care.
  Risk adjustment is used to set the expected cost of care for a patient panel. Pediatricians will be affected (especially pediatricians whose employers may already gain or lose revenue based on risk factor adjustment).
- Patient access to care may be affected when conditions are not documented or are documented in insufficient detail.
  If risk adjustment results in lower revenue for health plans, health plan coverage and benefits will undoubtedly be affected.

It is also important to know

- Like all health care payments, those based on HCCs are audited for accuracy. Documentation must support the *ICD-10-CM* codes used in assigning HCCs.

  Health plans may request medical records to validate *ICD-10-CM* codes supporting assigned HCCs.

- Pediatric HCC categories apply to children younger than 2 years (ie, before their second birthday) or to patients aged 2 through 20 years (ie, before their 21st birthday).

- Hierarchical condition category values are cumulative, making documentation of all diagnoses that affect management important for accurate calculation of risk.

Table 3-1. Examples of US Department of Health and Human Services Hierarchical Condition Categories and Weights[a] by Plan Type (2020)

Diagnosis Category	Health Plan Type				
	Platinum	Gold	Silver	Bronze	Catastrophic
Autistic Disorder	2.419	2.205	2.030	1.859	1.836
Cleft Lip/Cleft Palate	1.309	1.130	0.998	0.869	0.853
Central Nervous System Infections, Except Viral Meningitis	7.639	7.474	7.370	7.375	7.376
Quadriplegic Cerebral Palsy	2.136	1.935	1.829	1.823	1.824
Cerebral Palsy, Except Quadriplegic	0.189	0.141	0.109	0.080	0.076
Extremely Immature Severity Level 5 (Highest)	242.262	240.657	239.483	239.461	239.461
Extremely Immature Severity Level 4	148.994	147.251	145.979	145.799	145.783
Immature Severity Level 5 (Highest)	149.437	147.839	146.672	146.625	146.621
Asthma (It is important to capture severity.)	0.373	0.307	0.222	0.134	0.123

[a] Weights attributed to hierarchical condition categories (HCCs) are one of several factors in the calculation of a risk adjustment factor. Multiple HCCs may be supported for a single patient encounter, but only the highest-valued HCC describing a condition (eg, extremely immature or immature) can be assigned to a patient.

Healthcare Effectiveness Data and Information Set (HEDIS)

The National Committee for Quality Assurance (NCQA) describes HEDIS as a tool used by more than 90% of American health plans to measure performance on important dimensions of care and service. It is intended to allow purchasers and consumers to compare quality among health plans. The HEDIS measures are often incorporated in physician quality initiatives.

Altogether, HEDIS consists of more than 90 measures across 6 domains of care (effectiveness of care, access/availability of care, experience of care, utilization and risk-adjusted utilization, health plan descriptive information, and measures collected using electronic clinical data systems). To ensure HEDIS stays current, the NCQA has established an annual update to the measurement set.

The HEDIS measures address a broad range of important health issues. Among them are

- Children and Adolescents' Access to PCP (primary care physician/provider)
- Follow-up Care for Children Prescribed ADHD Medications
- Childhood and Adolescent Immunization Status
- Weight Assessment and Counseling for Nutrition and Physical Activity for Children and Adolescents

Each health plan reviews a select set of measures every year. Because so many plans collect HEDIS data and the measures are so specifically defined, it is important to become familiar with the HEDIS system as it relates to quality measures and pay for performance (P4P).

Why HEDIS Matters to Pediatricians

The Centers for Medicare & Medicaid Services (CMS) has directly linked payment for health care services to patient outcomes. Consequently, health plans and providers, including physicians, are being asked to close gaps in care and improve overall quality. This focus on quality outcomes can help patients and members get the most from their benefits, which ultimately means better use of limited resources.

There are large sums of money at stake for health plans. For example, for a health plan with just 100,000 members being evaluated by HEDIS, each quality measure could mean millions in payments from federal or state agencies. When you consider that there are 20 to 25 measures directly tied to payment (depending on the health plan and population served), this is a significant amount of money! Now consider what that might look like for larger managed care organizations that have 1 million or more members enrolled. This is what keeps health care plans running. However, they cannot do it without physicians.

A fundamental concept behind P4P quality initiatives is that the plans will pay the physicians to help them attain these funds from the CMS.

What Is a Pediatrician's Role in HEDIS?

You and your office staff can help facilitate HEDIS process improvement by
- Providing appropriate care within the designated time frames.

> Attention to the time frames for providing recommended screenings and services across the patient population is important.

Example

➤ **A practice uses a reminder system to track immunizations for children younger than 24 months to avoid failure to provide the recommended immunizations on or before the second birthday.**

If patients reach 25 months of age without receiving the recommended vaccines, this negatively affects the HEDIS score for the physician until the child turns 3 years old (ie, is no longer included in the patient count for the measure).
- Documenting all care in the patient's medical record.

> When a measure is met during an inpatient or observation stay (eg, newborn immunization during the birth admission), supporting documentation may be required in the record of the primary care physician even if the immunization was provided under supervision of a hospitalist or other physician or qualified health care professional.

- Watching payer guidelines for specific documentation requirements (eg, documentation of specific body mass index [BMI] percentile rather than a BMI value or percentile range).

> *International Classification of Diseases, 10th Revision, Clinical Modification (ICD-10-CM)* codes for pediatric body mass index (BMI) percentiles (Z68.51–Z68.54) are only reported in conjunction with physician documentation of a related condition (eg, overweight, obesity). See later in this chapter for an illustration of reporting BMI measurement in compliance with *ICD-10-CM* guidelines using *Current Procedural Terminology* Category II code **3008F** (BMI, documented).

- Not all patients will be included in a physician's patient count for HEDIS purposes, as continuous enrollment in the health plan without a gap of more than a specified number of days may be required for inclusion.

Example

➤ **The measure for appropriate prescribing for pharyngitis includes members continuously enrolled without a gap in coverage from 30 days prior to the encounter date through 3 days afterward (34 days total).**

●=New code   ▲=Revised code   #=Re-sequenced code   +=Add-on code

- Accurately coding all claims. Providing information accurately on a claim may reduce the number of records requested.

  Use a full spectrum of diagnosis, procedure, and National Drug Codes to show that each measure is met. Health plans typically produce educational resources giving examples of codes that indicate a measure has been met.
- Responding to a health plan's requests for medical records in a timely fashion (typically within a week). This is required under many health plan contracts.

  Health plans typically include a specific turnaround time for providing records. The time frames are set each year.
  — January to May 15: Medical record requests will come in from the plans. All data must be gathered by the plan by May 15, with no exceptions.
  — June: The plans must report their results to the NCQA.
  — July to October: The NCQA releases the new Quality Compass (a quality comparison tool) nationwide—commercial plans in July; Medicaid and Medicare in September and October.

Medical Record Requests

Some information cannot be captured through claims data, so requests for medical records related to health plan HEDIS surveys are necessary.

- The Health Insurance Portability and Accountability Act of 1996 allows disclosure of protected health information to a health plan for the plan's HEDIS purposes as long as the period for which information is needed overlaps with the period for which the patient is or was enrolled in the health plan.
- Health plans may contract with outside vendors to conduct HEDIS record reviews.
- Providers are notified of record requests.
- The request will include a member list, the measure that is being evaluated, and the minimum necessary chart information needed.
- Data collection may vary by plan but may include fax, mail, on-site visits for large requests, remote electronic health record access, and electronic data interchange via a secure web portal.

HEDIS Measures and Codes

In **Table 3-2**, some of the pediatric HEDIS measures for 2020 are listed, including the codes that may be used in HEDIS review (HEDIS 2021 measures were not finalized at time of publication). These include *ICD-10-CM,* Healthcare Common Procedure Coding System, and *CPT* codes. **Table 3-2** does not contain all measures applicable to the pediatric population.

Note that each measure includes a defined patient population (eg, children who turn 2 years of age during the measurement year).

Physicians and group practices may also report HEDIS measures as part of a pediatric medical home or other quality improvement initiative using data pulled from internal administrative data (eg, number of preventive medicine service *CPT* codes reported for population of patients 3–6 years old). Pediatric medical home and quality improvement initiatives vary by state or region and may include a combination of HEDIS and other nationally recognized quality measures.

Some measures include criteria that exclude a patient from the population for the measure. For example, hospice patients and adolescents with history of anaphylactic reaction to a vaccine or its components prior to their 13th birthday may be excluded from the measure for immunizations for adolescents. *ICD-10-CM* codes such as **Z28.04** (immunization not carried out because of patient allergy to vaccine or component), **Z87.892** (personal history of anaphylaxis), and **Z88.7** (allergy status to serum and vaccine status) may be reported to indicate this patient history.

Chapter 3. Coding to Demonstrate Quality and Value

Table 3-2. Healthcare Effectiveness Data and Information Set Pediatric Performance Measure Codes

Measure/Description	Codes
Weight Assessment and Counseling for Nutrition and Physical Activity for Children and Adolescents (WCC) Description: Percentage of members 3–17 years of age who had an outpatient visit with a PCP or an OB/GYN that included evidence of BMI documentation with corresponding height and weight (may be plotted on age-growth chart), counseling for nutrition, and/or counseling for physical activity *TIP: Documentation should be specific to the measure. Notations such as "well-nourished" or "health education" are typically not sufficient. Checklists may be used.*	**Diagnosis** (*ICD-10-CM*) Counseling: nutrition **Z71.3** Counseling for physical activity **Z71.82** **Procedure** Nutrition counseling—*CPT:* **97802–97804** HCPCS: **S9470, S9452, S9449, G0270, G0271,** or **G0447** Physical activity counseling—HCPCS: **S9451** or **G0447** BMI, documented—*CPT:* **3008F**, and if patient has a diagnosis related to BMI, **Z68.51–Z68.54**
Immunizations for Adolescents (IMA) Description: Percentage of adolescents 13 years of age (during the year) with appropriate immunizations Ages: HPV, 9–13 y; Tdap, 10–13 y; meningococcal, 11–13 y	**Procedure** (vaccine products) Meningococcal—*CPT:* **90734** (MenACWY-D or MenACWY-CRM) or **#90619** (MenACWY-TT) Tdap—*CPT:* **90715** Td—*CPT:* **90714** or **90718** Tetanus—*CPT:* **90703** Diphtheria—*CPT:* **90719** Human papillomavirus (complete series)—*CPT:* **90651** (9vHPV)
Follow-up Care for Children Prescribed ADHD Medications Percentage of children newly prescribed ADHD medication who had at least 3 follow-up care visits within a 10-month period, one of which was within 30 days of when the first ADHD medication was dispensed. Two rates are reported. 1. Initiation phase: The percentage of members 6–12 years of age as of the IPSD with an ambulatory prescription dispensed for ADHD medication, who had one follow-up visit with the practitioner with prescribing authority during the 30-day initiation phase. 2. Continuation and maintenance phase: The percentage of members 6–12 years of age as of the IPSD with an ambulatory prescription dispensed for ADHD medication, who remained on the medication for at least 210 days and who, in addition to the visit in the initiation phase, had at least 2 follow-up visits with a practitioner within 270 days (9 months) after the initiation phase ended. One of the 2 visits (during days 31–300) may be a telephone or telehealth visit with any practitioner.	**Procedure** *CPT* Stand-alone visits: **90804–90815, 96156–96159, 96164–96171, 98960–98962, 99078, 99202–99205, 99211–99215, 99217–99220, 99241–99245, 99341–99345, 99347–99350, 99381–99384, 99391–99394, 99401–99404, 99411, 99412, 99510** Telephone visits: **98966–98968, 99441–99443** *CPT* Telehealth Modifiers: **95, GT** Telehealth place of service: 02 HCPCS: **G0155, G0176, G0177, G0409–G0411, G0463, H0002, H0004, H0031, H0034–H0037, H0039, H0040, H2000, H2001, H2010–H2020, M0064, S0201, S9480, S9484, S9485, T1015** **Follow-up visits identified by the following *CPT* codes must be with a mental health practitioner:** *CPT* in most outpatient and partial hospitalization settings: **90791, 90792, 90801, 90802, 90816–90819, 90821–90824, 90826–90829, 90832–90834, 90836–90840, 90845, 90847, 90849, 90853, 90857, 90862, 90875, 90876** *CPT* in partial hospitalization or community mental health centers only: **99221–99223, 99231–99233, 99238, 99239, 99251–99255**

Abbreviations: ADHD, attention-deficit/hyperactivity disorder; BMI, body mass index; *CPT, Current Procedural Terminology*; HCPCS, Healthcare Common Procedure Coding System; HPV, human papillomavirus; *ICD-10-CM, International Classification of Diseases, 10th Revision, Clinical Modification*; IPSD, index prescription start date; OB/GYN, obstetrician/gynecologist; PCP, primary care physician; Td, tetanus, diphtheria; Tdap, tetanus, diphtheria toxoid, and acellular pertussis.

Chapter 3. Coding to Demonstrate Quality and Value

Examples

➤ **The parents of an established 13-month-old girl failed to keep her appointment for a 12-month preventive medicine service.** The pediatrician's administrative staff have identified that the girl has not received this service and contacted the patient's parents to schedule this appointment. The physician provides the age-appropriate preventive medicine service. A blood sample was collected for lead screening. Counseling for immunizations was provided by the pediatrician and vaccine/toxoids administered for measles, mumps, rubella, and varicella (separate MMR, VAR), and hepatitis A (HepA) vaccines are administered. Documentation does not support a separately identifiable evaluation and management (E/M) service but includes a diagnosis of mild acne vulgaris.

ICD-10-CM	CPT	Related HEDIS Measures
Z00.129 (encounter for routine child health examination without abnormal findings)	**99392** (periodic comprehensive preventive medicine reevaluation and management, age 1–4 years)	*Well-Child Visits in the First 15 Months of Life* Patients turning 15 months old during measurement year 6 or more comprehensive well-care visits completed during first 15 months after birth
Z00.129 **Z23** (encounter for immunization)	**90460** × 3 units (immunization administration, each initial component) **90461** × 2 units (immunization administration, each additional component) **90707** (MMR, live, for subcutaneous use) **90716** (VAR, live, for subcutaneous use) **90633** (HepA, pediatric/adolescent dosage, 2 dose schedule, for intramuscular use)	*Childhood Immunizations* *Patients turning 2 years old in the measurement year* ● 1-dose MMR *and* ● 1 dose VAR *and* ● 1 HepA vaccination series before the second birthday (in addition to 4 diphtheria, tetanus, acellular pertussis [DTaP]; 3 polio; 3 *Haemophilus influenzae* type b, 3 hepatitis B, 4 pneumococcal conjugate, 2 or 3 rotavirus, and 2 influenza) All of the above immunizations must be completed on or by the child's second birthday.
Z13.88 (encounter for screening for disorder due to exposure to contaminants)	**36416** (collection capillary blood specimen) **99000** (handling and/or conveyance of specimen)	*Lead Screening* Patients turning 2 years old in the measurement year At least one capillary or venous lead blood test completed on or before their second birthday

The physician in this scenario has proactively provided preventive care that is recommended for this patient and, in doing so, is able to report diagnosis and procedure codes demonstrating that quality measures have been met.

Healthcare Effectiveness Data and Information Set requires that measures be met within specific time frames (eg, before the second birthday). Catching up after the specified time will not be counted in the number of patients for whom the measure was met.

➤ **A physician sees an established patient (>3 months and <19 years old) for pharyngitis and other cold symptoms.** The caregiver requests an antibiotic but is instructed that the condition is viral and to use over-the-counter medicine as necessary for the child's comfort. No antibiotic is ordered.

ICD-10-CM	CPT	Related HEDIS Measures
J00 (acute nasopharyngitis)	**99213** (office or other outpatient visit for the E/M of an established patient [See full code descriptor in **Chapter 7**.])	*Appropriate Treatment for Children With Upper Respiratory Infection (URI)* Patients 3 mo–18 y with ● Diagnosis of URI (includes **J00**, **J06.0**, **J06.9**) *and* ● Not prescribed an antibiotic within 3 days of URI diagnosis

Because no antibiotic was ordered at this encounter, the HEDIS measure for appropriate treatment of infants and children 3 months and older with URI was met. The diagnosis of URI indicates this measure may apply. The health plan may measure this through comparison of medical claims data with prescription drug plan claims data.

Similar measures may apply for antibiotics appropriately prescribed for diagnosis of streptococcal pharyngitis following a positive laboratory test result for group A streptococcal infection.

Category II *Current Procedural Terminology* Codes: Pay for Performance Measures

Category II codes were developed and are used by physicians and hospitals to report performance measures and certain aspects of care not yet included in performance measures. Performance measures are developed by national organizations, including the NCQA and the Physician Consortium for Performance Improvement (PCPI), and based on quality indicators currently accepted and used in the health care industry.

As a member of the PCPI, the AAP is involved with the development of performance measures for pediatric diseases or conditions. The AAP policy statement, "A New Era in Quality Measurement: The Development and Application of Quality Measures" (http://pediatrics.aappublications.org/content/139/1/e20163442), includes recommendations to physicians and policy makers on adoption and use of quality measures. Any updated information on quality measures can be found at www.aap.org/en-us/professional-resources/quality-improvement/Pages/quality-measurement.aspx.

Reporting Category II codes allows internal monitoring of performance, patient compliance, and outcomes.

Performance Measure Codes

Performance measure codes
● Are intended for reporting purposes only.
● Describe clinical conditions (including complete performance measurements sets) and screening measures.
● Have no relative values on the Medicare Physician Fee Schedule (Resource-Based Relative Value Scale).
● Are reported on a voluntary basis.
● Are reported in addition to, *not in place of,* Category I *CPT* codes.
● Describe the performance of a clinical service typically included in an E/M code or the result that is part of a laboratory procedure/test.

Category II codes are included after the Category I procedure codes in the *CPT* manual and online at www.ama-assn.org/practice-management/cpt/category-ii-codes.

Codes are grouped within categories based on established clinical documentation methods (ie, history, physical findings, assessment, and plan). Each code identifies the specific clinical condition and performance measured. Categories are defined in **Table 3-3**.

Category II Modifiers

Category II modifiers (**1P, 2P, 3P,** and **8P**) are used to report services that were considered but not provided because of a medical reason(s), patient choice, or system reason. Modifier **8P** is equivalent to "action not performed, reason not otherwise specified." **Table 3-4** contains modifiers and examples.

Table 3-3. Performance Measure Codes

Category of Codes	Examples
Composite Measures—0000F Series Codes in the **0000F** range comprise several measures that are grouped to facilitate reporting of a clinical condition when all included components are performed.	Code **0012F** is reported when the assessment on an 18-year-old with community-acquired bacterial pneumonia includes all the following components: **1026F** Comorbid conditions assessed **2010F** Vital signs recorded **2014F** Mental status assessed **2018F** Hydration status assessed
Patient Management—0500F Series Codes in the **0500F** range are used to describe utilization measures or measures of patient care provided for specific clinical purposes (eg, prenatal care, presurgical and postsurgical care, referrals).	Code **0545F** is used to report that a plan for follow-up care was documented for a 15-year-old with a diagnosis of major depressive disorder.
Patient History—1000F Series Codes in the **1000F** range are used to describe measures for aspects of patient history and review of systems.	Code **1031F** is used to report that smoking status and exposure to secondhand smoke in the home were assessed in patients with asthma. Code **1050F** is used to report a patient history of new or changing moles.
Physical Examination—2000F Series Codes in the **2000F** range describe aspects of the physical examination or clinical assessment.	Code **2030F** is reported when the hydration status is documented as normally hydrated on a 2-month-old with acute gastroenteritis.
Diagnostic/Screening Processes or Results—3006F Series Codes in the **3006F** range are used to report results of clinical laboratory tests and radiologic or other procedural examinations.	Code **3008F** is reported when a patient's body mass index is documented.
Therapeutic, Preventive, or Other Interventions—4000F Series Codes in the **4000F** range are used to report pharmacologic, procedural, or behavioral therapies, including preventive services such as patient education and counseling.	Code **4015F** is reported when a preferred long-term control medication or an acceptable alternative treatment is prescribed for persistent asthma.
Follow-up or Other Outcomes—5005F Series Codes in the **5005F** range are used to describe the review and communication of test results to patients, patient satisfaction and experience with care, patient functional status, and patient morbidity and mortality.	Code **5250F** is reported to indicate that an asthma discharge plan was provided to a patient.
Patient Safety—6005F Series Codes in the **6005F** range are used to describe patient safety practices.	Code **6070F** is reported to indicate a patient was queried and counseled about antiepileptic drug side effects.
Structural Measures—7010F Series Codes in the **7010F** range are used to identify measures that address the setting or system of the delivered care and address aspects of the capabilities of the organization or health care professionals providing the care.	Code **7010F** is reported when patient information is entered into a recall system that includes a specified target date for the next examination of a patient with melanoma and a process to follow up with patients about missed or unscheduled appointments.
Non-measure Claims-Based Reporting—9001F Series Codes in the **9001F** range are used to identify certain aspects of care not currently represented by recognized performance measures but which may later be associated with measures approved by an appropriate quality improvement organization.	Code **9001F** is reported to identify the size of an abdominal aortic aneurysm less than 5.0 cm maximum diameter on centerline-formatted CT or minor diameter on axial-formatted CT.

Abbreviation: CT, computed tomography.

Table 3-4. Category II Modifiers	
Category II Modifier	**Examples**
Modifier 1P (performance measure exclusion modifier due to medical reasons) Used to report that one of the performance measures was not performed because it was not indicated (eg, already performed) or was contraindicated (eg, due to a patient's allergy)	Modifier **1P** is appended to code **6070F** (documentation that patient was queried and counseled about AED side effects) because the patient is not receiving an AED.
Modifier 2P (performance measure exclusion modifier due to patient choice) Used to report that the performance measure was not performed due to a patient's religious, social, or economic reasons; the patient declined (eg, noncompliance with treatment); or other specific reasons	Modifier **2P** is appended to code **3210F** (group A streptococcus test performed) when a physician considered the testing for streptococcus but the parent refused testing.
Modifier 3P (performance measure exclusion modifier due to system reasons) Used to report that the performance measure was not performed because the payer does not cover the service, the resources to perform the service are not available, or other reasons attributable to the health care delivery system Keep in mind that in the ED setting, appropriate medical screening and stabilization must be provided regardless of any consideration of payment. Providers are prohibited by federal statute from making treatment decisions in these circumstances based on payer coverage.	Modifier **3P** is appended to code **4062F** (patient referral for psychotherapy documented) when a 15-year-old with a diagnosis of major depressive disorder is not referred for psychotherapy because it is not available.
Modifier 8P (performance measure reporting modifier—action not performed, not otherwise specified) Used to allow the reporting of circumstances when an action described in a measure's numerator is not performed and the reason is not otherwise specified	Modifier **8P** would be appended to code **2001F** (weight recorded) when a 2-year-old with acute gastroenteritis is not weighed and, therefore, does not meet the performance measurement requirement.

Abbreviations: AED, antiepileptic drug; ED, emergency department.

Category II modifiers
- Are used only when allowed based on the specific reporting instructions for each performance measure.
- Are appended only to Category II *CPT* codes.
- Serve as a denominator exclusion from a performance measure (when measure allows).

The medical record should include written documentation of the reason that the service was ultimately not provided. Category II modifiers are only appended to Category II codes.

Reporting Performance Measures Applicable to Pediatrics

Many performance measures apply to the pediatric population. In addition, pediatric practices caring for patients 18 years or older may report Category II codes for conditions such as hypertension, diabetes mellitus, chronic kidney disease, gastroesophageal reflux disease, and community-acquired bacterial pneumonia as well as screening codes for tobacco use and cessation. Refer to the Alphabetical Clinical Topics Listing (ACTL) at www.ama-assn.org/practice-management/cpt/category-ii-codes for updated measures and reporting instructions.

The ACTL should be used in coordination with the Category II section in *CPT*.

Alphabetical Clinical Topics Listing

- Includes an alphabetical index of performance measures by clinical condition or topic
- Includes the measure developer (eg, PCPI), the performance measure, a description of the measure, and the associated Category II code
- Directs the reader to the measure developer's website to access the complete description of the measure (eg, specifications and requirements for reporting performance measures for asthma are located at www.aaaai.org/practice-resources/practice-tools/quality-measures)

Access the measure developer's website for the specification documents of the performance measure (ie, clinical measurement set, measurement set numerators and denominators, measure specifications, specifications for paper and electronic health records, an algorithm for measure calculation, data abstraction definitions, a medication table, and a retrospective data abstraction tool).

●=New code   ▲=Revised code   #=Re-sequenced code   +=Add-on code

The following websites provide information and resources:

- www.ncqa.org
- www.ama-assn.org/practice-management/cpt/category-ii-codes
- www.thepcpi.org

Each performance measure includes a symptom or activity assessment, numerator, denominator, percentage, and reporting instructions.

> A patient must meet the criteria specified in the denominator (diagnosis code) to be included in the numerator (Category II code) for a particular performance measure. Only the diagnosis code for the condition or disease will be linked to Category II *Current Procedural Terminology* codes.

Reporting measures to a payer (electronically or with a CMS-1500 claim form) is done the same way as reporting any *CPT* code. Report the appropriate E/M code (eg, **99202–99215, 99241–99245**) based on the level of service performed and documented with all the appropriate *diagnosis* codes that were addressed during the course of the visit. Report the Category II *CPT* code that relates to the performance measure with any applicable Category II modifier. Only the diagnosis code for the condition or disease will be linked to Category II *CPT* codes. Examples for some measures are included following the measures.

Acute Otitis Externa

These codes apply to patients aged 2 years and older with a diagnosis of acute otitis externa (AOE). Clinical components are reported to denote if pain was assessed, if topical therapy was prescribed, and if systemic antimicrobial therapy was avoided.

Category II *CPT* Codes: Acute Otitis Externa	Guidelines
1116F Auricular or periauricular pain assessed	Report at each encounter. Append modifier **1P** when the appropriate performance exclusion exists.
4130F Topical preparations (including over the counter) prescribed for acute otitis externa	If topical preparations are not prescribed, document the medical and/or patient reasons, and modifier **1P** or **2P** would be appended to code **4130F** or drug allergy or other adverse effects would be indicated by diagnosis codes.
4131F Systemic antimicrobial therapy prescribed **4132F** Systemic antimicrobial therapy not prescribed	Report code **4132F** when systemic antimicrobial therapy is not prescribed. Report code **4131F** with modifier **1P** with valid medical reason for prescribing systemic antimicrobial therapy. Exclusion modifiers cannot be reported with code **4132F**.

Example

➤ **A 4-year-old presents with acute onset of right ear pain.** The patient has been taking swimming lessons for the last 2 weeks. The diagnosis is AOE. The patient is sent home on topical antimicrobial and anti-inflammatory medication. All the criteria in the AOE measurement set as specified by the developer of the performance measurement are met and the ACTL is consulted for selection of appropriate *CPT* Category II codes.

ICD-10-CM	*CPT*
H60.331 (swimmer's ear, right ear)	**99213** (established patient; low-complexity medical decision-making) **1116F** (auricular or periauricular pain assessed) **4130F** (topical preparations [including over the counter] prescribed for AOE) **4132F** (systemic antimicrobial therapy not prescribed)

Acute Otitis Media With Effusion

These codes apply to patients aged 2 months through 12 years with a diagnosis of acute otitis media with effusion. Clinical components reported as part of this measure signify that an assessment of tympanic membrane mobility was performed using pneumatic otoscopy or tympanometry, that hearing testing was performed within 6 months prior to a tympanostomy tube insertion, and whether antihistamines, decongestants, or systemic steroids were avoided.

Category II *CPT* Codes: Acute Otitis Media With Effusion	Guidelines
2035F Tympanic membrane mobility assessed with pneumatic otoscopy or tympanometry	Reported at each encounter. Modifier **1P** or **2P** is appended when appropriate.
3230F Documentation that hearing test was performed within 6 months prior to a tympanostomy tube insertion	Reported at the time the tympanostomy tube insertion is performed. Documentation must reflect the performance and results of the test or, if the test is performed by another physician or provider, should include a copy of the test results. Modifiers **1P** or **3P** may be appended to code **3230F** as appropriate.
4131F Systemic antimicrobial therapy prescribed **4132F** Systemic antimicrobial therapy not prescribed **4133F** Antihistamines or decongestants prescribed or recommended **4134F** Antihistamines or decongestants neither prescribed nor recommended **4135F** Systemic corticosteroids prescribed **4136F** Systemic corticosteroids not prescribed	Used to report the absence or overuse of medications for each patient. Modifier **1P** is used with codes **4131F**, **4133F**, and **4135F** when appropriate. Modifiers **1P**, **2P**, and **3P** may not be reported with codes **4132F**, **4134F**, or **4136F**.

Asthma

This measure is applicable to all patients 5 to 50 years of age with a diagnosis of asthma.

Category II *CPT* Codes: Asthma	Guidelines
2015F Asthma impairment assessed **2016F** Asthma risk assessed	Used for each patient who was evaluated at least once for asthma control. Evaluation of asthma impairment and asthma risk must occur during the same medical encounter. There are no exclusions to the measures. Code **2016F** is also reported independently for each emergency department encounter or inpatient admission (with a diagnosis of acute asthma exacerbation). There are no performance exclusions for this measure.
1031F Smoking status and exposure to secondhand smoke in the home assessed	Report for each patient whose smoking status and exposure to secondhand smoke in the home was assessed. There are no performance exclusions.
1032F Current tobacco smoker OR currently exposed to secondhand smoke **1033F** Current tobacco nonsmoker AND not currently exposed to secondhand smoke **4000F** Tobacco use cessation intervention, counseling **4001F** Tobacco use cessation intervention, pharmacologic therapy	Report code **1032F** or **1033F** to indicate tobacco use status. If reporting code **1032F**, report **4000F** OR **4001F** to indicate type of tobacco use cessation intervention. There are no performance exclusions for this measure. Tobacco cessation interventions may be reported when provided to the patient's primary caregiver even if the caregiver is not the source of secondhand smoke in the home.
1038F Persistent asthma, mild, moderate, or severe **1039F** Intermittent asthma **4140F** Inhaled corticosteroids prescribed **4144F** Alternative long-term control medication prescribed	Report code **1038F** or **1039F** to indicate asthma severity. For patients with persistent asthma (**1038F**), report code **4140F**, **4144F**, or both. For patients with appropriate exclusion criteria, report code **4140F** or **4144F** with modifier **1P** or **2P**.
5250F Asthma discharge plan provided to patient	Report for each emergency department encounter or inpatient admission (with a diagnosis of acute asthma exacerbation) when an asthma discharge plan is provided to patient at time of discharge. There are no performance exclusions for this measure.

●=New code ▲=Revised code #=Re-sequenced code +=Add-on code

Chapter 3. Coding to Demonstrate Quality and Value

Example

➤ **A 10-year-old is seen with exacerbation of asthma.** His last exacerbation was 3 months ago. Asthma control test (ACT) is atypical at 19. Spirometry is performed and atypical for forced vital capacity (FVC), forced expiratory volume 1 (FEV_1), and FEV_1/FVC ratio. A nebulizer treatment with albuterol is administered. Examination following treatment shows decreased wheezing. Patient is sent home on albuterol and steroids administered by metered-dose inhaler with plan to follow up as necessary. Assessment of asthma status is documented as mild persistent. Category II codes for evaluation of asthma symptoms, persistent asthma, assessment of asthma status, and prescription of inhaled corticosteroids are reported. If documentation supports asthma risk (**2016F**), smoking status and exposure to second-hand smoke in the home (**1031F–1033F**), or tobacco use cessation intervention (**4000F, 4001F**), these may be additionally reported.

ICD-10-CM	CPT
J45.31 (mild persistent asthma with exacerbation)	**99214 25** (established patient; moderate-complexity medical decision-making) **94640** (aerosol treatment) **J7611** (albuterol, inhalation solution, US Food and Drug Administration–approved final product, non-compounded, administered through durable medical equipment concentrated form, 1 mg) **96160** ACT (administration of patient-focused health risk assessment instrument [eg, health hazard appraisal] with scoring and documentation, per standardized instrument) **1005F** (asthma symptoms evaluated) **1038F** (persistent asthma, mild, moderate, or severe) **2015F** (assessment of asthma status) **4140F** (inhaled corticosteroids prescribed)

If a payer follows Medicare and/or Medicaid National Correct Coding Initiative (NCCI) edits, spirometry (**94010**) is not separately reported during an encounter at which aerosol treatment (**94640**) is performed. Check payer guidelines for coverage of patient-focused health risk instrument administration and scoring (**96160**).

Pediatric Acute Gastroenteritis

The pediatric acute gastroenteritis measure applies to patients aged 1 month through 5 years with a diagnosis of acute gastroenteritis.

Category II *CPT* Codes: Pediatric Acute Gastroenteritis	Guidelines
4056F Appropriate oral rehydration solution recommended **4058F** Pediatric gastroenteritis education provided to caregiver	Used to report that the patient's caregiver was given a recommendation on an appropriate oral rehydration solution, diet education was performed, and the patient's caregiver was advised when to contact the physician. There are no performance exclusions.
2030F Hydration status documented, normally hydrated **2031F** Hydration status documented, dehydrated	Report when hydration status is documented in the medical record. When the patient is dehydrated and appropriate oral rehydration solution is recommended, report codes **4056F** and **2031F**. There are no performance exclusions.
2001F Weight recorded	Report when weight measurement is documented in the medical record. Modifiers **1P, 2P,** and **3P** may not be reported. Modifier **8P** may be reported.

Pediatric Pharyngitis and Upper Respiratory Infection

The pediatric pharyngitis measure applies to patients 2 to 18 years of age with a diagnosis of pharyngitis who were dispensed or prescribed antibiotic treatment and/or received a group A streptococcus test.

The URI measure applies to patients 3 years and older who were seen with a diagnosis of only URI and were appropriately not prescribed or dispensed an antibiotic.

Category II *CPT* Codes: Pediatric Pharyngitis and Upper Respiratory Infection	Guidelines
3210F Group A streptococcus test performed	Report when a patient is diagnosed with pharyngitis, is dispensed or prescribed an antibiotic, and received a group A streptococcus test. Modifier **1P** for medical exclusions or **2P** for patient exclusions may be used.
4120F Antibiotic prescribed or dispensed **4124F** Antibiotic neither prescribed nor dispensed	Report as appropriate for both performance measures (pediatric pharyngitis and URI). Modifier **1P**, **2P**, or **3P** may not be reported with code **4120F** or **4124F** for pharyngitis. Modifier **1P** is reported with code **4124F** when appropriate for URI. If a patient was dispensed or prescribed an antibiotic and received the group A streptococcus test, codes **3210F** and **4120F** would be reported.

Pediatric End-stage Renal Disease

This measure applies to patients aged 17 years and younger with a diagnosis of end-stage renal disease receiving hemodialysis, having clearance of urea/volume (Kt/V) measurements per the criteria listed in the codes, having received an influenza vaccine, and having a plan of care documented. This measure is reported during each calendar month that the patient is receiving hemodialysis.

Category II *CPT* Codes: End-stage Renal Disease	Guidelines
0505F Hemodialysis plan of care documented	Report when the hemodialysis plan of care is documented in the medical record on a patient aged 17 years or younger.
3082F Clearance of urea/volume (Kt/V) less than 1.2 **3083F** Kt/V greater than or equal to 1.2 and less than 1.7 **3084F** Kt/V greater than or equal to 1.7	Report code applicable to the corresponding Kt/V measurement. If the Kt/V is <1.2 (**3082F**) and the patient has a plan of care for inadequate hemodialysis, also report code **0505F**. There are no performance exclusions for this measure.
4274F Influenza immunization administered or previously received	Report when a patient aged 6 months through 17 years (with a diagnosis of end-stage renal disease and receiving dialysis) is seen between November 1 and February 15 and receives the influenza immunization or has received the influenza immunization from another provider. The medical record must support that the vaccine was administered. Modifier **1P**, **2P**, or **3P** may be used when appropriate.

Chapter 3. Coding to Demonstrate Quality and Value

●=New code   ▲=Revised code   #=Re-sequenced code   +=Add-on code

Epilepsy

This measure will be reported by the physician providing care to children and adults with a diagnosis of epilepsy.

Category II *CPT* Codes: Epilepsy	Guidelines
1200F Seizure type(s) and current seizure frequency(ies) documented **1205F** Etiology of epilepsy or epilepsy syndrome(s) reviewed and documented	Report when the seizure type(s) and current seizure frequency for each seizure type are documented in the medical record. Modifier **1P** or **2P** may be reported if appropriate. When the medical record documentation includes the etiology of epilepsy or the epilepsy syndrome(s) is reviewed and documented (if known) or documented as unknown or cryptogenic, code **1205F** is reported. There are no performance exclusions for code **1205F**.
3650F Electroencephalogram (EEG) ordered, reviewed, or requested **1119F** Initial evaluation for condition **1121F** Subsequent evaluation for condition	Code **3650F** is used to report whether the patient with a diagnosis of epilepsy seen for an initial evaluation had at least one EEG ordered or, if an EEG was performed previously, results were reviewed or requested. If code **3650F** is reported on the same day as a new patient E/M service (**99202–99205**), neither code **1119F** nor **1121F** is reported. If code **3650F** is reported on the same day as an established patient E/M visit (**99211–99215**) or office or outpatient consultation (**99241–99245**), code **1119F** is also reported to denote an initial evaluation for the condition or code **1121F** is reported to denote a subsequent evaluation. Modifier **1P**, **2P**, or **3P** may be reported with code **3650F** when appropriate.
3324F Magnetic resonance imaging (MRI) or computed tomography (CT) scan ordered, reviewed, or requested **1119F** Initial evaluation for condition **1121F** Subsequent evaluation for condition	When a patient with the diagnosis of epilepsy has MRI (preferred imaging) or CT ordered or if results are reviewed or requested of an MRI or a CT previously obtained, code **3324F** is reported. If code **3324F** is reported on the same day as a new patient E/M service (**99202–99205**), neither code **1119F** nor **1121F** is reported. If code **3324F** is reported on the same day as an established patient E/M visit (**99211–99215**) or office or outpatient consultation (**99241–99245**), code **1119F** is also reported to denote an initial evaluation for the condition or code **1121F** is reported to denote a subsequent evaluation. Modifier **1P**, **2P**, or **3P** may be reported with code **3324F**.
6070F Patient queried and counseled about antiepileptic drug (AED) side effects	Report when the patient is queried and counseled about AED side effects and the counseling is documented in the medical record. Modifier **1P** may be reported. This includes patients who are not taking an AED.
5200F Consideration of referral for a neurologic evaluation of appropriateness for surgical therapy for intractable epilepsy within the past 3 years	Report when a patient with a diagnosis of intractable epilepsy was considered for referral for a neurologic evaluation of appropriateness for surgical therapy within the past 3 years. There are no performance exclusions applicable.
4330F Counseling about epilepsy-specific safety issues provided to patient (or caregiver[s])	Report when counseling is provided to a patient and/or their caregiver(s) about context-specific safety issues appropriate to the patient's age, seizure type(s) and frequency(ies), and occupation and leisure activities (eg, injury prevention, burns, appropriate driving restrictions, bathing), at least once a year, and is documented in the medical record. Modifier **3P** may be reported when appropriate.
4340F Counseling for women of childbearing potential with epilepsy	Report whether or not a female of childbearing potential (12–44 years old) was counseled about how epilepsy and its treatment may affect contraception and pregnancy and the counseling is documented in the medical record. Modifier **1P** may be reported.

Major Depressive Disorder—Child and Adolescent

This measure is applicable for reporting care to all patients aged 6 through 17 years with a diagnosis of major depressive disorder (MDD).

Category II *CPT* Codes: Major Depressive Disorder	Guidelines
2060F Patient interviewed directly by evaluating clinician on or before date of diagnosis of MDD **1040F** *Diagnostic and Statistical Manual of Mental Disorders*, 5th Edition (*DSM-5*) criteria for MDD documented at the initial evaluation **3085F** Suicide risk assessed	Report code **2060F** when a patient is interviewed directly by the evaluating clinician on or before the date of diagnosis. Report code **1040F** when there is documented evidence that the patient met the *DSM-5* criteria—at least 5 elements with symptom duration of 2 weeks or longer, including depressed mood (can be irritable mood in children and adolescents) or loss of interest or pleasure—during the visit in which the new diagnosis or recurrent episode was identified. Code **3085F** is reported when an assessment for suicide risk is performed and documented. Modifiers **1P**, **2P**, **3P**, and **8P** may not be reported.
4060F Psychotherapy services provided **4062F** Patient referral for psychotherapy documented	Report code **4060F** when a patient receives psychotherapy during an episode of MDD and the service is documented in the medical record. Report code **4062F** when a patient is referred for psychotherapy and the referral is documented in the medical record. Modifier **1P**, **2P**, or **3P** may be reported.
4063F Antidepressant pharmacotherapy considered and not prescribed **4064F** Antidepressant pharmacotherapy prescribed	Used to report whether an antidepressant medication was considered or prescribed during an episode of MDD. Modifier **1P**, **2P**, or **3P** may not be reported.
0545F Plan for follow-up care for MDD, documented	Report when a plan for follow-up care is documented in the medical record. There are no performance exclusions for this measure.

Example

➤ **A 15-year-old new patient is seen with complaints of sleep disturbance and depressed mood.** The adolescent has not been eating well and has been increasingly irritable. A comprehensive history and detailed physical examination are performed. Three behavioral health assessment instruments to evaluate for depression, mood and feelings, and anxiety are completed and scored. The patient meets the *DSM-5* criteria for moderate MDD. Treatment options, including psychotherapy and antidepressant medications, are discussed. The patient chooses to pursue psychotherapy but refuses medication, and a referral is provided. The patient is scheduled for follow-up by phone call from a nurse in 1 week and appointment in 6 weeks. The physician's total time on the date of service was 45 minutes (not including time administering separately reported standardized instruments).

●=New code   ▲=Revised code   #=Re-sequenced code   +=Add-on code

Chapter 3. Coding to Demonstrate Quality and Value

ICD-10-CM	CPT
F32.1 (MDD single episode, moderate)	**99204** (new patient; 45–59 minutes total time on the date of the visit)
	96127 × first 2 standardized instruments (brief emotional/behavioral assessment [eg, depression inventory, attention-deficit/hyperactivity disorder (ADHD) scale], with scoring and documentation, per standardized instrument)
	96127 59 × third standardized instrument
	2060F (patient interviewed directly by evaluating clinician on or before date of diagnosis of MDD)
	1040F (criteria for MDD documented at the initial evaluation)
	3085F (suicide risk assessed)
	4062F (patient referral for psychotherapy documented)
	4063F (antidepressant pharmacotherapy considered and not prescribed)
	0545F (plan for follow-up care documented)

If a payer follows Medicaid NCCI Medically Unlikely Edits, a limit of 2 units of service per claim line is applied to code **96127**, but additional units (2 per claim line) may be reported on separate claim lines with modifier **59** (distinct procedure) when additional instruments are used in patient evaluation. There must be documentation in the medical record to support the use of more than 2 instruments. Payers may have a maximum number of units allowed by policy regardless of modifier use.

HIV/AIDS

This measure is reported by the physician providing ongoing HIV care to children and adults. There are 29 Category II codes used in this measure. Each measure has a different denominator that is specific to the patient's age. Measures include reporting cell counts, use of antiretroviral therapy, screening for opportunistic infections and high-risk behaviors, administration of vaccines, and use of *Pneumocystis jiroveci* pneumonia prophylaxis. Refer to the ACTL at www.ama-assn.org/practice-management/cpt/category-ii-codes for details on the requirements for reporting these codes.

Resources

AAP Policy Statement

"A New Era in Quality Measurement: The Development and Application of Quality Measures" (http://pediatrics.aappublications.org/content/139/1/e20163442)

CPT Category II Codes and Alphabetical Clinical Topics Listing

www.ama-assn.org/practice-management/cpt-category-ii-codes

Hierarchical Condition Categories

"Hierarchical Condition Categories: What They Are and Why They Matter to Pediatricians" July 2019 *AAP Pediatric Coding Newsletter™* (https://coding.solutions.aap.org/article.aspx?articleid=2736885; subscription required)

Quality Measures

Quality Measurement at the AAP (www.aap.org/en-us/professional-resources/quality-improvement/Pages/quality-measurement.aspx)

National Committee for Quality Assurance (www.ncqa.org)

Physician Consortium for Performance Improvement (www.thepcpi.org)

Test Your Knowledge!

1. **When does the Health Insurance Portability and Accountability Act of 1996 (HIPAA) allow disclosure of protected health information to a health plan for the plan's Healthcare Effectiveness Data and Information Set (HEDIS) purposes?**
   a. Only when the parents of the child sign an authorization to release the records
   b. Any health record may be disclosed for HEDIS.
   c. When the period for which information is needed overlaps with the period for which the patient is or was enrolled in the health plan
   d. HIPAA does not allow disclosure to provide health plans with information to support HEDIS reporting.

2. **Which of the following HEDIS measures does not apply to a patient who turns 3 years old during the measurement year?**
   a. Children 3 to 6 years of age who had 1 or more well-child visits with a primary care provider
   b. Percentage of children 2 years of age who had 1 or more capillary or venous lead blood test for lead poisoning on or by their second birthday
   c. Weight Assessment and Counseling for Nutrition and Physical Activity for Children and Adolescents (children and adolescents aged 3–17 years)
   d. Avoidance of Antibiotic Treatment for Acute Bronchitis/Bronchiolitis (ages 3 months and older)

3. **True or false? Modifier 8P is used to report that a measure was not performed because the resources to perform the service are not available.**
   a. True
   b. False

4. **Which of the following is not true of the Alphabetical Clinical Topics Listing?**
   a. Includes an alphabetical index of performance measures by clinical condition or topic
   b. Includes Category II *Current Procedural Terminology* codes for each measure
   c. Provides a complete description of each measure
   d. Includes the measure developer

The Business of Medicine: Working With Current and Emerging Payment Systems

Chapter 4. The Business of Medicine: Working With Current and Emerging Payment Systems

Contents

To maintain a viable practice, physicians and their staff must respond to changing payment systems and continually refine their practice management skills. This chapter's 3 sections address

- How services are currently valued and how assigned values may be used to guide practice management
- Guidelines and tools that may be used to monitor and manage charge accumulation, claims filing, review of payments, the appeals process, contract negotiations, and the use of audits to protect against lost revenue and incorrect billing practices
- Emerging payment methodologies and how these may affect traditional and newer practice models, such as accountable care organizations (ACOs)

Values Assigned to Physician Services

Connecting Codes to Payment and Budget

Before a claim is generated, a physician practice must establish fees for services that are greater than the cost of providing the service. A simple fee schedule methodology involves use of the Medicare Resource-Based Relative Value Scale (RBRVS). In 2020, most pediatric services are still valued and paid by Medicaid, Tricare, and commercial payers using a fee-for-service methodology based on the RBRVS. An understanding of how values are assigned to the codes for services, how the values relate to payment, and how this information contributes to a practice's finances is critical for the practice's financial viability and success.

The 3 components of the RBRVS are as follows:

1. *Physician work:* Physician work represents approximately 50% of the total relative value units (RVUs) assigned to most services. Work RVUs are commonly used in employment contracts as a factor in physician payment.
   - *Work* is described as time required to perform the service, mental effort and judgment, technical skill, physical effort, and psychological stress associated with concern about iatrogenic risk to the patient.
   - For most services, physician work is further broken down into *preservice, intraservice,* and *post-service* components. Correct coding requires understanding these components of work, as preservice and post-service components should not be separately reported.
     — *Preservice work:* For nonsurgical services, this preparatory non–face-to-face work includes typical review of records and communicating with other professionals. (Prolonged preservice work, such as extensive record review, may be separately reportable.) For surgical services, this includes physician work from the day before the service to the procedure but excludes the encounter that resulted in the decision for surgery or unrelated evaluation and management (E/M) services.
     — *Intraservice work:* For nonsurgical services, this includes time spent by the physician or other qualified health care professional (QHP) in direct patient care activities, such as obtaining history, examining the patient, and counseling the patient and/or caregivers. Surgical intraservice work begins with incision or introduction of instruments (eg, needle, scope) and ends with closure of the incision or removal of instruments.

       Certain services (eg, chronic care management) are inclusive only of intraservice time of physicians and/or clinical staff and are not valued to include pre- and post-service work.

> **New in 2021:** A physician's intraservice time on the date of an office or other outpatient evaluation and management service (99202–99205, 99212–99215) includes all time spent *on the date of the encounter* including pre-visit planning and post-visit work such as documenting the service provided.

     — *Post-service work:* For nonsurgical services, post-service work includes arranging for further services, reviewing and communicating test results, preparing written reports, and/or communicating by telephone or secure electronic means.
       - Separately reportable services, such as chronic care management or care plan oversight, are not included in post-service work.
       - For surgical services, post-service work includes typical work in the procedure or operating room after the procedure has ended, stabilization of the patient in the recovery area, communications with family or other health care professionals, and visits on the day of surgery. Surgical services are also valued to include typical follow-up care for the presenting problem during a defined global period (eg, 10 or 90 days after the service).

> **For more on the global period for surgery, see chapters 10 and 19.**

2. *Practice expense:* This component is an estimate of preservice, intraservice, and post-service clinical staff time; medical supplies; and procedure-specific and overhead equipment. Practice expense makes up about 44% of the total RVUs for most services. Practice expense varies by site of service (ie, facility vs non-facility). See the Place of Service Codes section later in this chapter for more information about how place of service affects payment.

3. *Professional liability:* This smallest component (about 4% of the total RVUs) is based on medical malpractice premium data.

Figure 4-1 illustrates the percent of total RVU for each component.

Each RVU component may be independently adjusted slightly upward or downward as a function of geographic area. The Centers for Medicare & Medicaid Services (CMS) calculates Medicare payment for a procedure code by multiplying total RVUs by a dollar conversion factor (CF) that is set annually.

Example

➤ **A payer uses the 2020 Medicare Physician Fee Schedule (MPFS) as a basis for physician payment with a CF or contracted fee schedule amount of $36 per RVU.** A physician submits established patient preventive medicine visit code **99392** to the payer.

The total non-facility RVUs (3.01) assigned to code **99392** are a combination of RVUs for physician work (1.50), non-facility practice expense (1.40), and professional liability (0.11). The total Medicare non-facility RVUs (3.01) are multiplied by the $36 CF to determine the allowed amount for the service.

(Total Medicare RVUs) × (Payer CF) = Allowed amount (3.01) × ($36) = $108.36

Actual payment may vary based on the patient's out-of-pocket obligation.

Medicaid fee schedules vary by state and, although often based on RVUs or the MPFS, state regulations may also designate amounts paid for specific services. Commercial payments for many procedure codes are often linked to a percentage of Medicare payment. Alternatively, payers may offer their own fee schedule for a practice's most used procedure codes.

Figure 4-1. Percent of Total Relative Value Units

■ Physician Work   ■ Practice Expense   ■ Professional Liability

- It is important to obtain the payer's fee schedule for all codes used or likely to be used by a practice (including codes for vaccines) and compare these with the MPFS and other published fee schedules. Although Medicare assigns a status of N (non-covered) to *Current Procedural Terminology* (*CPT*) codes **99381–99385** and **99391–99395** in the MPFS, component RVUs are published in the MPFS allowing calculation of Medicare equivalent payments.

- Medicaid and proposed commercial payments for pediatric preventive care can be evaluated in light of the Medicare equivalent payments.

- If a contract links payment to the MPFS, it is important to be specific about which year's fee schedule is used, as these change annually. Resetting payment based on the MPFS for the year of service may result in higher or lower payments.

Tip: When reviewing a payer's fee schedule, make sure the payer also fully discloses its policies for paying for services that it considers to be *bundled* (ie, payment for 2 or more codes during the same encounter may be less than the sum of the individual payments).

The RBRVS payment methodology may be used with practice- and physician-specific data generated from a practice's accounting and practice management systems to estimate an approximate cost of providing each service. This should result in a list of services that are each assigned a share of the practice's overhead costs as well as the margin and actual cost of providing the service.

- From the accounting system, an administrator may calculate the total practice expenses for a period, subtracting billable services that are not paid based on RVUs such as vaccines and medications.
- From the practice management system, reports may be generated to provide a total of the number of procedures billed by code, RVUs for each service, and total RVUs billed by the practice for the same period.
- By dividing total practice expenses by total RVUs, an administrator can calculate the practice cost per RVU.
- Additional calculations may be used to compare payment per RVU or per service among contracted payers. (Calculations should be viewed in context of other factors, such as history of timely and correct payment.)

Such calculations can be used to inform decisions on acceptance of contractual fee schedules, number of services necessary to break even or profit from provision of services, and return on investment potential for new equipment or services.

Keep in mind that some ACOs have financial agreements that require certain services be paid with a single lump payment that is then distributed among all providers of the service. To negotiate a fair portion of that lump payment, you need to know the cost of providing the service. (See the Accountable Care Organizations [ACOs] section later in this chapter.) More accurate cost estimates may be determined on an actual cost basis. However, RVU calculations are straightforward and typically provide a reasonably reliable result.

Participation in Relative Value Scale Update Committee Surveys

Pediatricians can also play a role in recommending values for services to the CMS by participation in American Academy of Pediatrics (AAP) surveys conducted through the American Medical Association/Specialty Society Relative Value Scale Update Committee (RUC). These surveys are conducted to estimate the time and complexity of performing a service in comparison with another service. American Academy of Pediatrics staff sends out requests for participation to AAP section members to allow completion by physicians who most typically perform the service being surveyed. To learn more about participation in RUC surveys, see the "Understanding the RUC Survey Instrument" video at www.youtube.com/watch?v=nu5unDX8VIs; for information on code valuation, RBRVS, and payment, see www.aap.org/en-us/professional-resources/practice-transformation/getting-paid/Coding-at-the-AAP/Pages/Code-Valuation-and-PaymentRBRVS.aspx.

Clean Claims to Correct Payment

Getting paid for services provided requires a practice-wide team effort. Opportunities for lost revenue can occur anywhere between patient scheduling and posting of health plan payments (or denials). **Figure 4-2** shows steps in the revenue cycle.

Even salaried physicians are affected by lost revenue and should take interest in the effectiveness of the practice's billing processes.

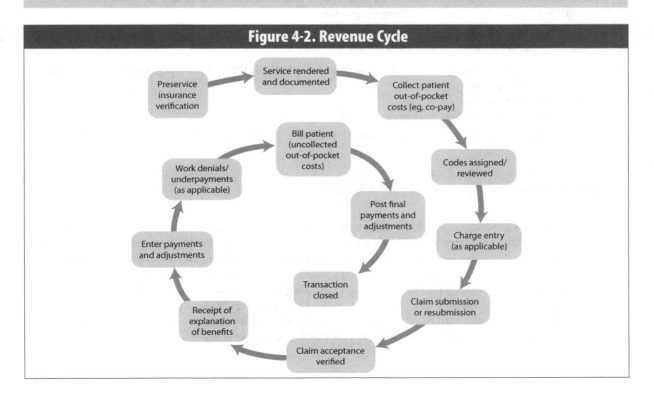

Figure 4-2. Revenue Cycle

●=New code   ▲=Revised code   #=Re-sequenced code   +=Add-on code

An effective charge accumulation system, accurate billing of procedure codes, and an efficient claims filing system are necessary but not sufficient to achieve clean claim submissions. Although the physician is ultimately responsible for the accuracy of codes selected and claims submitted, it typically takes a team effort to create and maintain an effective accounts receivable system, including

- Development and use of management tools.
  - Incorporation of claims processing tools for analysis of your claims processing procedures. A self-assessment tool for improving claims processing and payment can be found at www.aap.org/en-us/Documents/ImprovingClaimsProcessing.pdf.
  - Electronic health record (EHR) and/or billing systems may include automated tools to help identify errors prior to billing, alert you to payments that do not align with contracted fees, and provide data for monitoring the time lapse from provision of service to payment.
- Continuing provider and staff education with constant oversight and communication with staff, payers, and patients.
  - Policies and procedures support continuous monitoring of payer communications and dissemination of information on benefit policy changes that affect coding and payment.
  - Assurance that staff assigned with responsibilities related to correct coding and billing have access to authoritative resources on coding and documentation (eg, current Medicaid National Correct Coding Initiative [NCCI] edits and manual).

> **See chapters 2 and 5 for more information on code edits and compliant coding and billing.**

- Regularly performing audits to identify potential corrective actions required to remain compliant with billing standards, coding guidelines, and federal rules and regulations (eg, Health Insurance Portability and Accountability Act of 1996 [HIPAA], Anti-Kickback Statute, False Claims Act). Audits benefit the practice by identifying
  - The number of timely and correctly submitted claims, resulting in faster and more appropriate payments and reduced practice cost of obtaining payment
  - The need for physician and staff education on coding and documentation
  - Issues for payer contract negotiations
  - Incorrect coding and related potential risk for charges of fraud or abuse
  - Areas that need written office policies and procedures (eg, pre-authorization and referral processes, claims follow-up processes, control systems)
- Procedures for efficient review of payments and potentially inappropriate denials or reductions. Timely identification of payment errors is necessary to obtain redress because contracts often specify a time limit on appeals.
- Guidance for write-offs and initiation of appeals processes.

Capturing Charges in the Electronic Health Record

Many physicians now capture encounter and billing information in the EHR. The basics of charge capture in the EHR are
- Accurate listing of diagnoses
- Selection of complete codes
- Procedure code selection based on work performed and documented

While integrating charge capture into the encounter documentation should create efficiency, there are pitfalls to be avoided.

> **Compliant documentation and code selection are discussed in Chapter 5.**

When using an EHR, make sure that codes in the system are accurate and updated in accordance with code set updates. It is important to verify with your electronic system vendors how code updates are incorporated into the system. This might happen via scheduled upgrades that may or may not require system downtime, or it could occur via automated upgrades during night or weekend hours. It is important to make sure this information is outlined in your EHR contract.

- Code updates should be based on the effective date of changes (eg, deleted codes may be entered for charges with a date of service prior to the effective date of deletion even after the update has been made).
- Practice and billing managers must maintain contact with the system vendor's upgrade and support staff and verify what, if any, manual steps are required on the part of the practice in relation to code changes.

It is also important that code descriptors displayed in code selection are adequate for accurate code selection. Truncated descriptors may omit key information that differentiates one code from another (eg, hypertrophy of tonsils should provide options for hypertrophy of tonsils alone or hypertrophy of tonsils and adenoid and prompt reporting of a code for tonsillitis when both tonsillitis and hypertrophy are diagnosed).

Documentation of the diagnoses has been problematic in some EHR systems. As with the paper record, the physician must have the ability to fully describe patient diagnoses for each encounter.

Example

➤ 1. Attention-deficit/hyperactivity disorder (ADHD), predominately inattentive type, on parent and teacher scales with a positive family history of ADHD
2. Underachievement in school with grades dropping this semester
3. Disruption of family by separation and divorce, which is causing behavioral issues at home and school

- Systems should not use diagnosis codes for populating the physician's diagnostic statement or assessment. Code descriptors may be generalized and do not capture the physician's differential diagnoses (eg, delayed milestone in childhood—3 years old, late talker in speech therapy; possible autism spectrum disorder—little eye contact and likes to play alone).
- The EHR should not reorder diagnoses entered by the physician. An EHR that reorders documented diagnoses (eg, alphabetically) results in noncompliance with diagnosis coding guidelines.
  Physicians should list first the diagnosis and code most responsible for the encounter, followed by additional diagnoses, in compliance with coding guidelines.
- The patient problem list should not be pulled forward as the diagnoses for each encounter. Only those conditions addressed or that affected management or treatment of conditions addressed should be reported for that particular encounter.
  Follow payer guidelines for reporting diagnosis codes for chronic conditions that may be reported annually (eg, evaluating problems at preventive service visits) for purposes of risk stratification.

Automated code selection is also problematic. An EHR may be designed to determine the level of E/M service provided based on information documented. However, physicians must make the code determination based on the medically necessary services provided and documented and based on code selection criteria (ie, key components or time).

- Automatic population of records may result in documentation that overstates the level of work and intensity of the service provided.
- When EHR functionality includes automated E/M code suggestion, physicians must view the EHR code as a suggestion that must be confirmed or rejected based on documentation and medical necessity.
- Failure to override suggested codes when appropriate may be considered an abusive practice.

When encounter data is utilized to show performance of quality metrics, it is essential that the data are configured to correctly populate reports of the patients to whom the measure applies and whether there is documentation of the outcome or process of care specified in the measure (eg, all patients aged 3–17 years and the percentage of those patients who received counseling for diet and exercise).

See more on compliant electronic health record documentation in Chapter 5.

Encounter Forms and Other Coding Tools

Encounter forms are useful supplements to EHR-based code selection. They can also be used to convey codes to a billing office/system when systems are not integrated.

Designing and Reviewing the Encounter Form

The encounter form, whether computer generated or printed, should be designed to help physicians and clinical staff quickly find all codes for diagnoses and services common to the practice. An encounter form or superbill should prompt recognition of separately reported services and use of diagnosis codes that most accurately describe the patient presentation.

Chapter 4. The Business of Medicine: Working With Current and Emerging Payment Systems

When developing the encounter form

- Include all levels of service for each category of E/M services (eg, **99211–99215**, **99221–99223**) and ensure time is listed for coding based on time. List routine health examination codes by age and new or established patient.
- List procedures (eg, laboratory) in alphabetical order within the category of service. For example, group codes together in the order of your workflow (eg, visit codes followed by immunization, laboratory, respiratory, etc) to maximize efficiency and your workflow.
- The printed encounter form should prompt staff for specific details of a procedure when required for code verification. For example

  Code **120**_____ Simple repair loc* _____ size _____   (*Location)

- Include the most commonly reported diagnosis codes. Consider grouping diagnosis codes by organ system, and then alphabetically, within the system.
- Leave space on the printed form to allow the reporting of the specific diagnosis and full *International Classification of Diseases, 10th Revision, Clinical Modification (ICD-10-CM)* code.

Example

➤ **J45.2_**   *Asthma, mild intermittent*
  J45.3_   *Asthma, mild persistent*
  J45.4_   Asthma, moderate persistent
  J45.5_   *Asthma, severe, persistent*
      Add fifth character: 0, uncomplicated; 1, w/ (acute) exacerbation; 2, w/ status asthmaticus.

- Include the most frequently used modifiers.
- Leave space on printed forms to write in any services or diagnoses that are not included.
- Include add-on codes for prolonged and special services. For example
  +99356   Prolonged service in the inpatient or observation setting, first hour
  99058   Services provided on an emergency basis in the office, disrupting other scheduled services
- Develop a separate encounter form for hospital and outpatient hospital services. Make sure it includes all the services most commonly performed in the hospital setting.
      Access to a coding application or pocket-sized reference card with required key components and/or time of services also helps promote accurate code selection in facility settings.
- When quality initiatives are dependent on codes reported (eg, codes supporting Healthcare Effectiveness Data and Information Set [HEDIS] measures), be sure that these codes are clearly indicated on the encounter form, prompted by the EHR, or provided in an easily accessible quick reference.

  Encounter forms and other coding tools should be reviewed periodically and updated at the time of each code set update to ensure that most of, if not all, the services and procedures commonly performed in the practice are included and the codes are accurate.

See Chapter 1 for the timing of updates to code sets (eg, January, April, July, October).

Completing the Printed Encounter Form

Every practice should develop a written policy of the requirements needed to complete a form. Some points that should be part of the policy include

- The encounter form is *not* part of the medical record. Information such as the need for follow-up care, diagnostic tests, or referrals must always be documented in the medical record even if written on the encounter form.
- Services must be clearly identified (eg, circle procedure, use check mark).
- The person providing the service (eg, physician, laboratory technologist, medical assistant) should enter procedure codes or document that service on the encounter form to ensure only the procedures performed are reported. This ensures that only work that has been performed is reported.

Chapter 4. The Business of Medicine: Working With Current and Emerging Payment Systems

Example

➤ **Dr Good marks a urinalysis on the encounter form when she orders the test.** However, a specimen could not be obtained and the procedure may be billed inappropriately.

If the clinical staff (under supervision of the physician) had been responsible for reporting the service when performed, it would not have been reported because the urine was not obtained.

- The physician is ultimately responsible for the services reported and billed.
- The physician should identify the diagnosis as, for example, primary or secondary.
- Diagnoses and services or procedures must be numbered and linked to each other.

Example

➤ **An E/M service and removal of impacted cerumen from the right ear (69210) is performed.** The physician reports the primary diagnosis (**H66.001**, acute suppurative otitis media without spontaneous rupture of eardrum, right ear) (field 21A) and the secondary diagnosis (**H61.21**, impacted cerumen, right ear) (field 21B). *ICD-10-CM* pointer A (**H66.001**) is linked to the office visit (**99213 25**) in field 24E and pointer B (**H61.21**) is linked to the procedure (**69210**) in field 24 E of the respective service lines.

Table 4-1. Diagnosis Indicator on CMS-1500 Form

21. Diagnosis or nature of illness or injury (Relate A–L to service line below 24E)				ICD Ind. 0					
A. **H66.001**	B. **H61.21**	C.	D.						
E.	F.	G.	H.						
I.	J.	K.	L.						

24. A. Dates of service	B. POS	C. EMG	D. Procedures, services or supplies CPT/HCPCS	Modifier	E. Diagnosis Pointer	F. Charges	G. Days or units	H. EPSDT	I. ID Qual	J. Rendering Provider #
1/2/2021–1/2/2021	11		**99213** (E/M)	**25**	A	$$$	1		NPI	1234567890
1/2/2021–1/2/2021	11		**69210** (cerumen removal)		B	$$$	1		NPI	1234567890

Abbreviations: *CPT*, Current Procedural Terminology; E/M, evaluation and management; EMG, emergency; EPSDT, Early and Periodic Screening, Diagnostic, and Treatment; HCPCS, Healthcare Common Procedure Coding System; *ICD*, International Classification of Diseases; NPI, National Provider Identifier; POS, place of service.

- On a paper claim form, the linking of diagnoses to procedures would look like **Table 4-1.** An electronic claim form contains the same data in segments of loops 2300 and 2400.
- Procedures or diagnoses must be written on the form if they are not preprinted.
- A billing manager or clerk should only add or change a service or diagnosis with the agreement of the provider of service.
- A system should be instituted to monitor and ensure capture of charges for all of the day's patient encounters (eg, cross-reference to the patient check-in records).

Reviewing Assigned Codes

A staff member who understands correct coding and reporting guidelines should always review the assigned codes before the claim is submitted to ensure that all procedures and services are captured and accurate.

For example, the reviewer should look to see that

- An administration code is reported with vaccines and/or injections. Payer instructions for reporting National Drug Codes and units are followed.
- A venipuncture or finger stick is reported with a laboratory test. Clinical Laboratory Improvement Amendments number is included, when required.
- A handling fee is reported when the specimen is prepared and sent to an outside laboratory.

Chapter 4. The Business of Medicine: Working With Current and Emerging Payment Systems

- A modifier is appended when appropriate (eg, modifier **76** for repeat procedures or services).
- The office visit is reported using the correct new or established patient category of service.

> **See Chapter 6 for more information on new and established patients.**

- The diagnoses reported as primary and secondary are appropriate and are linked to the appropriate services or procedures.
- The documentation to support each service has been completed with required dates and signatures.

Place of Service Codes

The place of service is indicated on each claim by a *place of service code* (often integrated into billing systems without need for manual entry with each charge). The place of service may appear evident when reporting codes for services such as inpatient hospital care, but this is not always the case.

- When providing services in a facility such as a hospital outpatient clinic, it is important to report the correct place of service because differences in practice expense in a facility versus a non-facility setting affect physician payment.

Example

➤ **A procedure performed in a surgical center would be paid at a lower fee schedule amount than the same procedure performed in a physician's clinic (not hospital based) because the fee schedule takes into account the overhead or practice expense of providing services (eg, procedure room, supplies, clinical staff).**

If services provided in a facility setting are reported as if provided in a physician's clinic, an overpayment may occur. Physicians in provider-based practices (ie, those practices owned and operated as a part of a hospital) should be aware that the place of service code is especially important in this setting.

Physician and practice expense portions of the patient's charges are often billed separately in provider-based practices.

- The same services provided in a provider-based practice are often costlier than those provided in an independent (physician-owned) practice.
- Facility fees charged by the provider are often significantly higher than the non-facility fees charged in independent practices.
- The Medicare program created place of service code **19** to define an "off-campus" hospital practice to adopt site-neutral payment for many physician services provided at provider-based practices. The rules and payment modifications have not been universally adopted, but it is important to know how your office is classified to ensure proper billing regardless. When considering purchase by a hospital system, it is important to consider the effect of billing with a different place of service code.
- The increased number of high-deductible health plans has raised awareness of the greater costs to patients when services are rendered in provider-based facilities and has prompted Medicare and some states to take action to reduce the added costs. Practices should be aware of any such restrictions that apply to billing in their locality and under payer contracts.

Other place of service codes that may be commonly reported for pediatric services include **02**, telehealth; **03**, school; **11**, office; **12**, home; **14**, group home; **20**, urgent care facility; **21**, inpatient hospital; **22**, on campus—outpatient hospital; and **23**, emergency room—hospital.

Place of service codes are further discussed for certain E/M services in chapters dedicated to those sites of service. See a full list of place of service codes at www.cms.gov/Medicare/Coding/place-of-service-codes/Place_of_Service_Code_Set.html.

Submitting Clean Claims

Many states have enacted laws that require prompt payment of clean claims. In general, *clean claims* are those that contain sufficient and correct information for processing without further investigation or development by the payer (definitions may vary by state).

- Submitted claims must be accurate and in accordance with the process outlined in the executed carrier or health plan agreement. Knowing a payer's claim requirements will decrease chances of denied claims.

- Make sure the practice understands payer rules, for example, for billing for nonphysician services incident to a physician's or other QHP's service.

> **See chapters 6 and 13 for more information on billing for nonphysician services.**

- Be aware of any updates issued by the carrier that affect billing and claims submission.

Generally, a clean claim should have the following information:

- Practice information (name, address, phone, National Provider Identifier [NPI], group tax ID number)
- Patient information (patient name, birth date, policyholder, policy number, patient ID number, address)
- Codes (*CPT, ICD-10-CM*, Healthcare Common Procedure Coding System, place of service), modifiers, and service dates
- Carrier information
- Secondary and, when applicable, tertiary insurance information
- Referring physician name and NPI, if applicable
- Facility name and address, as appropriate

If additional information is necessary to support a service or explain an unusual circumstance (eg, unlisted procedure code, unusual procedure, complicated procedure)

- Use the attachments feature of the electronic claims system, clearinghouse, or other claim attachment procedure as directed by the payer (eg, submission of attachments by online portal).

Health plans may have specific instructions for submission of claims attachments (eg, inclusion of a unique identifier [2–50 characters] or internal control number linking the claim and attachment).

- If it is necessary, send a hard-copy claim with a cover letter and a narrative report or copy of the appropriate part of the medical record (eg, progress note, procedure note) to facilitate claim processing.
    — Any documentation (eg, coordination of benefits information, letter of medical necessity, clinical reports) should include the patient's name, service date, and policy number on each page in case the papers become separated.
    — Keep a copy of the claim and supporting information for follow-up of payment.
- When filing claims for patients with coordination of benefits, make certain all required information (ie, primary and secondary insurance information) has been obtained from the patient and claims are filed with the supporting information (eg, explanation of benefits [EOB] or electronic remittance advice information), according to plan requirements.

Claims should be submitted for payment as soon as possible and before the deadline for timely filing specified in the agreement.

- The optimum time for filing outpatient claims is on the day of or the day following the service but no more than 2 to 3 days from the date of service.
- Codes for services to patients with prolonged hospitalizations may be collected for 7 consecutive days before billing; in this case, claims should be filed within 2 to 3 days of the end of the service week. It is not necessary to withhold claims until the patient is discharged.

> **Practices should monitor lag time between completion of each service and submission of a claim for the service to identify and correct any cause of delayed submission. Timely finalization of documentation is necessary to make sure that codes are supported by the documentation before claims are submitted. Many practices adopt policies for timely completion of documentation.**

Policy should be adopted requiring completion of medical record documentation within a specified period to support prompt billing of services. Physicians must understand that timely completion of documentation is required for appropriate code selection, claim filing, and, ultimately, prompt payment.

Special Consideration for Medicare Claims

Many health plans receive Medicare claims automatically when they are the secondary payer. In this case, the explanation of Medicare benefits will indicate that the claim has been automatically crossed over for secondary consideration. Physicians and providers should look for this indication on their EOBs and should not submit a paper claim to the secondary payer.

●=New code   ▲=Revised code   #=Re-sequenced code   +=Add-on code

Monitoring Claim Status

An important aspect of billing operations is prompt and routine claim monitoring. A defined process for verifying that submitted claims were received and accepted by claim clearinghouses and/or payers should be included in the practice's or billing service's written billing procedures. Steps may include (see the last item in this list if billing is outsourced or centralized outside the practice)

- Identify each type of report and/or dashboard feature of the practice's billing system for use in verifying claim submission and acceptance for processing, assigning follow-up activities for unpaid claims, and tracking average time from date of service or submission to receipt of payment.
- Assign responsibilities for verifying that electronic claim submissions were received and accepted for processing as soon after transmission as possible.
  — Most clearinghouses will send a report indicating acceptance or rejection of a batch of claims within minutes of transmission and a report with individual claim-level detail within 24 hours of submission.
  — It is also necessary to log in to a payer's website or system to verify receipt of claims and monitor acceptance or rejection. Errors and omissions may occur in transmission.
- Electronic claim submission reports must be promptly reviewed for rejections or denials. All rejected or denied claims must be investigated to determine what corrections or payer contact is necessary to resubmit or return the claim for re-adjudication (eg, when a payer system error is corrected).
- Claims should not be resubmitted without investigation, as
  — Resubmission of a claim containing errors is unlikely to result in payment.
  — Resubmission of the claim with errors may reset the aging of the claim in the billing system and result in late follow-up or denial for lack of timely filing.

> Avoid potential denial of corrected claims due to duplicate charges. A claim frequency code, placed in box 22 of a CMS-1500 form or loop 2300 of an electronic 837 format, is used to indicate that a claim is a corrected (code 7) or voided (code 8) claim. Correcting or voiding a previously submitted claim typically results in either a complete replacement of a previously processed claim or voiding of the original claim from the health plan's record. See specific instructions from the health plan for full instructions when submitting a corrected claim.

- Identify staff responsible for claims follow-up and establish standards for timely follow-up on unpaid claims. System-generated reports are useful in identifying the age of claims.
- Policies and procedures should address communication with patients and responsible parties when a payer requests additional information prior to claims processing (eg, many payers will request information on other coverage and/or details of where and how an injury was sustained).
    Failure to respond to payer requests for information in a timely manner can result in delayed or denied claims payment.
- If centralized billing or an outsourced billing service is used, maintain oversight of performance by reviewing reports and taking action on any areas where potentially delayed or lost revenue are indicated. Examples of potential areas of concern include
  — Lag time between completion of documentation and submission of claims
  — Aging reports that show the average number of days since claim submission for unpaid claims
  — Amounts adjusted or written off

Monitoring Payments

Develop a process to monitor the timeliness of all payments. Tips for monitoring payments include

- Identify payers who do not pay clean claims within the time frame agreed on in your contract and follow up on all late payments with the payer.
  — Check the provisions of your state prompt pay law and know the provisions for clean claims, timely filing, and penalties.
  — Report a payer's practice of late or delinquent payments to the proper agency because your practice may be entitled to payment plus interest.
- Review each EOB and/or remittance advice (electronic or paper) carefully to determine if the payment is correct.
  — Familiarity with standard claim adjustment reason codes and remittance advice remark codes is essential to identifying denial reasons, such as a non-covered service, bundled payment, or provision of service not typical for physician specialty (not relevant for taxonomy code), and any patient responsibility for denied charges.
  — Find claim adjustment reason code and remittance advice remark code descriptions online at https://nex12.org/index.php/codes.

- Compare the EOBs and/or remittance advice to a spreadsheet listing your top 40 codes and their allowable payments by carrier to monitor contract compliance. Practice management software may also include the ability to add contractual allowances by payer. Make certain that the payment is consistent with the fee schedule, write-offs, and discounts agreed to by the practice and payer. Follow up with the payer on any discrepancies.

    Health plans may enter contracted fee schedules for each physician or provider individually, resulting in inaccurate payment for 1 or more providers in a practice.
- Identify any discrepancies, such as changes to codes, reduced payment, or denials.
- Review all payer explanations, particularly reasons for denials or down-coding. If the service provided is not a benefit covered by the plan, the patient should be billed directly (may need a signed waiver form).
  - Only bill patients for amounts deemed noncovered or patient responsibility by the payer and only in compliance with the health plan contract.
  - Do not bill patients for bundled services or other reduced payment due to the contract between your practice and the payer. Renegotiate your contract if payment is lower than costs of providing care.
- Make certain that any denials or reductions in payment are not due to practice billing errors (eg, incorrect modifiers, obsolete codes) or are incorrect applications of an NCCI edit that does not pertain to pediatrics. If so, correct the errors immediately and educate staff members as appropriate to ensure correct future claim submissions.
- One efficiency of many electronic systems is automatic application of payments and adjustments. However, systems may apply incorrect adjustments based on payer remark codes. Staff should monitor all denials and reduced payments as appropriate and appeal incorrect adjustments when applicable.
- Maintain a log of all denials or payment reductions. This can be used as a basis for future negotiations or education of the payer. (Identify 1 individual who has billing and coding expertise to monitor as well as accept or reject denials.)
- Review your fee schedule to see if your practice is paid at 100% of the billed charges. This is an indication that your fees are below the maximum amount established by the carrier. This excludes services that are always patient responsibility (eg, form fees, cosmetic services).
- Review your fees annually and understand the Medicare RBRVS, using it to value the services you provide. (For details on using the RBRVS, see "RBRVS: What Is It and How Does It Affect Pediatrics?" at https://downloads.aap.org/AAP/PDF/RBRVS.pdf, access code AAPCFP26.)

> Tracking vaccine acquisition cost is very important. Costs may change during the course of the contract. Review the carrier contract for mid-contract vaccine cost changes (eg, some contracts will default to a percentage of billed charges during vaccine price transitions).

- Review your payment to make sure it exceeds your cost of providing that service including time of clinical staff.
- When contracting with payers, be aware of payment options that may be specified (eg, paper checks, electronic fund transfers, virtual credit card payment). It is important to understand the pros and cons of each (eg, credit card processing fees typically apply to card-based payment).
- *Health plans must provide payment in compliance with electronic fund transfer standards of HIPAA rather than virtual card or wire transfer when requested by a physician.* Agreements to accept electronic fund transfers should not allow health plans to debit an account without notification and consent. Banks may offer additional protections against unauthorized withdrawals.

Filing Appeals

Do not assume that the carrier's denials or audits are accurate. Be prepared to challenge the carrier and request the specific policy on which the denial is based. If you are coding correctly and in compliance with coding conventions, you should appeal all inappropriately denied claims and carrier misapplication of *CPT* coding principles. Develop a system to monitor payer updates and any changes to the provider agreement so you are aware of the current payment policies and coding edits used by the payer.

> Appealing a claim denial requires confidence that the claim was correctly coded and supported in documentation. Ongoing coding education and internal compliance reviews are necessary to support compliant claim submissions. Learn more about coding compliance in Chapter 5.

- By accepting inappropriate claim denials, a practice may be setting itself up to charges of abusive billing practices.

    If a practice recodes claims as a result of inappropriate claim denials, the resubmitted claim may not actually reflect the treatment the patient received.

●=New code ▲=Revised code #=Re-sequenced code +=Add-on code

Here is a summary of basic guidelines and tips for appealing payments.
- When in contact with the payer, always document the date, name, and title of the payer representative with whom you have talked and a summary of the details of the conversation.
  - If a payer requests you submit a claim using codes or modifiers that are not consistent with clean coding standards, ask for written documentation of the direction (preferably via fax or email).
  - Address issues with the person who has the authority to make decisions to overturn denials or reductions in payment.
  - Keep an updated file with names and contact information of the appropriate personnel with each of your contracted payers.
  - Request an email or letter verifying the information provided and archive written correspondence containing payer representative advice and payer policies. If the carrier does not provide written documentation, prepare a summary and send it to your contact, stating that this will constitute the documentation of the discussion.
- Submit all appeals in writing.
  - Understand the payer's appeal process and appeal within its timeliness guidelines.
  - Format the letter to include the name of the patient, policy number, claim control number, and date of service(s) in question on each page of the letter.
  - The body of the letter should state the reason for the appeal and why you disagree with the payer's adjudication of the claim. Speak to the payer's rules/regulations regarding the decision and how your documentation supports payment.
  - Specify a date by which you expect the carrier to respond.
  - Support your case by providing medical justification and referencing *CPT* coding guidelines. If necessary, consult with the AAP Coding Hotline (https://form.jotform.com/Subspecialty/aapcodinghotline) for clarification of correct coding. It may be helpful to hire a certified coding expert with knowledge in pediatric coding to review your claims. (If hiring a full-time certified coding expert is not practical for a small practice, part-time employment or periodic consultation may be options for access to coding and compliance expertise.)
  - Consider sending correspondence to the carrier by certified mail to verify receipt. Document and retain copies of all communications with the carrier about the appeal.
- Maintain an appeals-pending file.
  - If there is no response from the payer within 4 weeks of the date of the letter, send a copy of the appeal letter stamped "Second Request."
  - If there is no response within 2 weeks, or if the matter continues to remain unresolved, contact the state department of insurance (or other appropriate agency in your state) to file a complaint or engage its assistance.
  - Contact your AAP chapter and pediatric council, if your chapter has one, to make them aware of the situation with the payer. American Academy of Pediatrics chapter pediatric councils meet with health plans to discuss carrier policies and practices affecting pediatrics and pediatricians.

The AAP has developed several sample appeal letters that may be used as templates in appealing payer decisions. The appeal letter templates can be found at www.aap.org/en-us/professional-resources/practice-transformation/getting-paid/Pages/Private-Payer-Advocacy-Templates-for-Appeal-Letters.aspx. Template topics include

- Bundling of services
- Immunization administration services (**90460**, **90461**; **90471–90474**)
- Modifier **25**
- Well-child care (**99381–99395**) and sick visit (**99202–99215**) reported on the same calendar day

In addition, the AAP has posted a narrative that explains the appropriateness of reporting certain circumstances based on NCCI edits.

When the AAP recognizes systemic issues with payer policies, it sends letters to payers on specific issues that need resolution or for information. These letters and carrier responses are posted on www.aap.org/en-us/professional-resources/practice-transformation/getting-paid/Pages/Private-Payer-Advocacy-Letters-to-Carriers.aspx.

Knowing when to appeal a payer denial is just as important as knowing how to properly appeal. Writing an effective appeal letter to payers requires knowledge of *CPT* guidelines, CMS policy, and payer policy. The AAP Private Payer Advocacy Advisory Committee has developed resources to effectively respond to inappropriate claim denials, handle requests for refunds, manage private payer contracts and denials, and respond to payer audits. (See www.aap.org/en-us/professional-resources/practice-transformation/getting-paid/pages/Oops-We-Overpaid-You-How-to-Respond-to-Payer-Audits.aspx.)

Negotiating With Payers

Payers need to be made aware and held accountable when their payment policies negatively affect the physician–carrier contractual arrangement. Previous class-action lawsuits against national carriers in response to payers' inappropriate down-coding and bundling of services have strengthened the position of physicians appropriately following *CPT* guidelines.

Negotiating payment with payers can be more successful if a practice is also prepared to provide quality of care data according to standard quality measures. Be prepared to demonstrate cost savings that may be recognized by the plan as well as the value the practice brings to the plan in terms of savings, quality of care data, and/or patient satisfaction.

The following suggestions can prepare physician participation in negotiations:

- Know a health plan's policies and procedures and their effect on pediatric services. Develop a system to monitor all updates and changes to the physician contract. Be aware of updates that are provided via periodic email bulletins or information posted on a payer website that practices have been instructed to review periodically. Practices must be aware that these alternative ways of disseminating payment information are often considered legal and binding.
- Know a health plan's processes to add new *CPT* codes/services and how each plan pays prior to determining payment policy and fee schedule amounts. (New codes are often paid at a percentage of charges if covered at all.)
- When adding new physicians to your practice, be aware of each payer's fee schedule policies. Do not assume that the same fee schedule will be applied across all physicians in the practice (eg, a payer may assign a reduced fee schedule to new physicians or carry forward a physician's contract from a previous practice).

  Be aware of the potential that patients may incur higher out-of-pocket costs (eg, co-pays) with services by different providers within the practice. When this occurs, discussion with a health plan should include the potential effect of delayed care when the patient/family opts to wait to see a provider for whom the out-of-pocket costs are lower.
- Be aware of any accountability (eg, penalties or other effect on shared savings) that a plan attributes to the practice when patients receive care outside their plan's network without referral by physicians within the practice.
- Know *CPT* codes and modifiers and the guidelines for their use.
- Understand how the NCCI adopted by some payers (including Medicaid) may relate to your practice.
- Understand and be able to describe the scope of services provided and the time requirements for the service.
- Be prepared to demonstrate cost savings that may be recognized by the plan as well as the value the practice brings to the plan in terms of savings, quality of care data, and/or patient satisfaction. *This is your leverage.*
- Monitor and know the use (distribution) of codes by each physician and, if in a group practice, for the practice as a whole.
- Identify your payer mix. Know how many patients you have in each plan and what percentage of your total patients that represents. In addition, know what percentage of RVUs each payer pays for your most frequently used codes and how they compare in payment with each other. Accurate information on payer mix and potential value/loss to the practice is essential in making participation decisions.
- Know and understand the payment basis and process.
- Have specific codes or issues to discuss, not generalities (agreement with general ideas may not address specific issues).

  In negotiations
- Try to negotiate for coverage and payment of services or, if payers refuse to cover services, get your contract amended to state that you can bill the service as non-covered. If the plan will allow for billing the patient for non-covered services, you must then advise your patients of this policy (usually requires a written notification prior to rendering the service).
- If the plan does agree to provide coverage for a particular service, make certain you understand how the carrier will cover and pay for the service and if there will be any restrictions or limitations.
- Keep notes during the discussion and be certain you understand answers to any of your questions. Any specific agreements should be in writing and signed by both parties.

  Seek assistance in negotiations.
- Engage parents or employers to work in partnership to help you negotiate with a plan. Encourage parents to work through their human resources department to communicate and appeal with payers. Petitions from parents can be very effective.
- Many AAP chapters have developed pediatric councils, which meet with payers to address pediatric issues. Advise your chapter pediatric council of specific issues you have experienced and see how it can work with the plan. (The AAP chapter pediatric councils are not forums for contract negotiation, setting fees, or discussing payments.)

  If your chapter does not have a pediatric council, this may be the right time to work with your chapter to begin developing one. To see if your state has a pediatric council or for more information, visit www.aap.org/en-us/professional-resources/practice-transformation/getting-paid/Pages/aap-pediatric-councils.aspx (AAP members only).

When Negotiations Fail

If the insurance company is not addressing your concerns satisfactorily, you should be willing to withdraw from its plan. Inform the payer (a formal notification process may be outlined in your contract), patients' families, and even the state insurance commission why continued participation is impossible.

— Some reasons for withdrawal might be slow payment, excessive documentation requirements, and substandard payment compared with other plans.

— Many times, negotiation begins when you walk away from the table.

Documentation and Coding Audits

Medicare, state Medicaid programs, and commercial payers will audit claims as well as monitor coding profiles (especially E/M coding). Physician practices should also adopt standards for conducting internal audits or reviews. Internal audits provide important information to inform practice policy and procedures, detect missed revenue, protect against erroneous billing, and avoid issues with payers and outside auditors. Some key benefits of internal auditing are

- Identification of negative billing and revenue trends, including
  - Increased lag time between encounter and billing (eg, delays in finalization of documentation, delayed coding or billing functions, technology issues)
  - Denial or underpayment of new services or new or revised procedure codes
  - Significant unexpected increase or decrease in revenue
  - Inappropriate adjustments or write-offs of unpaid or underpaid claims that should be appealed
- Charge verification (eg, number of charges is equal to or greater than number of encounters, with exception of unbilled visits included in a global period)
- Identification of incorrect billing and coding practices
- Identification of payment that does not align with payer contract
- Identification of electronic system or workflow issues
- Identification of areas where new or additional training is necessary

See Chapter 5 for more detailed information on conducting internal audits.

Tools for the Pediatric Practice

Working with third-party payers on coding and payment issues can be a difficult task because there is little uniformity between carriers and, frequently, great inconsistencies within the same umbrella organization of carriers. The AAP Private Payer Advocacy Advisory Committee is charged with enhancing systems for members and chapters to identify and respond to issues with private carriers.

To assist the pediatric practice, the AAP has several available resources to consider.

- American Academy of Pediatrics staff is available to provide clarification on coding issues. The AAP Coding Hotline can be accessed at https://form.jotform.com/Subspecialty/aapcodinghotline.
- Claims processing tools, a collection of template letters practices can use in appealing inappropriate carrier claim denials, and other tools are available through the AAP Resources for Payment site at www.aap.org/en-us/professional-resources/practice-transformation/getting-paid/Pages/resources-for-payment.aspx (AAP members only). Also, the AAP Coding Calculator allows physician practices to compare their actual E/M code use distribution to statistical norms and assess the potential effect on payment. It can be accessed at www.aap.org/en-us/professional-resources/practice-transformation/getting-paid/Coding-at-the-AAP/Pages/Coding-Calculator.aspx.
- For information on pediatric councils, go to www.aap.org/en-us/professional-resources/practice-transformation/getting-paid/Pages/aap-pediatric-councils.aspx (AAP members only).
- The AAP has created tools to assist practices with managed care contracting. These resources are available at www.aap.org/en-us/professional-resources/practice-transformation/getting-paid/Pages/resources-for-payment.aspx.
- Members of the AAP are encouraged to access the AAP Hassle Factor Form online to report health plan issues. The information submitted is used to assist the AAP and chapters in identifying issues and facilitating public and private payer advocacy related to health plans, including discussion topics with national carriers and at chapter pediatric council meetings with regional carriers. The Hassle Factor Form can be accessed at www.aap.org/en-us/professional-resources/practice-transformation/getting-paid/Pages/Hassle-Factor-Form-Concerns-with-Payers.aspx (AAP members only) and can be submitted electronically.
- American Academy of Pediatrics members and their staff are encouraged to attend AAP Coding Webinars, presented by pediatric coding experts. To obtain a list of scheduled webinars and to register, visit www.aap.org/webinars/coding.

- The *AAP Pediatric Coding Newsletter*™ provides articles on coding and documentation of specific services and supplies (eg, vaccines) with updates on new codes and emerging issues affecting coding and billing practices. Subscribers can access current and archived issues and coding resources at http://coding.aap.org.

Emerging Payment Methodologies

Many payers are in the process of transitioning from volume-based payments, such as fee for service, to value-based payment models that offer incentive payments to providers based on the quality of care, outcomes, and cost containment attributable to their practice. The intent is to promote patient value and efficiency, but some risk is shifted to physician practices and there could be a lack of clarity as to how payments are actually calculated.

> **Important Considerations in Value-Based Payment Models**
>
> In value-based programs, it is not always transparent to families how the value is calculated (ie, how much is quality and how much is cost). When discussing such programs with payers, practices should be aware of whether immunizations and preventive care are counted in the total cost of care, or they may find that if they improve well-visit and immunization rates, the costs of those services are counted against the practice in total cost of care calculations. In addition, some payers will preferentially drive patients to high-value practices or have tiered co-payments based on practice performance.

Under these emerging payment models, practice viability will depend on how well quality, cost, and efficiency are managed. Examples of some of these newer payment models include bundled payments, shared savings, and pay for performance. Physician payments may be based on a combination of fee for service and newer payment methodologies. Emerging forms of health care financing and delivery models include ACOs and integrated delivery systems.

- *Bundled payments:* These are a type of prospective payment in which health care providers (eg, hospitals, physicians, and other health care professionals) share 1 payment for a specified range of services as opposed to each provider being paid individually. The intent of bundled payment is to foster collaboration among multiple providers to coordinate services and control costs, thereby reducing unnecessary utilization.
- *Shared savings:* Under a shared savings arrangement, providers and payers seek to deliver care at a cost that is below current budgeted amounts. The resulting savings are shared among the payer(s) and providers.
  - The contractual arrangement among the payer(s) and providers will specify how the savings are calculated and distributed.
  - Shared savings models may include upside reward exclusively or upside reward and downside risk. In an upside-reward–only arrangement, the provider only shares in any savings and is not at risk for a loss. Under reward-and-risk arrangements, the practice shares a reward if costs are less than budgeted but also would share the loss should actual total costs exceed budgeted costs.
  - Shared savings should include an up-front agreement to continue additional payments for ongoing support of infrastructure for future years when the payer may want to cut back on the shared savings margin or reduce as those savings plateau.
  - Quality metrics are typically tied to payment of shared savings, with physicians not meeting established quality benchmarks not receiving a portion of savings.

> See Chapter 3 for more information on coding to support quality and performance measurement.

> For more information on shared savings, see www.aap.org/en-us/Documents/practicet_ gainsharing_and_ shared_savings.pdf or visit www.aap.org/cfp and enter password AAPCFP26.

- *Pay for performance:* In this arrangement, physician payments are based on a prospectively determined comparison of the provider's performance against acknowledged benchmarks. If the provider meets or exceeds those benchmarks, an enhanced payment or bonus is provided.
  - Benchmarks are often similar to the National Committee for Quality Assurance HEDIS quality metrics (some common metrics for pediatrics include rates of immunizations; rates of patient adherence to Early and Periodic Screening, Diagnostic, and Treatment visits; and rates of appropriate prescription of asthma medications).
  - Pay for performance arrangements often include the following 4 types of measures (**Figure 4-3**):
    - *Structure:* Measures use of staff capabilities, policies and procedures, and systems such as EHR and computerized physician order entry
    - *Process:* Determines the extent to which providers consistently give patients specific services that are consistent with recommended guidelines for care

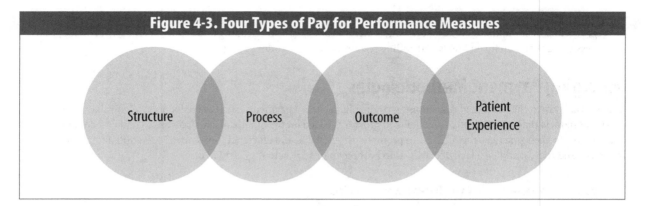

Figure 4-3. Four Types of Pay for Performance Measures

- *Outcome:* Measures the effects that 1 or more clinical interventions have had on patients' health, health status, and function
- *Patient experience:* Measures patient-reported experience of care

Each type of measure may include additional subtypes, and payers may use composite measures (ie, 2 or more measures that result in a single score).

In considering whether to participate in one of these newer payment models, a practice needs to determine expected costs and utilization and assess whether it can deliver services under the projected budget. Using *CPT* codes and their RVUs will aid in this assessment. Projections can be made using RVUs of the services currently provided and projected to be provided. With these types of data, the practice can assess the effect of new payment methodologies to its bottom line.

In some parts of the country, practices can earn additional incentives if the total cost of care for their patients compares favorably to geographically and specialty matched peers. In addition, some payers are incentivizing around "care efficiency measures." Both of these are often risk adjusted based on claims data about the overall patient population of the practice.

Preparing for New Payment Models

The new payment models discussed herein are already in place in some areas and will soon be adopted in others. Whether your practice provides primary or specialty care, there are steps that you should take to prepare for success. When payment is based on the costs of care and patient experience, practices must take responsibility for keeping costs low and quality of care and patient experience high. Steps that practices may take include

- Learning more about value-based payment options
- Generating and using reports of your costs, quality measurement, etc
- Learning who your active patients are and staying up to date through routine data analysis
  - Obtain lists of patients attributed to your practice by payers (patient panels) and reconcile to your active patient list.
  - Identify and agree on a methodology by which any disputes over attributed patient panels will be reconciled.

Assignment, Engagement, and Attribution of Patient Panels

Value-based payment may be based on the patients assigned and/or attributed to a practice (patient panel) by a payer. This may be limited to comparison of the cost of care for a physician's patient panel and other patients in a geographic area or other subset of patients. The cost of care for all attributed patients may lead to additional payment based on shared cost savings or may limit the amount of payments that the practice retains. It is important to understand the distinction between what you view as your practice panel and how the insurer views it.

It is important to differentiate assignment from engagement and attribution.

- *Assignment:* The patients the insurance company lists on your panel roster.

  For Medicaid managed care, every patient must be assigned to a provider (or provider practice) when patients are enrolled in the health plan. These patients may choose your practice or can be automatically assigned based on insurer algorithms.
- *Engagement:* Patients you have seen and with whom you have a medical home relationship.

  If you have an after-hours clinic and you see patients from other practices, it is essential you communicate to those patients that they are not part of your medical home (ie, they are part of another physician's or practice's panel).
- *Attribution:* Patients who fall into the denominator of a metric in which value (ie, payment) is assigned. Physicians should understand how health plans attribute patients to individual physicians and/or groups for purposes of performance measurement and cost of care.

— Factors such as time of continuous enrollment with the health plan and number of visits to a provider may affect how patients are attributed.
— The CMS has initiated voluntary reporting of modifiers **X1–X5**, which identify the provider–patient relationship for an episode of care. Because reporting these modifiers, which were created for Medicare, is not required, adoption by other payers and physicians may be slow.

> See Healthcare Common Procedure Coding System modifiers **X1–X5** in Chapter 2 for more information on these relationship modifiers.

To ensure you are engaging patients who are assigned to your practice, make sure you receive a panel roster monthly, preferably an Excel file, through the payer's portal. Identify new patients assigned to your practice and plan for what services they will need based on their age.

- Use the roster at check-in to make sure all patients seen in your medical home are assigned to you. This is just as important as identifying those you are not seeing on your roster. It will ensure you are getting credit for the quality work your office is providing.
- Know the insurer's rules for requesting a patient be removed from your roster. They may require specific documentation, such as number of outreach attempts by phone or mail, to fulfill your request.
- Track the number of patients assigned to your office each month. If there is a large increase, a group of patients from another practice may have been shifted to your practice. Consider including language in your contract that specifies that no panel transfers can be done without prior authorization of your practice.
- If the insurer is nonresponsive in working to ensure only patients who can be or are engaged are assigned, consider limiting the ages that can be assigned to your practice or closing your practice to auto-assignment altogether.

When considering overall cost of care or emergency department or hospital utilization, your full panel's costs will be assigned to your practice.

For HEDIS measures, patients must meet certain age-, utilization-, or encounter-based criteria to fall into your denominator. Knowing when they will be attributed (and show up on your "gaps in care" reports) is essential. See further discussion in **Chapter 3**.

Remember that your revenue comes from encounters with engaged patients regardless of assignment or attribution in a value-based payment model. Your practice will never have a 100% accurate assigned panel. The effort you put in to reaching this perfection must be balanced by what is being measured and how much payment is at risk.

Steps that may increase successful participation in value-based payment include

- Embracing automation and alternatives to paper handling and traditional office-based care.
- Seeking to remove inefficiencies by reviewing routine tasks and patient flow. Provide staff with incentives and an expectation to create consistency and efficiency.
- Learning about the communities of your patients—school and community resources, school schedules, average income and education of caregivers, urgent and emergency care utilization patterns—and using that information in providing care.
- Knowing the costs of the care you provide and order for your patients. Recognize that every provider within and outside of your practice must contribute to reducing the cost of care to reduce the practice's risk under new payment models.
  - Remember that care received in the emergency department and urgent care clinics and from subspecialists or qualified nonphysician health care professionals (eg, physical therapists) is included in the cost of care attributed to your cost to care for your patients.
  - Collaborate with subspecialists to ensure patients receive evidence-based and cost-effective care, including consideration of formulary and total cost of coordinated care.
- Considering options for adding nonphysician health care professionals, such as care coordinators, patient educators, and emotional/behavioral health specialists, to your practice. (These clinicians may also add separately reportable services under fee-for-service contracts.)
- Embedding clinical guidelines into care delivery through protocols and reminders.
- Configuring and using your EHR and other automated systems to promote efficiency (eg, display generic drugs first when brand name is entered).
- When considering an alternative payment model contract, seek expert consultation to help identify and, as necessary, negotiate points of concern within the contract.

Other considerations for pediatricians include

- Recognizing that, depending on how the payment model is set up, managing a healthy population of patients may not result in significant cost savings.

- The ability to access and monitor patient population and performance metric data is important to successful participation in new payment methodologies. Physicians must be aware of not only the patients they are seeing but those who are not receiving preventive and/or follow-up care.
- Physicians need to understand the links between new payment methodologies and data collection to support quality metrics (eg, failure to report codes for screening services performed may result in negative performance measurement and lost opportunity for enhanced payment).
- In states where the Children's Health Insurance Program (CHIP) operates independent of a state Medicaid program, children covered by CHIP may or may not be included in new payment methodologies and/or performance measurement.

See the *AAP News* article, "PPAAC: Chapter pediatric councils work with payers on medical home programs," at www.aappublications.org/news/2016/03/18/PPAAC031816 for examples of how AAP chapters and their pediatric councils advocate for developing adequate financing for pediatric medical homes under value-based payment methodologies.

Accountable Care Organizations (ACOs)

Most of the following content about ACOs is adapted with permission from the January 2011 AAP News *(www.aappublications. org/content/32/1/1.6). Information that has changed since publication of that article has been updated herein.*

As defined by the CMS, an ACO is an organization of health care professionals that agrees to be accountable for the quality, cost, and overall care of beneficiaries. In return, the ACO will receive incentive payments based on quality and cost containment instead of volume and intensity. Eligible providers are likely to be individual and group practices, hospitals, integrated delivery systems, and others who create a legal entity with a management structure able to deliver and report on evidence-based and informed care to a defined population, effectively engage patients, and receive and distribute shared savings.

The Patient Protection and Affordable Care Act of 2010 (PPACA) included a number of provisions that establish ACOs in Medicare, Medicaid, and CHIP. In October 2011, the CMS issued final regulations to assist physicians, hospitals, and other health care professionals in coordinating care through ACOs.

Interest in ACOs is accelerating, and the market continues to witness a growth in their numbers. As of 2018, the CMS has documented 561 Medicare Shared Savings Program (MSSP) ACOs. These approaches will evaluate the effectiveness of various payment models and how their approach can provide better care, work in conjunction with private payers, and reduce Medicare cost growth.

Beyond the federal government's push toward ACOs, commercial health insurers are also actively exploring the development of ACOs. One of the special features of commercially driven ACOs is their flexibility in implementing accountable care contracts. Many private ACOs emulate the CMS MSSP approach; however, the flexibility provided by market-driven ACOs permits them to undertake more creative approaches in modeling payment methodologies. Leavitt Partners LLC, a national health intelligence firm, reported in 2018 that there are more than 1,011 public and private ACOs covering 32.7 million patients across every state in the United States.

Pediatricians must be in a position to assess the ACO transition locally. More importantly, pediatricians need to be actively engaged in this transition to a new care model to ensure it best serves the needs of children and families and the pediatric health care delivery system.

The growing interest in ACOs as a principal driver in the reconfiguration of the US health care delivery system aligns with the Triple Aim espoused by former CMS administrator Don Berwick, MD. In the aggregate, the Triple Aim is designed to improve the individual experience of care, improve the health of populations, and reduce per capita costs of care for populations.

The Pediatric ACO Demonstration Project, legislated as part of the PPACA but unfunded, calls for participating state Medicaid programs to allow pediatric medical professionals to form ACOs and receive incentive payments. The US Department of Health and Human Services will develop quality guidelines that must be met. The applicant state and ACO must meet a certain level of savings or slow the rate of growth in health care costs to receive an incentive payment. However, if funded, it is anticipated the CMS will derive many of the ACO requirements on the basis of its MSSP.

American Academy of Pediatrics Resources for More Information on ACOs

In response to growing interest in the development of ACOs, in 2011, the AAP ACO Workgroup produced guidance for members on factors to consider in evaluating an opportunity to participate in an ACO (www.aap.org/en-us/professional-resources/practice-transformation/getting-paid/Pages/Accountable-Care-Organizations-and-Pediatricians-Evaluation-and-Engagement.aspx). The guidance was reevaluated in 2013 by a group of pediatrician experts in financing and economics and deemed to still be timely.

The AAP has since collaborated with Leavitt Partners to carry out a study of pediatric ACOs, including a series of 5 case studies of diverse pediatric models, a scan of Medicaid ACOs, and a summit of leaders in pediatric ACO development. These collaborative activities identified several issues in ACO formation and sustainability in pediatric settings and outlined a number of opportunities for the pediatric community in areas of organization, model change, and market dynamics; payment, financing, and contracting; quality and value; and use of new technologies. More information is available in the January 2017 *Pediatrics* article, "Pediatric Accountable Care Organizations: Insight From Early Adopters" (http://pediatrics.aappublications.org/content/early/2017/01/29/peds.2016-1840).

In addition, the CMS has published fact sheets that provide general information about ACOs and their operational and financial characteristics. They can be accessed at http://innovations.cms.gov/initiatives/ACO/index.html.

Resources

AAP Coding Assistance and Education

AAP Coding Hotline (https://form.jotform.com/Subspecialty/aapcodinghotline)

AAP Pediatric Coding Newsletter (https://coding.aap.org)

AAP Coding Webinars (www.aap.org/webinars/coding)

Charge Capture

AAP *Pediatric Office Superbill* (purchase at https://shop.aap.org/pediatric-office-superbill-2021)

Claims Processing

Improving Claims Processing and Payment: A Self-Assessment Tool for Physicians/Providers (www.aap.org/en-us/Documents/ImprovingClaimsProcessing.pdf)

Claim adjustment reason code and remittance advice remark code descriptions (https://nex12.org/index.php/codes)

"Codes Assigned by Payers: CARCs and RARCs," July 2019 *AAP Pediatric Coding Newsletter* (https://coding.solutions.aap.org/article.aspx?articleid=2736881; subscription required)

Coding Compliance

"Coding Compliance: Conducting Internal Audits"; "Planning Chart Audits"; and "Audit Tools: What You Need to Perform and Document Chart Audits," February 2019 *AAP Pediatric Coding Newsletter* (https://coding.solutions.aap.org/issues.aspx#issueid=937761; subscription required)

AAP Coding Calculator (www.aap.org/en-us/professional-resources/practice-transformation/getting-paid/Coding-at-the-AAP/Pages/Coding-Calculator.aspx)

Payment/Denial Advocacy

AAP Payer Advocacy Templates for Appeal Letters (www.aap.org/en-us/professional-resources/practice-transformation/getting-paid/Pages/Private-Payer-Advocacy-Templates-for-Appeal-Letters.aspx)

AAP Payer Advocacy: Letters to Carriers (www.aap.org/en-us/professional-resources/practice-transformation/getting-paid/Pages/Private-Payer-Advocacy-Letters-to-Carriers.aspx)

AAP Pediatric Councils (www.aap.org/en-us/professional-resources/practice-transformation/getting-paid/Pages/aap-pediatric-councils.aspx)

AAP Hassle Factor Form (www.aap.org/en-us/professional-resources/practice-transformation/getting-paid/Pages/Hassle-Factor-Form-Concerns-with-Payers.aspx; AAP members only)

AAP Oops We've Overpaid You: How to Respond to Payer Audits (www.aap.org/en-us/professional-resources/practice-transformation/getting-paid/pages/Oops-We-Overpaid-You-How-to-Respond-to-Payer-Audits.aspx)

Payment/Relative Value Units

AAP Resources for Payment (www.aap.org/en-us/professional-resources/practice-transformation/getting-paid/Pages/resources-for-payment.aspx)

AAP Managed Care Contracting (www.aap.org/en-us/professional-resources/practice-transformation/getting-paid/Pages/managed-care-contracting.aspx)

"Application of the Resource-Based Relative Value Scale System to Pediatrics" (http://pediatrics.aappublications.org/content/133/6/1158.full.pdf)

"2021 RBRVS: What Is It and How Does It Affect Pediatrics?" (www.aap.org/coding; access code AAPCFP26)

"Understanding the RUC Survey Instrument" video (www.youtube.com/watch?v=nu5unDX8VIs)

AAP Code Valuation and Payment RBRVS (www.aap.org/en-us/professional-resources/practice-transformation/getting-paid/Coding-at-the-AAP/Pages/Code-Valuation-and-PaymentRBRVS.aspx)

Place of Service Codes

Place of Service Code Set (www.cms.gov/Medicare/Coding/place-of-service-codes/Place_of_Service_Code_Set.html)

Value-Based Payment

AAP Value-Based Payment (www.aap.org/en-us/professional-resources/practice-transformation/getting-paid/Pages/value-based-payment.aspx)

AAP Webinar Series on Alternative Payment Models (www.aap.org/en-us/professional-resources/practice-transformation/getting-paid/Pages/alternative-payment-models.aspx; scroll down to webinar links)

Accountable Care Organizations (ACOs): General Information (http://innovations.cms.gov/initiatives/ACO/index.html)

"Accountable Care Organizations (ACOs) and Pediatricians: Evaluation and Engagement," *AAP News* (www.aappublications.org/content/32/1/1.6)

"Gainsharing and Shared Savings" (www.aap.org/en-us/Documents/practicet_gainsharing_and_shared_savings.pdf)

"Pediatric Accountable Care Organizations: Insight From Early Adopters," *Pediatrics* (http://pediatrics.aappublications.org/content/early/2017/01/29/peds.2016-1840)

"PPAAC: Chapter pediatric councils work with payers on medical home programs," *AAP News* (www.aappublications.org/news/2016/03/18/PPAAC031816)

Test Your Knowledge!

1. **What are the 3 components of the Resource-Based Relative Value Scale methodology?**
   a. Physician time, clinical staff time, and room time
   b. Preservice, intraservice, and post-service
   c. History, examination, and medical decision-making
   d. Physician work, practice expense, and professional liability

2. ***International Classification of Diseases, 10th Revision, Clinical Modification* codes selected in the electronic health record for an encounter should be placed in which order?**
   a. Alphabetical order
   b. Code number order
   c. Order of responsibility for the service(s) provided
   d. The order of the diagnosis codes is not important.

3. **How are services provided in a physician's office (not a hospital-based clinic) designated on a claim?**
   a. Place of service **11**
   b. The procedure code reported for the service
   c. A modifier appended to procedure codes
   d. A narrative statement on the claim

4. **Which of the following is an appropriate action in response to denial of a claim?**
   a. Immediately transfer the amount due to patient responsibility.
   b. Review claim adjustment reason and remittance advice remark codes.
   c. Change the codes on the claim to codes that are more likely to be paid.
   d. Refile the same claim without further investigation.

5. **Which of the following is true of reward-and-risk arrangements?**
   a. A bonus is given when the provider meets or exceeds performance benchmarks.
   b. Each of a patient's providers is paid a share of 1 payment for a specified range of services.
   c. The practice shares either reward or loss depending on actual total costs versus budgeted costs.
   d. The provider only shares in any savings and is not at risk for a loss.

CHAPTER 5

Preventing Fraud and Abuse: Compliance, Audits, and Paybacks

This chapter was contributed by the American Academy of Pediatrics Committee on Medical Liability and Risk Management.

Contents

Although most physicians work ethically, provide high-quality care, and submit appropriate claims for payment, unfortunately, there are some providers who exploit the health care system for personal gain. These few have necessitated an array of laws to combat fraud and abuse and protect the integrity of the health care payment system.

Just as patients put enormous trust in physicians, so do payers. Medicare, Medicaid, other federal health care programs, and private payers rely on physicians' medical judgment to treat patients with appropriate services. They depend on physicians to submit accurate and truthful claims for the services provided to their enrollees. And most physicians intend to do just that. However, the process is made more difficult by the complex and dynamic nature of payer coding and billing procedures, which, despite efforts to standardize variations, persist from carrier to carrier, policy to policy, state to state, and month to month.

This chapter outlines the importance of safeguarding the health care system from fraud and abuse, describes how compliance programs can protect medical practices from unintentional billing errors, and provides general considerations on how to respond to overpayment notices and inquiries from auditors.

Defining Medical Fraud and Abuse

The federal government has more than a dozen laws in its anti-fraud and anti-abuse arsenal. The 5 most important laws that apply to physicians are the

- False Claims Act
- Anti-Kickback Statute
- Physician Self-Referral Law (Stark)
- Exclusion Authorities
- Civil Monetary Penalties Law

Abiding by these laws is not just the right thing to do; violating them, even (for some) unwittingly, could result in criminal penalties, civil fines, exclusion from federal health care programs, or loss of a medical license from a state medical board. It all begins with understanding the definition of *fraud and abuse* in health care.

Fraud

Fraud is obtaining something of value through intentional misrepresentation or concealment of material facts. Examples of fraud in the physician's office may include

- Requiring that a patient return for a procedure that could have been performed on the same day
- Billing Medicare or Medicaid for services not provided, including no-shows
- Billing 1 member for services provided to another (non-covered) member
- Billing more than 1 party for the same service
- Billing services under a different National Provider Identifier (NPI) (except as allowed by payer guidance)
- Taking a kickback in money, in-kind, or other valuable compensation for referrals
- Completing a certificate of medical necessity for a patient who does not need the service or who is not professionally known by the provider

Abuse

Abuse includes any practice that is not consistent with the goals of providing patients with services that

- Are medically necessary
- Meet professionally recognized standards
- Are fairly priced

Examples of actions that will likely be considered abusive are

- Charging in excess for services or supplies
- Billing Medicare or Medicaid based on a higher fee schedule than for other patients
- Providing medically unnecessary services
- Submitting bills to Medicare or Medicaid that are the responsibility of another insurance plan
- Waiving co-payments or deductibles (except as permitted for financial hardship)
- Advertising for free services
- Coding all visits at the same level
- Unbundling claims (ie, billing separately for services that are correctly billed under 1 code)
- Billing claims under the wrong NPI

Kickbacks, Inducements, and Self-referrals

Business arrangements in which physician practices refer business to an outside entity (eg, hospitals, hospices, nursing facilities, home health agencies, durable medical equipment suppliers, vendors) should be on a fair market value basis. Whenever a physician practice intends to enter a business arrangement that involves making referrals, legal counsel familiar with anti-kickback and physician self-referral laws should review the arrangement.

Risk areas that may need to be addressed in policies and procedures include

- Offering inappropriate inducements to patients (eg, waiving coinsurance or deductible amounts without a good-faith determination that the patient is in financial need, failing to make reasonable efforts to collect the cost-sharing amount)
- Financial arrangements with outside entities to which the practice may refer federal health care program business
- Joint ventures with entities supplying goods or services to the physician practice or its patients
- Participation in an accountable care organization and/or compliance in the context of participation in a Medicaid Shared Savings Program
- Consulting contracts or medical directorships
- Laboratory payments based on volume of referred services
- Payments for services already covered by a federal health insurer (double-dipping)
- Office and equipment leases with entities to which the physician refers business
- Soliciting, accepting, or offering any gift or gratuity of more than nominal value to or from those who may benefit from a physician practice referral of federal health care program business

When considering whether to engage in a particular billing practice, enter into a particular business venture, or pursue an employment, consulting, or other personal services relationship, it is prudent to evaluate the arrangement for potential compliance problems. Use experienced health care lawyers to analyze the issues and provide a legal evaluation and risk analysis of the proposed venture, relationship, or arrangement.

> The state bar association may have a directory of local attorneys who practice in the health care field. The American Health Law Association is another resource (https://www.americanhealthlaw.org).

Evolving Safe Harbors and Exceptions

Rules proposed by the Office of Inspector General (OIG) and Centers for Medicare & Medicaid Services (CMS) in fall 2019 would add new safe harbors and exceptions to support value-based care arrangements and cybersecurity. Final rules were not yet available at the time of publication. Please consult a health lawyer for specific advice on business arrangements that may be affected.

Anti-fraud and Anti-abuse Activities

The battle against health care fraud and abuse is being waged on many fronts, including the federal and state levels of government as well as private payers. Increasingly, these groups are sharing information. This means that a provider under investigation by 1 government health care program will likely be contacted by another program and possibly by private payers.

- The US Department of Health and Human Services (HHS) OIG has several anti-fraud campaigns underway.
- Many states have enacted anti-fraud and anti-abuse legislation, and state Medicaid programs have established Medicaid fraud control units.
- The Patient Protection and Affordable Care Act (PPACA) introduced new Medicaid program integrity provisions, such as
  - Increased fraud detection methods
  - Terminating providers previously terminated from other government health care programs
  - Suspending future payments based on credible allegations of fraud
  - Adopting the National Correct Coding Initiative edits

> See Chapter 2 for more information on coding edits.

This all means that the momentum and resources for rooting out fraud and abuse at the federal and state levels have intensified. Physician practices are subject to several levels of scrutiny for possible fraudulent activity.

In addition, Medicaid auditors have a financial incentive to find fraud. The Medicaid Recovery Audit Contractors (RAC) program allows states to hire private contractors to audit Medicaid payments and keep a percentage of what they collect. Because it is Medicaid, pediatricians may be included in RAC audits.

- Contingency fees for these contractors vary by state and range from 5.25% to 17%, with most between 9% and 13%.
- Under some circumstances, there can be bonuses paid that increase these fees to more than 20%.
- The RAC program was established in provisions of the PPACA and modeled on a similar successful Medicare program.
- So far, the Medicare and Medicaid RAC programs have gone after larger organizations, but it is not inconceivable that they will eventually turn their attention to physician practices.

It is always better to be prepared. Information on the status of state Medicaid RAC programs is available through the CMS Medicaid website, www.medicaid.gov. This site includes the name and contact information for each state's RAC and medical directors as well as information on the look-back period for audits.

Areas of Specific Concern

Many findings and initiatives put physician practices under high scrutiny for miscoded services, failure to adequately document services, and operating in a manner that conflicts with anti-kickback and self-referral laws. Examples of audit and evaluation findings include

- Specific areas of concern that affect physicians include billing for a higher level of service than was provided, billing for services by clinical staff that do not meet incident-to provisions, and physician self-referral violations.
- Several cases in recent years involved inappropriate payments or other incentives paid by laboratory companies to physicians for sending business to their laboratories.
- Analysis of claims data is increasingly combined across payers and care settings to identify physicians and other providers who are outliers in their billing and referral patterns to identify potential fraud and abuse.

The fraud and abuse control units of HHS and the US Department of Justice also continue to cross-reference enrollment information for the physicians and providers when there is history of enrollment in multiple states and/or programs. By cross-referencing enrollment data, conflicting information and/or evidence of prior revocation of eligibility to participate in federal programs may be discovered.

Compliance Programs

Does your practice have a fraud and abuse prevention compliance program? For many years, compliance programs for small practices were voluntary. This is no longer the case; they are now required, even for small practices, but they can be scalable.

A compliance program establishes strategies to prevent, detect, and resolve conduct that does not conform to

- Federal and state law
- Federal, state, and private payer health care program requirements
- The practice's own ethical and business policies

Pediatric practices benefit from having compliance initiatives because they tighten billing and coding operations and documentation. Practices with written compliance programs report having better control on internal procedures, improved medical record documentation, and streamlined practice operations.

Section 6401(a) of the PPACA requires physicians and other providers and suppliers who enroll in Medicare, Medicaid, or the Children's Health Insurance Program to establish a compliance program with certain "core elements."

The 7 Elements of the Office of Inspector General Compliance Program

The 7 core elements described in the OIG guidance for compliance programs for small physician practices published in 2000 are

- Conduct internal monitoring and auditing.
- Implement written compliance and practice standards.
- Designate a compliance officer, contact, or committee.
- Conduct appropriate training and education.
- Respond appropriately to detected offenses and develop corrective action.
- Develop open lines of communication.
- Enforce disciplinary standards through well-publicized guidelines.

It is also useful to consult the *United States Sentencing Commission Guidelines Manual,* which makes it clear that an organization under investigation may be given more sympathetic treatment if a good compliance program is in place. Compliance programs not only help to prevent fraudulent or erroneous claims, but they also show that the physician practice is making a good-faith effort to submit claims appropriately. However, that would require the program to be integrated into the daily operations of the practice. It cannot be a set of policies and procedures merely kept in a binder or on a computer unrelated to actual business operations.

Here are some reasons cited by the *United States Sentencing Commission Guidelines Manual* to implement an effective compliance program.

- It may save the practice money if it prevents costly civil suits and criminal investigations.
- It sends an unambiguous message to employees that fraud and abuse will not be tolerated.
- It decreases the risk of employees suing the practice under the False Claims Act because employees will have an internal communication system for reporting questionable activities and resolving problems.
- It helps if an investigation occurs. Investigators may be more inclined to resolve the problem as a civil rather than a criminal matter, or it may lead to an administrative resolution rather than a formal false claim action.
- It may help reduce the range used for imposing fines under federal sentencing guidelines.
- It may influence an OIG decision on whether to exclude a provider from participation in federal health care programs.
- It frequently results in improved medical record documentation.
- It improves coding accuracy, reduces denials, and makes claims and payment processes more effective.
- It educates physicians and employees on their responsibilities for preventing, detecting, and reporting fraud and abuse.
- It should meet governmental requirements for practices to have a formal compliance plan.

Steps to Developing a Compliance Program

The CMS has described the steps to create an effective compliance and ethics program. A key aspect is that the organization exercises due diligence to prevent and detect criminal conduct and promotes a culture that encourages ethical conduct and a commitment to compliance with the law.

The CMS specifies that in creating the compliance program, the practice

1. Develop and distribute written policies, procedures, and standards of conduct to prevent and detect inappropriate behavior.
2. Designate a chief compliance officer and other appropriate bodies (eg, a corporate compliance committee) charged with the responsibility of operating and monitoring the compliance program and who report directly to high-level personnel and the governing body.
3. Use reasonable efforts not to include any individual in the substantial authority personnel whom the organization knew, or should have known, has engaged in illegal activities or other conduct inconsistent with an effective compliance and ethics program.
4. Develop and implement regular, effective education and training programs for the governing body; all employees, including high-level personnel; and, as appropriate, the organization's agents.
5. Maintain a process, such as a hotline, to receive complaints and adopt procedures to protect the anonymity of complainants and protect whistleblowers from retaliation. (In a small practice, a hotline could be replaced with an "anonymous fraud report box.")
6. Develop a system to respond to allegations of improper conduct and enforce appropriate disciplinary action against employees who have violated internal compliance policies, applicable statutes, regulations, or federal health care program requirements.
7. Use audits and/or other evaluation techniques to monitor compliance and assist in the reduction of identified problem areas.
8. Investigate and remediate identified systemic problems, including making any necessary modifications to the organization's compliance and ethics program.

Written Policies and Procedures

A compliance program should have written compliance standards and procedures that the practice follows. They should specifically describe the lines of responsibility for implementing the compliance program.

- Standards and procedures should reduce the likelihood of fraudulent activity while also helping to identify any incorrect billing practices.
- Policies and procedures should be updated periodically to address newly identified areas of risk, new regulations, or process changes in the practice.
- All staff should receive periodic education on policies and procedures to maintain up-to-date knowledge.

Coding and Billing

The following billing risk areas have been frequent areas of investigations and audits by the OIG and should be addressed in a good compliance program:

- Billing for items or services not provided or not provided as claimed
- Submitting claims for equipment, medical supplies, and services that are not reasonable and necessary
- Double billing
- Billing for non-covered services as if covered
- Known misuse of NPIs, which results in improper billing
- Billing separately for bundled services
- Misuse of modifiers
- Consistently under-coding or over-coding services
- Using only 1 evaluation and management (E/M) service code within a category of service

  Other areas that may trigger an audit include
- Profile of services reported differs from payer profiles of physicians of your specialty
- Repeated use of unspecified diagnosis codes or use of codes that are not consistent with the service or your specialty
- Surgical services not consistent with claims submitted by a facility
- Number of procedures or services reported exceed the hours in a day
- High numbers of denials

Medical Record Documentation

One of the most important physician practice compliance issues is the appropriate documentation of diagnosis and treatment. Patients and other providers must be able to trust that information within shared records is accurate and actionable for the care of the patient.

With most pediatricians now using electronic health records (EHRs) to document office-based services, compliant documentation must now encompass not only what should be documented but also what must be safeguarded from inaccuracies and potential noncompliant access to or disclosure of information.

The CMS has published guidance for physicians on detecting and responding to fraud, waste, and abuse associated with the use of EHRs (www.cms.gov/Medicare-Medicaid-Coordination/Fraud-Prevention/Medicaid-Integrity-Education/documentation-matters.html). The CMS instructs that physicians should apply the compliance program components previously discussed to take preventive action to deter the inappropriate use of EHR system features or inappropriate access to patient information. This includes a written compliance plan.

The written compliance plan should specify that medical record documentation should comply with the following documentation principles and guidelines:

- The medical record should be complete (and legible, when handwritten) and individualized for each patient encounter.
  - Do not allow cut-and-paste functionality in the EHR. Any use of copy and paste, copy forward, macros, or auto-population should be regulated by office policies that address maintenance of record integrity and supplementation via free text, where indicated.
  - Guidance from the CMS includes a decision table for ensuring proper use of EHR features and capabilities.
- Retain all signatures when there are multiple authors or contributors to a document so that individual contributions are unambiguously identified.
- All staff should receive initial and periodic education on compliant medical record documentation, including, as applicable, use of EHR functionality, use of individual sign-on, and appropriate access to records.
- Documentation should be completed at the time of service or as soon as possible afterward.
- The documentation of each patient encounter should include the reason for the encounter; any relevant history; physical examination findings; prior diagnostic test results, when pertinent; assessment, clinical impression, or diagnosis; plan of care; and date and legible identity of the observer.
- If not documented, the rationale for ordering diagnostic and other ancillary services should be easily inferred by an independent reviewer or third party.
- Past and present diagnoses and history should be accessible to the treating and/or consulting physician.
- Appropriate health risk factors should be identified. The patient's progress, patient's response to and any changes in treatment, and any revision in diagnosis should be documented.
- All pages in the medical record should include the patient name and an identifying number or birth date.
- Prescription drug management should include the name of the medication, dosage, and instructions.
- Clinically important telephone calls should be documented, including date, time, instructions, patient/parent understanding of and agreement with those instructions, and follow-up.

●=New code   ▲=Revised code   #=Re-sequenced code   +=Add-on code

- Anticipatory guidance, patient education, and counseling are best documented when performed.
- Any addenda should be identifiable with the author's signature and labeled with the date the addendum was made. The compliance plan should address what circumstances justify making changes to the EHR and identify who can make changes, requirements for amendments and corrections to an EHR, and what information cannot be changed (ie, author, date, and time of original note).
- Consent forms should be dated, the procedure documented, and the form signed by the patient or his or her legal representative. Documentation should include a summary of the discussion of the procedure and risks.
- All abbreviations used should be explicit.
- Patient noncompliance, including immunization refusal, should be documented as well as discussion of the risks and adverse consequences of noncompliance.
- Allergies and adverse reactions should be prominently displayed.
- Immunization and growth charts must be maintained and current.
- Problem and medication lists should be completed and current, including over-the-counter medications.
- The EHR audit log should always be enabled to ensure it creates an accurate chronological history of changes to the EHR. Practice procedures should describe any exceptions, including who can disable the log and under what circumstances this may be appropriate.

Coding Conundrum: Pitfalls of Electronic Health Record Coding

One advantage of using electronic health records (EHRs) is enhanced documentation of services. Documentation of an evaluation and management (E/M) service may be easier because of the use of templates or drop-down options, and legibility is not an issue. However, there are disadvantages to documenting in an EHR. When completing an audit, be aware of the following:

- Templates may not accurately describe pertinent patient history or abnormal findings on examination. Some EHRs do not allow free texting, thereby prohibiting more detailed, appropriate documentation. If a system does not allow free texting, work with the vendor to add this capability, or add any and all abnormal findings that might be pertinent in the template so documentation can be complete and accurate.
- Avoid templates and documentation tools that feature predefined text that may include information that is not relevant to the patient presentation and/or services rendered. Review and edit all defaulted data to ensure only patient-specific data are recorded for that visit while removing all other irrelevant data pulled in by the default template.
- Users should be familiar with the way the EHR constructs a note from the data entered into each field and how the system may be customized to enhance the final note.
- Only the history and physical examination that are pertinent to the problem or condition should be used in selection of an E/M code. Therefore, physicians should code each E/M service and override the EHR-assigned E/M code when appropriate.
- The EHR will usually capture all documentation, whether performed by ancillary staff or the provider. Make certain it is clear who documented each portion of a service. For example, if history of present illness (HPI) is documented by a nurse or medical assistant, the physician must document his or her agreement and any additional relevant history. (Electronic health record systems include audit trails that may be used to prove who entered specific elements of documentation. It is important to understand how the practice's EHR system creates and produces an audit trail.)
- The use of a scribe to enter information relayed by a physician or provider must be clearly entered in each record, when applicable. Most payers require identification of the scribe that includes a statement such as "acting as a scribe for Dr X." The physician or provider must review the note for accuracy and cosign indicating his or her words and actions were accurately recorded.
- If an EHR system automatically transfers the documented review of systems (ROS) and past, family, and social history from one encounter to the next or lists every medication that has been prescribed in the past, make certain the physician reviews the information to verify it is still accurate and documents his or her review of the pertinent copied information to support the level of history that was necessary and performed.
- The same information may be documented in the HPI and ROS (eg, HPI, "fever of 102°F"; ROS, "fever"). The repeated comment should only be used as HPI or ROS, not both, based on the context for which it was obtained (eg, description of problem, question to better define problem). The EHR system may not differentiate and will count the redundant information twice (or more), leading to a higher level of history.
- Most EHR systems have integrated an E/M coding system using standard guidance from *Current Procedural Terminology* or the Centers for Medicare & Medicaid Services, depending on the code set you are using. However, it is always important to verify the codes automatically selected are appropriate.
- If previous diagnoses are carried over from one encounter to the next, make sure only those that are pertinent to the current visit are considered when determining the complexity of the service provided.
- List the primary diagnosis first because the EHR may report the diagnoses in the order in which they are documented.
- To support management options, it may be necessary to document the diagnoses being considered. These suspected or ruled-out diagnoses should not be reported by the EHR system in the outpatient setting.
- Make certain that any separately reportable procedure or service has documentation to support that it was performed.
- Do not depend on the software vendor to add codes to the system. Review all new, deleted, and revised codes each year. Notify the vendor if codes have not been revised and educate physicians and billing staff on their appropriate use.

Retention of Records

Policies and procedures should be written to include the creation, distribution, retention, and destruction of documents. In designing a record-retention system, privacy concerns and federal and state regulatory requirements should be taken into consideration. In addition to maintaining appropriate and thorough medical records on each patient, the OIG recommends that the system include the following types of documents:

- All records and documentation (eg, billing and claims documentation) required for participation in federal, state, and private-payer health care programs
- All records necessary to demonstrate the integrity of the physician practice's compliance process and to confirm the effectiveness of the program

The following record-retention guidelines should be used:

- The length of time that a physician's medical record documentation is to be retained should be specified. Federal and state statutes should be consulted for specific time frames.
- Consulting with an attorney or risk management department of a medical liability insurer is prudent to determine the appropriate retention period.
  - At a minimum, pediatricians may want to retain records until patients obtain the age of majority plus the statute of limitations in their jurisdiction.
  - Longer retention periods may be prudent, depending on the circumstances.
- Medical records, including electronic correspondence, should be secured against loss, destruction, unauthorized access, unauthorized reproduction, corruption, and damage.
- Policies and procedures should stipulate the disposition of medical records in the event the practice is sold or closed.

The American Academy of Pediatrics (AAP) provides free Health Insurance Portability and Accountability Act of 1996 (HIPAA) privacy and security manuals with downloadable templates, policies, and procedures at www.aap.org/en-us/professional-resources/practice-transformation/managing-practice/Pages/HIPAA-Privacy-and-Security-Compliance-Manuals.aspx.

Document Advice From Payers

A physician practice should document its efforts to comply with applicable federal, state, and private health care program requirements. For example

- When requesting advice from a government agency charged with administering a federal or state health care program or from a private payer, document and retain a record of the request and of all written or oral responses.
- Maintain a log of oral inquiries between the practice and third parties.
- Keep copies of all provider manuals, provider bulletins, and communications from payers about coding and submission of claims.

Designate a Compliance Officer

To administer the compliance program, the practice should designate an individual responsible for overseeing the program. More than one employee may be designated with the responsibility of compliance monitoring, or a practice may outsource all or part of the functions of a compliance officer to a third party. Attributes and qualifications of a compliance officer include

- Independent position to protect against any conflicts of interest from "regular" position responsibilities and compliance officer duties
- Attention to detail
- Experience in billing and coding
- Effective communication skills (oral and written) with employees, physicians, and carriers

The primary responsibilities of a compliance officer include

- Overseeing and monitoring the implementation of the compliance program.
- Establishing methods, such as periodic audits, to improve the practice's efficiency and quality of services and reduce the practice's vulnerability to fraud and abuse.
- Revising the compliance program in response to changes in the needs of the practice or changes in the law and in the policies and procedures of government and private payer health plans.
- Developing, coordinating, and participating in a training program that focuses on the elements of the compliance program and seeks to ensure that training materials are appropriate.

●=New code   ▲=Revised code   #=Re-sequenced code   +=Add-on code

Chapter 5. Preventing Fraud and Abuse: Compliance, Audits, and Paybacks

- Checking the HHS OIG List of Excluded Individuals and Entities and the federal System for Award Management to ascertain whether any potential new hires, current employees, medical staff, or independent contractors are listed; advising management of findings; and seeing that appropriate action is taken as described in the compliance program.
- Informing employees and physicians of pertinent federal and state statutes, regulations, and standards and monitoring their compliance.
- Investigating any report or allegation concerning suspected unethical or improper business practices and monitoring subsequent corrective action, compliance, or both.
- Assessing the practice's situation and determining what best suits the practice in terms of compliance oversight.
- Maintaining records of compliance-related activities, including meetings, educational activities, and internal audits. Particular attention should be given to documenting violations found by the compliance program and documenting the remedial actions.

The Audit/Review Process

1. Obtain and review a productivity report from your billing system.
2. Calculate the percentage distribution of E/M codes within each category of service (new and established office or outpatient visits, initial observation or inpatient services, use of modifier **25**) for each physician in the practice. (Most billing software provides these calculations.) You might also use the AAP Coding Calculator (www.aap.org/ en-us/professional-resources/practice-transformation/getting-paid/Coding-at-the-AAP/Pages/Coding-Calculator.aspx) to help you profile your E/M code use and distribution.
3. Use data from a 12-month period to include seasonal trends and better reflect practice patterns.
4. Perform a comparative analysis of the distribution with each physician in the practice. Remember that data only reflect the billing patterns and not if one is more correct than another. More frequent oversight and monitoring is necessary for services provided by physicians who are new to the practice and may use documentation or coding guidance that conflicts with practice policy.
5. Review the report to ensure that all procedures performed are being captured and reported appropriately. For example, are discharge visits (**99238** and **99239**) being billed and is the number proportionate to the number of newborn and other hospital admissions performed?
6. Review the practice encounter form or code selection application to ensure that *Current Procedural Terminology* (*CPT*®) and *International Classification of Diseases, 10th Revision, Clinical Modification* (*ICD-10-CM*) codes are correct and match the corresponding description.
7. Review the actual encounter and claim form with the medical record to ensure the claim is submitted with the appropriate codes and/or modifiers. (See the Documentation and Coding Audits section later in this chapter.)
8. Review each medical record and encounter form (as applicable) with the following questions in mind:
   - Are the patient's name, identification number, and/or date of birth on every page in the medical record?
   - Does the medical record contain updated demographic information?
   - Are allergies noted and prominently displayed?
   - Is the date of service documented?
   - Was the service medically necessary?
   - Does the documentation support the level of E/M service based on the code descriptor and/or type of service (eg, consultation, preventive medicine service)?
   - Are all the services and/or procedures documented/captured on the encounter form?
   - Does the documentation for the preventive medicine visit meet the requirements of the Medicaid Early and Periodic Screening, Diagnostic, and Treatment program when applicable?
   - Does the documentation support the procedure billed (eg, administration of injection, catheterization, impacted cerumen removal)?
   - Does the documentation support the diagnosis code(s) billed?
   - If using an EHR, does the documentation support physician review and personal documentation? For example, if the EHR always brings up the patient's history, is there a notation that the physician reviewed it? If not, it should not be counted as part of the service.
   - Is there a completed growth chart and immunization record?
   - Is the documentation legible?
   - Does any order for medication include the specific dosage and use?
   - Is there documentation of a follow-up plan?
   - Are diagnostic reports (eg, laboratory tests, radiograph) signed and dated to reflect review?

●=New code   ▲=Revised code   #=Re-sequenced code   +=Add-on code

- Does documentation include the name and credentials of each contributing author in a manner that reflects each author's individual contributions?
- Was an appropriate modifier reported with sufficient documentation?
- Is the documentation in compliance with Physicians at Teaching Hospitals guidelines and/or incident-to provisions as appropriate?

Documentation and Coding Audits

Medicare, state Medicaid programs, and commercial payers will audit claims as well as monitor E/M coding profiles. While the specialty-specific E/M profiles published by the CMS provide helpful information, keep in mind that these distributions only reflect code use and not code accuracy. An atypical code distribution may be the result of care for a more complex patient population than average (eg, patients with chronic diseases or with social and economic challenges). Correct coding appropriately identifies the risk stratification for your patients and may directly affect your payments.

Also, just because you got paid does not mean that payers will not retrospectively audit and demand repayment or withhold future payments, particularly if claims were processed incorrectly or in error according to your contract. Practices are advised to become familiar with state laws addressing retrospective audits and repayments and with payer procedures for repayment. Your AAP chapter or state medical society may be able to help you understand your state-specific laws.

Preparing for the Audit

Before using documentation and coding audits to reduce the practice's vulnerability to fraud and abuse, it is important to consider how your practice can best conduct and use findings of an internal audit. Individual practices must consider how to conduct audits in a manner that offers the most benefit and least disruption to the practice. **Figure 5-1** offers steps to consider when developing a chart audit process.

Performing the Audit

Make certain that the reviewer has all appropriate and necessary tools, which may include
- The CMS *Documentation Guidelines for Evaluation and Management Services* (1995 and/or 1997) that are used by the practice or physician.

> Use *Current Procedural Terminology* documentation and code selection guidelines in lieu of 1995 or 1997 when reviewing office and other outpatient evaluation and management services (99202–99215) with dates of service on and after January 1, 2021. See Chapter 7 for more information.

- Current *CPT, ICD-10-CM,* and Healthcare Common Procedure Coding System manuals.
- Access to or copies of all payer newsletters or information bulletins that outline coding and/or payment policies.
- An audit worksheet. This may be one designed by your practice, or one of many published templates may be used. Note that the CMS has never endorsed any specific audit form or coding template. Make certain the audit form used includes appropriate requirements for selection of an E/M service.
- A general documentation checklist of elements of documentation applicable to all records (eg, having patient identification, date, and page numbers on each page of a record), which can help with identification of missing nonclinical documentation and record authentication (see **Table 5-1**; a printable version can be found online at www.aap.org/cfp [use access code AAPCFP26]).
- A log to document findings for each provider (**Table 5-2**). This log should include a summary detail of findings for each encounter reviewed. The log and E/M audit worksheets can be used as teaching tools at the conclusion of the audit.
- Audit summary reporting forms—results by individual provider with encounter details (eg, levels of history, examination, and medical decision-making assigned versus audit finding); results by individual with codes and variances (eg, level of service and/or relative value unit variances); and report of key findings (eg, practice accuracy rates; strengths; areas of concern, including historical comparisons; recommendations for correction/improvement).

Figure 5-1. Preparing and Planning Medical Chart Audits

Focus
Focus audits on documentation and coding of the most commonly performed services, adherence to medical record standards, appropriate reporting of diagnosis codes, use of modifiers, and adherence to coding and federal guidelines (eg, Physicians at Teaching Hospitals guidelines, physician self-referral laws).

Agree
Make certain all physicians in the practice are in agreement with how any audit will be conducted and how results will be used.

Auditor
The auditor (eg, physician, physician extender, coder or other administrative employee, outside consultant, a combination thereof) must be proficient at coding, understand payer guidelines and requirements, and know medical terminology. Consider a team approach (eg, nurse and coder). If a physician is not actually performing record reviews, one should be available to assist as necessary.

Legal
• Determine if audits should be performed under the direction of a health care attorney who may offer assistance with developing an audit process and provide guidance on any internal compliance concerns discovered in the process.
• Attorney–client privilege may apply when audits are directed by an attorney.

Timing
• Determine if your audit will be retrospective (ie, performed on paid claims and services) or prospective (ie, performed on services and claims that have not yet been billed).
• Prospective reviews are recommended because any necessary corrections can be made before a claim is filed. Although a prospective review will delay claims submission and introduce additional practice expense, this practice may have a net positive financial effect.

Services
• Select the types of services to be included in the audit. For example, if the review will include only office or outpatient services, include services most frequently reported (eg, a sampling of new and established patient problem-oriented and preventive medicine visits, documentation of nebulizer treatments).
• Include newborn care, critical care, initial and subsequent observation, and inpatient services when performing an audit of inpatient services.

Number
Determine how many records or encounters will be included in the audit. Most coding consultants recommend at least 10 records per physician or provider per baseline or subsequent review (may be less for part-time providers). If a more focused review is required, the sample size may need to be increased. Medical records should be randomly selected for each evaluation and management level of service and from different dates of service.

Schedule
Determine the frequency of audits. Large practices might consider conducting audits on a rotating schedule of 1 physician or provider per week or 1 physician or provider per month throughout the year.

Table 5-1. General Documentation Checklist	
Applicable to All Records (1 = completed, 0 = incomplete/unsatisfactory)	**Points**
Documentation was readily available.	
All pertinent information was included/accessible (eg, orders, test results).	
Patient identification on each page of record	
Date of service on each page of record	
Page numbers are provided for each episode of care.	
Demographics were updated/verified to be correct.	
HIPAA notice provided	
Insurance verification on file	
Provider identification is distinct for each record entry (eg, ancillary staff and physician notes).	
Corrections and addendums are clearly identified and appropriate.	
Signature/electronic authentication is complete and timely (per practice or payer specification).	
Total	
General documentation recommendations:	
Abbreviation: HIPAA, Health Insurance Portability and Accountability Act of 1996.	

Table 5-2. Sample Audit Log[a]					
Physician:		**Date:**		**Auditor:**	
Patient Name	**Patient ID/ DOB**	**Date of Service**	**Reported Code**	**Audited Code**	**Comments**
Jane	5/1/15	6/3/21	99214	99213	Total physician time not documented; medical decision-making = **99213**; history carried forward conflicts with current history of present illness
			J30.89; J34.89	J30.89	Rhinorrhea (**J34.89**) is inherent to perennial allergic rhinitis (**J30.89**).
Zach	2/4/16	6/4/21	69210	0	Cerumen not documented as impacted
Gracie	11/12/13	6/4/21	99212	99202	Patient was last seen 4 years ago by pediatrician in same group practice. Patient is new.

Abbreviations: DOB, date of birth; ID, identification.

[a] Also available at www.aap.org/cfp; use access code AAPCFP26.

Following the Audit

- Discuss audit findings with each provider.
- Educate providers and staff as necessary.
- If a problem is encountered (eg, inappropriate use of modifiers, miscoding), a more focused retrospective review should be conducted to determine how long the error has been occurring and its effect. This is especially important when reviewing claims for physicians new to the practice or when a particular coding guideline or code has changed.

Chapter 5. Preventing Fraud and Abuse: Compliance, Audits, and Paybacks

- If overpayments have occurred due to miscoding or billing errors, the errors should be corrected and education of appropriate staff performed. The errors may need to be disclosed and incorrect payments refunded.

  Always refer to payer contracts and agreements to understand their requirements and policies for overpayments and disclosure. Always seek advice from the practice's attorney prior to disclosure or repayment.

- If necessary, document a corrective action plan with deadlines for completion (eg, completion of education, attainment of a specified accuracy rate) and administrative sign-off verifying completion.

- Schedule follow-up audits, if indicated, to determine if problems have been resolved (eg, improved documentation, capturing procedures, correct use of modifiers).

- Determine if audits need to be performed on a quarterly or annual basis and follow through with audits on a routine basis.

- If changes need to be made to the EHR system, contact the vendor and discuss how these might be accomplished. Educate physicians and providers on the changes made or need for additional physician documentation.

- Establish or update written policies and procedures.

- Maintain records of your compliance efforts and training.

- As illustrated in **Figure 5-2**, audits are not one-time events. Depending on your practice's resources for conducting audits and education, your practice may choose to conduct small audits monthly (eg, 5 charts per provider), larger audits quarterly (eg, 10 charts per provider), or continuous prospective audit of a small number of charts weekly. There may be a period of trial and error to find what works best for your practice.

Figure 5-2. Audit Cycle

Plan an audit. → Conduct audit. → Report findings. → Educate and correct. → Document audit and corrective actions.

Do Not Get Caught Without a Plan

Most practices will never have to deal with demands for paybacks or fraud audits. Nevertheless, all practices should have a plan just in case they occur. Because time is of the essence in responding to these communications, it would be a calamity to have a letter sit on someone's desk while precious days tick away. Often, a response must be received within 30 days of the date of the request, and the paperwork demanded is not insignificant.

The first communication may be a request for repayment based on payer software analysis of claims history to detect claims paid in conflict with payment policies. It is important for all staff to be trained to recognize these requests and know to get them to the compliance officer immediately. Then, qualified staff tasked with receiving all requests for paybacks can determine the veracity of the request and, if inaccurate, act in accordance with the payer's rebuttal and appeal processes in a timely manner. Likewise, requests for records must be handled carefully and expeditiously.

Responding to Repayment Demands

In an effort to control costs and stamp out fraud, carrier claims processing and special investigative units use sophisticated software programs to identify providers with atypical coding patterns that could indicate erroneous coding and potential overpayments. For example, some carriers may flag providers considered outliers in frequently reporting high-level E/M codes or frequent use of modifiers. They then extrapolate the alleged overpayments over several years and demand across-the-board repayments. Worse, carriers will reduce payments on future claims to correct alleged overpayments on past claims. These requests require a swift and skilled response. Usually, several thousand dollars are involved. Given the compressed timeline and dollars at stake, seeking legal advice is invaluable in these situations.

Here is some general guidance for your consideration.

- If it is truly due to a billing error by the practice, take action to correct the problem and demonstrate to the carrier how it has or will be corrected and the measures implemented to avoid the problem in the future.

- Reply in writing to inform the carrier you are willing to work with it and ask that it identify each of the claims in question as well as the specific criteria or standards it is applying to the audit.

- Make sure the practice and the carrier consistently apply current *CPT* guidelines. Reference *CPT* coding guidelines and have appropriate documentation for support. The AAP Coding Hotline can be a resource to you as well (https://form.jotform.com/Subspecialty/aapcodinghotline).

- Review your carrier contract's clauses on audits and dispute resolution as well as applicable state laws on audits and repayments with your attorney.
- Focus any overpayment recovery efforts on a case-by-case basis. Avoid unilateral take-backs by not allowing the carrier to extrapolate repayments on any or all future claims.
- Have the carrier provide documentation as proof of overpayment for each contested claim.
- Obtain and secure written documentation of all contacts with the carrier on this issue. Should a carrier payment policy require reporting that varies from *CPT* guidelines, obtain written, dated documentation from the carrier to verify that is the case. Keep this documentation permanently.
- Use legal counsel skilled in carrier contracting when negotiating contracts and confronted with repayment demands.

The AAP Payer Advocacy Advisory Committee has a resource for AAP members on responding to retrospective audit and carrier take-back. To access it, go to www.aap.org/cfp (use access code AAPCFP26).

What if Your Practice Is Audited?

- Contact legal counsel as soon as possible. Make sure the attorney or legal practice has experience with audits. If it is a Medicaid audit, it is preferable to have an attorney with Medicaid audit experience. An audit is a complex legal process with significant consequences. It is unwise to attempt to maneuver through this process without sound legal advice.
- Designate 1 physician or staff member to serve as the primary contact with the attorney and auditors. However, keep in mind that all physicians and staff members may need to work with auditors to some extent.
- Request that the auditor provide you with an opening and closing conference. At the initial meeting, ask for the individual's credentials and job title and ask him or her to summarize the purpose of the review or audit.
- Know how far back auditors may conduct reviews, the number of records a contractor may request, the amount of time allowed to respond to each request, any rebuttal process in place, and steps necessary to appeal adverse findings.
- If the time requirements for producing copies or gathering medical records are unmanageable, contact the auditing entity and request an extension in writing. Provide a clear justification for the extension request.
- Keep copies of all written communication (eg, letters, directives, memos, emails). Keep the postmarked envelopes of all letters, including the original notice.
- Fully document all verbal communication, including time, date, persons involved, substance of the discussion, and conclusions and agreements.
- In response to requests for information, provide only the information requested and maintain copies of what you provide auditors. Before providing files, remove any information unrelated to the audit. For example, in a Medicaid audit, you could exclude information related to services provided when the patient was covered under a commercial plan or was uninsured.
- Do not alter any documents or medical records.
- Respond only to questions from the auditors; do not try to engage them in any conversations. If the auditors are conducting the review in your office, try to place them in a separate office away from patients, staff, and business operations.
- Be prepared to respond promptly to each request received. Keep a log of requests received by date, response due date, requesting party, any communication with the requestor, date of response, and outcome.
- Know HIPAA privacy regulations, documentation principles, coding guidelines, and payment policies, and verify that all supporting documentation is included in each response.
- If legibility of the record is questionable, include a transcribed copy with attestation by the author of the original document stating that the transcription is accurate and provided to ensure legibility. Any unsigned entry should also be accompanied by a separate attestation by its author.
- Copied or scanned medical records should be carefully reviewed to be sure that all pages were legibly copied (front and back, if applicable) and are straight and within the margins on the page.
- Any questions about the sufficiency of medical record documentation should be addressed with the physician or provider who ordered or documented the service prior to responding to the request for records.
  - Any corrections to an entry should be performed in a manner that maintains legibility of the original content (eg, single-line strike-through) and should be signed and dated.
  - A summary of the service provided may be included to provide more information but should be distinctly labeled as such and not as part of the original record.
- Include any policy or correspondence from the payer that was used to guide your billing and coding practices related to the service. (Archived payer manuals supportive of claims from previous years may be available on state Medicaid websites.) Clinical practice guidelines, policy statements, textbooks, and manuals may also be supportive of medical necessity.
- Send records in a manner that allows for confirmation of receipt.

- Secure a copy of auditors' contact information in case you need to follow up.
- Obtain, in writing, the expected date of a written summary of findings.

Can This Really Happen?

Conventional wisdom says that auditors will probably go after big organizations when it comes to investigating fraud and abuse, but the OIG has said repeatedly that it has zero tolerance for fraud, so, technically, everyone is at risk. Because most of the software programs used to detect unusual coding and billing patterns are based on adult services, pediatricians may be identified as outliers. As a result, valid pediatric coding may be tagged as improper and honest providers may have to respond to inappropriate recoupment requests or audits. The AAP works hard to minimize these problems and help chapters respond when state Medicaid programs target pediatric coding as inappropriate. This is an ongoing challenge.

Unfortunately, there are instances of fraud involving pediatricians. A review of past OIG reports to Congress and press releases revealed the following cases:

- A New Jersey pediatrician was found guilty of 48 counts of health care claims fraud and 1 count of Medicaid fraud for billing for more than 24 hours of services per day on 48 days despite her office being open only 3 days per week for 8 hours per day. The pediatrician was sentenced to 3 years in prison.
- A Tennessee pediatrician pleaded guilty to fraud for knowingly up-coding and billing for services that his practice had no equipment to provide. As a result, he was excluded from participating in federal health care programs for 20 years.
- A Pennsylvania pediatrician pleaded guilty to charges of health care fraud, mail fraud, and forfeiture. The pediatrician was sentenced to 8 years' incarceration and ordered to pay $7 million in restitution for submitting fraudulent claims to Medicaid, TRICARE, and private insurance companies for services not rendered.
- A Connecticut pediatrician pleaded guilty to charges of health care fraud for billing Medicaid and other insurance programs for childhood vaccines received free of charge from the joint federal/state Vaccines for Children program.
- A New York pediatrician was jailed for 37 months and fined $75,000 dollars for accepting bribes for laboratory test referrals. This was part of a $100 million fraud scheme in which 22 physician defendants have pleaded guilty.

Explore the Need for Additional Insurance

Many medical liability insurers and insurance brokers offer products to provide additional coverage for the consequences of billing errors and omissions. Pediatric practices may want to contact their insurers to see whether their current medical liability policies cover any of the following problems. If they do not, it might be worthwhile to explore insurance options for obtaining that additional protection.

- Defense coverage for a Medicaid audit
- Qui tam action (False Claims Act)
- Unintentional billing errors and omissions
- Physician Self-Referral Law (Stark) violations
- Unintentional release of medical or financial data
- Breach of computers or network security
- Data recovery
- HIPAA fines or investigation costs

Summary

These are interesting times for pediatric practices and require thoughtful preparation and ongoing concern. Learn about the fraud and abuse enforcement climate in your state. Implement an effective compliance program and follow it. Be sure your staff knows what a demand for repayment or audit notice looks like and what they need to do with it just on the off chance that something should happen. Have a response plan in place should an auditor knock on your door or a recoupment letter come in the mail. Consult with an attorney when needed. Think about the need for insurance for billing errors and omissions. Keep current with coding and billing updates.

Resources

AAP Coding Calculator

www.aap.org/en-us/professional-resources/practice-transformation/getting-paid/Coding-at-the-AAP/Pages/Coding-Calculator.aspx

Documentation

Program Integrity: Documentation Matters Toolkit (www.cms.gov/Medicare-Medicaid-Coordination/Fraud-Prevention/Medicaid-Integrity-Education/documentation-matters.html)

"What Does Your EHR Documentation Say?" March 2017 *AAP Pediatric Coding Newsletter*™ (https://coding.solutions.aap.org/article.aspx?articleid=2606145; subscription required)

Health Insurance Portability and Accountability Act

AAP HIPAA privacy and security compliance manuals (www.aap.org/en-us/professional-resources/practice-transformation/managing-practice/Pages/HIPAA-Privacy-and-Security-Compliance-Manuals.aspx; member log-in required)

Legal Advice

American Health Law Association (https://www.americanhealthlaw.org)

Payer Audits

Payer Contract Negotiations and Payment Resources (www.aap.org/en-us/professional-resources/practice-transformation/getting-paid/Pages/payer-contract-negotiations-and-payment-resources.aspx; access code AAPCFP26)

Medicaid RAC program (www.medicaid.gov)

Test Your Knowledge!

1. **Which of the following is an example of potential abuse?**
   a. Coding all services at the same level
   b. Taking a kickback in money, in-kind, or other valuable compensation for referrals
   c. Billing 1 member for services provided to another (non-covered) member
   d. Billing for services not provided

2. **Which of the following is recommended in a practice's record retention policy?**
   a. Privacy concerns and federal and state regulatory requirements
   b. Record retention as recommended by the electronic health record vendor
   c. Retention of records does not require a policy.
   d. State that records may never be destroyed.

3. **Which of the following is a desired attribute or qualification of a compliance officer?**
   a. Must be a physician or other qualified health care professional
   b. Puts practice profitability above all other concerns
   c. Uses a compliance program developed to hide any compliance concerns
   d. Experience in billing and coding

4. **Which of the following is a recommended first step if your practice is audited?**
   a. Cancel your contract with the payer who is auditing your practice.
   b. Review documentation and alter to meet the payer's requirements.
   c. Call and argue your case with the auditor.
   d. Contact legal counsel as soon as possible.

Evaluation and Management Documentation Guidelines Other Than Office and Other Outpatient Services

Contents

Evaluation and Management (E/M) Documentation and Coding Guidelines

This chapter outlines the evaluation and management (E/M) guidelines for all E/M services *except* office and other outpatient E/M services (office E/M, **99202–99205, 99211–99215**). *Current Procedural Terminology* (*CPT*®) introduces a distinct set of guidelines in 2021 that apply only to codes **99202–99205** and **99211–99215**. Please see **Chapter 7** for guidelines for code selection and documentation of office E/M services.

For all E/M services other than office E/M services, 3 versions of E/M documentation guidelines exist, including *CPT* and the 1995 and 1997 guidelines published by the Centers for Medicare & Medicaid Services (CMS). Most Medicaid and private payers allow use of either the 1995 or 1997 CMS guidelines in E/M code selection but include elements of the *CPT* guidelines for E/M services (eg, guidelines for distinguishing between new and established patients).

> **Separate Guidelines for Office Visits**
>
> Please see Chapter 7 for distinct documentation guidelines applicable only to office and other outpatient evaluation and management services (99202–99205, 99211–99215). Codes for these services are selected based on the level of medical decision-making alone or the physician's or other qualified health care professional's total time on the date of service with no rule regarding the amount of time spent in counseling and/or coordination of care.

Current Procedural Terminology Guidelines

- The vaguest of all guidelines; defines the components of E/M services and provides general guidance on selecting levels of history, examination, and medical decision-making (MDM) or code selection based on time.
- Includes specialty-specific clinical examples in Appendix C of the American Medical Association *CPT 2021*.
- Provides expanded guidelines for topics such as distinguishing new patients from established patients, use of time in E/M code selection, and distinguishing between physicians and other qualified health care professionals (QHPs) and clinical staff.

> American Medical Association clinical examples are only examples and should not be used as a basis for coding patient encounters with the same diagnosis because the selection of a code must be based on the medically necessary services performed and documented and may include clinical variations.

Centers for Medicare & Medicaid Services *Documentation Guidelines for Evaluation and Management Services*

- Two sets of guidelines, 1995 and 1997 (see in this chapter or online at www.aap.org/cfp, access code AAPCFP26).
- Followed by the Medicare program, most private payers, and state Medicaid programs.
- Go beyond the *CPT* definitions and guidance for selecting levels of service providing specific documentation guidance. For example
  - The chief complaint (CC), review of systems (ROS), and past, family, and social history (PFSH) may be listed as separate elements of history, or they may be included in the description of history of present illness (HPI).
  - Specific abnormal and relevant negative findings of the examination of the affected or symptomatic body area(s) or organ system(s) should be documented. A notation of "abnormal" without elaboration is insufficient.
- The CMS documentation guidelines were based on the adult population because few children are covered under the Medicare program. However, the 1995 and 1997 guidelines state that a history and/or examination performed on a pediatric patient may vary from the adult standard and yet be appropriate when considering the selection of an E/M code. As noted in the 1997 guidelines, under Section III, Documentation of E/M Services, paragraph 5:

> "These Documentation Guidelines for E/M services reflect the needs of the typical adult population. For certain groups of patients, the recorded information may vary slightly from that described here. Specifically, the medical records of infants, children, adolescents, and pregnant women may have additional or modified information recorded in each history and examination area.

> "As an example, newborn records may include under history of the present illness (HPI) the details of mother's pregnancy, and the infant's status at birth; social history will focus on family structure; family history will focus on congenital anomalies and hereditary disorders in the family. In addition, the content of a pediatric examination will vary with the age and development of the child. Although not specifically defined in these documentation guidelines, these patient group variations on history and examination are appropriate."

- The key difference between the 1995 and 1997 E/M guidelines is the physical examination component.
  - The 1997 guideline includes specific physical examination elements for a general multisystem examination and for single-system examinations (eg, cardiovascular, respiratory, skin).
  - See more in the 1995 Guidelines for Documentation of Examination and 1997 Guidelines for Documentation of Examination sections later in this chapter.

> Pediatric clinical vignettes are presented throughout this manual. These, too, are only examples, and the associated *Current Procedural Terminology* codes should not be used for every patient with the same diagnosis.

Coding E/M Services From a Clinical Perspective

The definitions of the levels of service and requirements for each key component (ie, history, physical examination, and MDM) are ambiguous, and the steps defined in the requirements for selection of the code are not consistent with a physician's approach to addressing and treating an illness or problem. A physician does not enter a room and perform first a history, and then a physical examination, and finally MDM. Rather, the key components of an E/M service are performed in conjunction with one another. The MDM typically supports the level of history and/or physical examination medically necessary and is derived from the following obtained information:

- The documented CC helps to formulate the presenting problem or nature of the patient presentation.
- The level of history obtained and documented is based on the nature of the patient presentation. Concurrently, the physician is forming his or her impression of the problem's severity, possible diagnoses, other factors that require consideration in patient management, and a potential plan of care.
- The level of the performed physical examination is based on the presenting problem(s) and history. From the moment the physician observes the patient and while obtaining the history, the physician simultaneously is starting his or her physical assessment and examination (eg, general appearance). Additional history may be obtained concurrently with the examination. While performing the examination, the physician again is determining the severity or risk, need for diagnostic testing, differential diagnosis(es), and treatment plan.
- The documentation of the history, physical examination, ordered and performed diagnostic studies, assessment, and plan infer and support the complexity of MDM.

Categories of E/M Codes

There are 26 categories of E/M codes (eg, office or outpatient services, consultations, prolonged physician services, newborn care). Specific guidelines for reporting codes within these categories are described in detail in chapters of this manual devoted to E/M services provided in specific settings (eg, office, emergency department) and type of service (eg, critical care).

Many E/M codes require the performance and documentation of key components. Those E/M services that do not require the key components as the basis for code selection include those services that are

- Bundled as a daily care code (eg, pediatric and neonatal critical care)
- Bundled as a period of care (eg, transitional care management)
- Based on specific guidelines (eg, office and other outpatient, normal newborn care, preventive medicine visits)
- Based on time (eg, hourly critical care, discharge services, prolonged service)

E/M Code Components

Key Components

Most E/M services require performance and documentation of 2 or 3 of the key components (ie, history, physical examination, and MDM).

Seven Components Are Considered When Selecting the Level of Evaluation and Management Service Code

Key components: used to select a level of evaluation and management (E/M) service, using all 3 or 2 of 3

1. History
2. Examination
3. Medical decision-making

Contributory factors: may contribute to but are not required for the selection of a code. However, these usually affect the extent of the key components that are performed.

4. Counseling
5. Coordination of care
6. Nature of presenting problem

Explicit component: used to select a level of E/M service when time is the controlling factor

7. Time

Contributory Factors

CPT defines a *presenting problem* as "a disease, condition, illness, injury, symptom, sign, finding, complaint or other reason for encounter, with or without a diagnosis being established at the time of the encounter." This may be better described as patient presentation and may include psychosocial issues or ethical considerations determined by the physician or other QHP to require consideration in patient management. The nature of the patient presentation may be more extensive or different from the patient's CC (eg, adolescent girl states her reason for visit is headaches but also presents with anxiety about possible unwanted pregnancy). The nature of the presenting problem generally determines the level of history and physical examination performed and documented and supports MDM. For example, an infant with high fever and wheezing warrants a more comprehensive history and/or examination to determine the diagnosis or condition than an infant presenting with a diaper rash. This does not mean that all elements of examination, for example, require individual justification.

> The nature of the presenting problem is defined by severity, risk, and probability of functional impairment.

Levels of presenting problems are defined in the Risk of Significant Complications, Morbidity, and/or Mortality section later in this chapter.

Explicit Component: Time

Time shall be used as the key or controlling factor in the selection of some E/M services (those that are assigned a typical time) when more than 50% of the physician face-to-face patient and/or family encounter is spent in counseling and/or coordination of care.

See separate time instructions for services such as office or other outpatient services and critical care services.

> See Chapter 1 for more on time-based billing.

1995 and 1997 Documentation Guidelines for Evaluation and Management Services

It is important to note that history, MDM, and time do not vary between the 1995 and 1997 guidelines. The physical examination element is the only difference.

I.   Introduction

What is documentation and why is it important?

Medical record documentation is required to record pertinent facts, findings, and observations about an individual's health history including past and present illnesses, examinations, tests, treatments, and outcomes. The medical record chronologically documents the care of the patient and is an important element contributing to high-quality care. The medical record facilitates

---

●=New code   ▲=Revised code   #=Re-sequenced code   +=Add-on code

- The ability of the physician and other health care professionals to evaluate and plan the patient's immediate treatment, and to monitor his/her health care over time
- Communication and continuity of care among physicians and other health care professionals involved in the patient's care
- Accurate and timely claims review and payment
- Appropriate utilization review and quality of care evaluations
- Collection of data that may be useful for research and education

An appropriately documented medical record can reduce many of the "hassles" associated with claims processing and may serve as a legal document to verify the care provided, if necessary.

What do payers want and why?

Because payers have a contractual obligation to enrollees, they may require reasonable documentation that services are consistent with the insurance coverage provided. They may request information to validate

- The site of service
- The medical necessity and appropriateness of the diagnostic and/or therapeutic services provided
- That services provided have been accurately reported

II.   General Principles of Medical Record Documentation

The principles of documentation listed below *are applicable to all types of medical and surgical services in all settings*. For E/M services, the nature and amount of physician work and documentation varies by type of service, place of service, and the patient's status. The general principles listed below may be modified to account for these variable circumstances in providing E/M services.

1. The medical record should be complete and legible.
2. The documentation of each patient encounter should include
   - Reason for the encounter and relevant history, physical examination findings, and prior diagnostic test results
   - Assessment, clinical impression, or diagnosis
   - Plan for care
   - Date and legible identity of the observer
3. If not documented, the rationale for ordering diagnostic and other ancillary services should be easily inferred.
4. Past and present diagnoses should be accessible to the treating and/or consulting physician.
5. Appropriate health risk factors should be identified.
6. The patient's progress, response to and changes in treatment, and revision of diagnosis should be documented.
7. The *CPT* and *ICD-10-CM* codes reported on the health insurance claim form or billing statement should be supported by the documentation in the medical record.

III.   Documentation of E/M Services

This publication provides definitions and documentation guidelines for the three key components of E/M services and for visits that consist predominantly of counseling or coordination of care. The three key components—history, examination, and medical decision making—appear in the descriptors for hospital observation services, hospital inpatient services, consultations, emergency department services, nursing facility services, domiciliary care services, and home services. While some of the text of *CPT* has been repeated in this publication, the reader should refer to *CPT* for the complete descriptors for E/M services and instructions for selecting a level of service. **Documentation guidelines are identified by the symbol •DG.**

The descriptors for the levels of E/M services recognize seven components that are used in defining the levels of E/M services. These components are

- History
- Examination
- Medical decision making
- Counseling
- Coordination of care
- Nature of presenting problem
- Time

The first three of these components (ie, history, examination, and medical decision making) are the **key** components in selecting the level of E/M services. An exception to this rule is the case of visits that consist predominantly of counseling or coordination of care; for these services time is the key or controlling factor to qualify for a particular level of E/M service when the service is assigned a typical time.

For certain groups of patients, the recorded information may vary slightly from that described here. Specifically, the medical records of infants, children, adolescents, and pregnant women may have additional or modified information recorded in each history and examination area.

As an example, newborn records may include under history of the present illness (HPI) the details of mother's pregnancy and the infant's status at birth; social history will focus on family structure; family history will focus on congenital anomalies and hereditary disorders in the family. In addition, information on growth and development and/or nutrition will be recorded. Although not specifically defined in these documentation guidelines, these patient group variations on history and examination are appropriate.

A. Documentation of History

While the history requirements for both sets of documentation guidelines are nearly identical, the 1995 History of Present Illness (HPI) section does not state that the status of at least 3 chronic or inactive conditions supports an extended HPI. However, the CMS has published guidance stating that this is allowed.

The levels of E/M services are based on four types of history (problem focused, expanded problem focused, detailed, and comprehensive.) Each type of history includes some or all of the following elements:

- Chief complaint (CC)
- History of present illness (HPI)
- Review of systems (ROS)
- Past, family, and/or social history (PFSH)

The extent of history of present illness; review of systems; and past, family, and/or social history that is obtained and documented is dependent upon clinical judgment and the nature of the presenting problem(s). Refer to **Table 6-1** for further descriptions.

Table 6-2 *shows the progression of the elements required for each type of history. To qualify for a given type of history, all 3 elements in the table must be met. (A CC is indicated at all levels.)*

- **•DG:** *The CC, ROS, and PFSH may be listed as separate elements of history, or they may be included in the description of the history of the present illness.*
- **•DG:** *A ROS and/or a PFSH obtained during an earlier encounter does not need to be rerecorded if there is evidence that the physician reviewed and updated the previous information. This may occur when a physician updates his or her own record or in an institutional setting or group practice where many physicians use a common record. The review and update may be documented by*
  - *Describing any new ROS and/or PFSH information or noting there has been no change in the information*
  - *Noting the date and location of the earlier ROS and/or PFSH*
- **•DG:** *The ROS and/or PFSH may be recorded by ancillary staff or on a form completed by the patient. To document that the physician reviewed the information, there must be a notation supplementing or confirming the information recorded by others. The CMS now allows ancillary staff, patients, and medical students to complete documentation of any portion of the history and examination. Individual payer policies may be consistent with 1995/1997 guidelines.*
- **•DG:** *If the physician is unable to obtain a history from the patient or other source, the record should describe the patient's condition or other circumstance that precludes obtaining a history.*

Definitions and specific documentation guidelines for each of the elements of history are listed below.

Chief Complaint (CC)

The CC is a concise statement describing the symptom, problem, condition, diagnosis, physician-recommended return, or other factor that is the reason for the encounter.

•DG: *The medical record should clearly reflect the chief complaint.*

Examples: Patient is here for follow-up of attention-deficit/hyperactivity disorder following medication initiation 3 weeks ago.

Patient presents for a refill on her asthma medication.

History of Present Illness (HPI)

The HPI is a chronological description of the development of the patient's present illness from the first sign and/or symptom or from the previous encounter to the present. It includes the following elements:

- Location (*right ear, big toe, head, right lower abdomen*)
- Duration (*2 days, since last night, 1 week*)
- Timing (*persistent, occasionally, twice a week, recurrent, daily, 15 minutes after…*)

Table 6-1. The Elements of History

History Components	Description	Elements
Chief complaint (CC)	The stated purpose or reason for the encounter (usually a quote of the patient's or parent's words)	Although not a defined element, a CC is required as part of the history documentation for all levels.
History of present illness (HPI)	Description of the development of the present illness from the onset of the problem or symptom or from the previous encounter to the present; described with 8 specified elements or a summary of the status of 3 or more chronic or inactive conditions	• Location (specific anatomic site) • Duration (period from onset of sign/symptom to present) • Timing (number or frequency of occurrences of sign/symptom within the time that patient has experienced the sign/symptom) • Quality (characterizations of sign/symptom) • Severity (acuteness or intensity of sign/symptom) • Context (circumstances or situation in which sign/symptom occurred) • Modifying factors (effort taken to change the sign/symptom and its effect) • Associated signs and symptoms (other related or additional signs/symptoms) *Alternatively,* Status of each of 3 or more chronic or inactive conditions (stated in 1997 guidelines; allowed under either guideline)
Review of systems (ROS)	A series of questions asked to identify signs or symptoms experienced by the patient and to more clearly define the problem to help in establishing a diagnosis(es) and management options	• Constitutional (eg, fever, weight loss) • Eyes • Ears, nose, mouth, and throat • Cardiovascular • Respiratory • Gastrointestinal • Genitourinary • Musculoskeletal • Integumentary (skin or breast) • Neurologic • Psychiatric • Endocrine • Hematologic/lymphatic • Allergic/immunologic
Past, family, and social history (PFSH)	Review of medical/surgical history Review of medical events in the patient's family that may place a patient at risk Age-appropriate review of activities	Illnesses, injuries, treatments, surgeries, hospitalizations, current medications, allergies, age-appropriate immunization status, age-appropriate feeding or dietary status, pregnancy and birth history (weight, Apgar score), developmental history Health status or cause of death of family members, specific diseases of family members, hereditary disorders in the family Living arrangements; use of drugs, alcohol, and tobacco by patient or caregiver; education level; sexual history; domestic violence; other relevant social factors

Table 6-2. Progression of Elements Required for Each Type of History			
History of Present Illness (HPI)	Review of Systems (ROS)	Past, Family, and/or Social History (PFSH)	Type of History
Brief (1–3 elements)	N/A	N/A	Problem focused
Brief (1–3 elements)	Problem pertinent (at least 1 system)	N/A	Expanded problem focused
Extended (4 elements or status of 3 chronic conditions)	Extended (2–9 systems)	Pertinent (1 item related to patient presentation)	Detailed
Extended (4 elements or status of 3 chronic conditions)	Complete (at least 10 of 14 systems)	Complete[a]	Comprehensive

Abbreviation: N/A, not applicable.

[a] One item from 2 areas required for established patient domiciliary and home visits, subsequent nursing home visits, or emergency department visits. One item from 3 areas required for new patient domiciliary home visits, initial nursing facility visits, observation, initial inpatient hospital visits, consultations, or comprehensive nursing facility assessments.

- Quality (*dull, clear, cloudy, thick, throbbing*)
- Severity (*moderate, pain scale [1–10], low grade, progressive, improving, worsening*)
- Context (*occurred when awoke from nap, while playing soccer, fell from tree*)
- Modifying factors (*took acetaminophen without relief, improved with albuterol treatment*)
- Associated signs and symptoms (*blurred vision with headache, coughing with runny nose, nausea with vomiting*)

Brief and **extended** HPIs are distinguished by the amount of detail needed to accurately characterize the clinical problem(s).

A **brief** HPI consists of one to three elements of the HPI.

•**DG:**   *The medical record should describe one to three elements of the present illness (HPI).*

An **extended** HPI consists of four or more elements of the HPI or the status of at least three chronic or inactive conditions. *(Applies for 1995 and 1997 documentation guidelines.)*

•**DG 1995:** *The medical record should describe four or more elements of the present illness (HPI) or associated co-morbidities. The CMS has stated that the status of at least 3 chronic or inactive conditions also supports an extended HPI for 1995 documentation guidelines.*

•**DG 1997:** *The medical record should describe at least four elements of the present illness (HPI), or the status of at least three chronic or inactive conditions.*

- *Pediatricians must review and confirm the accuracy and completeness of HPI documented by others.*
- *If the HPI summarizes the status of chronic conditions, include information such as current medications and their effects, a description of the patient's present condition (eg, stable intermittent asthma, autism spectrum disorder with improved attention and communication skills), and patient compliance with treatment plans.*

Review of Systems (ROS)

A ROS is an inventory of body systems obtained through a series of questions seeking to identify signs and/or symptoms that the patient may be experiencing or has experienced.

For purposes of ROS, the following systems are recognized:

- Constitutional symptoms (eg, fever, weight loss)
- Eyes
- Ears, nose, mouth, throat
- Cardiovascular
- Respiratory
- Gastrointestinal
- Genitourinary
- Musculoskeletal
- Integumentary (skin and/or breast)

- Neurological
- Psychiatric
- Endocrine
- Hematologic/lymphatic
- Allergic/immunologic

A **problem-pertinent** ROS inquires about the system directly related to the problem(s) identified in the HPI.

•**DG:**   *The patient's positive responses and pertinent negatives for the system related to the problem should be documented.*

An **extended** ROS inquires about the system directly related to the problem(s) identified in the HPI and a limited number of additional systems.

•**DG:**   *The patient's positive responses and pertinent negatives for two to nine systems should be documented.*

A **complete** ROS inquires about the system(s) directly related to the problem(s) identified in the HPI plus all additional body systems.

•**DG:**   *At least 10 organ systems must be reviewed. Those systems with positive or pertinent negative responses must be individually documented. For the remaining systems, a notation indicating all other systems are negative is permissible. In the absence of such a notation, at least 10 systems must be individually documented.*

- *Documentation should clarify any conflicting information between the ROS completed by the patient, family, or ancillary staff and the physician's documentation of the patient presentation (eg, ROS is negative for musculoskeletal complaints, but HPI says patient has pain in right knee).*
- *Appropriate documentation for a complete ROS (at least 10 of 14 systems) might include a checklist with documentation of "negative" or the pertinent response for each system. If a checklist is not used, documentation might indicate pertinent responses and "otherwise negative or unremarkable for all systems," pertinent responses and "all other systems reviewed and negative," or "complete ROS unchanged from previous review dated _____." Documentation of "ROS negative" is not sufficient.*
- *An ROS does not have to be recorded again on a subsequent encounter if there is documentation that the physician reviewed or updated a previous version. Documentation to reflect the subsequent review might be "ROS unchanged from most recent visit dated _____." (Tip: When history is pulled forward in the electronic health record [EHR] from a previous encounter, physicians must attest that the information has been reviewed and updated. Inconsistencies between the history pulled forward and the remainder of the encounter note may fail to represent the patient presentation and level of E/M service provided.)*
- *If a separate patient history form is used (eg, new patient history), the physician must sign and date the form to reflect his or her review. Pertinent responses to the ROS or PFSH may be documented on a separate history form, a progress note, or the signed history form.*
- *If the physician is unable to obtain a history, the record must describe the circumstance that prevents obtaining the history. In that circumstance, the history may be considered comprehensive. For example, a child is transferred to the emergency department of a children's hospital and her parents are transferred to another facility following an automobile accident. In this case, if the accepting physician documents this limitation as well as any history obtained from available past medical records or the medical transport team, the history is considered comprehensive.*
- *The distinction between an HPI and ROS is often confusing. The HPI and ROS are obtained for different reasons and both contribute to the level of history performed in the selection of an E/M service code.*
- *Documentation guidelines do not directly state that a comment made under the HPI cannot be counted again in the ROS when it is repeated. However, coders and payers may refer to this as double-dipping.*

Example: HPI: "abdominal pain for 3 days"; ROS: "abdominal pain." Think about the context in which the information was obtained. If the information was gathered as a description of the development of the problem, consider it as location in the HPI. If the information was obtained to help further define the scope of the problem, consider the information as part of the ROS. Example: HPI: "location: lower abdominal pain; duration: 3 days; signs/symptoms: without nausea, vomiting, constipation; timing: not associated with eating or exercise"; ROS: "GU [genitourinary]: intermittent dysuria; constitutional: denies fever."

Past, Family, and/or Social History (PFSH)

The PFSH consists of a review of three areas

- Past history (the patient's past experiences with illnesses, operations, injuries, and treatments)
- Family history (a review of medical events in the patient's family, including diseases that may be hereditary or place the patient at risk)

- Social history (an age-appropriate review of past and current activities)
- *Like the ROS, the PFSH may be recorded by the patient or caregiver, clinical staff, or physician (or medical student if a payer follows Medicare policy). When recorded by someone other than the physician, the physician should review the documented information and correct, clarify, or supplement it as needed.*
- *The PFSH is considered a single element of the overall history.*
- *Notation of allergies without current complaint and current medications are counted as past history.*

For the categories of subsequent hospital care, follow-up inpatient consultations and subsequent nursing facility care, *CPT* requires only an "interval" history. It is not necessary to record information about the PFSH.

A **pertinent** PFSH is a review of the history area(s) directly related to the problem(s) identified in the HPI.

•DG: *At least one specific item from* **any** *of the three history areas must be documented for a pertinent PFSH.*

A *complete* PFSH is a review of two or all three of the PFSH history areas, depending on the category of the E/M service. A review of all three history areas is required for services that by their nature include a comprehensive assessment or reassessment of the patient. A review of two of the three history areas is sufficient for other services.

•DG: *At least one specific item from* **two** *of the three history areas must be documented for a complete PFSH for the following categories of E/M services: emergency department; subsequent nursing facility care; domiciliary care, established patient; and home care, established patient.*

•DG: *At least one specific item from* **each** *of the three history areas must be documented for a complete PFSH for the following categories of E/M services: hospital observation services; hospital inpatient services, initial care; consultations; comprehensive nursing facility assessments; domiciliary care, new patient; and home care, new patient.*

Establishing the Level of History Performed

The patient history may be problem focused, expanded problem focused, detailed, or comprehensive. **Table 6-2** *lists required documentation elements for each level of history. To select a particular level of history, all elements of CC, HPI, ROS, and PFSH required for that level must be met.*

For example, consider a 13-year-old established patient.

- *Problem focused: "Here for stomachache. Left upper quadrant pain for 2 days."*
  - *CC: left upper quadrant*
  - *HPI: location—left upper stomachache, duration—2 days*
- *Expanded problem focused: "Here for stomachache. Generalized abdominal pain has hurt for 2 days. No diarrhea or constipation."*
  - *CC: stomachache*
  - *HPI: location—abdomen, right lower quadrant, duration—2 days*
  - *ROS: gastrointestinal (GI)*
- *Detailed: "Here for stomachache with generalized abdominal pain. Stomach has hurt on and off for a few months. Pain occurs primarily after eating, worsening over the last few days. No fever, diarrhea, or vomiting; last menstrual period 2 weeks ago and normal. Takes no medication; no known allergies."*
  - *CC: stomachache*
  - *HPI: location—abdomen, timing—on and off, duration—few months, context—after eating, severity—worsening*
  - *ROS: constitutional, GI, GU*
  - *PFSH: past medical—no medications, no allergies*
- *Comprehensive: "Here for stomachache. Complains of generalized abdominal pain on and off for a few months. Pain occurs primarily after eating, worsening over the last few days. No fever, diarrhea, or vomiting; last menstrual period 2 weeks ago and normal; no rashes; no injuries; all other systems reviewed and negative. Takes no medication, no known allergies, no exposure to illness, has excellent grades and enjoys school. Family history negative for abdominal problems or headaches."*
  - *CC: stomachache*
  - *HPI: location—abdomen, timing—on and off, duration—few months, context—after eating, severity—worsening*
  - *ROS: constitutional, GI, GU, skin, all others negative (indicates review of at least 10 of 14 systems)*
  - *PFSH: medical—no medications, no allergies, no exposure to illness; family—negative for abdominal or headache; social—excellent grades, enjoys school*

B. Documentation of Examination

The main distinction between the 1995 and 1997 documentation guidelines lies in the documentation of examination.
Table 6-3 outlines the differences.

Table 6-3. Comparison of 1995 and 1997 Levels of Physical Examination		
Level of Examination	**1995 Guidelines**	**1997 Guidelines**
Problem focused	Limited examination of the affected area or system	Performance and documentation of 1–5 elements identified by a bullet (●) in 1 or more areas or systems
Expanded problem focused	Limited examination of the affected body area or organ system and other symptomatic or related organ system(s)	Performance and documentation of at least 6 elements identified by a bullet (●) in 1 or more areas or systems
Detailed	Extended examination of the affected body area(s) and other symptomatic or related organ system(s)	Multisystem examination—Performance and documentation of at least 2 elements identified by a bullet (●) in at least 6 areas or systems or at least 12 elements identified by a bullet (●) in at least 2 areas or systems Single organ system examination—at least 12 elements identified by a bullet (●) (Eye and psychiatric examinations require only 9.)
Comprehensive	General multisystem examination (requires 8 or more organ systems) or a complete examination of a single organ system	Multisystem examination—Examination of at least 9 organ systems or body areas with performance of all elements identified by a bullet (●) in each area/system examined Documentation is expected for at least 2 elements identified by a bullet (●) of each area(s) or system(s). Single organ system examination—Performance of all elements identified by a bullet (●) and documentation of every element in each box with a shaded border and at least one element in a box with an unshaded border

1995 Guidelines for Documentation of Examination

The levels of E/M services are based on four types of examination that are defined as follows:

- **Problem Focused**—a limited examination of the affected body area or organ system.
- **Expanded Problem Focused**—a limited examination of the affected body area or organ system and other symptomatic or related organ system(s).
- **Detailed**—an extended examination of the affected body area(s) and other symptomatic or related organ system(s).
- **Comprehensive**—a general multisystem examination or complete examination of a single organ system.

  For purposes of examination, the following **body areas** are recognized:
- Head, including face
- Neck
- Chest, including breasts and axillae
- Abdomen
- Genitalia, groin, buttocks
- Back, including spine
- Each extremity

  For purposes of examination, the following **organ systems** are recognized:
- Constitutional (eg, vital signs, general appearance)
- Eyes
- Ears, nose, mouth, throat
- Cardiovascular
- Respiratory
- Gastrointestinal

- Genitourinary
- Musculoskeletal
- Skin
- Neurological
- Psychiatric
- Hematologic/lymphatic/immunologic

The extent of examinations performed and documented is dependent upon clinical judgment and the nature of the presenting problem(s). They range from limited examinations of single body areas to general multisystem or complete single organ system examinations.

- **•DG:** *Specific abnormal and relevant negative findings of the examination of the affected or symptomatic body area(s) or organ system(s) should be documented. A notation of "abnormal" without elaboration is insufficient.*
- **•DG:** *Abnormal or unexpected findings of the examination of the unaffected or asymptomatic body area(s) or organ system(s) should be described.*
- **•DG:** *A brief statement or notation indicating "negative" or "normal" is sufficient to document normal findings related to unaffected area(s) or asymptomatic organ system(s).*
- **•DG:** *The medical record for a general multisystem examination should include findings about eight or more of the 12 organ systems.*

There is no clear guidance on the distinction between a limited examination versus an extended examination. Unfortunately, this leaves room for subjectivity. The CMS does not offer guidance on this issue; however, some audit programs have attempted to quantify this.

1997 Guidelines for Documentation of Examination

The levels of E/M services are based on four types of examination

- **Problem Focused**—a limited examination of the affected body area or organ system.
- **Expanded Problem Focused**—a limited examination of the affected body area or organ system and any other symptomatic or related body area(s) or organ system(s).
- **Detailed**—an extended examination of the affected body area(s) or organ system(s) and any other symptomatic or related body area(s) or organ system(s).
- **Comprehensive**—a general multisystem examination or complete examination of a single organ system and other symptomatic or related body area(s) or organ system(s).

These types of examinations have been defined for general multisystem and the following single organ systems:

- Cardiovascular
- Ears, nose, mouth, throat
- Eyes
- Genitourinary (female)
- Genitourinary (male)
- Hematologic/lymphatic/immunologic
- Musculoskeletal
- Neurological
- Psychiatric
- Respiratory
- Skin

A general multisystem examination or a single organ system examination may be performed by any physician regardless of specialty. The type (general multisystem or single organ system) and content of examination are selected by the examining physician and are based upon clinical judgment, the patient's history, and the nature of the presenting problem(s).

The content and documentation requirements for each type and level of the 1997 examination are summarized below and described in detail in tables beginning on page <?>. In the tables, organ systems and body areas recognized by *CPT* for purposes of describing examinations are shown in the left column. The content, or individual elements, of the examination pertaining to that body area or organ system are identified by bullets (●) in the right column.

Parenthetical examples, "(eg, ...)", have been used for clarification and to provide guidance regarding documentation. Documentation for each element must satisfy any numeric requirements (such as "Measurement of *any three of the following seven...")* included in the description of the element. Elements with multiple components but with no specific numeric requirement (such as "Examination of *liver* and *spleen*") require documentation of at least one component. It is possible for a given examination to be expanded beyond what is defined here. When that occurs, findings related to the additional systems and/or areas should be documented.

•**DG:**   *Specific abnormal and relevant negative findings of the examination of the affected or symptomatic body area(s) or organ system(s) should be documented. A notation of "abnormal" without elaboration is insufficient.*

•**DG:**   *Abnormal or unexpected findings of the examination of any asymptomatic body area(s) or organ system(s) should be described.*

•**DG:**   *A brief statement or notation indicating "negative" or "normal" is sufficient to document normal findings related to unaffected area(s) or asymptomatic organ system(s).*

General Multisystem Examinations

General multisystem examinations are described in detail in **Table 6-4.**

Table 6-4. General Multisystem Examination—1997 Documentation Guidelines	
System/Body Area	**Elements of Examination**
Constitutional	• Measurement of **any three of the following seven** vital signs: 1) sitting or standing blood pressure, 2) supine blood pressure, 3) pulse rate and regularity, 4) respiration, 5) temperature, 6) height, 7) weight (may be measured and recorded by ancillary staff) • General appearance of patient (eg, development, nutrition, body habitus, deformities, attention to grooming)
Eyes	• Inspection of conjunctivae and lids • Examination of pupils and irises (eg, reaction to light and accommodation, size and symmetry) • Ophthalmoscopic examination of optic discs (eg, size, C/D ratio, appearance) and posterior segments (eg, vessel changes, exudates, hemorrhages)
Ears, Nose, Mouth, and Throat	• External inspection of ears and nose (eg, overall appearance, scars, lesions, masses) • Otoscopic examination of external auditory canals and tympanic membranes • Assessment of hearing (eg, whispered voice, finger rub, tuning fork) • Inspection of nasal mucosa, septum, and turbinates • Inspection of lips, teeth, and gums • Examination of oropharynx: oral mucosa, salivary glands, hard and soft palates, tongue, tonsils, and posterior pharynx
Neck	• Examination of neck (eg, masses, overall appearance, symmetry, tracheal position, crepitus) • Examination of thyroid (eg, enlargement, tenderness, mass)
Respiratory	• Assessment of respiratory effort (eg, intercostal retractions, use of accessory muscles, diaphragmatic movement) • Percussion of chest (eg, dullness, flatness, hyperresonance) • Palpation of chest (eg, tactile fremitus) • Auscultation of lungs (eg, breath sounds, adventitious sounds, rubs)
Cardiovascular	• Palpation of heart (eg, location, size, thrills) • Auscultation of heart with notation of abnormal sounds and murmurs Examination of: • Carotid arteries (eg, pulse amplitude, bruits) • Abdominal aorta (eg, size, bruits) • Femoral arteries (eg, pulse amplitude, bruits) • Pedal pulses (eg, pulse amplitude) • Extremities for edema and/or varicosities
Chest (Breasts)	• Inspection of breasts (eg, symmetry, nipple discharge) • Palpation of breasts and axillae (eg, masses or lumps, tenderness)

Table 6-4 (*continued*)

System/Body Area	Elements of Examination
Gastrointestinal (Abdomen)	• Examination of abdomen with notation of presence of masses or tenderness • Examination of liver and spleen • Examination for presence or absence of hernia • Examination (when indicated) of anus, perineum, and rectum, including sphincter tone, presence of hemorrhoids, rectal masses • Obtain stool sample for occult blood test when indicated
Genitourinary	*Male* • Examination of the scrotal contents (eg, hydrocele, spermatocele, tenderness of cord, testicular mass) • Examination of the penis • Digital rectal examination of prostate gland (eg, size, symmetry, nodularity, tenderness) *Female* • Pelvic examination (with or without specimen collection for smears and cultures) including • Examination of external genitalia (eg, general appearance, hair distribution, lesions) and vagina (eg, general appearance, estrogen effect, discharge, lesions, pelvic support, cystocele, rectocele) • Examination of urethra (eg, masses, tenderness, scarring) • Examination of bladder (eg, fullness, masses, tenderness) • Cervix (eg, general appearance, lesions, discharge) • Uterus (eg, size, contour, position, mobility, tenderness, consistency, descent, or support) • Adnexa/parametria (eg, masses, tenderness, organomegaly, nodularity)
Lymphatic	Palpation of lymph nodes in **two or more** areas: • Neck • Axillae • Groin • Other
Musculoskeletal	• Examination of gait and station • Inspection and/or palpation of digits and nails (eg, clubbing, cyanosis, inflammatory conditions, petechiae, ischemia, infections, nodes) Examination of joints, bones, and muscles of **one or more of the following six areas:** 1) head and neck; 2) spine, ribs, and pelvis; 3) right upper extremity; 4) left upper extremity; 5) right lower extremity; and 6) left lower extremity. The examination of a given area includes: • Inspection and/or palpation with notation of presence of any misalignment, asymmetry, crepitation, defects, tenderness, masses, effusions • Assessment of range of motion with notation of any pain, crepitation, or contracture • Assessment of stability with notation of any dislocation (luxation), subluxation, or laxity • Assessment of muscle strength and tone (eg, flaccid, cog wheel, spastic) with notation of any atrophy or abnormal movements
Skin	• Inspection of skin and subcutaneous tissue (eg, rashes, lesions, ulcers) • Palpation of skin and subcutaneous tissue (eg, induration, subcutaneous nodules, tightening)
Neurological	• Test cranial nerves with notation of any deficits • Examination of deep tendon reflexes with notation of pathological reflexes (eg, Babinski) • Examination of sensation (eg, by touch, pin, vibration, proprioception)
Psychiatric	• Description of patient's judgment and insight Brief assessment of mental status including: • Orientation to time, place, and person • Recent and remote memory • Mood and affect (eg, depression, anxiety, agitation)

To qualify for a given level of 1997 multisystem examination, the following content and documentation requirements should be met:

- **Problem-Focused Examination**—should include performance and documentation of one to five elements identified by a bullet (●) in one or more organ system(s) or body area(s).
- **Expanded Problem-Focused Examination**—should include performance and documentation of at least six elements identified by a bullet in one or more organ system(s) or body area(s).
- **Detailed Examination**—should include at least six organ systems or body areas. For each system/area selected, performance and documentation of at least two elements identified by a bullet is expected. Alternatively, a detailed examination may include performance and documentation of at least 12 elements identified by a bullet in two or more organ systems or body areas.
- **Comprehensive Examination**—should include at least nine organ systems or body areas. For each system/area selected, all elements of the examination identified by a bullet should be performed, unless specific directions limit the content of the examination. For each of nine areas/systems, documentation of at least two elements identified by a bullet is expected.

Single Organ System Examinations

The single organ system examinations recognized by *CPT* are described in detail (see **tables 6-5 through 6-14**). Variations among these examinations in the organ systems and body areas identified in the left columns and in the elements of the examinations described in the right columns reflect differing emphases among specialties. To qualify for a given level of single organ system examination, the following content and documentation requirements should be met:

- **Problem-Focused Examination**—should include performance and documentation of one to five elements identified by a bullet, whether in a shaded or unshaded area.
- **Expanded Problem-Focused Examination**—should include performance and documentation of at least six elements identified by a bullet, whether in a shaded or unshaded area.
- **Detailed Examination**—examinations other than the eye and psychiatric examinations should include performance and documentation of at least 12 elements identified by a bullet, whether in a shaded or unshaded area.
  — Eye and psychiatric examinations should include the performance and documentation of at least 9 elements identified by a bullet, whether in a shaded or unshaded area.
- **Comprehensive Examination**—should include performance of all elements identified by a bullet, whether in a shaded or unshaded area. Documentation of every element in a shaded area and at least one element in each category in each unshaded area is expected.

Table 6-5. Cardiovascular Examination	
System/Body Area	**Elements of Examination**
Constitutional	• Measurement of **any three of the following seven** vital signs: 1) sitting or standing blood pressure, 2) supine blood pressure, 3) pulse rate and regularity, 4) respiration, 5) temperature, 6) height, 7) weight (may be measured and recorded by ancillary staff) • General appearance of patient (eg, development, nutrition, body habitus, deformities, attention to grooming)
Eyes	• Inspection of conjunctivae and lids (eg, xanthelasma)
Ears, Nose, Mouth, and Throat	• Inspection of teeth, gums, and palate • Inspection of oral mucosa with notation of presence of pallor or cyanosis
Neck	• Examination of jugular veins (eg, distension; a, v, or cannon a waves) • Examination of thyroid (eg, enlargement, tenderness, mass)
Respiratory	• Assessment of respiratory effort (eg, intercostal retractions, use of accessory muscles, diaphragmatic movement) • Auscultation of lungs (eg, breath sounds, adventitious sounds, rubs)

System/Body Area	Elements of Examination
Table 6-5 (continued)	
Cardiovascular	• Palpation of heart (eg, location, size, and forcefulness of the point of maximal impact; thrills; lifts; palpable S3 or S4) • Auscultation of heart including sounds, abnormal sounds, and murmurs • Measurement of blood pressure in two or more extremities when indicated (eg, aortic dissection, coarctation) Examination of • Carotid arteries (eg, waveform, pulse amplitude, bruits, apical-carotid delay) • Abdominal aorta (eg, size, bruits) • Femoral arteries (eg, pulse amplitude, bruits) • Pedal pulses (eg, pulse amplitude) • Extremities for peripheral edema and/or varicosities
Gastrointestinal (Abdomen)	• Examination of abdomen with notation of presence of masses or tenderness • Examination of liver and spleen • Obtain stool sample for occult blood from patients who are being considered for thrombolytic or anti-coagulant therapy
Musculoskeletal	• Examination of the back with notation of kyphosis or scoliosis • Examination of gait with notation of ability to undergo exercise testing and/or participation in exercise programs • Assessment of muscle strength and tone (eg, flaccid, cog wheel, spastic) with notation of any atrophy and abnormal movements
Extremities	• Inspection and palpation of digits and nails (eg, clubbing, cyanosis, inflammation, petechiae, ischemia, infections, Osler's nodes)
Skin	• Inspection and/or palpation of skin and subcutaneous tissue (eg, stasis dermatitis, ulcers, scars, xanthomas)
Neurological/ Psychiatric	Brief assessment of mental status including: • Orientation to time, place, and person • Mood and affect (eg, depression, anxiety, agitation)

System/Body Areas Not Required: Head and Face, Chest (Breasts), Genitourinary (Abdomen), and Lymphatic

System/Body Area	Elements of Examination
Table 6-6. Ear, Nose, and Throat Examination	
Constitutional	• Measurement of **any three of the following seven** vital signs: 1) sitting or standing blood pressure, 2) supine blood pressure, 3) pulse rate and regularity, 4) respiration, 5) temperature, 6) height, 7) weight (may be measured and recorded by ancillary staff) • General appearance of patient (eg, development, nutrition, body habitus, deformities, attention to grooming) • Assessment of ability to communicate (eg, use of sign language or other communication aids) and quality of voice
Head and Face	• Inspection of head and face (eg, overall appearance, scars, lesions, and masses) • Palpation and/or percussion of face with notation of presence or absence of sinus tenderness • Examination of salivary glands • Assessment of facial strength
Eyes	• Test ocular motility including primary gaze alignment

Chapter 6. Evaluation and Management Documentation Guidelines Other Than Office and Other Outpatient Services

Table 6-6 (continued)

System/Body Area	Elements of Examination
Ears, Nose, Mouth, and Throat	• Otoscopic examination of external auditory canals and tympanic membranes including pneumo-otoscopy with notation of mobility of membranes • Assessment of hearing with tuning forks and clinical speech reception thresholds (eg, whispered voice, finger rub) • External inspection of ears and nose (eg, overall appearance, scars, lesions, and masses) • Inspection of nasal mucosa, septum, and turbinates • Inspection of lips, teeth, and gums • Examination of oropharynx: oral mucosa, hard and soft palates, tongue, tonsils, and posterior pharynx (eg, asymmetry, lesions, hydration of mucosal surfaces) • Inspection of pharyngeal walls and pyriform sinuses (eg, pooling of saliva, asymmetry, lesions) • Examination by mirror of larynx including the condition of the epiglottis, false vocal cords, true vocal cords, and mobility of larynx (use of mirror not required in children) • Examination by mirror of nasopharynx including appearance of the mucosa, adenoids, posterior choanae, and eustachian tubes (use of mirror not required in children)
Neck	• Examination of neck (eg, masses, overall appearance, symmetry, tracheal position, crepitus) • Examination of thyroid (eg, enlargement, tenderness, mass)
Respiratory	• Inspection of chest including symmetry, expansion, and/or assessment of respiratory effort (eg, intercostal retractions, use of accessory muscles, diaphragmatic movement) • Auscultation of lungs (eg, breath sounds, adventitious sounds, rubs)
Cardiovascular	• Auscultation of heart with notation of abnormal sounds and murmurs • Examination of peripheral vascular system by observation (eg, swelling, varicosities) and palpation (eg, pulses, temperature, edema, tenderness)
Lymphatic	• Palpation of lymph nodes in neck, axillae, groin, and/or other location
Neurological/ Psychiatric	• Test cranial nerves with notation of any deficits Brief assessment of mental status including: • Orientation to time, place, and person • Mood and affect (eg, depression, anxiety, agitation)

System/Body Areas Not Required: Chest (Breasts), Gastrointestinal (Abdomen), Genitourinary, Musculoskeletal, Extremities, and Skin

Table 6-7. Eye Examination

System/Body Area	Elements of Examination
Eyes	• Test visual acuity (does not include determination of refractive error) • Gross visual field testing by confrontation • Test ocular motility including primary gaze alignment • Inspection of bulbar and palpebral conjunctivae • Examination of ocular adnexae including lids (eg, ptosis or lagophthalmos), lacrimal glands, lacrimal drainage, orbits, and preauricular lymph nodes • Examination of pupils and irises including shape, direct and consensual reaction (afferent pupil), size (eg, anisocoria), and morphology • Slit lamp examination of the corneas including epithelium, stroma, endothelium, and tear film • Slit lamp examination of the anterior chambers including depth, cells, and flare • Slit lamp examination of the lenses including clarity, anterior and posterior capsule, cortex, and nucleus • Measurement of intraocular pressures (except in children and patients with trauma or infectious disease) Ophthalmoscopic examination through dilated pupils (unless contraindicated) of: • Optic discs including size, C/D ratio, appearance (eg, atrophy, cupping, tumor elevation), and nerve fiber layer • Posterior segments including retina and vessels (eg, exudates and hemorrhages)

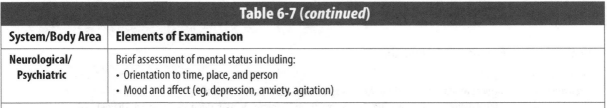

System/Body Area	Elements of Examination
Neurological/ Psychiatric	Brief assessment of mental status including: • Orientation to time, place, and person • Mood and affect (eg, depression, anxiety, agitation)

System/Body Areas Not Required: Constitutional; Head and Face; Ears, Nose, Mouth, and Throat; Neck; Respiratory; Cardiovascular; Chest (Breasts); Genitourinary; Lymphatic; Musculoskeletal; Extremities; and Skin Extremities and Skin

Table 6-8. Genitourinary Examination

System/Body Area	Elements of Examination
Constitutional	• Measurement of **any three of the following seven** vital signs: 1) sitting or standing blood pressure, 2) supine blood pressure, 3) pulse rate and regularity, 4) respiration, 5) temperature, 6) height, 7) weight (may be measured and recorded by ancillary staff) • General appearance of patient (eg, development, nutrition, body habitus, deformities, attention to grooming)
Neck	• Examination of neck (eg, masses, overall appearance, symmetry, tracheal position, crepitus) • Examination of thyroid (eg, enlargement, tenderness, mass)
Respiratory	• Assessment of respiratory effort (eg, intercostal retractions, use of accessory muscles, diaphragmatic movement) • Auscultation of lungs (eg, breath sounds, adventitious sounds, rubs)
Cardiovascular	• Auscultation of heart with notation of abnormal sounds and murmurs • Examination of peripheral vascular system by observation (eg, swelling, varicosities) and palpation (eg, pulses, temperature, edema, tenderness)
Chest (Breasts)	[See Genitourinary (female)]
Gastrointestinal (Abdomen)	• Examination of abdomen with notation of presence of masses or tenderness • Examination for presence or absence of hernia • Examination of liver and spleen • Obtain stool sample for occult blood test when indicated
Genitourinary	*Male* • Inspection of anus and perineum Examination (with or without specimen collection for smears and cultures) of genitalia including: • Scrotum (eg, lesions, cysts, rashes) • Epididymides (eg, size, symmetry, masses) • Testes (eg, size, symmetry, masses) • Urethral meatus (eg, size, location, lesions, discharge) • Penis (eg, lesions, presence or absence of foreskin, foreskin retractability, plaque, masses, scarring, deformities) Digital rectal examination including: • Prostate gland (eg, size, symmetry, nodularity, tenderness) • Seminal vesicles (eg, symmetry, tenderness, masses, enlargement) • Sphincter tone, presence of hemorrhoids, rectal masses

	Table 6-8 (*continued*)
System/Body Area	**Elements of Examination**
Genitourinary (*continued*)	*Female* Includes **at least seven of the following 11** elements identified by bullets: • Inspection and palpation of breasts (eg, masses or lumps, tenderness, symmetry, nipple discharge) • Digital rectal examination including sphincter tone, presence of hemorrhoids, rectal masses Pelvic examination (with or without specimen collection for smears and cultures) including: • External genitalia (eg, general appearance, hair distribution, lesions) • Urethral meatus (eg, size, location, lesions, prolapse) • Urethra (eg, masses, tenderness, scarring) • Bladder (eg, fullness, masses, tenderness) • Vagina (eg, general appearance, estrogen effect, discharge, lesions, pelvic support, cystocele, rectocele) • Cervix (eg, general appearance, lesions, discharge) • Uterus (eg, size, contour, position, mobility, tenderness, consistency, descent, or support) • Adnexa/parametria (eg, masses, tenderness, organomegaly, nodularity) • Anus and perineum
Lymphatic	• Palpation of lymph nodes in neck, axillae, groin, and/or other location
Skin	• Inspection and/or palpation of skin and subcutaneous tissue (eg, rashes, lesions, ulcers)
Neurological/ Psychiatric	Brief assessment of mental status including: • Orientation (eg, time, place, and person) • Mood and affect (eg, depression, anxiety, agitation)
System/Body Areas Not Required: Head and Face; Eyes; Ears, Nose, Mouth, and Throat; Musculoskeletal; and Extremities	

Table 6-9. Hematologic/Lymphatic/Immunologic Examination	
System/Body Area	**Elements of Examination**
Constitutional	• Measurement of **any three of the following seven** vital signs: 1) sitting or standing blood pressure, 2) supine blood pressure, 3) pulse rate and regularity, 4) respiration, 5) temperature, 6) height, 7) weight (may be measured and recorded by ancillary staff) • General appearance of patient (eg, development, nutrition, body habitus, deformities, attention to grooming)
Head and Face	• Palpation and/or percussion of face with notation of presence or absence of sinus tenderness
Eyes	• Inspection of conjunctivae and lids
Ears, Nose, Mouth, and Throat	• Otoscopic examination of external auditory canals and tympanic membranes • Inspection of nasal mucosa, septum, and turbinates • Inspection of teeth and gums • Examination of oropharynx (eg, oral mucosa, hard and soft palates, tongue, tonsils, posterior pharynx)
Neck	• Examination of neck (eg, masses, overall appearance, symmetry, tracheal position, crepitus) • Examination of thyroid (eg, enlargement, tenderness, mass)
Respiratory	• Assessment of respiratory effort (eg, intercostal retractions, use of accessory muscles, diaphragmatic movement) • Auscultation of lungs (eg, breath sounds, adventitious sounds, rubs)
Cardiovascular	• Auscultation of heart with notation of abnormal sounds and murmurs • Examination of peripheral vascular system by observation (eg, swelling, varicosities) and palpation (eg, pulses, temperature, edema, tenderness)
Gastrointestinal (Abdomen)	• Examination of abdomen with notation of presence of masses or tenderness • Examination of liver and spleen
Lymphatic	• Palpation of lymph nodes in neck, axillae, groin, and/or other location

Table 6-9 (continued)

System/Body Area	Elements of Examination
Extremities	• Inspection and palpation of digits and nails (eg, clubbing, cyanosis, inflammation, petechiae, ischemia, infections, nodes)
Skin	• Inspection and/or palpation of skin and subcutaneous tissue (eg, rashes, lesions, ulcers, ecchymoses, bruises)
Neurological/ Psychiatric	Brief assessment of mental status including: • Orientation to time, place, and person • Mood and affect (eg, depression, anxiety, agitation)

System/Body Areas Not Required: Chest (Breasts), Genitourinary, and Musculoskeletal

Table 6-10. Musculoskeletal Examination

System/Body Area	Elements of Examination
Constitutional	• Measurement of **any three of the following seven** vital signs: 1) sitting or standing blood pressure, 2) supine blood pressure, 3) pulse rate and regularity, 4) respiration, 5) temperature, 6) height, 7) weight (may be measured and recorded by ancillary staff) • General appearance of patient (eg, development, nutrition, body habitus, deformities, attention to grooming)
Cardiovascular	• Examination of peripheral vascular system by observation (eg, swelling, varicosities) and palpation (eg, pulses, temperature, edema, tenderness)
Lymphatic	• Palpation of lymph nodes in neck, axillae, groin, and/or other location
Musculoskeletal	• Examination of gait and station Examination of joint(s), bone(s), and muscle(s)/tendon(s) of **four of the following six** areas: 1) head and neck; 2) spine, ribs, and pelvis; 3) right upper extremity; 4) left upper extremity; 5) right lower extremity; and 6) left lower extremity. The examination of a given area includes: • Inspection, percussion, and/or palpation with notation of any misalignment, asymmetry, crepitation, defects, tenderness, masses, or effusions • Assessment of range of motion with notation of any pain (eg, straight leg raising), crepitation, or contracture • Assessment of stability with notation of any dislocation (luxation), subluxation, or laxity • Assessment of muscle strength and tone (eg, flaccid, cog wheel, spastic) with notation of any atrophy or abnormal movements *Note:* For the comprehensive level of examination, all four of the elements identified by a bullet must be performed and documented for each of four anatomic areas. For the three lower levels of examination, each element is counted separately for each body area. For example, assessing range of motion in two extremities constitutes two elements.
Extremities	[See Musculoskeletal and Skin]
Skin	• Inspection and/or palpation of skin and subcutaneous tissue (eg, scars, rashes, lesions, cafe-au-lait spots, ulcers) in **four of the following six** areas: 1) head and neck, 2) trunk, 3) right upper extremity, 4) left upper extremity, 5) right lower extremity, and 6) left lower extremity. *Note:* For the comprehensive level, the examination of all four anatomic areas must be performed and documented. For the three lower levels of examination, each body area is counted separately. For example, inspection and/or palpation of the skin and subcutaneous tissue of two extremities constitutes two elements.
Neurological/ Psychiatric	• Test coordination (eg, finger/nose, heel/knee/shin, rapid alternating movements in the upper and lower extremities, evaluation of fine motor coordination in young children) • Examination of deep tendon reflexes and/or nerve stretch test with notation of pathological reflexes (eg, Babinski) • Examination of sensation (eg, by touch, pin, vibration, proprioception) Brief assessment of mental status including: • Orientation to time, place, and person • Mood and affect (eg, depression, anxiety, agitation)

System/Body Areas Not Required: Head and Face; Eyes; Ears, Nose, Mouth, and Throat; Neck; Respiratory; Chest (Breasts); Gastrointestinal (Abdomen); and Genitourinary

Table 6-11. Neurological Examination	
System/Body Area	**Elements of Examination**
Constitutional	• Measurement of **any three of the following seven** vital signs: 1) sitting or standing blood pressure, 2) supine blood pressure, 3) pulse rate and regularity, 4) respiration, 5) temperature, 6) height, 7) weight (may be measured and recorded by ancillary staff) • General appearance of patient (eg, development, nutrition, body habitus, deformities, attention to grooming)
Eyes	• Ophthalmoscopic examination of optic discs (eg, size, C/D ratio, appearance) and posterior segments (eg, vessel changes, exudates, hemorrhages)
Cardiovascular	• Examination of carotid arteries (eg, pulse amplitude, bruits) • Auscultation of heart with notation of abnormal sounds and murmurs • Examination of peripheral vascular system by observation (eg, swelling, varicosities) and palpation (eg, pulses, temperature, edema, tenderness)
Musculoskeletal	• Examination of gait and station Assessment of motor function including: • Muscle strength in upper and lower extremities • Muscle tone in upper and lower extremities (eg, flaccid, cog wheel, spastic) with notation of any atrophy or abnormal movements (eg, fasciculation, tardive dyskinesia)
Extremities	[See Musculoskeletal]
Neurological	Evaluation of higher integrative functions including: • Orientation to time, place, and person • Recent and remote memory • Attention span and concentration • Language (eg, naming objects, repeating phrases, spontaneous speech) • Fund of knowledge (eg, awareness of current events, past history, vocabulary) Test the following cranial nerves: • 2nd cranial nerve (eg, visual acuity, visual fields, fundi) • 3rd, 4th, and 6th cranial nerves (eg, pupils, eye movements) • 5th cranial nerve (eg, facial sensation, corneal reflexes) • 7th cranial nerve (eg, facial symmetry, strength) • 8th cranial nerve (eg, hearing with tuning fork, whispered voice, and/or finger rub) • 9th cranial nerve (eg, spontaneous or reflex palate movement) • 11th cranial nerve (eg, shoulder shrug strength) • 12th cranial nerve (eg, tongue protrusion) • Examination of sensation (eg, by touch, pin, vibration, proprioception) • Examination of deep tendon reflexes in upper and lower extremities with notation of pathological reflexes (eg, Babinski) • Test coordination (eg, finger/nose, heel/knee/shin, rapid alternating movements in the upper and lower extremities, evaluation of fine motor coordination in young children)
System/Body Areas Not Required: Head and Face; Ears, Nose, Mouth, and Throat; Neck; Respiratory; Chest (Breasts); Gastrointestinal (Abdomen); Genitourinary; Lymphatic; Skin; and Psychiatric	

Table 6-12. Psychiatric Examination

System/Body Area	Elements of Examination
Constitutional	• Measurement of **any three of the following seven** vital signs: 1) sitting or standing blood pressure, 2) supine blood pressure, 3) pulse rate and regularity, 4) respiration, 5) temperature, 6) height, 7) weight (may be measured and recorded by ancillary staff) • General appearance of patient (eg, development, nutrition, body habitus, deformities, attention to grooming)
Musculoskeletal	• Assessment of muscle strength and tone (eg, flaccid, cog wheel, spastic) with notation of any atrophy and abnormal movements • Examination of gait and station
Psychiatric	• Description of speech including: rate, volume, articulation, coherence, and spontaneity with notation of abnormalities (eg, perseveration, paucity of language) • Description of thought processes including: rate of thoughts (eg, logical vs. illogical, tangential), abstract reasoning, and computation • Description of associations (eg, loose, tangential, circumstantial, intact) • Description of abnormal or psychotic thoughts including hallucinations, delusions, preoccupation with violence, homicidal or suicidal ideation, and obsessions • Description of the patient's judgment (eg, concerning everyday activities and social situations) and insight (eg, concerning psychiatric condition) Complete mental status examination including: • Orientation to time, place, and person • Recent and remote memory • Attention span and concentration • Language (eg, naming objects, repeating phrases) • Fund of knowledge (eg, awareness of current events, past history, vocabulary) • Mood and affect (eg, depression, anxiety, agitation, hypomania, lability)

System/Body Areas Not Required: Head and Face; Eyes; Ears, Nose, Mouth, and Throat; Neck; Respiratory; Cardiovascular; Chest (Breasts); Gastrointestinal (Abdomen); Genitourinary; Lymphatic; Extremities; Skin; and Neurological

Table 6-13. Respiratory Examination

System/Body Area	Elements of Examination
Constitutional	• Measurement of **any three of the following seven** vital signs: 1) sitting or standing blood pressure, 2) supine blood pressure, 3) pulse rate and regularity, 4) respiration, 5) temperature, 6) height, 7) weight (may be measured and recorded by ancillary staff) • General appearance of patient (eg, development, nutrition, body habitus, deformities, attention to grooming)
Ears, Nose, Mouth, and Throat	• Inspection of nasal mucosa, septum, and turbinates • Inspection of teeth and gums • Examination of oropharynx (eg, oral mucosa, hard and soft palates, tongue, tonsils, and posterior pharynx)
Neck	• Examination of neck (eg, masses, overall appearance, symmetry, tracheal position, crepitus) • Examination of thyroid (eg, enlargement, tenderness, mass) • Examination of jugular veins (eg, distension; a, v, or cannon a waves)
Respiratory	• Inspection of chest with notation of symmetry and expansion • Assessment of respiratory effort (eg, intercostal retractions, use of accessory muscles, diaphragmatic movement) • Percussion of chest (eg, dullness, flatness, hyper-resonance) • Palpation of chest (eg, tactile fremitus) • Auscultation of lungs (eg, breath sounds, adventitious sounds, rubs)
Cardiovascular	• Auscultation of heart including sounds, abnormal sounds, and murmurs • Examination of peripheral vascular system by observation (eg, swelling, varicosities) and palpation (eg, pulses, temperature, edema, tenderness)

Chapter 6. Evaluation and Management Documentation Guidelines Other Than Office and Other Outpatient Services

Table 6-13 (*continued*)

System/Body Area	Elements of Examination
Gastrointestinal (Abdomen)	• Examination of abdomen with notation of presence of masses or tenderness • Examination of liver and spleen
Lymphatic	• Palpation of lymph nodes in neck, axillae, groin, and/or other location
Musculoskeletal	• Assessment of muscle strength and tone (eg, flaccid, cog wheel, spastic) with notation of any atrophy and abnormal movements • Examination of gait and station
Extremities	• Inspection and palpation of digits and nails (eg, clubbing, cyanosis, inflammation, petechiae, ischemia, infections, nodes)
Skin	• Inspection and/or palpation of skin and subcutaneous tissue (eg, rashes, lesions, ulcers)
Neurological/ Psychiatric	Brief assessment of mental status including: • Orientation to time, place, and person • Mood and affect (eg, depression, anxiety, agitation)

System/Body Areas Not Required: Head and Face, Eyes, Chest (Breasts), and Genitourinary

Table 6-14. Skin Examination

System/Body Area	Elements of Examination
Constitutional	• Measurement of **any three of the following seven** vital signs: 1) sitting or standing blood pressure, 2) supine blood pressure, 3) pulse rate and regularity, 4) respiration, 5) temperature, 6) height, 7) weight (may be measured and recorded by ancillary staff) • General appearance of patient (eg, development, nutrition, body habitus, deformities, attention to grooming)
Eyes	• Inspection of conjunctivae and lids
Ears, Nose, Mouth, and Throat	• Inspection of lips, teeth, and gums • Examination of oropharynx (eg, oral mucosa, hard and soft palates, tongue, tonsils, posterior pharynx)
Neck	• Examination of thyroid (eg, enlargement, tenderness, mass)
Cardiovascular	• Examination of peripheral vascular system by observation (eg, swelling, varicosities) and palpation (eg, pulses, temperature, edema, tenderness)
Gastrointestinal (Abdomen)	• Examination of liver and spleen • Examination of anus for condyloma and other lesions
Lymphatic	• Palpation of lymph nodes in neck, axillae, groin, and/or other location
Extremities	• Inspection and palpation of digits and nails (eg, clubbing, cyanosis, inflammation, petechiae, ischemia, infections, nodes)

System/Body Area	Elements of Examination
Table 6-14 (*continued*)	
Skin	• Palpation of scalp and inspection of hair of scalp, eyebrows, face, chest, pubic area (when indicated), and extremities Inspection and/or palpation of skin and subcutaneous tissue (eg, rashes, lesions, ulcers, susceptibility to and presence of photo damage) in **eight of the following 10** areas: • Head, including face • Neck • Chest, including breasts and axillae • Abdomen • Genitalia, groin, buttocks • Back • Right upper extremity • Left upper extremity • Right lower extremity • Left lower extremity *Note:* For the comprehensive level, the examination of at least eight anatomic areas must be performed and documented. For the three lower levels of examination, each body area is counted separately. For example, inspection and/or palpation of the skin and subcutaneous tissue of the right upper extremity and the left upper extremity constitutes two elements. • Inspection of eccrine and apocrine glands of skin and subcutaneous tissue with identification and location of any hyperhidrosis, chromhidroses, or bromhidrosis
Neurological/ Psychiatric	Brief assessment of mental status including: • Orientation to time, place, and person • Mood and affect (eg, depression, anxiety, agitation)

System/Body Areas Not Required: Head and Face, Respiratory, Chest (Breasts), Genitourinary, and Musculoskeletal

C. Documentation of the Complexity of Medical Decision-making

The levels of E/M services recognize four types of medical decision-making (straightforward, low complexity, moderate complexity, and high complexity). Medical decision-making refers to the complexity of establishing a diagnosis and/or selecting a management option as measured by

1. The number of possible diagnoses and/or the number of management options that must be considered
2. The amount and/or complexity of medical records, diagnostic tests, and/or other information that must be obtained, reviewed, and analyzed
3. The risk of significant complications, morbidity, and/or mortality, as well as co-morbidities, associated with the patient's presenting problem(s), the diagnostic procedure(s), and/or the possible management options.

   Table 6-15 shows the progression of the elements required for each level of medical decision-making. To qualify for a given type of decision-making, **two of the three elements in the table must be either met or exceeded.**

Table 6-15. Determining Medical Decision-making

Number of Diagnoses or Management Options	Amount and/or Complexity of Data to Be Reviewed	Risk of Significant Complications, Morbidity, and/or Mortality	Type of Decision-Making
Minimal	Minimal or none	Minimal	Straightforward
Limited	*Limited*	Low	Low complexity
Multiple	Moderate	*Moderate*	*Moderate complexity*
Extensive	Extensive	High	High complexity

Each of the elements of medical decision-making is described below.

Number of Diagnoses or Management Options

The number of possible diagnoses and/or the number of management options that must be considered is based on the number and types of problems addressed during the encounter, the complexity of establishing a diagnosis, and the management decisions that are made by the physician.

Generally, decision-making with respect to a diagnosed problem is easier than that for an identified but undiagnosed problem. The number and type of diagnostic tests employed may be an indicator of the number of possible diagnoses. Problems that are improving or resolving are less complex than those that are worsening or failing to change as expected. The need to seek advice from others is another indicator of complexity of diagnostic or management problems.

- **•DG:**   *For each encounter, an assessment, clinical impression, or diagnosis should be documented. It may be explicitly stated or implied in documented decisions regarding management plans and/or further evaluation.*
  - For a presenting problem with an established diagnosis the record should reflect whether the problem is: (a) improved, well controlled, resolving, or resolved; or (b) inadequately controlled, worsening, or failing to change as expected.
  - For a presenting problem without an established diagnosis, the assessment or clinical impression may be stated in the form of a differential diagnoses or as "possible," "probable," or "rule out" (R/O) diagnoses.
- **•DG:**   *The initiation of, or changes in, treatment should be documented. Treatment includes a wide range of management options including patient instructions, nursing instructions, therapies, and medications.*
- **•DG:**   *If referrals are made, consultations requested, or advice sought, the record should indicate to whom or where the referral or consultation is made or from whom the advice is requested.*

Amount and/or Complexity of Data to Be Reviewed

The amount and/or complexity of data to be reviewed is based on the types of diagnostic testing ordered or reviewed. A decision to obtain and review old medical records and/or obtain history from sources other than the patient increases the amount and complexity of data to be reviewed.

Discussion of contradictory or unexpected test results with the physician who performed or interpreted the test is an indication of the complexity of data being reviewed. On occasion the physician who ordered a test may personally review the image, tracing, or specimen to supplement information from the physician who prepared the test report or interpretation; this is another indication of the complexity of data being reviewed.

- **•DG:**   *If a diagnostic service (test or procedure) is ordered, planned, scheduled, or performed at the time of the E/M encounter, the type of service (eg, lab or x-ray) should be documented.*
- **•DG:**   *The review of lab, radiology, and/or other diagnostic tests should be documented. An entry in a progress note such as "WBC elevated" or "chest x-ray unremarkable" is acceptable. Alternatively, the review may be documented by initialing and dating the report containing the test results.*
- **•DG:**   *A decision to obtain old records or to obtain additional history from the family, caretaker, or other source to supplement that obtained from the patient should be documented.*
- **•DG:**   *Relevant findings from the review of old records and/or the receipt of additional history from the family, caretaker, or other source should be documented. If there is no relevant information beyond that already obtained, that fact should be documented. A notation of "old records reviewed" or "-additional history obtained from family" without elaboration is insufficient.*
- **•DG:**   *The results of discussion of laboratory, radiology, or other diagnostic tests with the physician who performed or interpreted the study should be documented.*
- **•DG:**   *The direct visualization and independent interpretation of an image, tracing, or specimen previously or subsequently interpreted by another physician should be documented.*

Risk of Significant Complications, Morbidity, and/or Mortality

The risk of significant complications, morbidity, and/or mortality is based on the risks associated with the presenting problem(s), the diagnostic procedure(s), and the possible management options.

- **•DG:**   *Co-morbidities/underlying diseases or other factors that increase the complexity of medical decision making by increasing the risk of complications, morbidity, and/or mortality should be documented.*
- **•DG:**   *If a surgical or invasive diagnostic procedure is ordered, planned, or scheduled at the time of the E/M encounter, the type of procedure (eg, laparoscopy) should be documented.*

•*DG:* *If a surgical or invasive diagnostic procedure is performed at the time of the E/M encounter, the specific procedure should be documented.*

•*DG:* *The referral for or decision to perform a surgical or invasive diagnostic procedure on an urgent basis should be documented or implied.*

Table 6-16 may be used to help determine whether the risk of significant complications, morbidity, and/or mortality is **minimal, low, moderate,** or **high.** Because the determination of risk is complex and not readily quantifiable, the table includes common clinical examples rather than absolute measures of risk. The assessment of risk of the presenting problem(s) is based on the risk related to the disease process anticipated between the present encounter and the next one. The assessment of risk of selecting diagnostic procedures and management options is based on the risk during and immediately following any procedures or treatment. *The highest level of risk in **any one category** (presenting problem(s), diagnostic procedure(s), or management options) determines the overall risk.*

Table 6-16. CMS Table of Risk			
Level of Risk	**Presenting Problem(s)**	**Diagnostic Procedure(s) Ordered**	**Management Options Selected**
Minimal	• One self-limited or minor problem (eg, cold, insect bite, tinea corporis)	• Laboratory tests requiring venipuncture • Chest x-rays • EKG/EEG • Urinalysis • Ultrasound, eg, echocardiography • KOH prep	• Rest • Gargles • Elastic bandages • Superficial dressings
Low	• Two or more self-limited or minor problems • One stable chronic illness (eg, well-controlled hypertension, non–insulin-dependent diabetes, cataract, benign prostatic hyperplasia) • Acute uncomplicated illness or injury (eg, cystitis, allergic rhinitis, simple sprain)	• Physiologic tests not under stress (eg, pulmonary function tests) • Non-cardiovascular imaging studies with contrast (eg, barium enema) • Superficial needle biopsies • Clinical laboratory tests requiring arterial puncture • Skin biopsies	• Over-the-counter drugs • Minor surgery with no identified risk factors • Physical therapy • Occupational therapy • Intravenous fluids without additives
Moderate	• One or more chronic illnesses with mild exacerbation, progression, or side effects of treatment • Two or more stable chronic illnesses • Undiagnosed new problem with uncertain prognosis (eg, lump in breast) • Acute illness with systemic symptoms (eg, pyelonephritis, pneumonitis, colitis) • Acute complicated injury (eg, head injury with brief loss of consciousness)	• Physiologic tests under stress (eg, cardiac stress test, fetal contraction stress test) • Diagnostic endoscopies with no identified risk factors • Deep needle or incisional biopsy • Cardiovascular imaging studies with contrast and no identified risk factors (eg, arteriogram, cardiac catheterization) • Obtain fluid from body cavity (eg, lumbar puncture, thoracentesis, culdocentesis)	• Minor surgery with identified risk factors • Elective major surgery (open, percutaneous, or endoscopic) with no identified risk factors • Prescription drug management • Therapeutic nuclear medicine • Intravenous fluids with additives • Closed treatment of fracture or dislocation without manipulation

CPT copyright 2020 American Medical Association. All rights reserved.   ●=New code   ▲=Revised code   #=Re-sequenced code   +=Add-on code

| Table 6-16 (continued)		
Level of Risk	**Presenting Problem(s)**	**Diagnostic Procedure(s) Ordered**	**Management Options Selected**

Level of Risk	Presenting Problem(s)	Diagnostic Procedure(s) Ordered	Management Options Selected
High	• One or more chronic illnesses with severe exacerbation, progression, or side effects of treatment • Acute or chronic illnesses or injuries that pose a threat to life or body function (eg, multiple trauma, acute myocardial infarction, pulmonary embolus, severe respiratory distress, progressive severe rheumatoid arthritis, psychiatric illness with potential threat to self or others, peritonitis, acute renal failure) • An abrupt change in neurologic status (eg, seizure, transient ischemic attack, weakness, sensory loss)	• Cardiovascular imaging studies with contrast with identified risk factors • Cardiac electrophysiologic tests • Diagnostic endoscopies with identified risk factors • Discography	• Elective major surgery (open, percutaneous, or endoscopic) with identified risk factors • Emergency major surgery (open, percutaneous, or endoscopic) • Parenteral controlled substances • Drug therapy requiring intensive monitoring for toxicity • Decision not to resuscitate or to deescalate because of poor prognosis

An encounter resulting in multiple diagnoses/management options, limited data, and moderate risks leads to overall moderate complexity for MDM (see **Table 6-15***).*

D. **Documentation of an Encounter Dominated by Counseling or Coordination of Care**

For E/M services that are assigned a typical time of service, time (face-to-face or unit/floor) is considered the key or controlling factor in code selection when counseling and/or coordination of care dominates (more than 50%) the physician/patient and/or family encounter. Please see other chapters for discussion of the use of time for each type of E/M service.

•**DG:**   *If the physician elects to report the level of service based on counseling and/or coordination of care, the total length of time of the encounter (face-to-face or floor time, as appropriate) should be documented and the record should describe the counseling and/or activities to coordinate care.*

As of 2021, this no longer applies to **99202–99205** *or* **99212–99215.** *See* **Chapter 7.**

Split/Shared E/M Services

A split/shared E/M service is one in which a physician and a QHP from the same group practice each personally perform a medically necessary and substantive portion of 1 or more face-to-face E/M encounters on the same date. A portion of the key components of the service must be provided face-to-face by the physician to report under the physician's National Provider Identifier. Split/shared services were defined and implemented for services to Medicare beneficiaries. Private payers may adopt the same or a similar policy. The split/shared concept is applied differently for inpatient services than for services in the office or clinic setting (see **Chapter 7***).*

- When a hospital inpatient/hospital outpatient (on-campus outpatient hospital or off-campus outpatient hospital) or emergency department E/M is shared between a physician and an NPP from the same group practice and the physician provides any face-to-face portion of the E/M encounter with the patient, the service may be billed under either the physician or the NPP.
  - Payment will be made at the appropriate physician fee schedule rate based on the reporting provider entered on the claim.
  - If there was no face-to-face encounter between the patient and the physician (eg, even if the physician participated in the service by only reviewing the patient's medical record), then the service may only be billed under the NPP. Payment will be at the NPP rate (eg, 85% of physician fee schedule amount).

The following conditions apply to all split/shared services:
- *The physician and QHP must document and sign their portion of the service. A physician cannot merely sign off on the documentation of the QHP's work.*
- *If the E/M service is reported based on counseling and/or coordination of care, only the physician's time is used to select the level of service. The physician must document his or her total time spent in counseling and/or coordination of care and a summary of the issues discussed or coordination of care provided.*

- *Critical care is never a split/shared service because critical care services reflect the work of only 1 individual.*
- *Split/shared billing does not apply in the nursing or skilled nursing facility settings.*

More E/M Documentation and Coding Tips

- When using an EHR system, it is important that the documentation for each encounter is unique and reflects the purpose and activity of that encounter. Use of documentation features, such as carryforward of prior history, copy and paste, and auto-completion, may lead to inaccurate documentation and wrong code assignment.

> See "Coding Conundrum: Pitfalls of Electronic Health Record Coding" in Chapter 5 for more on electronic health record documentation.

- Ideally, physicians in a group practice should be consistent in their documentation policies. However, if documentation practices differ among physicians, have those differences documented in the practice's written policies.
- The code selected for a new patient will often be 1 level lower than for an established patient for the same amount of work. However, the Medicare relative value units are higher for new patient visits, compensating the physician for the extra work required.
- The American Academy of Pediatrics (AAP) has developed forms that promote good documentation of office or outpatient visits. Examples can be ordered from the AAP by calling 888/227-1770 or visiting http://shop.aap.org.

Teaching Physician Guidelines for Reporting E/M Services

> Refer to Chapter 19 for the teaching physician guidelines for billing surgical, high-risk, or other complex procedures.

- A teaching physician may bill for resident or fellow services if the teaching physician personally performs the key components (ie, history, physical examination, and MDM) of the service, performs the key components jointly with a resident, or personally observes the resident performing the key or critical components.
- The level of service billed will be dependent on the level of work performed and documented by the resident and the teaching physician in combination or by the teaching physician if seen independent of the resident.
- The teaching physician, resident, or nurse must document that he or she was physically present (ie, in the same room as the patient) during the key or critical portions of the service performed by the resident and participated in the management of the patient. The selected key or critical portion of the visit is at the discretion of the physician.

  Medicare requires that modifier **GC** (service performed in part by a resident under the direction of a teaching physician) be reported for each service, unless the service is furnished under the primary care exception (reported with modifier **GE**). Other payers may or may not require a modifier.
- Time-based services (eg, face-to-face prolonged services, critical care, hospital discharge management) can only be billed when the teaching physician is present for the time required by the description of the service.

  This also applies to E/M visits when time is considered the key component in the selection of the E/M code (>50% of the total face-to-face visit was spent counseling and/or coordinating care). The total time spent by the teaching physician must be documented.
- The teaching physician must document the key or critical part of the service personally performed, link his or her documentation back to the resident's note, and document that the care plan was reviewed and approved. It is not necessary to repeat the resident's documentation.

> When a resident admits a patient to the hospital without the teaching physician present and the teaching physician sees the patient later, including on the next day, the teaching physician's date of service is the day he or she saw the patient. The code reported is based on his or her personal work of obtaining a history, performing a physical examination, and participating in medical decision-making regardless of whether the combination of the teaching physician's and resident's documentation satisfies criteria for a higher level of service. For payment, the composite of the teaching physician's entry and the resident's entry must support the medical necessity of the billed service and the level of the service billed by the teaching physician.

- The teaching physician documentation must be linked to the resident's note and all exceptions to the resident's findings must be documented. A signature alone is not acceptable documentation.

- Medicare guidelines stipulate that when documenting in an EHR, the teaching physician may use a macro (eg, predetermined text) as the required personal documentation if it is personally entered by the teaching physician. The resident or teaching physician must enter customized information to support medical necessity. If the resident and teaching physician use only macros, the documentation is not sufficient. See **Table 6-17** for minimal documentation required.

Table 6-17. Unacceptable and Minimal Acceptable Documentation by a Teaching Physician

Unacceptable	Minimal Acceptable Documentation Required *Substitute the resident's name for Dr Resident.*
Countersignature	"I performed a history and physical exam of the patient. Findings are consistent with Dr Resident's note. Discussed patient's management with Dr Resident and agree with the documented findings and plan of care." Signature
"Agree with above." Signature "Rounded, reviewed, agree." Signature	"I saw and evaluated the patient. I agree with the findings and the plan of care as documented in Dr Resident's note." Signature
"Patient seen with resident and evaluated." Signature "Seen and agree." Signature	"I saw the patient with Dr Resident and agree with Dr Resident's findings and plans as written." Signature
"Discussed with resident." Signature	"I was present with Dr Resident during the history and exam. I discussed the case with Dr Resident and agree with the findings and plan as documented in Dr Resident's note." Signature

Examples

➤ **A resident admits a 2-month-old at 10:30 pm.** The teaching physician's initial visit is performed the following morning at 8:00 am. The teaching physician reports an initial hospital care service based on the work personally performed that morning. The teaching physician documents, "I saw and evaluated the patient. Discussed with resident and agree with the findings and plan as documented in Dr Resident's note except as per my addendum and edits within Dr Resident's note." *Note:* Edits should be distinguishable in the note.

➤ **The teaching physician sees the same patient for follow-up inpatient care subsequent to the resident's visit.** The teaching physician documents, "I saw and evaluated the patient. Discussed with Dr Resident and agree with Dr Resident's findings and plan as documented in the resident's note."

➤ **The teaching physician and resident jointly admit on the same patient.** The teaching physician documents, "I was present with Dr Resident during the history and exam. I discussed the case with Dr Resident and agree with the findings and plan as documented in Dr Resident's note."

➤ **The teaching physician and resident jointly provide a subsequent hospital visit.** The teaching physician documents, "I saw the patient with the resident and agree with Dr Resident's findings and plan."

Medical Student Documentation

- Any contribution and participation of a student to the performance of a billable service (other than the ROS and/or PFSH, which are not separately billable but are taken as part of an E/M service) must be performed in the physical presence of a teaching physician or a resident in a service meeting the requirements set forth in this section for teaching physician billing.
- Students may document services in the medical record. However
  - The teaching physician must verify in the medical record all student documentation or findings, including history, physical examination, and/or MDM.

— The teaching physician must personally perform (or re-perform) the physical examination and MDM activities of the E/M service being billed but may verify any student documentation in the medical record, rather than re-documenting this work.

Primary Care Exception Rule

The primary care exception rule (PCER) in the teaching physician guidelines allows teaching physicians to bill for services provided by residents under their supervision who have completed at least 6 months of approved graduate medical education (GME).

- To qualify for this exception, services must be provided in a teaching hospital ambulatory care center or clinic. If the services are provided outside a hospital, there must be a written agreement with the teaching hospital that includes a contract outlining the payment for the teaching services or written documentation that the services will be "donated." In general, this exception cannot be applied in a private physician's office.
- Preventive medicine visit codes are not included in the Medicare exception at this time. Some state Medicaid programs have granted the exemption for preventive medicine services to established patients.
- No more than 4 residents can be supervised at a time by a teaching physician. This may include residents with fewer than 6 months in a GME-approved residency program in the mix of 4 residents under the teaching physician's supervision. However, the teaching physician must be physically present for the critical or key portions of services furnished by the resident with fewer than 6 months in a GME-approved residency program. That is, the primary care exception does not apply in the case of the resident with fewer than 6 months in a GME-approved residency program.
- Patients seen should consider this practice as their primary location for health care.
- The teaching physician
  - Must be physically present in the clinic or office and immediately available to the residents and may not have other responsibilities (including supervising other personnel or seeing patients).
  - Must review the care provided (ie, history, findings on physical examination, assessment, and treatment plan) during or immediately after each visit. The documentation must reflect the teaching physician's participation in the review and direction of the services performed.

Example

➤ **The teaching physician is supervising a second-year resident in the clinic under the PCER.** An established patient is diagnosed with acute otitis media.

Unacceptable	Acceptable
Countersignature	"I reviewed Dr Resident's note and agree with Dr Resident's findings and plans as written." Signature "I reviewed Dr Resident's note and agree but will refer to ENT for consultation." Signature

- May only report codes **99202** and **99203** for new patient visits or **99211–99213** for established patient visits. If a higher-level E/M service is necessary and performed, the teaching physician must personally participate in the care of the patient as outlined in the guidelines. As always, code selection is based on the E/M code descriptions and documentation guidelines.
- Modifier **GE** (service performed by a resident without the presence of a teaching physician under the primary care exception) may be required by a payer that follows Medicare guidelines for teaching physician services.

The AAP continues to advocate for the preventive medicine service codes (99381–99385 and 99391–99395) to be included under the PCER. In some instances, state Medicaid plans already consider preventive medicine service codes as part of their primary care exception, so be sure to check with your payers. Look for updates in the AAP Pediatric Coding Newsletter™.

You can access the updated guidelines addressing the PCER at www.aap.org/cfp (access code AAPCFP26) or www.cms.gov/Outreach-and-Education/Medicare-Learning-Network-MLN/MLNProducts/MLN-Publications-Items/CMS1243499.html?DLPage=1&DLEntries=10&DLFilter=teaching%20physician&DLSort=0&DLSortDir=descending.

Chapter 6. Evaluation and Management Documentation Guidelines Other Than Office and Other Outpatient Services

Resources

Documentation Guidelines for Evaluation and Management Services

1995 and 1997 guidelines (See in this chapter or online at www.aap.org/cfp, access code AAPCFP26.)

Evaluation and Management Coding

American Academy of Pediatrics *Pediatric Evaluation and Management: Coding Quick Reference Card* (https://shop.aap.org/pediatric-evaluation-and-management-coding-quick-reference-card-2021)

Teaching Physician and Primary Care Exception

Medicare Learning Network *Guidelines for Teaching Physicians, Interns, and Residents* booklet (www.cms.gov/Outreach-and-Education/Medicare-Learning-Network-MLN/MLNProducts/MLN-Publications-Items/CMS1243499)

Test Your Knowledge!

1. **Which evaluation and management (E/M) services are subject to guidelines other than the general *Current Procedural Terminology*, 1995, and 1997 guidelines?**
   a. Hospital E/M services
   b. All E/M services except hospital services
   c. Office consultation codes **99241–99245**
   d. Office and other outpatient E/M services **99202–99205** and **99211–99215**

2. **Which of the following is a key component of an E/M service?**
   a. Nature of the presenting problem
   b. History
   c. Counseling
   d. Coordination of care

3. **Which of the following might be described as information gathered as a description of the development of the problem?**
   a. Review of systems
   b. History of present illness
   c. Family history
   d. Past medical history

4. **Under the 1997 documentation guidelines, an expanded problem-focused general multisystem examination should include how many elements identified by a bullet?**
   a. 6
   b. 12
   c. 8
   d. 18

5. **Which level of risk is supported by one minor illness, no diagnostic procedures ordered, and instruction to use an over-the-counter medication?**
   a. Minimal
   b. Low
   c. Moderate
   d. High

Part 2

Primarily for the Office and Other Outpatient Settings

Part 2: Primarily for the Office and Other Outpatient Settings

CHAPTER 7

Office and Other Outpatient Evaluation and Management Services

Contents

This chapter provides information on reporting office and other outpatient evaluation and management (E/M) codes **99202–99205** and **99211–99215** as revised in *Current Procedural Terminology* (*CPT®*) *2021*.

Please see **Chapter 6** *for guidelines applicable to other categories of E/M service.*

Physicians who report codes **99202–99205** and **99211–99215** for services provided on and after January 1, 2021, must understand and use the new guidelines for code selection. Although these changes are intended to reduce the complexity of code selection and reduce documentation burden, the new guidelines and code descriptors introduce a completely new code selection methodology (not applicable to other E/M services at this time) and new definitions that are key to appropriate code selection.

> For background information on how and why these changes took place, please see "Office E/M 2021: The Why and How of Changes to Office and Other Outpatient Evaluation and Management Services" in the January 2020 *AAP Pediatric Coding Newsletter*™ (https://coding. solutions.aap.org/article.aspx?articleid=2758025; subscription required).

This chapter includes coding for E/M services in a pediatric office or outpatient clinic setting as well as in urgent care facilities. For information on other services provided in office and other outpatient settings (eg, consultations, critical care, testing, and procedures), see **chapters 8 through 14**.

Overview of Office and Other Outpatient Evaluation and Management (E/M) Codes

2021 brings not only revisions to the code descriptors for office E/M services but also separate guidelines that apply only to office E/M services. Important changes include

- Deletion of code **99201** (level 1 new patient visit)
- Revised code descriptors for **99202–99205** and **99212–99215**
  - History and physical examination are no longer used as criteria in code selection.
  - Code selection based on either medical decision-making (MDM) *alone* or total time *spent by the physician or other qualified health care professional (QHP)* on the date of service.
  - Allow time-based reporting regardless of the amount of time spent in counseling and coordination of care.
  - Allow code selection based on all of a physician's or other QHP's time on the day of service.
  - The same level of MDM is required for new or established patient visits at each level of service (eg, level 2, **99202** and **99212**) in 2021. However, when selecting a code based on time, more time is required for new patient codes than for established patient codes.

> **Why Is 99201 Deleted in 2021?**
>
> Prior to 2021, codes 99201 and 99202 required straightforward medical decision-making (MDM) in addition to differing levels of history and/or examination. With only MDM required for code selection in 2021, code 99201 was redundant to code 99202.

Table 7-1 provides an overview of the requirements for selection of each level of E/M service other than code **99211**. (Code **99211** is not included here because MDM and time are not used in support of this code.)

New Versus Established Patients

New and established patients are defined the same for office E/M services as other E/M services that designate new or established patient. The criteria are as follows:

- *New patients* have not received a face-to-face professional service from the physician or QHP, or any physician or QHP of the same group practice and same exact specialty and subspecialty (eg, primary care, allergist), in the prior 3 years.
- *Established patients* have received, and a claim has been submitted for, a face-to-face professional service from a physician or QHP of the same group practice and same exact specialty within the past 3 years.
- Per *CPT,* a QHP working with a physician(s) and who may report E/M services is considered to be working in the exact same specialty and subspecialty as the physician(s). (Medicare assigns different specialty designations to QHPs and does not consider the specialty of the physician providing supervision when determining whether a patient is new. Medicaid and private plans may follow either *CPT* or Medicare practices.)

●=New code   ▲=Revised code   #=Re-sequenced code   +=Add-on code

Table 7-1. Code Selection Overview for Office Evaluation and Management Service Levels 2 Through 5

Code		Level of Medical Decision-making	Time Spent on the Date of the Encounter[a] (minutes)
New Patient	99202	Straightforward	15–29
	99203	Low	30–44
	99204	Moderate	45–59
	99205	High	60–74
Established Patient	99212	Straightforward	10–19
	99213	Low	20–29
	99214	Moderate	30–39
	99215	High	40–54

[a] Does not include time of clinical staff. Include only time spent by the physician or other qualified health care professional directed to the individual patient's care on the date of the encounter.

Telemedicine services (delivered via real-time audiovisual technology) are face-to-face services, even though the physician is present only by audiovisual technology.

Examples

➤ **If a physician of a different specialty is covering for another physician (eg, pediatrician covering for a family physician) and has the first face-to-face contact with the other physician's established patient, the encounter is considered new.**

If a physician is covering for another physician of the same specialty, the patient's encounter is coded as it would have been by the physician who is not available. For example, an established patient for a pediatrician is seen by the on-call pediatrician. The on-call pediatrician should report that patient as established.

> Per *Current Procedural Terminology*, if a physician is covering for another physician of the same specialty, the patient's encounter is reported as it would have been by the physician who is not available.

➤ **If the physician has moved to a different location or changed his or her tax identification number, patients would still be considered established if they were established patients before these changes took place.**

When a new physician joins a group of other pediatricians, patients who follow the physician to the new practice are considered to be established patients to any of the pediatricians in the new practice because the patients were seen by a physician of the same specialty in the group within the past 3 years.

➤ **When a newborn or child is examined in the hospital (eg, nursery or emergency department [ED] care) and is subsequently examined in the office by the same physician or member of the same group and same specialty, the newborn or child is considered an established patient.**

E/M Services in Urgent Care Facilities

Urgent care facilities are not EDs as defined in *CPT* (ie, an organized hospital-based facility for the provision of unscheduled episodic services to patients who present for immediate medical attention and are available 24 hours a day).

The Centers for Medicare & Medicaid Services describes an *urgent care facility* as a location, distinct from a hospital ED, an office, or a clinic, the purpose of which is to diagnose and treat illness or injury for unscheduled, ambulatory patients seeking immediate medical attention.

● Codes **99281–99285** are not reported for urgent care E/M services.

- *CPT* does not include codes specific to E/M services provided at an urgent care facility. Office E/M codes (**99202–99215**) are typically reported.
- The site of service is differentiated by the place of service code (eg, 20 for urgent care facility; 11 for office).
- Other E/M codes that may be applicable to services in an urgent care facility include
  - After-hours service codes discussed later in this chapter.
  - Healthcare Common Procedure Coding System (HCPCS) code **S9088** (services provided in an urgent care center) may be listed in addition to the codes for other services provided.
  - Some urgent care clinics also contract to bill all services under code **S9083** (global fee urgent care centers).

Some physician practices operate as a primary care pediatric practice and an urgent care center in the same location but with different tax identification numbers and insurance contracts for each. Physicians should consult a health care attorney for assistance in establishing an urgent care practice and contracting with payers to cover the additional overhead costs often applicable to urgent care (eg, extended staffing, radiology, procedural services).

It is imperative to know your contractual agreements for coding and billing as an urgent care facility or clinic versus a primary care practice, as rates of payment are typically higher for urgent care facilities and so, too, are patient co-payments. Billing and payment also vary for those urgent care facilities owned by hospitals, and guidance on billing and coding for these locations should be obtained from the compliance officer or other administrative personnel.

Visits Not Requiring a Physician's or Qualified Health Care Professional's Presence

▲99211   Office or other outpatient visit for the evaluation and management of an established patient, that may not require the presence of a physician or other qualified health care professional. Usually, the presenting problem(s) are minimal.

Services by clinical staff, such as **99211** visits, are considered incidental to a physician's or QHP's services and are reported under the supervising physician's or QHP's name and National Provider Identifier (NPI).

Per *Current Procedural Terminology*, a *clinical staff member* is a person working under the supervision of a physician or other qualified health care professional and who is allowed by law, regulation, and facility policy to perform or assist in the performance of a specified professional service but who does not individually report that professional service.

Code **99211**
- Is not reported on the same date as an office E/M service by a physician or QHP of the same group practice.
- Services are provided based on a physician's or QHP's order.
- Is reported for clinical staff assessments and other follow-up care not included in services described by other procedure codes (eg, face-to-face patient education not included in time billed as chronic care management services).
- Is reported only for established patients.
- Does not require the presence of a physician or QHP.
- Does not require MDM by a physician or QHP.
- Is not a time-based service.

Do not report **99211** for non-E/M services such as venipuncture (**36415**, **36416**), or injections (**96372**) or for demonstration or teaching use of an inhalation device (**94664**). Do not report **99211** in conjunction with administration of immunizations (**90471–90474**) without separate and distinct nursing assessment and management.

Examples

➤ **An established patient presents for weight check.**
   History: The patient is here for weight check per Dr Good's order. There are no concerns, and the patient is having fewer symptoms of attention-deficit/hyperactivity disorder (ADHD). The patient has a normal appetite.
   Physical assessment: The patient's height is 121.1 cm (47.7 inches) and weight is 22.4 kg (49.4 lb).
   Plan: Discussed with Dr Good. The patient is to continue current prescription, with recheck in 1 month.
   Codes reported are **99211** linked to **F90.1** (ADHD, predominantly hyperactive type) and **Z79.899** (other long term [current] drug therapy).

➤ **An established patient is provided education on use of self-injectable epinephrine by a nurse.** The supervising pediatrician reports **99211**.

➤ **An established patient is seen for evaluation of reaction to a tuberculosis skin test.** A medical assistant assesses the site of the injection and finds no signs of reaction. The supervising pediatrician reports **99211**.

Many payers follow Medicare policy for reporting services that are incident to a physician's service, which requires all of the following conditions:

- Clinical staff providing incident-to services must be directly or contractually employed by the practice of the reporting physician/QHP.
- The services performed are within the scope of practice of the performing clinical staff.
- The services are to an established patient in continuation of the physician's plan of care for an established problem.
- The services are provided with the supervising physician or QHP in the office suite at the time of service.

For health plans that pay for **99211** only when provided in compliance with incident-to policy, do not report **99211** when

- The patient presents with a new problem (eg, urinary tract infection) or a problem that requires new management.
- There is no supervising pediatrician or QHP in the office suite or clinic at the time of service.
- The patient is a new patient to the supervising physician or QHP.

Check for individual health plan guidance for reporting services by clinical staff.

> **Learn more about the Medicare incident-to policy in Chapter 13.**

Office E/M Guidelines

The following guidelines *apply only to office E/M codes* **99202–99205** and **99212–99215**. Unlike other categories of E/M codes (eg, home visits, hospital care), office E/M codes are not chosen based on 3 key components. Use of time for code selection is also different for office E/M codes. For both new and established patient visits, the level of service is determined by either of the following:

- The level of MDM alone
- The total amount of time (face-to-face and non–face-to-face) spent by a pediatrician or other QHP on the date of service directed to care of the patient.

See **Table 7-2** for an overview of the key guidelines for code selection for office E/M services.

Office E/M Terms and Concepts

To correctly select a level of service for office E/M services, it is important to understand the meanings of the terms used in the code descriptors and the table used to select the level of MDM. Included in the new guidelines for office E/M codes are definitions of these terms.

Appropriate source: Professionals who are not health care professionals but may be involved in the management of the patient. Examples include a lawyer, case manager, or teacher. *Family or informal caregivers are not appropriate sources,* although they may be independent historians.

Discussion of management with appropriate sources is a data element in moderate- or high-complexity MDM.

Chronic condition: A problem with an expected duration of at least 1 year or until the death of the patient. Conditions are treated as chronic whether or not stage or severity changes (eg, uncontrolled diabetes and controlled diabetes are a single chronic condition).

Data: Divided into the following 3 categories:

1. Tests, documents, orders, or independent historian(s) (Each unique test, order, or document is counted to meet a threshold number specified in *CPT*.)
2. Independent interpretation of tests that are not separately reported (eg, interpretation of an electrocardiogram reported with **93000** would not count toward data reviewed and analyzed)
3. Discussion of management or test interpretation with external physician or other QHP or appropriate source

Table 7-2. Key Office Evaluation and Management Coding Guidelines 2021

History and examination: Code selection is *not* based on the extent of history and examination. Each service includes a medically appropriate history and/or physical examination, when performed. Information supplied directly by the patient/caregiver or obtained by the care team may be reviewed and expanded on (as necessary) rather than redocumented.

Code selection: Select a code based either on MDM or the pediatrician's or QHP's total time on the date of the visit.

MDM: Four types of MDM are recognized: straightforward, low, moderate, and high.

Determine the level of MDM based on the highest 2 of 3 elements of MDM.

1. Number and complexity of problems addressed. Include problems addressed or managed by the reporting pediatrician/QHP as part of the encounter.
2. Amount and/or complexity of data reviewed and analyzed. Data include
   - Tests, documents, orders, or independent historian(s)
   - Independent interpretation of tests
   - Discussion of management/test interpretation with external physician, QHP, or appropriate source
3. Risk of complications, morbidity, and/or mortality of patient management decisions made at the visit, associated with the patient's problem(s), and the diagnostic procedure(s), treatment(s) including possible management options selected and those considered but not selected.

Time: May be used to select a code level whether or not counseling and/or coordination of care dominates the service.
- Time includes the total time on the date of the encounter (face-to-face and non–face-to-face) personally spent by the physician and/or QHP focused on the care of *1 patient.*
  — Do not include time in activities performed or normally performed by clinical staff (eg, rooming the patient).
  — Time does not need to be continuous. Total all time on 1 date.
- Include the time of the following activities when performed by the reporting pediatrician/QHP:
  — Preparing to see the patient (eg, review of previous tests)
  — Obtaining and/or reviewing separately obtained history
  — Performing a medically appropriate examination and/or evaluation
  — Counseling and educating the patient/family/caregiver
  — Ordering medications, tests, or procedures
  — Referring/communicating with other QHPs (when not separately reported)
  — Documenting clinical information in the electronic or other health record
  — Independently interpreting results (when not separately reported) and communicating results to patient/family/caregiver
  — Coordinating care (when not separately reported)

Abbreviations: MDM, medical decision-making; QHP, qualified health care professional.

Chapter 7. Office and Other Outpatient Evaluation and Management Services

The differentiation between single or multiple unique tests is defined in accordance with the *Current Procedural Terminology* code set. For instance, where a single code represents a panel of laboratory tests, the panel is counted as 1 test. Do not count each test in the panel as a unique test.

- Data include
  — Medical records, tests, and/or other information that must be obtained, ordered, reviewed, and analyzed for the encounter
  — Information obtained from multiple sources or interprofessional communications that are not separately reported

Drug therapy requiring intensive monitoring for toxicity: A prescribed therapeutic agent with the potential to cause serious morbidity or death is monitored for assessment of these adverse effects and not primarily for assessment of therapeutic efficacy.
- The monitoring may be by a laboratory test, a physiological test, or imaging. Monitoring by history or examination does not qualify.
- When long-term, monitoring is usually quarterly.
- Monitoring should be that generally accepted for the agent but may be patient-specific in some cases.

External records, communications, and/or test results: Those from an external physician, QHP, facility, or health care organization.

External physician or other QHP: An individual who is not in the same group practice or is of a different specialty or subspecialty including licensed professionals who are practicing independently. It may also be a facility or organizational provider such as a hospital, nursing facility, or home health care agency.

Independent historian(s): An individual (eg, parent, guardian, surrogate, witness) who provides a history in addition to a history provided by a patient who is unable to provide a complete or reliable history (eg, due to developmental stage, loss of consciousness) or because a confirmatory history is judged to be necessary.

In the case where there may be conflict or poor communication between multiple historians and more than 1 historian(s) is needed, the independent historian(s) requirement is met.

Independent interpretation: The interpretation of a test for which there is a *CPT* code and an interpretation or report is customary. This does not apply when the same physician or QHP is reporting or has previously reported interpretation and report for the service.

An interpretation should be documented but need not conform to the usual standards of a complete report for the test (ie, notation of pertinent findings from review of an image or tracing is sufficient rather than the typical documentation completed by the radiologist or cardiologist providing an interpretation and report).

Medical decision-making: Work of establishing diagnoses, assessing the status of a condition, and/or selecting a management option. Medical decision-making in the office and other outpatient services code set is defined by the following 3 elements:

1. The number and complexity of problem(s) that are addressed during the encounter
2. The amount and/or complexity of data to be reviewed and analyzed
3. The risk of complications, morbidity, and/or mortality of patient management decisions made at the visit, associated with the patient's problem(s), the diagnostic procedure(s), and treatment(s)

   Four types of MDM are recognized: straightforward, low, moderate, and high.

Morbidity: A state of illness or functional impairment that is expected to be of substantial duration during which function is limited, quality of life is impaired, or there is organ damage that may not be transient despite treatment.

Problem: A disease, condition, illness, injury, symptom, sign, finding, complaint, or other matter addressed at the encounter, with or without a diagnosis being established at the time of the encounter.

Risk: The probability and/or consequences of an event. For the purposes of MDM, level of risk is based on consequences of the problem(s) addressed at the encounter when appropriately treated. Risk also includes MDM related to the need to initiate or forego further testing, treatment, and/or hospitalization.

- Definitions of risk are based on the usual behavior and thought processes of a physician or QHP in the same specialty.
- Trained clinicians apply common meanings to terms such as *high, medium, low,* or *minimal* risk and do not require quantification for these definitions (quantification may be provided when evidence-based medicine has established probabilities).
- The assessment of the level of risk is affected by the nature of the event under consideration. For example, a low probability of death may be high risk, whereas a high chance of a minor, self-limited adverse effect of treatment may be low risk.
- Risk includes the possible management options selected, and those considered but not selected, after shared MDM with the patient and/or family. For example, a decision about hospitalization includes consideration of alternative levels of care.

Shared MDM: Eliciting patient and/or family preferences and patient and/or family education and explaining risks and benefits of management options.

Shared or split visit: A visit in which a physician and QHP jointly provide the face-to-face and non–face-to-face work related to the visit.

Social determinants of health: Economic and social conditions that influence the health of people and communities. Examples may include food or housing insecurity.

Test: Imaging, laboratory, psychometric, or physiological data. A clinical laboratory is a single test panel (eg, basic metabolic panel [**80047**]). The differentiation between single or multiple unique tests is defined in accordance with the *CPT* code assignment.

Time Guidelines and Application

Time may be used to select a code level in office E/M services *whether or not* counseling and/or coordination of care dominates the service.

- **The total time should be documented in the medical record when it is used as the basis for code selection. No specific verbiage is required by *CPT*.**
- Time is the physician's and/or QHP's total time on the date of service.

- Both face-to-face and non–face-to-face time spent on the date of service are included in the time of the encounter. **Figure 7-1** illustrates the time included in the physician's or QHP's total time.
- No time spent by clinical staff or time spent by a physician or QHP in activities typically performed by clinical staff is included.
- For shared or split visits, each minute of time is counted only once. When the pediatrician and a QHP meet with a patient/caregiver at the same time, only the reporting individual's time is counted.

See **Table 7-1** for time ranges assigned to each office E/M code.

> Because the primary goals of the 2021 code changes are simplification of code selection and reduced documentation burden, there is no requirement for documentation of each segment of time spent on the date of service or any specific format of documentation. The physician must, however, document the total amount of time spent on the date of the encounter and be able to account for the time spent.

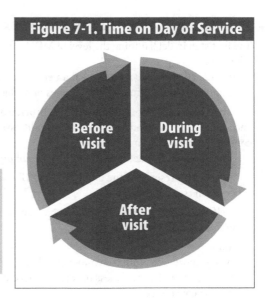

Figure 7-1. Time on Day of Service

Examples

➤ **A nurse practitioner sees an established patient for a follow-up visit due to parent concerns about resolution of otitis media.** Five minutes are spent reviewing the patient chart, and it is noted that the child is unimmunized for measles, mumps, and rubella due to parent's fear of autism spectrum disorder. After a brief examination finding resolving otitis media and counseling the parents (10 minutes), the nurse practitioner consults the pediatrician, who joins the practitioner in answering questions and counseling the parents for another 10 minutes. The parents again refuse immunization. The nurse practitioner spends another 5 minutes documenting the encounter for a total time on the date of the visit of 30 minutes.

Code **99214** (30–39 minutes) is reported. Only 10 minutes is counted for the time spent jointly by the pediatrician and the nurse practitioner.

A payer may allow physician reporting of split/shared visits only when following an established plan of care (ie, established problem with order for follow-up) and otherwise require reporting by the nurse practitioner.

➤ **A pediatrician spends 10 minutes reviewing laboratory results and consultation reports prior to a visit on the same date.** Later that day, a face-to-face visit with the patient and caregivers lasts 20 minutes. After the visit but on the same date, the pediatrician spends 10 minutes in discussion with a consulting subspecialist and another 10 minutes in follow-up with the caregiver and in documentation. The total time on the date of service is 50 minutes.

If the patient is a new patient, code **99204** (45–59 minutes) is reported. If the patient is established, code **99215** (40–54 minutes) is reported.

Medical Decision-making (MDM): Guidelines for Selecting a Level

As previously noted, MDM is determined by assessing the level at which 2 of 3 elements of MDM are supported in the documentation of an encounter. The 3 elements of MDM are
1. The number and complexity of problem(s) that are addressed during the encounter
2. The amount and/or complexity of data to be reviewed and analyzed
3. The risk of complications, morbidity, and/or mortality of patient management decisions made at the visit, associated with the patient's problem(s), the diagnostic procedure(s), and treatment(s)

Four types of MDM are recognized: straightforward, low, moderate, and high. Each level of MDM is based on the same criteria whether the patient is new or established. (Time and other factors considered in valuing codes differentiate new versus established patient office E/M services.)

Chapter 7. Office and Other Outpatient Evaluation and Management Services

Number and Complexity of Problems Addressed

The first step in determining the level of MDM for an encounter is identification of the number and complexity of problems addressed.

- Include all problems addressed at an encounter in the number and complexity of problems.
- Complexity is determined by the types of problems addressed.

The guidelines for office E/M services provide definitions of the types of problems that are typically addressed at these encounters. See the "Coding Conundrum: Addressed or Not Addressed" box later in this chapter for guidance on problems considered to have been addressed.

The following are definitions for the types of problems identified in the level of MDM from *CPT 2021:*

Minimal: Presence of the physician or QHP is not required, but the service is provided under the physician's or QHP's supervision (see code **99211**).

Self-limited or minor: A problem that runs a definite and prescribed course, is transient in nature, and is not likely to permanently alter health status.

Low

- Two or more self-limited or minor problems.
- Acute, uncomplicated illness or injury. A recent or new short-term problem with low risk of morbidity for which treatment is considered.
  - Little to no risk of mortality with treatment and full recovery without functional impairment is expected.
  - May be a self-limited or minor problem that is not resolving consistently with a definite and prescribed course.
  - Examples may include cystitis, allergic rhinitis, or a simple sprain.
- Stable chronic illness. A problem with an expected duration of at least 1 year or until the death of the patient where the risk of morbidity is significant without treatment.
  - *Stable* is defined by the individual patient's specific treatment goals. A patient who is not at his or her treatment goal is not stable, even if the condition has not changed and there is no short-term threat to life or function.
  - Examples of stable chronic illness may include well-controlled ADHD, asthma, or cystic fibrosis.

Moderate

- Two stable chronic illnesses.
- Chronic illness with exacerbation, progression, or side effects of treatment. Acutely worsening, poorly controlled, or progressing with an intent to control progression; *requiring additional supportive care or requiring attention to treatment for side effects* but not consideration of hospital level of care.

   Examples include non-severe exacerbation of asthma, generalized anxiety disorder now with school avoidance, and ADHD with tics secondary to treatment.
- Acute, complicated injury. Requires evaluation of body systems that are not directly part of the injured organ, extensive injury, multiple treatment options, and/or association with risk of morbidity (eg, head injury with brief loss of consciousness).
- Acute illness with systemic symptoms. An illness causing systemic symptoms and with high risk of morbidity without treatment.
  - For systemic general symptoms (eg, fever, body aches, fatigue) in a minor illness that may be treated to alleviate symptoms, shorten the course of illness, or prevent complications, see the definitions of *self-limited or minor* or *acute, uncomplicated illness.*
  - Systemic symptoms may not be general but may be single system (eg, juvenile oligoarticular arthritis with only musculoskeletal symptoms).
  - Examples may include pyelonephritis or bacterial gastroenteritis.
- Undiagnosed new problem with uncertain prognosis. A problem in the differential diagnosis that represents a condition likely to result in a high risk of morbidity without treatment.

   Examples may include unexplained bruising, anterior neck mass, unexpected weight loss, and school failure.

High

- Chronic illness with severe exacerbation, progression, or side effects of treatment. Severe exacerbation or progression of chronic illness or severe side effects of treatment with significant risk of morbidity and may require hospital level of care.
- Acute or chronic illness or injury posing a threat to life or bodily function. Acute illness with systemic symptoms or an acute complicated injury, or a chronic illness or injury with exacerbation and/or progression or side effects of treatment, that poses a threat to life or bodily function in the near term without treatment.

Examples may include severe respiratory distress, psychiatric illness with potential threat to self or others, acute renal failure, or an abrupt change in neurologic status.

See Table 7-3 for the levels of problems in medical decision-making.

Table 7-3. Defining Levels of Problems in Medical Decision-making

Level	Type of Problem
NA	**Minimal**: Presence of the physician or QHP is not required, but the service is provided under the physician's or QHP's supervision (see **99211**).
SF	**Self-limited or minor**: A problem that runs a definite and prescribed course, is transient in nature, and is not likely to permanently alter health status
Low	**≥2 self-limited or minor problems** **Acute, uncomplicated illness or injury**: A recent or new short-term problem with low risk of morbidity for which treatment is considered Little to no risk of mortality with treatment and full recovery without functional impairment is expected. May be a self-limited or minor problem that is not resolving consistent with a definite and prescribed course. Examples may include cystitis, allergic rhinitis, or a simple sprain. **Stable chronic illness**: A problem with an expected duration of at least 1 year or until the death of the patient where the risk of morbidity is significant without treatment. *Stable* is defined by the individual patient's specific treatment goals. A patient that is not at his or her treatment goal is not stable, even if the condition has not changed and there is no short-term threat to life or function. Examples of stable chronic illness may include well-controlled ADHD, asthma, or cystic fibrosis.
Moderate	**2 stable chronic illnesses** **Chronic illness with exacerbation, progression, or side effects of treatment**: Acutely worsening, poorly controlled, or progressing with an intent to control progression *and requiring additional supportive care or requiring attention to treatment for side effects*, but no consideration of hospital level of care. Examples include non-severe exacerbation of asthma, generalized anxiety disorder now with school avoidance, ADHD with tics secondary to treatment. **Acute, complicated injury**: Requires evaluation of body systems that are not directly part of the injured organ, extensive injury, multiple treatment options, and/or associated with risk of morbidity (eg, head injury with brief LOC). **Acute illness with systemic symptoms**: An illness causing systemic symptoms and with high risk of morbidity without treatment. For systemic general symptoms (eg, fever, body aches or fatigue) in a minor illness that may be treated to alleviate symptoms, shorten the course of illness, or prevent complications, see "Self-limited or minor" or "Acute, uncomplicated illness or injury." Systemic symptoms may not be general but may be single system (eg, juvenile oligoarticular arthritis with only musculoskeletal symptoms). Examples may include pyelonephritis or bacterial gastroenteritis. **Undiagnosed new problem with uncertain prognosis**: A problem in the differential diagnosis that represents a condition likely to result in a high risk of morbidity without treatment. Examples may include unexplained bruising, anterior neck mass, unexpected weight loss, and school failure.
High	**Chronic illness with severe exacerbation, progression, or side effects of treatment**: Severe exacerbation/progression of chronic illness or severe side effects of treatment with significant risk of morbidity and may require hospital level of care. **Acute/chronic illness or injury posing a threat to life or bodily function**: Acute illness with systemic symptoms, an acute complicated injury, a chronic illness or injury with exacerbation and/or progression, or side effects of treatment that pose a threat to life or bodily function in the near term without treatment. Examples may include severe respiratory distress, psychiatric illness with potential threat to self or others, acute renal failure, or an abrupt change in neurologic status.

Abbreviations: ADHD, attention-deficit/hyperactivity disorder; LOC, loss of consciousness; NA, not applicable; QHP, qualified health care professional; SF, straightforward.

●=New code ▲=Revised code #=Re-sequenced code +=Add-on code

Chapter 7. Office and Other Outpatient Evaluation and Management Services

---

Coding Conundrum: Addressed or Not Addressed

A problem is addressed or managed when it is evaluated or treated at the encounter by the physician or other qualified health care professional (QHP) reporting the service.

- This includes consideration of further testing or treatment that may not be elected by virtue of risk to benefit analysis or patient, parent, guardian, or surrogate choice.
- Notation in the patient's medical record that another professional is managing the problem without additional assessment or care coordination documented does not qualify as being addressed or managed by the physician or QHP reporting the service.
- Referral without evaluation (by history, examination, or diagnostic study[ies]) or consideration of treatment does not qualify a problem as being addressed or managed by the physician or QHP reporting the service.
- Do not include problems simply listed in the medical record when determining code level if those problems were not addressed.

Determination of the type of problem addressed may require a pediatrician's clinical judgement. Coding staff should query the pediatrician when unsure of the appropriate types of problems addressed at an encounter (eg, self-limited vs acute, uncomplicated illness).

Examples

➤ **A patient presents for follow-up after treatment of otitis media.** The patient appears well, and parents have no complaints. Tympanic membrane is white with evidence of mild effusion. The physician explains that effusion is expected to resolve without further treatment. Patient is to return as needed or at next scheduled preventive visit.

> The patient presented with a resolving problem of otitis media with effusion.
> Level of problems addressed ⅲ➡ Self-limited or minor

➤ **A patient presents for follow-up after treatment of otitis media that has occurred 3 times after removal of ear tubes 9 months ago.** Adenoids were removed at the time of prior ear tube placement. The patient also frequently complains of chest pain after eating. Diagnoses are chronic otitis media with effusion, gastroesophageal reflux, and perennial allergies.

> *Plan:* See otolaryngologist for unresolved effusion. Continue fluticasone propionate and loratadine. Add nizatidine to be given twice daily. Underweight at the fifth percentile despite parent's report of healthy appetite and good eating habits at home.
>
> The pediatrician addressed several problems, including chronic otitis media with effusion despite prior ear tubes and adenoidectomy, perennial allergies, and a new problem of gastroesophageal reflux in an underweight child.
> Level of problems addressed ⅲ➡ Moderate
> **Teaching Point:** There is no severe exacerbation, progression, or side effect of treatment and no immediate threat to life or bodily function; the number and complexity of problems is not high.

Amount and/or Complexity of Data to Be Reviewed and Analyzed

Data are divided into the following 3 categories:
1. Tests, documents, orders, or independent historian(s) (Each unique test, order, or document is counted to meet a threshold number.)
2. Independent interpretation of tests that are not separately reported
3. Discussion of management or test interpretation with external physician or other QHP or appropriate source

When data are used in support of low, moderate, or high MDM, the requirements for either 1 or 2 categories of data must be met. Instructions are provided for each level of data. Minimal or no data are required for straightforward MDM. **Table 7-4** shows the data requirements for low, moderate, and extensive data.

Examples

➤ **A 16-year-old boy presents with a fishhook in his finger.** After examination, a pediatrician clips the barb and removes the hook, cleans and bandages the wound, and orders a diphtheria and tetanus immunization.

> Level of data reviewed and analyzed ⅲ➡ Minimal or none
> **Teaching Point:** Medical decision-making will likely be based on the problem addressed and risk.

Table 7-4. Defining Data Required by Level of Medical Decision-making	
Limited *(Must meet the requirements of 1 of the 2 categories)*	**Category 1: Tests and documents** Any combination of 2 from the following: • Review of prior external note(s) from each unique source[a] • Review of the result(s) of each unique test[a] • Ordering of each unique test[a]
	Category 2: Assessment requiring an independent historian(s)
Moderate *(Must meet the requirements of 1 out of 3 categories)*	**Category 1: Tests, documents, or independent historian(s)** Any combination of 3 from the following: • Review of prior external note(s) from each unique source[a] • Review of the result(s) of each unique test[a] • Ordering of each unique test[a] • Assessment requiring an independent historian(s)
	Category 2: Independent interpretation of tests performed by another physician/other qualified health care professional (not separately reported)
	Category 3: Discussion of management or test interpretation with external physician/other qualified health care professional/appropriate source (not separately reported)
Extensive *(Must meet the requirements of at least 2 out of 3 categories)*	**Category 1: Tests, documents, or independent historian(s)** Any combination of 3 from the following: • Review of prior external note(s) from each unique source[a] • Review of the result(s) of each unique test[a] • Ordering of each unique testa • Assessment requiring an independent historian(s)
	Category 2: Independent interpretation of tests performed by another physician/other qualified health care professional (not separately reported)
	Category 3: Discussion of management or test interpretation with external physician/other qualified health care professional/appropriate source (not separately reported)
[a] Each unique test, order, or document is counted.	

➤ **A 6-year-old patient presents for follow-up after treatment of otitis media that has occurred 3 times after removal of ear tubes 9 months ago.** Although the patient can provide some history, due to her developmental status, her parents provide details such as frequency, timing, and modifying factors related to the patient's history of otitis media, allergies, and a new complaint of frequent chest pain after meals. No external notes are reviewed, and no tests are ordered or reviewed.

    Level of data reviewed and analyzed ⅢⅢ➡ Low

    Teaching Point: Data are low based on assessment requiring an independent historian.

➤ **A 6-year-old new patient presents with fever, cough, and vomiting for 2 days.** Parents provide past history of pre-term birth, congenital heart defect (repaired), and failure to thrive in addition to history of the present illness. A chest radiograph and influenza test are ordered. The pediatrician contacts the child's former pediatrician and discusses the child's history before determining a diagnosis and plan of care.

    Level of data reviewed and analyzed ⅢⅢ➡ Extensive

    Teaching Point: This is based on orders for 2 unique tests, assessment requiring an independent historian, and discussion of management with an external physician.

➤ **A 6-year-old new patient presents with fever, cough, and vomiting for 2 days.** Parents provide past history of preterm birth, congenital heart defect (repaired), and failure to thrive in addition to history of the present illness. A chest radiograph and influenza test are ordered. The physician accesses, views, and documents an impression of the chest radiographic image(s), but a radiologist has or will interpret and produce a formal report of findings from the image(s).

　　　Level of data reviewed and analyzed ⅢⅢ➡ Extensive

　　　Teaching Point: This is based on 2 unique tests ordered, assessment requiring an independent historian, and independent interpretation of a test by a physician not reporting a code for the interpretation and report of the findings.

Risk of Complications and/or Morbidity or Mortality of Patient Management

For the purposes of MDM, the level of risk is based on consequences of the problem(s) addressed at the encounter when appropriately treated. Risk also includes MDM related to the need to initiate or forego further testing, treatment, and/or hospitalization. Risk levels are minimal, low, moderate, and high. **Table 7-5** provides examples of each level of risk.

Table 7-5. Examples of Levels of Risk[a]	
Minimal	Rest and drink plenty of fluids. Diaper ointment. Superficial wound dressing.
Low	Over-the-counter medication(s) Removal of sutures Physical, language, or occupational therapy
Moderate	Prescription drug management Decision about minor surgery with identified patient or procedure risk factors Decision about elective major surgery without identified patient or procedure risk factors Diagnosis or treatment significantly limited by social determinants of health
High	Drug therapy requiring intensive monitoring for toxicity Decision about hospitalization Decision about emergency major surgery Decision not to resuscitate or to de-escalate care because of poor prognosis

[a] Examples are subject to clinical judgment for each individual patient and encounter.

Examples

➤ **A patient presents for follow-up after treatment of otitis media.** The patient appears well, and parents have no complaints. Tympanic membrane is white with evidence of mild effusion. The physician explains that effusion is expected to resolve without further treatment. The patient is to return as needed or at next scheduled preventive visit.

　　　Risk ⅢⅢ➡ Minimal to none

➤ **A 16-year-old boy presents with a fishhook in his finger.** After examination, a pediatrician clips the barb and removes the hook, cleans and bandages the wound, and orders a diphtheria and tetanus immunization. The patient is instructed to keep the wound clean and apply over-the-counter antibiotic ointment until healed.

　　　Risk ⅢⅢ➡ Low

➤ **A pediatric otolaryngologist sees a 6-year-old patient who presents for follow-up after treatment of otitis media that has occurred 3 times after removal of ear tubes 9 months ago.** Repeat bilateral myringotomy with tube insertion under general anesthesia is recommended, and parents agree to proceed with the procedure.

　　　Risk ⅢⅢ➡ Moderate

　　　Teaching Point: Decision for major surgery equals moderate risk level.

➤ **A 14-year-old presents for follow-up after implementing behavior changes to reduce migraine frequency.** The intervention has not significantly reduced the frequency and a prophylactic medication is prescribed.

> Risk ⅢⅢ➡ Moderate

➤ **A 6-month-old patient presents with fever, cough, listlessness, and poor feeding.** After examination, the pediatrician recommends hospitalization for evaluation of possible bacterial or viral infection and treatment of dehydration and respiratory distress.

> Risk ⅢⅢ➡ High
>
> **Teaching Point:** The risk associated with the decision to hospitalize the ill infant is high.

Selection of Level 2 Through 5 Codes

To select a code for office E/M services, you must determine which code is supported by 2 of 3 elements of MDM or the physician's or QHP's total time on the date of service. Refer to **Table 7-6** for an at-a-glance reminder of the levels of MDM or time required for each level of office E/M service.

The following pages provide an overview of a level of office E/M service with time and MDM reporting criteria and examples of each level of service. Key point to remember in code selection are as follows:

- Examples given are not clinical recommendations and levels of service supported may vary based on documentation and patient presentation (eg, ill appearance beyond what is typical for complaint).
- Select a code based on either total physician/QHP time on the date of service or MDM.
- The use of new versus established patient codes is based on whether the patient has received any face-to-face professional service from the same physician or a physician in the same group practice of the same exact specialty and subspecialty in the 3 years prior to the date of service.
- When selecting a code based on time, the total physician and/or QHP time spent devoted to the single patient's care must be documented.
- When selecting a code level based on MDM as described by *CPT*, the documentation should include the medically appropriate history and examination findings and all problems, diagnoses, management, and treatment options considered.

Office E/M Level 2 (99202, 99212)

★▲**99202**   Office or other outpatient visit for the evaluation and management of a new patient, which requires a medically appropriate history and/or examination and straightforward medical decision making
       When using time for code selection, 15–29 minutes of total time is spent on the date of the encounter.

★▲**99212**   Office or other outpatient visit for the evaluation and management of an established patient, which requires a medically appropriate history and/or examination and straightforward medical decision making
       When using time for code selection, 10–19 minutes of total time is spent on the date of the encounter.

Level 2 (99202, 99212) Medical Decision-making Requirements	
Documentation must support at least 2 of 3 elements (problems, data, risk).	
Problems addressed—number and complexity	**Minimal**—1 self-limited or minor problem
Data—amount/complexity to be reviewed and analyzed	**Minimal** or none
Risk of complications and/or morbidity or mortality of patient management	**Minimal** risk of morbidity from additional diagnostic testing or treatment

Time Requirements (in Lieu of MDM)

- **99202**: 15–29 minutes total physician and/or QHP time spent on the date of the encounter
- **99212**: 10–19 minutes total physician and/or QHP time spent on the date of the encounter

Table 7-6. Code Selection Requirements for Office Evaluation and Management Service Levels 2 Through 5

Level/Codes/ Total Time (min)[a]	Medical Decision-making (2 of 3 required: data,[b] problems, risk)		
	Problems Addressed	Data Reviewed and Analyzed[c]	Risk
Straightforward *New patient* **99202** (15–29) *Established patient* **99212** (10–19)	1 self-limited or minor	Minimal or none	Minimal *Examples* • Rest and drink plenty of fluids. • Diaper ointment. • Superficial wound care.
Low *New patient* **99203** (30–44) *Established patient* **99213** (20–29)	Low—*Any 1 of* ≥2 self-limited or minor 1 stable chronic illness 1 acute, uncomplicated illness or injury	Limited (*Meet 1 of 2 categories*) Category 1: Tests and documents (*Any 2*) • Review of prior external note(s)—each unique source • Review of the result(s) of each unique test • Ordering of each unique test Category 2: Assessment requiring an independent historian(s)	Low *Examples* • Over-the-counter medication(s) • Removal of sutures • Physical, language, or occupational therapy
Moderate *New patient* **99204** (45–59) *Established patient* **99214** (30–39)	Moderate—*Any 1 of* ≥1 chronic illnesses with exacerbation, progression, or side effects of treatment ≥2 stable chronic illnesses 1 undiagnosed new problem with uncertain prognosis 1 acute illness with systemic symptoms 1 acute complicated injury	Moderate (*Meet 1 out of 3 categories*) Category 1 (*Meet any 3*) • Review of prior external note(s)—each unique source • Review of the result(s) of each unique test • Ordering each unique test • Assessment requiring an independent historian(s) Category 2: Independent interpretation of a test performed by another physician/ other QHP[c] Category 3: Discussion of management or test interpretation with external physician/ other QHP/appropriate source	Moderate *Examples* • Prescription drug management • Decision about minor surgery with identified patient or procedure risk factors • Decision about elective major surgery without identified patient or procedure risk factors • Diagnosis or treatment significantly limited by social determinants of health
High *New patient* **99205** (60–74) *Established patient* **99215** (40–54)	High—*1 of* ≥1 chronic illnesses with severe exacerbation, progression, or side effects of treatment 1 acute or chronic illness or injury that poses a threat to life or bodily function	Extensive (*Meet 2 out of 3 categories*) Category 1: (*Meet any 3*) • Review of prior external note(s) from each unique source • Review of the result(s) of each unique test • Ordering of each unique test • Assessment requiring an independent historian(s) Category 2: Independent interpretation of a test performed by another physician/ other QHP Category 3: Discussion of management or test interpretation with external physician/ other QHP/appropriate source[c]	High • Drug therapy requiring intensive monitoring for toxicity • Decision about elective major surgery with identified patient or procedure risk factors • Decision about emergency major surgery • Decision about hospitalization • Decision not to resuscitate or to de-escalate care because of poor prognosis

Abbreviation: QHP, qualified health care professional.

[a] Does not include time of clinical staff. Include only time spent by the physician or QHP directed to the individual patient's care on the date of the encounter.

[b] Each unique test, order, or document contributes to the combination of 2 or combination of 3 in Category 1.

[c] Do not count data review or communications reported with other codes (eg, test interpretation, interprofessional consultation).

Examples

➤ **A 16-year-old new patient who is working as a volunteer at a child care center was recently exposed to chicken-pox and is unsure if she needs any vaccines.** Review of old records and the state immunization registry shows she is fully vaccinated. Total time of the visit is 15 minutes.

International Classification of Diseases, 10th Revision, Clinical Modification (ICD-10-CM): **Z20.820** (contact with and [suspected] exposure to varicella)

CPT: **99202** (total time 15–29 minutes) is supported by the total time of 15 minutes.

➤ **A patient presents for a follow-up visit for recurrent nonsuppurative left otitis media.** Parents note the patient has no symptoms of ongoing illness. The examination is normal. Diagnosis is resolved otitis media.

ICD-10-CM: **Z09** (follow-up after completed treatment for conditions other than malignant neoplasm) and **Z86.69** (personal history of other diseases of the nervous system and sense organs)

Because the infection is no longer present, a follow-up code (**Z09**) and history code (**Z86.69**) are reported.

CPT: The resolved problem with minimal data and risk supports **99212**.

➤ **Parents of a 2-year-old new patient present with concerns about their child having tantrums.** Parents are counseled on normal versus abnormal behavior and response to tantrums. Diagnosis is need for counseling on management of tantrums. Total time of service, including time before and after the visit, is 20 minutes.

ICD-10-CM: **Z71.89** (other specified counseling)

CPT: **99202** is supported by the total time of 20 minutes.

Office E/M Level 3 (99203, 99213)

★▲**99203**   Office or other outpatient visit for the evaluation and management of a new patient, which requires a medically appropriate history and/or examination and low level of medical decision making

       When using time for code selection, 30–44 minutes of total time is spent on the date of the encounter.

★▲**99213**   Office or other outpatient visit for the evaluation and management of an established patient, which requires a medically appropriate history and/or examination and low level of medical decision making

       When using time for code selection, 20–29 minutes of total time is spent on the date of the encounter.

Time Requirements (in Lieu of MDM)

- **99203**: 30–44 minutes total physician and/or QHP time spent on the date of the encounter
- **99213**: 20–29 minutes total physician and/or QHP time spent on the date of the encounter

Level 3 (99203, 99213) Medical Decision-making Requirements	
Documentation must support at least 2 of 3 elements (problems, data, risk).	
Problems addressed—number and complexity	**Low** (*Any 1 of the following*) ≥2 self-limited or minor problems 1 stable chronic illness 1 acute, uncomplicated illness or injury
Data—amount/complexity to be reviewed and analyzed	**Limited** (*Must meet the requirements of 1 of the 2 categories*) **Category 1:** Tests and documents (*Any combination of 2 from the following*) • Review of prior external note(s) from each unique source • Review of the result(s) of each unique test • Ordering of each unique test **Category 2:** Assessment requiring an independent historian(s)
Risk of complications and/or morbidity or mortality of patient management	**Low** *Examples* • Over-the-counter medication(s) • Removal of sutures • Physical, language, or occupational therapy

Examples

➤ **A 6-year-old new patient presents for complaint of sore throat for 2 days.** Parents report complaints of headache and abdominal pain today. Strep test result is positive. An antibiotic is prescribed.
> *ICD-10-CM:* **J02.0** (streptococcal pharyngitis)
> *CPT:* **99203**. Low MDM is supported by the acute uncomplicated illness, data (order/review of strep test and need for independent historian), and moderate risk (prescription drug management).
> Prescription drug management alone supports moderate risk but not moderate MDM.

➤ **A 6-year-old new patient presents with recurrent bed-wetting.** Parents are counseled on techniques to address it. Time spent managing the problem, which includes reviewing old records prior to the visit and documenting the encounter, is 35 minutes.
> *ICD-10-CM:* **N39.44** (nocturnal enuresis)
> *CPT:* 35 minutes of physician time on the date of service supports **99203**.

➤ **An established patient presents for asthma follow-up.** Asthma control test and symptom log indicate good control on current medication. The patient has no complaints. It is decided to continue the current plan and follow up in 3 months. Prescription is refilled. The diagnosis is intermittent asthma.
> *ICD-10-CM:* **J45.20** (mild intermittent asthma, uncomplicated)
> *CPT:* **99213** (low MDM based on 1 chronic condition addressed, low data [symptom log], and moderate risk [prescription drug management]) and **96160** (administration of patient-focused health risk assessment instrument [eg, health hazard appraisal] with scoring and documentation, per standardized instrument [for asthma control test])

Office E/M Level 4 (99204, 99214)

★▲**99204**   Office or other outpatient visit for the evaluation and management of a new patient, which requires a medically appropriate history and/or examination and moderate level of medical decision making
> When using time for code selection, 45–59 minutes of total time is spent on the date of the encounter.

★▲**99214**   Office or other outpatient visit for the evaluation and management of a new patient, which requires a medically appropriate history and/or examination and moderate level of medical decision making
> When using time for code selection, 30–39 minutes of total time is spent on the date of the encounter.

Level 4 (99204, 99214) Medical Decision-making Requirements
Documentation must support at least 2 of 3 elements (problems, data, risk).

Problems—number and complexity of problems addressed: Moderate (*Any 1 of the following*)	
≥1 chronic illnesses with exacerbation, progression, or side effects of treatment ≥2 stable chronic illnesses	1 undiagnosed new problem with uncertain prognosis 1 acute illness with systemic symptoms 1 acute complicated injury

Data—amount/complexity to be reviewed and analyzed: Moderate (*Must meet the requirements of at least 1 out of 3 categories*)	
Category 1 (*Any combination of 3*) • Review of prior external note(s) from each unique source • Review of the result(s) of each unique test • Ordering of each unique test • Assessment requiring an independent historian(s)	**Category 2:** Independent interpretation of a test performed by another physician/other QHP (not separately reported) **Category 3:** Discussion of management or test interpretation with external physician/other QHP/appropriate source (not separately reported)

Risk of complications and/or morbidity or mortality of patient management: Moderate
• Prescription drug management • Decision about minor surgery with identified patient or procedure risk factors • Decision about elective major surgery without identified patient or procedure risk factors • Diagnosis or treatment significantly limited by social determinants of health

Chapter 7. Office and Other Outpatient Evaluation and Management Services

Time Requirements (in Lieu of MDM)

- **99204**: 45–59 minutes total physician and/or QHP time spent on the date of the encounter
- **99214**: 30–39 minutes total physician and/or QHP time spent on the date of the encounter

Examples

➤ **A new 8-year-old patient presents with history of a recent ED visit for asthma.** The pediatrician reviews the hospital and prior pediatrician's records prior to the visit (same day). The patient is new to the community and has not established care with a pediatrician. The patient has no current complaints. Parents confirm history of poor compliance with daily asthma medication due to concern about overmedication. Parents and patient are counseled about the importance of medication, and a care plan is developed with shared decision-making. Total time of the visit is 50 minutes.

ICD-10-CM: **J45.30** (mild persistent asthma, uncomplicated) and **Z91.14** (patient's other noncompliance with medication regimen)

CPT: Time spent on the date of the encounter was 50 minutes or moderate MDM, which supports **99204**.

Code **99204** is supported by either the time of 50 minutes or any 2 of the following: a chronic condition that is not stable (ie, not controlled); data (eg, hospital record, prior pediatrician's records, independent historians); and risk (ie, prescription medication management).

➤ **An established patient with asthma presents with shortness of breath unrelieved by home inhalation treatment.** The patient stabilizes after an inhalation treatment in the office. New medication is prescribed. The diagnosis is exacerbation of mild persistent asthma.

ICD-10-CM: **J45.31** (mild persistent asthma with [acute] exacerbation)

CPT: Moderate MDM (exacerbation of a chronic condition with prescription drug management) supports **99214**. Spirometry and inhalation treatment are separately billed.

➤ **An established patient presents with concern of influenza.** Influenza test result is negative and nasopharyngitis is diagnosed. The child is under-immunized due to parents' fear of harmful effects of immunization. The pediatrician spends 15 minutes counseling the parents on the need for and safety of immunization. After the encounter, the pediatrician spends 10 minutes documenting details of the discussion about immunization and emailing additional educational information on immunizations to the parents. The pediatrician's total time on the date of service is 35 minutes.

ICD-10-CM: **J00** (acute nasopharyngitis [common cold]), **Z28.3** (under-immunization), and **Z28.82** (immunization not carried out because of caregiver refusal)

CPT: **99214** is supported by the physician's total time of 35 minutes.

All of the physician's time spent in care of the 1 patient on the date of the encounter is included in the time used to select the level of service for the office visit. There is no requirement that more than 50% of that time be spent in counseling and/or coordination of care.

Office E/M Level 5 (99205, 99215)

★▲**99205** Office or other outpatient visit for the evaluation and management of a new patient, which requires a medically appropriate history and/or examination and high level of medical decision making

When using time for code selection, 60–74 minutes of total time is spent on the date of the encounter.

(For services 75 minutes or longer, see prolonged services code **99417**.)

★▲**99215** Office or other outpatient visit for the evaluation and management of an established patient, which requires a medically appropriate history and/or examination and high level of medical decision making

When using time for code selection, 40–54 minutes of total time is spent on the date of the encounter.

(For services 55 minutes or longer, see prolonged services code **99417**.)

Time Requirements (in Lieu of MDM)

- **99205**: 60–74 minutes total physician and/or QHP time spent on the date of the encounter
- **99215**: 40–54 minutes total physician and/or QHP time spent on the date of the encounter

Examples

➤ **A new 3-month-old patient presents for an urgent appointment with a primary care pediatrician.** The infant's presentation is consistent with possible sepsis. The decision is made to arrange for direct hospital admission by an intensivist.

> *ICD-10-CM:* Diagnosis codes are reported for the child's symptoms.
> *CPT:* **99205** is supported by the acute illness that poses a threat to life or bodily function and decision to hospitalize.

➤ **A pediatrician reviews records of a new patient with complex medical history and later that day sees the patient and assists the parents with establishing subspecialty care.** The physician's total time on the date of the visit is 60 minutes.

> *ICD-10-CM:* Appropriate codes for the diagnoses addressed at the encounter are reported.
> *CPT:* **99205** is reported based on the physician's total time on the date of the encounter.

➤ **An established patient presents with symptoms of diabetes with ketoacidosis.** Laboratory tests ordered and reviewed are a urine dipstick and basic metabolic panel. The decision is made to hospitalize for new onset type 1 diabetes with ketoacidosis.

> *ICD-10-CM:* **E10.10** is reported for type 1 diabetes with ketoacidosis without coma.
> *CPT:* **99215** is supported by the problems addressed (ie, illness with threat to life or bodily function) and risk (ie, hospitalization).

➤ **An established patient presents with history of having had a complex seizure yesterday followed by care in the ED.** While in the office, the child experiences another seizure. The seizure continues for more than 5 minutes. Less than 30 minutes are spent by the pediatrician caring for the child before an ambulance team assumes management.

> *ICD-10-CM:* **G40.909** (epilepsy, unspecified, not intractable, without status epilepticus) or code for more specific diagnosis, when known
> *CPT:* **99205** is supported by the problems addressed (ie, illness with threat to life or bodily function) and risk (ie, hospitalization).

➤ **An established patient presents for follow-up of depression.** Just before seeing the patient, the pediatrician spends 5 minutes reviewing records of the last 3 encounters with the patient. The pediatrician then spends a total of 25 minutes counseling the patient followed by 10 minutes sending an electronic prescription refill and referral request to a local psychiatrist and another 10 minutes documenting the encounter. Time spent on the date of the encounter is 50 minutes.

> *ICD-10-CM:* **F32.1** (major depressive disorder, single episode, moderate)
> *CPT:* **99215** is supported by the total time of 50 minutes that was spent on the date of the encounter.

Prolonged Office E/M Service

Prolonged Service by a Physician or Other Qualified Health Care Professional

Prolonged service *on the date of an office E/M service* is reported with code **99417**. Codes **99354** and **99355** are not used in conjunction with codes **99202–99205** and **99211–99215**.

★+●**99417**   Prolonged office or other outpatient evaluation and management service(s) beyond the minimum required time of the primary procedure which has been selected using total time, requiring total time with or without direct patient contact beyond the usual service, on the date of the primary service, each 15 minutes of total time

> (List separately in addition to codes **99205**, **99215** for office or other outpatient evaluation and management services)
> (Use **99417** in conjunction with **99205**, **99215**)
> (Do not report **99417** on the same date as **99354–99355**, **99358–99359**, **99415–99416**)
> (Do not report **99417** for any time unit less than 15 minutes)

- Report code **99417**
  - Only when the office E/M code has been selected based on time *and only* after the minimum total time of the highest-level service (ie, **99205** or **99215**) has been exceeded by a full 15 minutes
  - When 15 minutes or more of additional time has been attained with 1 unit for each full 15 minutes beyond the minimum total time on the date of the visit
- Do not report **99417**
  - For prolonged service of less than 15 minutes on the date of the office E/M service
  - For any additional time increment of less than 15 minutes
  - For time spent performing separately reported services other than the E/M service with 1 unit for each full 15 minutes beyond the minimum total time on the date of the visit
  - In addition to **99202–99204** or **99211–99214**
  - On the same date as **99354** and **99355**, **99358** and **99359**, or **99415** and **99416**

Table 7-7 provides the required times for reporting units of **99417** in addition to either **99205** or **99215**. See note pertaining to **99417** on page IV.

Table 7-7. Times Supporting Prolonged Service With Codes 99205 and 99215[a]			
Reporting With 99205		**Reporting With 99215**	
Time (min)	**Codes Reported**	**Time (min)**	**Codes Reported**
60–74	**99205**	40–54	**99215**
75–89	**99205 + 99417** × 1	55–69	**99215 + 99417** × 1
90–104	**99205 + 99417** × 2	70–84	**99215 + 99417** × 2
≥105	**99205 + 99417** × 3 plus 1 unit for each full 15-minute period beyond the first 74 minutes	≥85	**99215 + 99417** × 3 plus 1 unit for each full 15-minute period beyond 119 minutes

[a] The times in this table are based on current *Current Procedural Terminology* (*CPT*) recommendations. The Centers for Medicare & Medicaid Services (CMS) has proposed different thresholds for prolonged services. The American Academy of Pediatrics will update this publication at www.aap.org/coding if *CPT* is revised or we learn payers are adopting CMS policy.

For E/M services that require prolonged clinical staff time and may include face-to-face services by the physician or QHP, see codes **99415** and **99416**.

Examples

➤ **A new patient is referred following discharge from observation care for asthma.** The patient has no usual source of care and has been seen in 3 EDs for a total of 4 visits in the past year. The pediatrician spends 30 minutes prior to the face-to-face visit, on the same date, reviewing observation and ED records for the child. At the visit, the pediatrician spends 45 minutes evaluating the patient, who also has behavioral issues in school; developing a plan of care; and counseling the patient and caregiver on the plan. After the visit, the pediatrician spends 15 minutes on the same date providing instructions to the school nurse about the patient's use of a rescue inhaler and arranging for teachers to complete rating scales for ADHD. The pediatrician reports codes **99205** and **99417** × 2 for the 90 minutes devoted to the patient's care on the date of the encounter.

➤ **An established adolescent patient and her parents meet with a pediatrician to discuss newly diagnosed idiopathic scoliosis.** Because the parents do not speak fluent English, an interpreter is required. The pediatrician spends 75 minutes discussing the diagnosis and management options and coordinating care. Code **99417** × 2 units is reported in addition to **99215**.

Prolonged service by a physician or QHP on a date before or after the date of a face-to-face office E/M service (in-person or telehealth) is reported with code **99358**.

Prolonged Clinical Staff Service (99415, 99416)

+▲99415　　　Prolonged clinical staff service (the service beyond the highest time in the range of total time of the service) during an evaluation and management service in the office or outpatient setting, direct patient contact with physician supervision; first hour

+▲99416　　　each additional 30 minutes

　　　Codes **99415** and **99416** are used to report 30 minutes or more of prolonged clinical staff time spent face-to-face providing care to a patient under the supervision of a physician or other QHP who has provided an office or other outpatient E/M service at the same session. See time requirements in **Table 7-8**.

● Report prolonged clinical staff service **99415** and **99416** in addition to office or other outpatient E/M codes **99202–99215**.

● *Never report both* prolonged office E/M service by a physician or other QHP (**99417**) and prolonged clinical staff services together.

Table 7-8. Level 2 Through 5 Office Evaluation and Management Times and Start of Prolonged Clinical Staff Time			
Code		**Assigned Time (min)**	**Minimum Time Required for Reporting 99415** (minutes of face-to-face clinical staff time)
New Patient	99202	15–29	59
	99203	30–44	74
	99204	45–59	89
	99205	60–74	104
Established Patient	99212	10–19	49
	99213	20–29	59
	99214	30–39	69
	99215	40–54	84

● Codes **99415** and **99416** were assigned relative value units (RVUs) based only on clinical staff's intraservice time, as the preservice and post-service times were considered to be included in the value of the related E/M service. Relative value units (2020 non-facility practice expense only) assigned are 0.28 for **99415** and 0.12 for **99416**. When paid at a conversion rate of $36.0896 per RVU, code **99415** would be valued at $10.11 (0.28 × 36.0896) and code **99416** would be valued at $4.33 per unit (0.12 × 36.0896).

　　　The following guidelines apply to reporting of prolonged clinical staff services:

● A physician or other QHP must supervise the duration of prolonged clinical staff service.

● Prolonged clinical staff services are reported only when the face-to-face time spent by clinical staff is 30 minutes or more beyond the highest total time of the related E/M service on the same date.

● Do not report prolonged service of less than 30 minutes beyond the highest total time of the related E/M service.

● The total time of and medical necessity for the service must be documented.

● Time spent providing separately reported services, such as intravenous medication administration or inhalation treatment, is not counted toward the time of prolonged service.

● When not continuous, document the face-to-face time of each episode of clinical staff time.

● Report code **99416** for each additional 30 minutes of clinical staff time beyond the first hour and for the last 15 to 30 minutes of prolonged clinical staff service. Do not report **99416** for less than 15 minutes beyond the first hour or last 30-minute period.

　　　Table 7-9 shows the calculation of units of service for codes **99415** and **99416**.

Table 7-9. How to Code Prolonged Clinical Staff Services	
Minutes Beyond End Time of Office E/M Code	**Code(s)**
<30	Not reported separately
30–74	**99415** × 1
75–104	**99415** × 1 AND **99416** × 1
≥105 (≥1 h 45 min)	**99415** × 1 AND **99416** × 2 (and additional units for each full 30 minutes or the last 15–30 minutes)
Abbreviation: E/M, evaluation and management.	

Examples

➤ **A child is seen for diarrhea and concerns of dehydration.** The physician diagnoses moderate dehydration due to viral gastroenteritis. Oral rehydration is ordered. The physician completes her documentation and selects code **99214** for service. The physician remains in the office suite while a nurse delivers and monitors a time-based oral rehydration plan using an electrolyte solution. The nurse's total direct care time is 2 hours.

   ICD-10-CM: **A08.4** (viral intestinal infection, unspecified) and **E86.0** (dehydration)

   CPT: E/M service by physician is reported with **99214** (includes 39 minutes); prolonged clinical staff time is reported with **99415** × 1 (first hour) and **99416** × 1 (final 30-minute period).

   Teaching Point: In this scenario, with clinical staff time of 120 minutes, the physician service includes 39 minutes, so prolonged clinical staff time is 81 minutes. The final 21 minutes is reported with code **99416** because 15 to 30 minutes beyond the previous period is separately reported.

   CPT instructs that prolonged clinical staff time begins after the typical time of the E/M service provided by the physician and is not reported if the prolonged clinical staff time is less than 45 minutes. When a physician reports code **99214** (includes 39 minutes), prolonged clinical staff time is not reported unless clinical staff have spent at least 69 minutes in face-to-face patient care.

➤ **A new patient who has been vomiting for 2 days is seen in the physician's office.** After evaluation by a physician, she is given antipyretics and fluids and then monitored and assessed by clinical staff for a total face-to-face clinical staff time of 104 minutes. After the monitoring period, the physician returns to the examination room and provides final instruction to the mother before releasing the child. The physician service includes moderate-complexity MDM (**99204**) based on key components. The physician's total time on the date of service was 45 minutes.

   ICD-10-CM: **K52.9** (gastroenteritis, unspecified)

   CPT: **99204** (includes 45–59 minutes) and **99415** × 1 (first hour of prolonged clinical staff time)

   Teaching Point: Prolonged service by clinical staff under physician supervision is reported rather than the physician's prolonged service, as the physician's total time did not exceed the time of code **99205** (includes 60–74 minutes). Code **99415** is reported because clinical staff time of 104 minutes was more than 30 minutes beyond the 59 minutes included in code **99204**.

➤ **A physician provides treatment to an established patient with acute exacerbation of moderate persistent asthma.** Over the course of 2 hours, the patient is given fluids (oral) for mild dehydration and oxygen as needed, oral steroids, and 3 inhaled bronchodilators. Documentation supports moderate-complexity MDM and total time by the physician of 70 minutes. Clinical staff also document 60 minutes of direct patient care (eg, providing nebulizer treatments) following the physician's E/M service.

   ICD-10-CM: **J45.41** (acute exacerbation of moderate persistent asthma) and **E86.0** (dehydration)

   CPT: **99215** (includes 40–54 minutes), **99417** (additional 15 minutes), and **94640 76** × 3 (nebulizer treatments)

   Teaching Point: The physician's service described includes code **99215**, office or other outpatient encounter, and 1 unit of prolonged office E/M service (**99417**). Prolonged clinical staff service is not reported on the same date as prolonged service by a physician or QHP, and time spent providing separately reported services (eg, nebulizer treatment) is not included in any prolonged service time.

Supplies related to services such as nebulizer treatment (**94640**) are included in the practice expense RVUs assigned to each code. If a payer does not base payment on RVUs, supplies may be separately reported with code **99070** (supplies and materials [except spectacles], provided by the physician or other QHP over and above those usually included with the office visit or other services rendered [list drugs, trays, supplies, or materials provided]) or specific HCPCS codes (eg, **A7003**, administration set, with small volume nonfiltered pneumatic nebulizer, disposable).

Split/Shared Office E/M Services

A *split/shared E/M service* is one in which a physician and a QHP from the same group practice each personally perform a medically necessary and substantive portion of 1 or more face-to-face E/M encounters on the same date. *A portion of the key components of the service must be provided face-to-face by the physician to report under the physician's NPI.*

By reporting under the physician's NPI, a higher fee schedule amount may be paid for the service (eg, 100% vs 85% of fee schedule). Split/shared services were defined and implemented for services to Medicare beneficiaries. Private payers may adopt the same or a similar policy. The split/shared concept is applied differently for inpatient services than for services in the office setting (see **Chapter 6**).

- In the non-facility office setting (place of service 11), split/shared E/M services must meet incident-to requirements for the service to be reported under the physician's NPI.

   Incident-to services require the physician's presence in the office suite at the time of the QHP service and that the QHP provides care only in accordance with a physician's established care plan for the patient.

> **See Chapter 13 for more information on incident-to services.**

- The physician and QHP must document and sign their portion of the service. A physician cannot merely sign off on the documentation of the QHP's work.
- If the E/M service is reported based on time the physician and QHP must each document his or her total time spent in care of the patient on the date of the encounter. Each minute of time must be attributed to either the physician or QHP, but not both.
- Critical care is never a split/shared service because critical care services reflect the work of only one individual.

Example

➤ **The patient history and a portion of the examination are provided in the office by a nurse practitioner for an established patient in continuation of a physician's previously documented plan of care for irritable bowel syndrome.** The physician is consulted about concerns of increased gastrointestinal symptoms, sees the patient face-to-face, performs a more detailed examination, and documents the assessment and plan of care.

   The total service may be reported under the physician's NPI because incident-to provisions have been met and both professionals provided face-to-face services.

After-hours Services (99050–99058)

Codes **99050–99058** are used to report services that are provided after hours or on an emergency basis and are always reported in addition to the primary service (eg, E/M service).
- Third-party payers will have specific policies for coverage and payment.
  - Some carriers pay practices for extended hours because they recognize the cost benefit realized from decreased urgent care and ED visits.
  - Communicate with individual payers to understand their definition or interpretation of the service and their coverage and payment policies.
  - As part of this negotiation and education process, it is important to demonstrate the cost savings recognized by the payer for these adjunct services.
- If appropriate, more than 1 adjunct code may be reported on the same day of service (eg, **99058** and **99051**).

   Many payers will pay only for the use of a single special services code per encounter and may manually review, question, or deny payment for a claim with multiple after-hours codes.

After-hours service codes are used by physicians or other QHPs (under their state scope of practice and when billing with their own NPI) to identify the services that are adjunct to the basic services rendered. These codes

- Describe the special circumstances under which a basic service is provided.
- Are only reported in addition to an associated basic service (eg, E/M, fracture care).
- Are reported without a modifier appended to the basic service because they only further describe the services provided.

Services Provided When the Office Is Normally Closed

99050   Service(s) provided in office at times other than regularly scheduled office hours, or days when the office is normally closed (eg, holidays, Saturday, Sunday), in addition to basic service

- Office hours must be posted. *CPT* does not define a holiday or posted office hours. While most commonly applied to evening, weekend, or holiday hours, code **99050** could be applied to services provided at the patient request on a weekday if the office is typically closed on that day.
- Code **99050** is *not* reported when a physician or other QHP is behind schedule and sees patients after posted office hours.
- The service must be requested by the patient, and the physician or other QHP must agree to see the patient.
- Documentation must indicate the time and date of the encounter and the request to be seen outside of normal posted hours.

Services Provided During Regularly Scheduled Evening, Weekend, or Holiday Hours

99051   Service(s) provided in the office during regularly scheduled evening, weekend, or holiday office hours, in addition to basic service

- Regularly scheduled office hours must be posted.
- Documentation must include the time and date of the encounter.
- Evenings and holidays are not defined by *CPT,* but holidays can generally refer to national and/or state holidays, and evenings are generally 6:00 pm and later. Check with payers for coverage and/or ability to bill patients these charges under the health plan contract.

Example

➤ **A pediatric clinic offers urgent care appointments 3 evenings a week with staffing by nonphysician QHPs (ie, nurse practitioners, physician assistants) working under general supervision.** A patient who has been seen at the clinic by Dr A within the last year is seen in the evening clinic by a nurse practitioner who documents an expanded problem-focused history and examination with low-complexity MDM with diagnosis of upper respiratory infection.

    ICD-10-CM: **J06.9** (acute upper respiratory infection, unspecified)

    CPT: **99213** (established office E/M) and **99051** (service provided in office during regularly scheduled weekend hours)

    Teaching Point: Because the office offers regularly scheduled evening hours, code **99051** is reported. The patient is established because *CPT* instructs that QHPs are considered to be of the same specialty as the physicians with whom they work in a group practice.

Services Provided on an Emergency Basis in the Office

99058   Service(s) provided on an emergency basis in the office, which disrupts other scheduled office services, in addition to basic service

- Report when an office patient's condition, in the clinical judgment of the physician, warrants the physician interrupting care of another patient to deal with the emergency.
- Code **99058** may not be reported when patients are simply fit into the schedule or for walk-ins.
- Document that the patient was seen immediately and the reason for the emergent care.

Example

➤ **A child is seen for severe exacerbation of moderate persistent asthma on a Saturday at 9:00 am.** The child arrives 30 minutes prior to the scheduled time and is immediately taken to an examination room by the triage nurse, and the physician disrupts his schedule to see the child urgently. The office is open on Saturday mornings from 8:00 am to 12:00 noon.

ICD-10-CM: **J45.41** (moderate persistent asthma with acute exacerbation)

CPT: **99202–99215** (new or established office E/M), **99058** (service provided on an emergency basis in office, disrupting other scheduled services), and **99051** (service provided in office during regularly scheduled weekend hours)

Teaching Point: If the Saturday hours were for walk-in visits only (ie, no scheduled appointments), code **99058** would *not* be reported. Note that if the patient is admitted to observation or inpatient hospital care on the same date by the same physician or a physician or other QHP of the same specialty and same group practice who later sees the patient in the facility setting on the same date, all services on that date are included in the code selection for initial observation or initial hospital care.

Continuum Models: Asthma, Attention-Deficit/Hyperactivity Disorder, and Otitis Media

Continuum Model for Asthma			
Code selection at any level above **99211** *may be based on complexity of MDM or the total time spent on the date of service by the reporting physician or other qualified health care professional.*			
The extent of history and examination documented does not affect code selection.			
***CPT* Code and Vignette**	**MDM (2 of 3 elements required)**		
99211 Nurse visit for a well 10-year-old established patient	*Time and MDM do not apply. Must indicate continuation of physician's plan of care, medical necessity, assessment, and/or education provided.* CC: Asthma care plan review Documentation of medications, peak expiratory flow, education topics reviewed, and questions answered		
***CPT* Code With Total Physician Time and Vignette**	**Number and Complexity of Problems Addressed**	**Amount and/or Complexity of Data Reviewed and Analyzed**	**Risk of Complications and/or Morbidity or Mortality of Patient Management**
99212 (Time: 10–19 min) An 8-year-old with stable asthma presents to get the influenza vaccine and parent has a question about effectiveness of control medication.	**SF:** 1 self-limited or minor problem	**SF:** None	**SF:** Minimal risk of morbidity from treatment
99213 (Time: 20–29 min) A 7-year-old with stable persistent asthma who is using a metered-dose steroid inhaler with β-agonist as needed returns for follow-up with complaint of watery eyes.	**Low:** 1 stable chronic illness 1 self-limited or minor problem	**Low:** Assessment requiring an independent historian(s)—mother provides history of asthma symptoms and medication compliance since last visit	**Moderate:** Prescription drug management
99214 (Time: 30–39 min) An 8-year-old with unstable asthma is examined because of an acute exacerbation of the disease; already receiving inhaled albuterol and inhaled steroids by metered-dose inhaler.	**Moderate:** 1 or more chronic illnesses with exacerbation, progression, or side effects of treatment	**Low:** Assessment requiring an independent historian(s)—mother provides history *Note: Spirometry and pulse oximetry provided are separately reported and not counted toward data reviewed and analyzed.*	**Moderate:** Prescription drug management

Continuum Model for Asthma (*continued*)

CPT Code With Total Physician Time and Vignette	Number and Complexity of Problems Addressed	Amount and/or Complexity of Data Reviewed and Analyzed	Risk of Complications and/or Morbidity or Mortality of Patient Management
99215 (Time: 40–54 min) A 1-year-old known to have recurrent wheezing following respiratory syncytial virus bronchiolitis has had increasingly frequent attacks during the past 2 months. New infiltrates are revealed by chest radiograph (film interpreted, not separately reported). Cystic fibrosis is suspected. A sweat test is ordered.	**High:** 1 acute or chronic illness or injury that poses a threat to life or bodily function	**High:** Review of prior external note(s) from recent ED visit; order sweat test; assessment requiring independent historians (parents) and independent interpretation of radiograph performed by another physician (not separately reported)	**Moderate:** Assumes prescription drug management

Abbreviations: CC, chief complaint; *CPT, Current Procedural Terminology*; ED, emergency department; MDM, medical decision-making; SF, straightforward.

Continuum Model for Attention-Deficit/Hyperactivity Disorder

Code selection at any level above 99211 may be based on the complexity of MDM or the total time spent by the physician or other qualified health care professional on the date of the encounter. (Code 99211 is not included due to lack of indication for follow-up by clinical staff.)

CPT Code With Total Physician Time and Vignette	MDM (2 of 3 elements required)		
	Number and Complexity of Problems Addressed	Amount and/or Complexity of Data Reviewed and Analyzed	Risk of Complications and/or Morbidity or Mortality of Patient Management
99211 Nurse visit to check growth or blood pressure prior to renewing prescription for psychoactive drugs	*Time and MDM do not apply. Must indicate continuation of physician's plan of care, medical necessity, assessment, and/or education provided.* CC: Check growth or blood pressure. Documentation: Height, weight, and blood pressure. Existing medications and desired/undesired effects. Assessment: Doing well. Obtained physician approval for prescription refill. Keep appointment with physician in 1 month.		
99212 (Time: 10–19 min) 4-year-old whose parents are concerned about ADHD symptoms	**Minimal:** 1 self-limited problem	**Limited:** Assessment requiring an independent historian	**Minimal:** Parent education
99213 (Time: 20–29 min) Initial follow-up after initiation of medication, patient responding well	**Low:** 1 stable chronic illness	**Limited:** Assessment requiring an independent historian	**Moderate:** Prescription drug management, delayed prescribing
99214 (Time: 30–39 min) Follow-up recent weight loss in patient with established ADHD otherwise stable on stimulant medication	**Moderate:** 1 chronic illness with side effects of treatment	**Limited:** Assessment requiring an independent historian	**Moderate:** Prescription drug management

Continuum Model for Attention-Deficit/Hyperactivity Disorder (*continued*)

CPT Code With Total Physician Time and Vignette	MDM (2 of 3 elements required)		
	Number and Complexity of Problems Addressed	Amount and/or Complexity of Data Reviewed and Analyzed	Risk of Complications and/or Morbidity or Mortality of Patient Management
99215 (Time: 40–54 min) Initial evaluation of patient with ADHD and new onset of suicidal ideation. Patient and mother refuse hospitalization due to cost. *Tip:* Add **99417** if time on the date of service is ≥55 minutes. Add **99058** if service(s) are provided on an emergency basis in the office, which disrupts other scheduled office services.	**High:** 1 acute or chronic illness or injury that poses a threat to life or bodily function	**Moderate:** Assessment requiring an independent historian; discussion with behavioral health specialist; psychiatric testing	**High:** Decision regarding hospitalization

Abbreviations: ADHD, attention-deficit hyperactivity disorder; CC, chief complaint; *CPT, Current Procedural Terminology*; MDM, medical decision-making.

Continuum Model for Otitis Media

*Code selection at any level above **99211** may be based on the complexity of MDM or the total time spent by the physician or other qualified health care professional on the date of the encounter. (Code **99211** is not included due to lack of indication for follow-up by clinical staff.)*

CPT Code With Total Physician Time and Vignette	MDM (2 of 3 elements required)		
	Number and Complexity of Problems Addressed	Amount and/or Complexity of Data Reviewed and Analyzed	Risk of Complications and/or Morbidity or Mortality of Patient Management
99212 (Time: 10–19 min) Follow-up otitis media, uncomplicated	**Minimal:** Follow-up otitis media, evaluation of effusion and hearing	**Limited:** Tympanometry, audiometry, and/or assessment requiring an independent historian	**Minimal:** Risk associated with diagnostic testing and treatment
99213 (Time: 20–29 min) 2-year-old presents with tugging at her right ear. Afebrile. Mild otitis media.	**Low:** 1 acute, uncomplicated illness or injury	**Limited:** Assessment requiring an independent historian	**Moderate:** Prescription drug management, delayed prescribing
99214 (Time: 30–39 min) Infant presents with fever and cough and suspected third episode of otitis media within 3 months.	**Moderate:** 1 acute illness with systemic symptoms	**Limited:** Assessment requiring an independent historian	**Moderate:** Prescription drug management
99215 (Time: 40–54 min) 6-month-old presents with high fever, vomiting, and irritability. After tests, antipyretics, and fluid, infant is stable.	**High:** 1 acute illness that poses a threat to life or bodily function	**Moderate:** Orders and/or review of laboratory tests, chest radiograph, and possible lumbar puncture. Assessment requiring an independent historian.	**High:** Decision about hospitalization (Hospitalization discussed with parents and decision made for care at home with strict instructions and close follow-up.)

Abbreviations: *CPT, Current Procedural Terminology*; MDM, medical decision-making.

Resources

Documentation

American Academy of Pediatrics Initial History Questionnaire Documentation Form for office or outpatient visits (available for purchase at http://shop.aap.org)

Examples of Office E/M Code Levels

"Office E/M 2021: Level 2 Visits" (August 2020 *AAP Pediatric Coding Newsletter*ˉ) (https://coding.solutions.aap.org/article. aspx?articleid=2765198; subscription required)

"Office E/M 2021: Level 3 Visits" (September 2020 *AAP Pediatric Coding Newsletter*) (https://coding.solutions.aap.org/article. aspx?articleid=2765216; subscription required)

"Office E/M 2021: Level 4 Visits" (October 2020 *AAP Pediatric Coding Newsletter*) (https://coding.aap.org; subscription required)

"Office E/M 2021: Requirements, Examples, and Use of the Prolonged Service Code" (November 2020 *AAP Pediatric Coding Newsletter*) (https://coding.aap.org; subscription required)

Medical Decision-making

"Office E/M 2021: An Overview of Medical Decision-making" (February 2020 *AAP Pediatric Coding Newsletter*) (https://coding.solutions. aap.org/article.aspx?articleid=2759684; subscription required)

"Office E/M 2021: Determining the Number and Complexity of Problems Addressed" (April 2020 *AAP Pediatric Coding Newsletter*) (https://coding.solutions.aap.org/article.aspx?articleid=2763373; subscription required)

"Office E/M 2021: Determining Levels of Amount and/or Complexity of Data" (May 2020 *AAP Pediatric Coding Newsletter*) (https://coding.solutions.aap.org/article.aspx?articleid=2765177; subscription required)

"Office E/M 2021: Determining the Level of Risk" (June 2020 *AAP Pediatric Coding Newsletter*) (https://coding.solutions.aap.org/article. aspx?articleid=2765184; subscription required)

"Office E/M 2021: Determining the Level of Medical Decision-making" (July 2020 *AAP Pediatric Coding Newsletter*) (https://coding. solutions.aap.org/article.aspx?articleid=2765191; subscription required)

Overview of Office E/M Changes

"Office E/M 2021: The Why and How of Changes to Office and Other Outpatient Evaluation and Management Services" (January 2020 *AAP Pediatric Coding Newsletter*) (https://coding.solutions.aap.org/article.aspx?articleid=2758025; subscription required)

"Questions and Answers and Tips for Adopting the New Coding Guidelines" (December 2020 *AAP Pediatric Coding Newsletter*) (https:// coding.aap.org; subscription required)

Time-Based Code Selection for Office E/M

"Office E/M 2021: An Overview of Time-Based Code Selection" (March 2020 *AAP Pediatric Coding Newsletter*) (https://coding.solutions. aap.org/article.aspx?articleid=2761969; subscription required)

Prolonged Services in Conjunction With Office Visits

"Office E/M 2021: An Overview of Time-Based Code Selection" (March 2020 *AAP Pediatric Coding Newsletter*) (https://coding.solutions. aap.org/article.aspx?articleid=2761969; subscription required)

Test Your Knowledge!

1. **Which of the following would be a new patient per *Current Procedural Terminology* instruction?**
   a. A patient is seen for the first time by an allergist in the same group practice as the patient's primary care pediatrician.
   b. A patient was seen by the same pediatrician in another practice 2 years ago.
   c. A patient is seen for the first time in the office setting after the same physician provided hospital care.
   d. All of the above

2. **Which of the following are appropriate sources as defined for office evaluation and management (E/M)?**
   a. A patient
   b. A patient's parent or primary caregiver
   c. A physician's clerical staff
   d. A schoolteacher

3. **Which is correctly included when selecting an office E/M code based on time?**
   a. All of the physician's and clinical staff's time spent face-to-face with the patient
   b. All of the physician's or other qualified health care professional's (QHP's) time spent face-to-face with the patient
   c. All of the physician's or QHP's time on the date of service spent on care of the patient
   d. Office E/M codes are not selected based on time.

4. **When data are used in support of low, moderate, or high medical decision-making (MDM), which of the following is a requirement for office E/M services?**
   a. Instructions are provided for each level of data.
   b. The data categories are the same for each level of MDM. 2 of 3 data categories are required for each level of MDM.
   c. 1 of 3 data categories is required for each level of MDM.

5. **How many elements of MDM must be met to support a level of office E/M service?**
   a. All 3 elements must be met for each code.
   b. Any 2 of 3 elements must be met.
   c. The amount and/or complexity of data alone supports the level of service.
   d. At least 1 element of MDM must be met.

Consultations and Residential Evaluation and Management Services

Contents

Selecting the Appropriate Evaluation and Management Codes

This chapter includes information on coding for evaluation and management (E/M) services provided in nonhospital settings (other than office E/M services [**99202–99205, 99211–99215**]). Included here are codes for reporting

- Office and outpatient consultations (**99241–99245**)
- Home care services (**99341–99350**)
- Domiciliary, rest home, or custodial care services (**99324–99337**)
- Nursing facility care (**99304–99310, 99315, 99316, 99318**)
- Out-of-office service add-on codes (**99056–99060**)
- Telephone services (**99441–99443, 98966–98968**)
- Prolonged services (**99354–99359**)
- Critical care (**99291, 99292**)

> **See Chapter 7 for information on office and other outpatient evaluation and management services (99202–99205, 99211–99215).**

Note: All E/M code descriptors and their specific instructions reflect the exclusion of references to provider/professional type, when nonessential, throughout the code set. When the word "physician" is included in a code descriptor, a qualified health care professional (QHP) working within his or her scope of practice may also provide the service.

When codes are provided for new and established patient E/M services, a new patient is one who has not received any *face-to-face* professional services within the past 3 years from the physician or another physician of the same specialty who belongs to the same group practice.

Time may be used as the key controlling factor in the selection of the code, in lieu of key components, when appropriate. To report based on time for E/M services provided in the sites of service discussed in this chapter, counseling and/or coordination of care must account for more than 50% of the face-to-face time with the patient.

- Billing based on time requires documentation of the total face-to-face time (may be approximate) and the percentage or number of minutes spent in counseling and/or coordination of care.
- *Current Procedural Terminology* (*CPT*®) instructs that time is met when the midpoint is passed unless code descriptors or prefatory instructions indicate otherwise. Other payers may require that the typical time specified for a service be met or exceeded.

> **See also Chapter 6 for a detailed description of evaluation and management guidelines, documentation requirements, and tips. See Chapter 12 for guidelines for reporting chronic care management and other non–face-to-face services provided to manage complex and/or chronic conditions.**

Table 8-1 provides the key components and specific details on required elements within each level of history and physical examination (eg, problem focused, expanded) and medical decision-making (MDM) (eg, straightforward, moderate) for most E/M codes. Refer to this table for more information on key components when using some of the other tables in this chapter to assign codes to examples. These tables can be downloaded at www.aap.org/cfp (access code AAPCFP26).

The examples included throughout this chapter are based on the 1995 E/M documentation guidelines. Each section includes a table illustrating key components of each type of service. Medical decision-making is listed before history and physical examination because some payers place greater emphasis on MDM than history and examination. Some payers require that the level of MDM be 1 of the 2 key components met to support the level of service for an established patient encounter.

Medical necessity for the extent of history, examination, and MDM should be evident in the documentation for each encounter. Consider only clinically indicated services when selecting the level of E/M service.

Chapter 8. Consultations and Residential Evaluation and Management Services

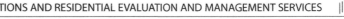

Table 8-1. Evaluation and Management Key Components				
History (must meet or exceed HPI, ROS, and PFSH)	**Problem Focused** HPI: 1–3 elements ROS: 0 PFSH: 0	**Expanded** HPI: 1–3 elements ROS: 1 PFSH: 0	**Detailed** HPI: 4+ elements or status of 3 chronic or inactive conditions ROS: 2–9 PFSH: 1	**Comprehensive** HPI: 4+ elements or status of 3 chronic or inactive conditions ROS: 10+ PFSH: 2 (established patient) or 3 (new patient)
Physical Examination	**Problem Focused** 1995: 1 body area/organ system 1997: Performance and documentation of 1–5 elements identified by a bullet (●) in ≥1 areas or systems	**Expanded** 1995: Limited examination—affected body area/organ system and 1–6 other related areas/systems 1997: Performance and documentation of at least 6 elements identified by a bullet (●) in ≥1 areas or systems	**Detailed** 1995: Extended examination—affected body area(s) and 1–6 other symptomatic or related organ system(s) 1997: Performance and documentation of at least 2 elements identified by a bullet (●) in at least 6 areas or systems or at least 12 elements identified by a bullet (●) in at least 2 areas or systems	**Comprehensive** 1995: 8+ organ systems or complete examination of a single organ system 1997: <u>Multisystem examination</u>—9 systems or areas with performance of all elements identified by a bullet (●) in each area/system examined Documentation of at least 2 elements identified by a bullet (●) of each area(s) or system(s) <u>Single organ system examination</u>—Performance of all elements identified by a bullet (●) and documentation of every element in box with shaded border and at least 1 element in box with unshaded border
Medical Decision-making	Straightforward	Low complexity	Moderate complexity	High complexity
(Must meet 2 of diagnoses/options, data, and risk.)				
Presenting Problem	Usually self-limited or minor severity	Usually moderate severity	Usually moderate to high severity	Usually moderate to high severity
No. of D/M Options	Minimal	Limited	Multiple	Extensive
Data	Minimal	Limited	Moderate	Extensive
Risk	Minimal	Low	Moderate	High

Abbreviations: D/M, diagnosis and management; HPI, history of present illness; PFSH, past, family, and social history; ROS, review of systems.

Office and Outpatient Consultations (99241–99245)

Codes **99241–99245** are used to report consultations provided in a pediatric office or outpatient clinic, a patient's home, a domiciliary, a rest home, or a custodial care home.

See codes **99251–99255** in **Chapter 16** for information on reporting consultations in nursing facility settings.

Consultations are defined by *CPT* as services provided by a physician at the request of another physician or "other appropriate source" to provide advice or opinion about the management or evaluation of a specific problem or to determine whether to accept responsibility for ongoing management of the patient's entire care or for the care of a specific condition/problem.

The "other appropriate source" is not explicitly defined in *CPT*. It may mean any interested source who seeks a medical opinion (eg, schools, juvenile court, attorney, psychologist, dentist, physician extender, occupational therapist).

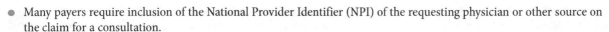

- Many payers require inclusion of the National Provider Identifier (NPI) of the requesting physician or other source on the claim for a consultation.
- When the source requesting a consultation does not have an NPI (eg, school counselor, teacher, attorney), verify payers' coding and billing requirements for the consultation. Claims for consultation services submitted without the NPI of the requestor may be rejected.

> **Do not report a consultation code for an encounter requested by a patient, parent, or guardian.**

Guidelines for reporting consultations include
- A physician or other appropriate source must request the consultation for opinion and/or advice (ie, with a question).
- Documentation must include
  - The request (written or verbal from the consultant; if verbal, still must be documented).
  - Name of the requesting physician or other appropriate source who requested the consultation.
  - Reason or need for the consultation (advice or opinion requested).
  - Opinion, recommendations, and services performed or ordered.
  - Written report back to the requesting physician or other appropriate source. A copy of the report must be maintained in the medical record.

> **A consultation report may be in letter form, a copy of the progress note, or a completed form (eg, preoperative form, consultation template). In a large group practice with shared medical records, it is acceptable to include the consultant's report as part of the documentation. A separate letter or report is not required.**

  - The requesting physician or other appropriate source must also document the request (even if it is a verbal request) for consultation in his or her patient medical record. This is not required by *CPT*, but some payers have adopted this policy to assist in review of records when it is unclear that consultation (ie, advice or opinion) was requested in lieu of a transfer of care for a particular problem.
- The consultant may initiate diagnostic or therapeutic services at the same or at a subsequent visit. Any identifiable procedures performed on or after the date of initial consultation (eg, endoscopy, cardiac catheterization, biopsy) should be reported separately.
- The management of the patient remains with the requesting or attending physician and is released in whole or in part only by the written notation of the requesting or attending physician in the medical record.
- Physicians in a group practice can provide consultations at the request of another member of the same practice if they are a different specialty or have an expertise in a specific medical area. For example, a primary care pediatrician may refer a patient to a partner, who is an allergist.
- Consultations for preoperative clearance may be reported when the surgeon requests an opinion and/or advice and a written report is sent to the requesting physician. Be aware of Medicaid program and commercial payer guidelines—some do not allow preoperative clearance consultations.
- Follow-up visits that are initiated by the physician consultant are reported using codes for established patients appropriate to the place of service (eg, office, home, domiciliary, rest home, custodial care).
- If an additional request for an opinion or advice on the same or a new problem is received from the attending physician and documented, the consultation codes may be used again.
- Consultations mandated by a third party (eg, payer, regulatory authority) are reported with modifier **32**.

Three of 3 key components must be met or exceeded when selecting the level of service for consultation services. A summary of key components for each level is in **Table 8-2**.

Codes do not distinguish between new or established patients. Face-to-face time with the patient may be used to select the level of service when more than 50% was spent in counseling and/or coordination of care.

●=New code   ▲=Revised code   #=Re-sequenced code   +=Add-on code

Table 8-2. New or Established Office/Outpatient Consultation Codes (99241–99245)

Key Components (For a description of key components, see Table 8-1.)
3 of 3 key components must be performed to at least the degree specified under the code.

CPT Code/ Time[a]	Medical Decision-making	History[b]	1995 Examination[c]
99241 15 min	Straightforward PP: Usually self-limited or minor	HPI: 1–3; ROS: 0; PFSH: 0	1 body area/system
99242 30 min	Straightforward PP: Usually low to moderate severity	HPI: 1–3; ROS: 1; PFSH: 0	2–7 limited
99243 40 min	Low complexity PP: Usually moderate severity	HPI: ≥4 or 3 CC; ROS: 2–9; PFSH: 1/3	2–7 detailed
99244 60 min	Moderate complexity PP: Usually moderate to high severity	HPI: ≥4 or 3 CC; ROS: ≥10; PFSH: 3/3	≥8 body areas/systems
99245 80 min	High complexity PP: Usually moderate to high severity	HPI: ≥4 or 3 CC; ROS: ≥10; PFSH: 3/3	≥8 body areas/systems

Abbreviations: CC, chronic condition; CPT, *Current Procedural Terminology;* HPI, history of present illness; PFSH, past, family, and social history; PP, presenting problem; ROS; review of systems.

[a] Typical time is an average and represents a range of times that may be higher or lower depending on clinical circumstances. The presenting problem is considered to be a contributory factor and does not need to be present to the degree specified.

[b] A chief complaint is required for all levels of history.

[c] Number of body areas or organ systems examined; see **Table 8-1** for details.

Guidelines Used by Payers That Follow Medicare Consultation Guidelines

It is important to check with major payers to determine if they have adopted the Medicare policy to not pay consultation codes, or if they have established their own policies and guidelines for reporting consultations. The American Academy of Pediatrics position on Medicare consultation policy is available at www.aap.org/cfp (access code AAPCFP26).

- If the payer does not pay for consultation codes, the consulting physician reports codes for the appropriate site of service based on the performance and documentation of the required key components or time, if appropriate (**Table 8-3**).
- Documentation of the request for consultation and a report of the results back to the referring physician are required as discussed earlier in this chapter.

Table 8-3. Coding Consultations Under Medicare Rules

New Patient	Established Patient
99202–99205 (office, outpatient hospital, observation)	**99212–99215** (office, outpatient hospital, observation)
99341–99345 (home visit)	**99347–99350** (home visit)
99324–99328 (domiciliary or rest home visit)	**99334–99336** (domiciliary or rest home visit)
99304–99306 (initial nursing facility care)	**99307–99310** (subsequent nursing facility care)

Use **tables 8-2 and 8-3** to determine the appropriate consultation codes in the following examples:

Examples

➤ **A primary care pediatrician consults a pediatrician specializing in diagnosis and treatment of cystic fibrosis for advice on management of a neonate with a positive immunoreactive trypsinogen screening test result but negative DNA screening result.** The patient is new to the consulting pediatrician, who reviews and summarizes the neonate's birth record and test results. A comprehensive history and detailed examination are performed and documented. A sweat test is ordered to confirm or rule out cystic fibrosis.

Chapter 8. Consultations and Residential Evaluation and Management Services

Assessment/plan: Abnormal newborn screening; possible cystic fibrosis. A report is transmitted to the primary care pediatrician outlining the plan for sweat testing and, if indicated, follow-up appointments to assume management of cystic fibrosis.

MDM: High complexity (new problem with additional workup; old record reviewed/summarized, laboratory tests reviewed, and medical test ordered) *History:* Comprehensive *Physical examination:* Detailed	***International Classification of Diseases, 10th Revision, Clinical Modification (ICD-10-CM)*** **P09** (abnormal findings on neonatal screening)
	CPT **99243** or, if payer does not recognize consultations, **New Patient Office E/M** **99204** (moderate MDM—moderate number and complexity of problems and moderate amount and complexity of data reviewed and analyzed)

Teaching Point: The detailed examination limits the consultation code to **99243** because a comprehensive examination is required for **99244**. However, if a payer requires reporting an office or other outpatient E/M service in lieu of an outpatient consultation, code **99204** is supported based on a moderate level of MDM because an undiagnosed new problem with uncertain prognosis was addressed and a moderate amount and complexity of data was analyzed (ie, review of external notes and laboratory tests and order of a sweat test).

Because the code selection guidelines for office E/M services differ from those for consultations, the level of MDM supported for the consultation is high, but the level of MDM for the office visit is moderate. Medical decision-making alone is used in support of **99204**.

➤ **A 13-year-old boy who has obesity and Down syndrome (new patient) is referred to a cardiologist for evaluation of a murmur.** Past medical records and laboratory test results are reviewed and summarized by the cardiologist prior to the visit. A comprehensive history and physical examination are performed. Electrocardiogram (ECG) and echocardiogram are performed and interpreted.

Assessment/plan: Down syndrome. Patient with mitral valve prolapse with minimal regurgitation—will evaluate again in 6 months and start medication, if indicated. Obesity—dietary changes and increased exercise were recommended. A written report is sent back to the referring physician. Total face-to-face time of the consultation service was 30 minutes. Total physician time on the date of service was 60 minutes, not including time spent in interpretation and report of tests.

MDM: Moderate complexity (1 new problem with no additional workup and 1 stable chronic condition; review of laboratory test results and review and summarization of medical records) *History:* Comprehensive *Physical examination:* Comprehensive	***ICD-10-CM*** **I34.1** (nonrheumatic mitral [valve] prolapse) **E66.9** (obesity, unspecified) **Q90.9** (Down syndrome)
	CPT **99244** or, if payer does not recognize consultations, **New Patient** **99205** (60–74 minutes total time)

Teaching Point: The cardiologist evaluated the patient's murmur and addressed obesity. A cardiologist billing for interpretation and report of an ECG and/or echocardiogram will not count the test toward the data analyzed in determining the level of MDM. Where a payer requires an office E/M code in lieu of a consultation code, code **99205** is supported by the cardiologist's total time (60 minutes) on the date of the encounter. If time were used in selection of a consultation code, code **99242** would be reported for 30 minutes of face-to-face time.

➤ **A pediatrician is consulted for a 14-year-old boy who lives in a group home.** The boy has become withdrawn and disinterested in activities that he previously enjoyed. The social worker for the group home is concerned that he may need medical management of depression.

●=New code   ▲=Revised code   #=Re-sequenced code   +=Add-on code

The pediatrician visits the patient at the group home and uses a standardized screening instrument to assess for depression. The score indicates moderate depression. The pediatrician obtains history and conducts an examination (10 minutes) before spending 20 minutes counseling the patient. After the visit, the pediatrician spends 10 minutes on the phone coordinating care with the social worker. The pediatrician spends another 5 minutes with the group home staff to advise of the treatment plan and address their questions about caring for the patient. Diagnosis is moderate major depressive disorder, single episode. Total time is documented as 30 minutes spent face-to-face with more than 50% spent in counseling and/or coordination of care.

ICD-10-CM	CPT
F32.1 (major depressive disorder, single episode, moderate)	The consultant reports **99242** (based on typical time of 30 minutes) or, if the payer does not recognize consultation codes, **99335** (based on typical time of 25 minutes)

Teaching Point: Levels of key components were not provided in this scenario. Time is documented with an indication that more than 50% was spent in counseling and/or coordination of care. Time on the phone with the social worker and in the office of the group home discussing care with the staff would not be attributed to the face-to-face time of the consultation service. Based on the total face-to-face time of 30 minutes, code **99242** is reported.

Coding for visits in a group home is discussed more later in this chapter.

Home Care Services (99341–99350)

- For purposes of reporting home visits, *CPT* defines *home* as a private residence, temporary lodging, or short-term accommodation (eg, hotel, campground, hostel, cruise ship).
- Home visits are typically reported with place of service code **12** (home location, other than hospital or other facility, where patient receives care in a private residence).
- Place of service code **16** (temporary lodging—hotel, campground, hostel, cruise ship, or resort) may also be reported in conjunction with codes **99341–99350**.

Table 8-4. Home Visits for New Patients

Key Components (For a description of key components, see Table 8-1.)
3 of 3 key components must be performed to at least the degree specified under the code.

CPT Code/Time[a]	Medical Decision-making	History[b]	1995 Examination[c]
99341 20 min	Straightforward PP: Usually low severity	HPI: 1–3; ROS: 0; PFSH: 0	1 body area/system
99342 30 min	Low complexity PP: Usually moderate severity	HPI: 1–3; ROS: 1; PFSH: 0	2–7 limited
99343 45 min	Moderate complexity PP: Usually moderate to high severity	HPI: ≥4 or 3 CC; ROS: 2–9; PFSH: 1/3	2–7 detailed
99344 60 min	Moderate complexity PP: Usually moderate to high severity	HPI: ≥4 or 3 CC; ROS: ≥10; PFSH: 3/3	≥8 body areas/systems
99345 75 min	High complexity PP: Usually patient is unstable or has developed a new problem requiring immediate physician attention.	HPI: ≥4 or 3 CC; ROS: ≥10; PFSH: 3/3	≥8 body areas/systems

Abbreviations: CC, chronic condition; *CPT, Current Procedural Terminology;* HPI, history of present illness; PFSH, past, family, and social history; PP, presenting problem; ROS, review of systems.

[a] Typical time is an average and represents a range of times that may be higher or lower depending on clinical circumstances. The presenting problem is considered to be a contributory factor and does not need to be present to the degree specified.

[b] A chief complaint is required for all levels of history.

[c] Number of body areas or organ systems examined; see **Table 8-1** for details.

Table 8-5. Home Visits for Established Patients

Key Components (For a description of key components, see Table 8-1.)
2 of 3 key components must be performed to at least the degree specified under the code. Some payers may require medical decision-making as 1 of the 2 components performed and documented.

CPT Code/Time[a]	Medical Decision-making	History[b]	Examination[c]
99347 15 min	Straightforward PP: Usually self-limited or minor	HPI: 1–3; ROS: 0; PFSH: 0	1 body area/system
99348 25 min	Low complexity PP: Usually low to moderate severity	HPI: 1–3; ROS: 1; PFSH: 0	2–7 limited
99349 40 min	Moderate complexity PP: Usually moderate to high severity	HPI: ≥4 or 3 CC; ROS: 2–9; PFSH: 1/3	2–7 detailed
99350 60 min	Moderate to high complexity PP: Usually moderate to high severity	HPI: ≥4 or 3 CC; ROS: ≥10; PFSH: 2/3	≥8 body areas/systems

Abbreviations: CC, chronic condition; *CPT, Current Procedural Terminology;* HPI, history of present illness; PFSH, past, family, and social history; PP, presenting problem; ROS, review of systems.

[a] Typical time is an average and represents a range of times that may be higher or lower depending on clinical circumstances. The presenting problem is considered to be a contributory factor and does not need to be present to the degree specified.

[b] A chief complaint is required for all levels of history.

[c] Number of body areas or organ systems examined; see **Table 8-1** for details.

- Medicaid plans may vary in sites of service reported as home visits.
- Do not report home visit codes for visits to patients in residential facilities or group homes. See codes for domiciliary, rest home, or custodial care services (**99324–99328** and **99334–99337**).
- Code selection is based on the performance and documentation of the required key components or on time if more than 50% of the time is spent in counseling and/or coordination of care, as seen in **tables 8-4 and 8-5.**
- Travel time to and from a patient's home is assumed to be in the level of care, just as travel time to and from the hospital is included in hospital care codes and is not counted in the time spent. However, if escorting a patient to a medical facility becomes necessary, code **99082** (unusual travel) is available.
- Services provided by a nonphysician provider who does not have his or her own NPI may not be billed unless the physician provides direct supervision. Refer to **Chapter 13**, Qualified Nonphysician Health Care Professional Services.
- Any procedures performed by the physician may be separately reported.
- Payers may have varied policies on coverage and reporting requirements for home visits and may not use Medicare incident-to guidelines. Check with them prior to reporting this service.

Example

➤ **A pediatrician agrees to provide a home visit to a 6-year-old with symptoms of influenza or other upper respiratory illness.** The child was immunized against influenza 1 week ago during a new patient well-child (health supervision) visit. A problem-focused history and examination are documented in addition to results of a point-of-care influenza test that is positive for influenza A. The pediatrician prescribes oseltamivir. The parents are concerned that the immunization did not protect their child. The pediatrician spends 13 minutes counseling the parents about the time from immunization administration to development of immunity and potential for exposure. The total face-to-face time of the visit is 25 minutes.

ICD-10-CM	CPT
J11.1 (influenza due to unidentified influenza virus with other respiratory manifestations)	**99348** (typical time 25 minutes)

Teaching Point: 13 of 25 minutes of the face-to-face visit were spent in counseling and/or coordination of care, supporting code selection based on the total face-to-face time.

Many payers require documentation of medical necessity for provision of services in the home rather than the office. Inclusion of codes that limit the patient's ability to be seen in the office or outpatient clinic may help demonstrate medical necessity.

●=New code   ▲=Revised code   #=Re-sequenced code   +=Add-on code

Domiciliary, Rest Home, or Custodial Care Services (99324–99337)

Table 8-6. Domiciliary, Rest Home, or Custodial Care Services: New Patient

Key Components (For a description of key components, see Table 8-1.)
3 of 3 key components must be performed to at least the degree specified under the code.

CPT Code/Time[a]	Medical Decision-making	History[b]	Examination[c]
99324 20 min	Straightforward PP: Usually low severity	HPI: 1–3; ROS: 0; PFSH: 0	1 body area/ system
99325 30 min	Low complexity PP: Usually moderate severity	HPI: 1–3; ROS: 1; PFSH: 0	2–7 limited
99326 45 min	Moderate complexity PP: Usually moderate to high severity	HPI: ≥4 or 3 CC; ROS: 2–9; PFSH: 1/3	2–7 detailed
99327 60 min	Moderate complexity PP: Usually high severity	HPI: ≥4 or 3 CC; ROS: ≥10; PFSH: 3/3	≥8 body areas/ systems
99328 75 min	High complexity PP: Usually patient is unstable or has developed a new problem requiring immediate physician attention.	HPI: ≥4 or 3 CC; ROS: ≥10; PFSH: 3/3	≥8 body areas/ systems

Abbreviations: CC, chronic condition; *CPT, Current Procedural Terminology*; HPI, history of present illness; PFSH, past, family, and social history; PP, presenting problem; ROS, review of systems.

[a] Typical time is an average and represents a range of times that may be higher or lower depending on clinical circumstances. The presenting problem is considered to be a contributory factor and does not need to be present to the degree specified.

[b] A chief complaint is required for all levels of history.

[c] Number of body areas or organ systems examined; see **Table 8-1** for details.

Table 8-7. Domiciliary, Rest Home, or Custodial Care Services: Established Patient

Key Components (For a description of key components, see Table 8-1.)
2 of 3 key components must be performed to at least the degree specified under the code. Some payers may require medical decision-making as 1 of the 2 components performed and documented.

CPT Code/Time[a]	Medical Decision-making	History[b]	Examination[c]
99334 15 min	Straightforward PP: Usually self-limited to minor	HPI: 1–3; ROS: 0; PFSH: 0	1 body area/system
99335 25 min	Low complexity PP: Usually low to moderate severity	HPI: 1–3; ROS: 1; PFSH: 0	2–7 limited
99336 40 min	Moderate complexity PP: Usually moderate to high severity	HPI: ≥4 or 3 CC; ROS: 2–9; PFSH: 1/3	2–7 detailed
99337 60 min	Moderate to high complexity PP: Usually moderate to high severity; patient may be unstable or develop new problem requiring immediate attention.	HPI: ≥4 or 3 CC; ROS: ≥10; PFSH: 2/3	≥8 body areas/systems

Abbreviations: CC, chronic condition; *CPT, Current Procedural Terminology*; HPI, history of present illness; PFSH, past, family, and social history; PP, presenting problem; ROS, review of systems.

[a] Typical time is an average and represents a range of times that may be higher or lower depending on clinical circumstances. The presenting problem is considered to be a contributory factor and does not need to be present to the degree specified.

[b] A chief complaint is required for all levels of history.

[c] Number of body areas or organ systems examined; see **Table 8-1** for details.

- These services are provided in a facility that provides room and board and other personal assistance services (eg, assisted living facility).
- Codes **99324–99337** are not reported for patients residing in a private residence (see codes **99341–99350**).

- Codes **99324–99328** and **99334–99337** are reported for services provided in facilities assigned the following place of service codes: **13** (assisted living), **14** (group home), **33** (custodial care facility), and **55** (residential substance abuse facility).
- Prolonged services provided in a domiciliary, rest home, or custodial care are reported with codes **99354** and **99355**.

Use **tables 8-6 and 8-7** to select codes for the following example:

Example

➤ **A pediatrician agrees to provide medically necessary services at the infirmary of a youth ranch where the patient lives.** The established patient presents with complaint of a foreign body in his right foot. The pediatrician examines the patient's foot and removes a splinter without making an incision. Documentation includes a problem-focused history and examination and straightforward MDM.

ICD-10-CM	CPT
S90.851A (superficial foreign body, right foot, initial encounter)	99334

Teaching Point: No procedure code is reported because the foreign body was removed without an incision.

The place of service on this claim could be a group home (**14**) or a custodial care facility (**33**). It is important to verify the appropriate place of service for reporting, as it may affect payment and coverage.

Nursing Facility Care

Nursing facility care is provided to patients who require medical, nursing, or rehabilitative services above the level of custodial care but not at the level of care available in a hospital. Place of service codes for nursing facility care were created by Medicare to differentiate between skilled nursing facility care and nursing facility care because Medicare benefits are different for patients requiring skilled nursing care. Medicaid and private payer plans may offer specific instructions on the appropriate places of service for reporting physician services provided in nursing facilities.

Examples of nursing facility services that may be provided during one admission are included in **Table 8-8**. Place of service codes for physician services provided to patients in a nursing facility are described in **Table 8-9**.

Table 8-8. Examples of Nursing Facility Evaluation and Management Services

Service Provided	Procedure Code(s)
A pediatrician accepts management of a child's care following discharge from a rehabilitation hospital for brain injury due to near-drowning and provides initial care in a nursing facility. 60 minutes are spent reviewing the child's history; examining the patient; ordering physical, occupational, and speech-language therapies; obtaining a consultation for possible hyperbaric oxygen therapy; and explaining management plans to the parents.	**99306** (initial nursing facility care, per day requiring a comprehensive history; comprehensive examination; and MDM of high complexity or 45 minutes are spent at the bedside and on the patient's facility floor or unit)
The pediatrician conducts an established patient nursing facility visit to follow the child's progress since the last visit and orders changes to the plan of care based on reports from therapists and clinical staff of the facility. Detailed interval history, detailed examination, and moderate-complexity MDM are documented.	**99309** (subsequent nursing facility care, per day requiring a detailed interval history; detailed examination; and MDM of moderate complexity or 25 minutes are spent at the bedside and on the patient's facility floor or unit)
The pediatrician performs an annual assessment of the child, whose stay in the nursing facility has lasted 1 year. Documentation supports a detailed history, comprehensive examination, and MDM of moderate complexity.	**99318** (annual nursing facility assessment, which requiring a detailed interval history; a comprehensive examination; and MDM of low to moderate complexity and 30 minutes are spent at the bedside and on the patient's facility floor or unit)
The pediatrician spends 45 minutes in discharge management activities to order home health and outpatient therapies for the child, who can now be cared for in the parent's home.	**99316** (nursing facility discharge day management; >30 minutes)
Abbreviation: MDM, medical decision-making.	

Chapter 8. Consultations and Residential Evaluation and Management Services

Table 8-9. Nursing Facility Place of Service Codes	
Place of Service Code	**Description**
31	A facility which primarily provides inpatient skilled nursing care and related services to patients who require medical, nursing, or rehabilitative services but does not provide the level of care or treatment available in a hospital
32	A facility which primarily provides to residents skilled nursing care and related services for the rehabilitation of injured, disabled, or sick persons, or, on a regular basis, health-related care services above the level of custodial care to other than individuals with intellectual disabilities

Initial Nursing Facility Care (99304–99306)

- Services are reported for a new or an established patient.
- The level of service reported is dependent on performance and documentation of the 3 key components (ie, history, physical examination, and MDM) or time if more than 50% of the floor or unit time is spent in counseling and/or care coordination (**Table 8-10**).
- The nursing facility care level of service reported by the admitting physician should include services related to the admission he or she provided in the other sites of service (eg, hospital emergency department, physician's office) on the same date.
  - Do not separately report E/M services performed in other sites of service by the same physician or physicians of the same specialty and same group practice on the same date.
  - *Exception:* When a patient is discharged from hospital inpatient or observation status on the same date of nursing facility admission or readmission, hospital discharge services (**99238**, **99239**, or **99217**) should be reported in addition to the initial nursing facility care. (For a patient admitted and discharged from observation or inpatient status on the same date, see codes **99234–99236**.)
- For nursing facility care discharge, see codes **99315** and **99316** (discussed later in this chapter).

Table 8-10. Initial Nursing Facility Care: New or Established Patient			
Key Components (For a description of key components, see Table 8-1.) 3 of 3 key components must be performed to at least the degree specified for each code.			
CPT Code/Time[a]	**Medical Decision-making**	**History[b]**	**Examination[c]**
99304 25 min	Straightforward or low PP: Usually low severity	HPI: ≥4 or 3 CC; ROS: 2–9; PFSH: 1/3	2–7 detailed
99305 35 min	Moderate complexity PP: Usually moderate severity	HPI: ≥4 or 3 CC; ROS: ≥10; PFSH: 3/3	≥8 body areas/systems
99306 45 min	High complexity PP: Usually high severity	HPI: ≥4 or 3 CC; ROS: ≥10; PFSH: 3/3	≥8 body areas/systems

Abbreviations: CC, chronic condition; *CPT, Current Procedural Terminology;* HPI, history of present illness; PFSH, past, family, and social history; PP, presenting problem; ROS, review of systems.

[a] Typical time is an average and represents a range of times that may be higher or lower depending on clinical circumstances. The presenting problem is considered to be a contributory factor and does not need to be present to the degree specified.

[b] A chief complaint is required for all levels of history.

[c] Number of body areas or organ systems examined; see **Table 8-1** for details.

- Prolonged service provided in conjunction with a face-to-face nursing facility service is reported with codes **99356** and **99357**. For more information on these codes, see **Chapter 16**, Noncritical Hospital Evaluation and Management Services.

Subsequent Nursing Facility Care (99307–99310)

- Codes are used to report services provided to residents of nursing facilities who do not require a comprehensive assessment and/or who have not had a major, permanent change of status.
- Code selection is based on the performance and documentation of 2 of the 3 key components or time if more than 50% of the floor or unit time is spent in counseling and/or coordination of care (**Table 8-11**).

- All levels of service include reviewing the medical record and results of diagnostic studies, noting changes in the resident's status and response to management since the last visit, and reviewing and signing orders.
- An interval history, not requiring past, family, or social history, is used in selecting the level of history.

Table 8-11. Subsequent Nursing Facility Care

Key Components (For a description of key components, see Table 8-1.)

2 of 3 key components must be performed to at least the degree specified for each code. Some payers may require medical decision-making as 1 of the 2 components performed and documented.

CPT Code/Time[a]	Medical Decision-making	History[b]	Examination[c]
99307 10 min	Straightforward PP: Usually stable, recovering, or improving	HPI: 1–3; ROS: 0; PFSH: 0	1 body area/system
99308 15 min	Low complexity PP: Usually responding inadequately to therapy or minor complication	HPI: 1–3; ROS: 1; PFSH: 0	2–7 limited
99309 25 min	Moderate complexity PP: Usually patient develops significant complication or new problem.	HPI: ≥4 or 3 CC; ROS: 2–9; PFSH: 0	2–7 detailed
99310 35 min	High complexity PP: Usually patient is unstable or has a new problem requiring immediate attention.	HPI: ≥4 or 3 CC; ROS: ≥10; PFSH: 0	≥8 body areas/systems

Abbreviations: CC, chronic condition; *CPT, Current Procedural Terminology;* HPI, history of present illness; PFSH, past, family, and social history; PP, presenting problem; ROS, review of systems.

[a] Typical time is an average and represents a range of times that may be higher or lower depending on clinical circumstances. The presenting problem is considered to be a contributory factor and does not need to be present to the degree specified.

[b] A chief complaint is required for all levels of history.

[c] Number of body areas or organ systems examined; see **Table 8-1** for details.

Nursing Facility Discharge Services (99315, 99316)

- The nursing facility discharge day management codes (**Table 8-12**) are used to report the total time spent by a physician for the final nursing facility discharge of a patient, even if the time spent by the physician on that date is not continuous.
- The codes include, as appropriate, final patient examination and discussion of the nursing facility stay. Instructions are given to all relevant caregivers for continuing care, preparation of discharge records, prescriptions, and referral forms.
- If the work of performing the discharge management is more than 30 minutes, the total time must be documented in the medical record.

Table 8-12. Nursing Facility Discharge Services

99315	Nursing facility discharge day management; 30 minutes or less
99316	more than 30 minutes

Annual Nursing Facility Assessment (99318)

Code **99318** is used to report a comprehensive annual assessment that includes a detailed interval history, comprehensive physical examination, and minimum data set or resident assessment instrument evaluation. The patient's and family's goals for care and preferences for medical interventions are assessed, including, if applicable, reassessment of advance directives and updates of contact information for surrogate decision-makers. **Table 8-13** describes the 3 key components for code **99318**.

Chapter 8. Consultations and Residential Evaluation and Management Services

Table 8-13. Annual Nursing Facility Assessment

Key Components (For a description of key components, see Table 8-1.)
3 of 3 key components must be performed to at least the degree specified under the code.

CPT Code/Time[a]	Medical Decision-making	History[b]	Examination[c]
99318 30 min	Low to moderate complexity PP: Usually stable, recovering, or improving	HPI: ≥4 or 3 CC; ROS: 2–9; PFSH: 0	≥8 body areas/systems

Abbreviations: CC, chronic condition; CPT, *Current Procedural Terminology*; HPI, history of present illness; PFSH, past, family, and social history; PP, presenting problem; ROS, review of systems.

[a] Typical time is an average and represents a range of times that may be higher or lower depending on clinical circumstances. The presenting problem is considered to be a contributory factor and does not need to be present to the degree specified.

[b] A chief complaint is required for all levels of history.

[c] Number of body areas or organ systems examined; see **Table 8-1** for details.

Out-of-Office Service Add-on Codes (99056–99060)

Codes **99056–99060** are used to report services that are provided after hours or on an emergency basis and are an adjunct to the basic E/M service provided.

Third-party payers will have specific policies for coverage and payment. Communicate with individual payers to understand their definition or interpretation of the service and their coverage and payment policies. As part of this negotiation and education process, it is important to demonstrate the cost savings recognized by the payer for these adjunct services. After-hours service codes are used by physicians or other QHPs (under their state scope of practice and when billing with their own NPI) to identify the services that are adjunct to the basic services rendered. These codes

- Describe the special circumstances under which a basic procedure is performed.
- Are only reported in addition to an associated basic service (eg, home visit).
- Are reported without a modifier appended to the basic service because they only further describe the services provided.

99056   Service(s) typically provided in the office, provided out of the office at request of patient, in addition to basic service

Documentation should include the patient's request to be seen outside of the office.

99060   Service(s) provided on an emergency basis, out of the office, which disrupts other scheduled office services, in addition to basic service

Documentation should indicate that the physician was called away during scheduled office hours to attend to a patient in another location (eg, nursing facility).

Example

➤ **A 10-year-old is seen in her home for exacerbation of moderate persistent asthma at the request of the parents.** The pediatrician evaluates the patient, who is improved after a self-administered inhalation treatment. The child has had 2 urgent visits for exacerbation of asthma in the past 4 months. The parents and child are counseled about medication compliance and control of allergens in the home and given an action plan for home and school. The total time of the visit is 25 minutes, including 15 minutes spent in counseling. The diagnosis is exacerbation of moderate persistent asthma.

ICD-10-CM	CPT
J45.41 (moderate persistent asthma with acute exacerbation)	**99348** (established home E/M with typical time of 25 minutes) **99056** (service[s] typically provided in the office, provided out of the office at request of patient, in addition to basic service)

    Teaching Point: Payers may or may not allow payment for code **99056** when services are rendered in the patient's home. The level of home visit was determined by time because more than 50% of the visit was spent in counseling and/or coordination of care.

Telephone Services (99441–99443, 98966–98968)

99441	Telephone E/M service by a physician or other qualified health care professional who may report evaluation and management services provided to an established patient, parent, or guardian not originating from a related E/M service provided within the previous 7 days nor leading to an E/M service or procedure within the next 24 hours or soonest available appointment; 5–10 minutes of medical discussion
99442	11–20 minutes of medical discussion
99443	21–30 minutes of medical discussion
98966	Telephone assessment and management services provided by a qualified nonphysician health care professional to an established patient, parent, or guardian not originating from a related assessment and management service provided within the previous 7 days nor leading to an assessment and management service or procedure within the next 24 hours or soonest available appointment; 5–10 minutes of medical discussion
98967	11–20 minutes of medical discussion
98968	21–30 minutes of medical discussion

Codes **99441–99443** may be reported when

- The call was initiated by an established patient or guardian of an established patient.
- They include physician management of a new problem that does not result in an office visit within 24 hours from the telephone call or at the next available urgent visit appointment.
- They include physician management of an existing problem for which the patient was not seen in a face-to-face encounter in the previous 7 days from the telephone call (physician requested or unsolicited patient follow-up) or within the postoperative period of a performed and reported procedure.
- The physician documentation of telephone calls includes the date of the call, name and telephone number of the patient, name of person and relationship of the caller, type of service provided (eg, provide consultation or medical management, initiate or adjust therapy, report results), and the time spent in the encounter.

Codes **99441–99443** are *not* reported when

- The call results in a face-to-face encounter within 24 hours.
- There was a face-to-face encounter related to the problem in the previous 7 days from the telephone call.
- The call occurs within the postoperative period of a reported procedure.
- The call occurs within 7 days of a previously reported telephone management service.
- Care plan oversight (**99339, 99340, 99374–99380**), care management (**99487–99490**), or transitional care management (**99495, 99496**) services are reported and the calls are included as part of these services.
- Non–face-to-face communication is between the physician and other health care professionals. If applicable, the services may be reported using non–face-to-face prolonged physician service codes **99358** and **99359** or as part of care plan oversight or care management services (**99339, 99340; 99374–99380; 99487–99490; 99495, 99496**).
- Performed by a provider who may not report E/M services. (See codes **98966–98968** for services by QHPs who may not report E/M services.)

Telephone services (**99441–99443**) are non–face-to-face E/M services provided to a patient using the telephone by a physician or other QHP who may report E/M services.

Codes **98966–98968** are used to report telephone assessment and management services by health care professionals who may not report E/M services (eg, occupational therapists, speech-language pathologists).

Guidelines for reporting of telephone assessment and management services are the same as those for physician and QHP telephone E/M services.

Prolonged Services

Prolonged Service With Direct Patient Contact (99354–99357)

+★▲**99354**	Prolonged service(s) in the outpatient setting requiring direct patient contact beyond the time of the usual service; first hour
+**99355**	each additional 30 minutes
+**99356**	Prolonged service in the inpatient or observation setting, requiring unit/floor time beyond the usual service; first hour
+**99357**	each additional 30 minutes

Chapter 8. Consultations and Residential Evaluation and Management Services

Prolonged service codes **99354** and **99355** are used to report 30 minutes or more of a physician's or QHP's prolonged face-to-face E/M service provided on the same date as designated E/M services that have a typical or designated time published in *CPT* or for prolonged service in conjunction with psychotherapy of 60 minutes or more (**90837**).

Prolonged service codes **99356** and **99357** are used to report 30 minutes or more of a physician's or QHP's prolonged unit/floor time of an E/M service provided on the same date as nursing facility services. See **Chapter 16** for more information on these codes.

Prolonged Service Without Direct Patient Contact (99358, 99359)

99358   Prolonged evaluation and management service before and/or after direct patient care; first hour

+99359   each additional 30 minutes (Use in conjunction with code **99358**.)

Prolonged service without direct patient contact (ie, non–face-to-face) is reported when a physician provides prolonged service that does not involve face-to-face care. The prolonged service must relate to a service and patient where direct (face-to-face) patient care has occurred or will occur and to ongoing patient management.

Only time spent by a physician or other QHP may be counted toward the time of prolonged service. Prolonged service of less than 30 minutes on a given date is not separately reported. Report code **99359** for 15 or more minutes beyond the first hour or the last full 30-minute period of prolonged service. See **Chapter 12**, Outpatient Management of Chronic and Complex Conditions, for more information and a coding example.

Critical Care (99291, 99292)

Regardless of the patient's age, critical care services provided in outpatient settings are reported with hourly critical care codes (**99291, 99292**).

> See Chapter 18 for reporting guidelines for critical care services.

If the same patient requires outpatient and inpatient critical care services on the same day, the physician or a physician of the same group and specialty would report his or her services based on where the services were provided as well as the patient's age. Refer to **Figure 8-1** for information on coding when critical care occurs in the outpatient setting.

Examples

➤ **A 3-year-old girl with moderate persistent childhood asthma is seen in her home with complaints of shortness of breath and wheezing.** The patient goes into respiratory failure with hypoxia, and her vital signs are deteriorating. The physician initiates critical care. An ambulance is called, and the physician continues critical care services until the transport team accepts care of the patient. The total time for critical care services provided in the child's home was 35 minutes. The patient is admitted to the pediatric intensive care unit under a pediatric intensivist. The pediatrician provides no more hands-on care for the patient that day and reports outpatient critical care services with a diagnosis of respiratory failure due to status asthmaticus. Documentation includes the critical nature of the patient's condition, the care provided, and the total time spent in critical care dedicated to this patient.

ICD-10-CM	CPT
J96.01 (acute respiratory failure with hypoxia) **J45.42** (moderate persistent asthma with status asthmaticus)	**99291** (critical care, first 30–74 minutes)

Teaching Point: If the same physician or physician of the same specialty and group practice provided outpatient and inpatient critical care services on the same calendar date, due to the patient's age, only the per-day critical care code (**99475**, initial inpatient pediatric critical care, per day, for the E/M of a critically ill infant or young child, 2–5 years of age) would be reported. Had the patient been 6 years or older, the time spent in outpatient critical care would be combined with time spent providing critical care in the inpatient setting.

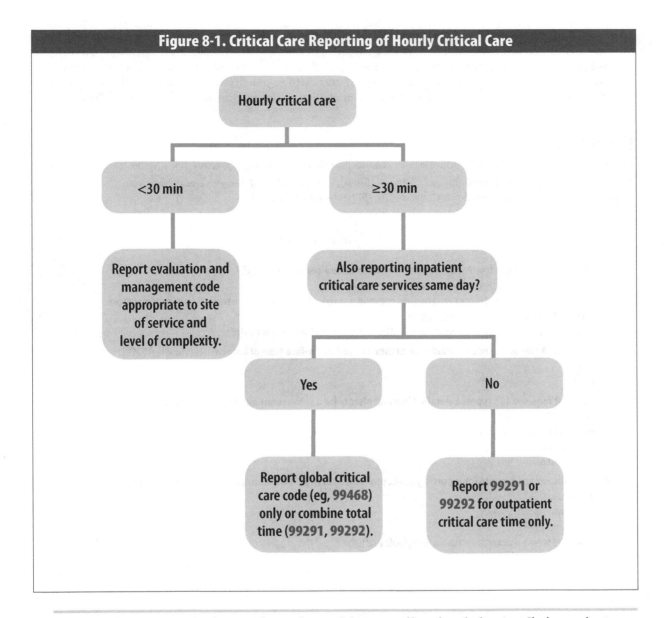

Figure 8-1. Critical Care Reporting of Hourly Critical Care

➤ **A 3-year-old girl is seen in her home with complaints of shortness of breath and wheezing.** She has moderate persistent childhood asthma. During the physician's examination, the patient goes into respiratory failure with hypoxia, and vital signs are deteriorating. The physician initiates critical care. An ambulance is called, and the physician continues critical care services until the transport team accepts care of the patient. The total time for critical care services provided in the child's home was 25 minutes. The patient is admitted to the pediatric intensive care unit at the local university hospital under a pediatric intensivist. The pediatrician provides no more hands-on care for the patient that day and reports a home visit with a diagnosis of respiratory failure due to status asthmaticus. Documentation includes a detailed history, comprehensive examination, and high-complexity MDM due to the critical nature of the patient's condition and the care provided.

ICD-10-CM	CPT
J96.01 (acute respiratory failure with hypoxia) **J45.42** (moderate persistent asthma with status asthmaticus)	**99350**

●=New code   ▲=Revised code   #=Re-sequenced code   +=Add-on code

Teaching Point: Critical care of less than 30 minutes is reported with an E/M code appropriate to the place of service—in this case, home visit E/M. Code **99350** is supported by a new problem (respiratory failure) requiring additional workup and high risk of morbidity/mortality due to organ failure. If the home visit was requested by the patient's parent/caregiver in lieu of care in an office or other outpatient setting, code **99056** (service[s] typically provided in the office, provided out of the office at request of patient, in addition to basic service) may be reported in addition to **99350**.

Resources

American Academy of Pediatrics position on Medicare consultation policy (www.aap.org/cfp; access code AAPCFP26)

"Consultations: Aligning With Payer Guidelines (Online Exclusive), " January 2018 *AAP Pediatric Coding Newsletter™* (https://coding.solutions.aap.org/article.aspx?articleid=2667610; subscription required)

Test Your Knowledge!

1. **Which of the following is true for outpatient consultation services 99241–99245?**
   a. The request for consultation must be documented.
   b. Codes **99241–99245** and office evaluation and management codes (**99202–99205**) have the same key components.
   c. Codes distinguish new or established patients.
   d. Codes **99241–99245** may be selected based on the physician's total time on the date of service.

2. **True or false? A physician should include travel time in the face-to-face time of home visits (99341–99350).**
   a. True
   b. False

3. **Which is not required to support a detailed interval history for a subsequent nursing facility visit?**
   a. Review of 2 to 9 systems
   b. Past, family, and social history
   c. A chief complaint
   d. A history of present illness

4. **Which codes are appropriate for reporting direct prolonged service on the unit/floor of a nursing facility?**
   a. **99356** and **99357**
   b. **99354** and **99355**
   c. **99358** and **99359**
   d. Prolonged service is not reported in a nursing facility setting.

CHAPTER 9

Preventive Services

Contents

Preventive Care

Preventive care is the hallmark of pediatrics. The Patient Protection and Affordable Care Act (PPACA) recognized the importance of preventive care for children and includes a critical provision that ensures that most health care plans cover, *without cost sharing*, the criterion standard of pediatric preventive care—the American Academy of Pediatrics (AAP) *Bright Futures: Guidelines for Health Supervision of Infants, Children, and Adolescents*, 4th Edition.

Coverage of and appropriate payment for these pediatric preventive services should, at a minimum, reflect the total relative value units (RVUs) outlined for the current year under the Medicare Resource-Based Relative Value Scale Physician Fee Schedule (PFS), inclusive of all separately reported codes for these services. Section 2713 of the PPACA includes the following 2 sets of services that must be provided to children without cost sharing:

1. The standard set of immunizations recommended by the Advisory Committee on Immunization Practices (ACIP) of the Centers for Disease Control and Prevention (CDC) with respect to the individual involved
2. Evidence-informed preventive care and screenings provided for in the comprehensive guidelines supported by the Health Resources and Services Administration (HRSA), which include
   - Bright Futures recommendations for preventive pediatric health care
   - Recommendations of the Advisory Committee on Heritable Disorders in Newborns and Children

The Bright Futures periodicity schedule, "Recommendations for Preventive Pediatric Health Care," is a great tool to identify recommended age-appropriate services; in addition, it can be used to identify those services that can and should be reported with their own *Current Procedural Terminology* (*CPT*®) or Healthcare Common Procedure Coding System code, and it identifies appropriate diagnosis coding. This tool can be found as an insert in this book and can be accessed online at www.aap.org/periodicityschedule.

Although all recommended preventive services are covered, physicians and practice managers should be aware of health plan policies that may affect payment.

- Specific diagnosis codes may be required to support claims adjudication under preventive medicine benefits. Be sure to link the appropriate diagnosis to each service provided (eg, code **Z71.3**, dietary counseling, may be linked to code **99401** for a risk-factor reduction counseling visit).
- Some payers bundle certain services when the services are provided on the same date. For instance, some plans will not allow separate payment for obesity counseling on the same date as a well-child examination (health supervision visit) but will cover obesity counseling when no other evaluation and management (E/M) service is provided on the same date.
  - It is beneficial to monitor and maintain awareness of the payment policies of the plans most commonly billed by your practice.
  - Most policies are available on payers' websites with notification of changes provided in payer communications, such as electronic newsletters.

Preventive Medicine Evaluation and Management Services

Well-child or preventive medicine services are a type of E/M service and are reported with codes **99381–99395**. Most health plans provide a 100% benefit (no patient out-of-pocket cost) for the 31 recommended preventive medicine service encounters when provided by in-network providers. The selection of the pediatric-specific codes **99381–99395** is based simply on the age of the patient and whether the patient is new or established to the practice (**Table 9-1**).

Table 9-1. New and Established Preventive Medicine Codes		
Code Description **Comprehensive preventive medicine evaluation and management**	**New Patient Code**	**Established Patient Code**
infant (age <1 year)	99381	99391
early childhood (age 1–4 years)	99382	99392
late childhood (age 5–11 years)	99383	99393
adolescent (age 12–17 years)	99384	99394
age 18–39 years	99385	99395

●=New code ▲=Revised code #=Re-sequenced code +=Add-on code

In brief, an established patient has been seen (face-to-face, including via real-time audiovisual telehealth) by the physician or another physician of the same specialty and group practice within the last 3 years. Generally, other qualified health care professionals (QHPs) are considered to be working in the same specialty as the physicians with whom they work. Refer to **Chapter 7**, Office and Other Outpatient Evaluation and Management Services, for more information about *new* versus *established* patients.

- Most health plans will limit the benefits for preventive medicine E/M services covered in a year based on the patient's age. See **Figure 9-1** for an illustration of recommended preventive visits by age.

Figure 9-1. Preventive Visits by Patient Age as Recommended by the American Academy of Pediatrics/Bright Futures Periodicity Schedule

6 Visits
- 3–5 days
- 1, 2, 4, 6, and 9 months

3 Visits
- 12, 15, and 18 months

2 Visits
- 24 and 30 months

1 Visit
- Ages 3 to 21 years (per year/per 12 months)

- Immunizations, laboratory tests, and other special procedures or screening tests (eg, vision, hearing, developmental screening) that have their own specific *CPT* codes are reported separately *in addition to* preventive medicine E/M services.
- Most payers will require reporting modifier **25** with the preventive medicine service when immunizations or other services are also performed and reported.
- A comprehensive history and physical examination must reflect an age- and a gender-appropriate history and examination and are *not* synonymous with the "comprehensive" history and examination described in the E/M documentation guidelines from the Centers for Medicare & Medicaid Services (CMS) (see **Chapter 6**, Evaluation and Management Documentation Guidelines Other Than Office and Other Outpatient Services).
- The comprehensive history performed as part of a preventive medicine visit does not require a chief complaint or history of present illness. It does require a comprehensive age-appropriate review of systems (ROS) with an updated past, family, and social history. The history should also include a comprehensive assessment or history of age-pertinent risk factors.

Generally, the ROS of a preventive medicine service is not a list of systems with pertinent positive and negative responses but, rather, a list of inquiries and patient responses for those areas of risk identified in preventive medicine guidelines as pertinent for patients of that age and gender. However, some payers may require review of all systems regardless of age and gender (eg, required by some Medicaid plans under Early and Periodic Screening, Diagnostic, and Treatment [EPSDT] benefits).

- Routine management of contraception is considered part of the comprehensive preventive medicine E/M service when it is provided during the well-care health supervision visit.
- A comprehensive physical examination is a multisystem examination that may include a routine pelvic and breast examination (when performed in the absence of specific symptoms of a separate problem) depending on the age of the patient and/or sexual history. If the pelvic examination is performed because of a gynecologic problem during a routine preventive medicine service, it may be appropriate to report a problem-oriented E/M service in addition to the preventive medicine service when additional physician work and required key components of the E/M code are met.
- State Medicaid programs have requirements for performing, documenting, and reporting certain services in their EPSDT programs. Review your state Medicaid policies for the specific documentation and reporting requirements for services to patients in these programs.

ICD-10-CM Codes for Preventive Care Visits

International Classification of Diseases, 10th Revision, Clinical Modification (ICD-10-CM) well-care diagnosis codes should be linked to the appropriate preventive medicine code (**99381–99395**). *ICD-10-CM* codes for well-child examinations include developmental, hearing, and vision screening.

Z00.110	Health supervision for newborn <8 days
Z00.111	Health supervision for newborn 8–28 days old
Z00.121	Routine child health examination (≥29 days) with abnormal findings
Z00.129	Routine child health examination (≥29 days) without abnormal findings
Z00.00	Encounter for general adult medical examination without abnormal findings
Z00.01	Encounter for general adult medical examination with abnormal findings

- For the purpose of assigning codes from this category, an *abnormal finding* is a newly discovered condition on a screen or a known or chronic condition that requires attention (eg, uncontrolled, acutely exacerbated). Assign additional codes for any abnormal findings. A stable chronic condition is not considered an abnormal finding.
- *ICD-10-CM* does not specify an age at which codes **Z00.00** and **Z00.01** are reported in lieu of codes **Z00.121–Z00.129**. The age of majority varies by state and payers, who may or may not adopt the Medicare Outpatient Code Editor assignment of age limitations (29 days–17 years) to codes **Z00.121–Z00.129**, as indicated in many *ICD-10-CM* references.
- Code **Z23** (encounter for immunization) must be reported in addition to the routine health examination codes (eg, **Z00.129**) when immunizations are administered at the preventive medicine encounter. *ICD-10-CM* instructs to code **Z00** first, followed by code **Z23**.
- When an existing problem is addressed at the preventive medicine service but is not a newly discovered condition or a known or chronic condition that has increased in severity, report a routine child health examination without abnormal findings and also code the condition addressed.

Examples

➤ **A 2-year-old is seen for an established patient preventive medicine service.** The child was seen 1 week ago for acute otitis media of the left ear. Parents report no fever or signs of further illness or pain. On examination, the tympanic membrane is improved from the prior encounter. An age- and a gender-appropriate preventive service is provided and documented. Parents are reassured that the ear infection is resolving as expected and instructed to follow up if new concerns arise. Diagnoses are resolving otitis media of the left ear (**H65.192**) and well-child visit.

ICD-10-CM	CPT
Z00.129 (routine child health exam without abnormal findings) **H65.192** (other acute nonsuppurative otitis media, left ear)	**99392** (preventive medicine visit; age 1–4)

Teaching Point: Because the otitis media is not newly identified or failing to respond adequately to treatment, this is not an abnormal finding. However, it is appropriate to report the code for the otitis media that is still present in addition to code **Z00.129**. In this example, the work of noting the improved otitis media did not equate to a significant, separately identifiable E/M service.

➤ **A 3-year-old was diagnosed 1 week ago with recurrent bilateral otitis media with effusion (H65.196).** The child presents today for a scheduled preventive service and follow-up visit. On examination, the eardrums are still inflamed, and the child complains of intermittent pain. A different class of antibiotic is prescribed and after discussion with the parents, referral to an otolaryngologist is made. The age- and gender-appropriate preventive service is also provided and documented. The diagnoses are well-child visit with abnormal findings (**Z00.121**) and recurrent bilateral otitis media.

ICD-10-CM	CPT
Z00.121 (routine child health exam with abnormal findings) **H65.196** (other acute nonsuppurative otitis media, recurrent, bilateral)	**99392** (preventive medicine visit; age 1–4)
H65.196	**99213 25**

●=New code   ▲=Revised code   #=Re-sequenced code   +=Add-on code

Chapter 9. Preventive Services

Teaching Point: Because the otitis media was inadequately controlled, the routine health examination included an abnormal finding. If the otitis media had resolved, code **Z00.129** (routine child health exam without abnormal findings) would be reported. See more on reporting problem-oriented E/M services in conjunction with a preventive service later in this chapter. Code **H65.916** is reported once on the claim but linked to each procedure code.

Quality Initiatives and Preventive Care

Quality initiatives and measurement are becoming standard practice in health care. Many physicians have participated in quality measurement through programs such as the CMS Promoting Interoperability Programs and medical home recognition programs. In pediatrics, many quality measures are associated with preventive care (eg, provision of one meningococcal vaccine on or between the patient's 11th and 13th birthdays).

Quality measurement is also required of health plans funded by government programs or offered through health exchanges created to support health insurance adoption under the PPACA. These health plans must collect and submit Quality Rating System measure data to the CMS. This entails collecting clinical quality measures, including a subset of the National Committee for Quality Assurance Healthcare Effectiveness Data and Information Set (HEDIS) measures and a Pharmacy Quality Alliance measure. Physicians contracting with these plans may be asked to provide evidence that quality measures were met through claims data or medical records. It is important to note that a request for medical records is less likely when claims are submitted with procedure and diagnosis codes associated with pediatric quality measures. Examples of HEDIS measures related to preventive care include

- Percentage of members 12 to 21 years of age who had at least 1 comprehensive well-care visit with a primary care provider or obstetrician-gynecologist during the measurement year
- Percentage of members who were 3, 4, 5, or 6 years of age who received 1 or more well-child visits with a primary care provider during the measurement year
- Percentage of members who turned 15 months old during the measurement year and who had 6 or more well-child visits with a primary care provider during the first 15 months after birth
- Members 3 to 17 years of age who had an outpatient visit with a primary care provider and who had the following services in the current year:
  — Body mass index (BMI) percentile documentation
  — Counseling for nutrition
  — Counseling for physical activity

Certain preventive services, such as anticipatory guidance on healthy diet and exercise, are components of the preventive medicine service and require no additional procedure coding for payment purposes. However, associated diagnosis and procedure codes may be reported to support quality reporting initiatives.

> It is important to note that a request for medical records is less likely when claims are submitted with procedure and diagnosis codes associated with pediatric quality measures.

Example

➤ **A group practice participates in a quality improvement program that requires documentation of counseling for nutrition and for physical activity at all well-child visits for children and teens aged 3 to 17 years.** A preventive service is provided to an established patient (aged 14 years), including documentation of the teen's BMI and counseling for healthy diet and exercise.

ICD-10-CM	CPT
Z00.129 (routine child health exam without abnormal findings)	**99394**
Z71.3 (dietary counseling) **Z71.82** (exercise counseling)	**3008F** (BMI, documented)

Teaching Point: *ICD-10-CM* codes for BMI percentiles (**Z68.51–Z68.54**) are reported *only in conjunction with diagnosis of a related condition* (eg, underweight, overweight, obesity), which is official guidance from *Coding Clinic.*

Certain procedure codes also support quality measurement. For example, submission of claims containing codes for meningococcal (**90734**, **#90619**); tetanus, diphtheria, and acellular pertussis (Tdap) (**90715**); and 2 or 3 doses of human papillomavirus (HPV) vaccine (**90649–90651**) provided to an adolescent before the patient's 13th birthday is indicative of meeting the measure for the immunization of adolescents.

Codes **Z13.41** (encounter for autism screening) and **Z13.42** (encounter for screening for global developmental delays [milestones]) may be used to track developmental screening measures of the Child Core Set for patients receiving benefits through their state Medicaid and Children's Health Insurance Program. Use of the Child Core Set is optional for state programs and physicians. Codes **Z13.41** and **Z13.42** may be reported at any encounter where screening is performed (eg, with or without a preventive E/M service).

> See Chapter 3, Coding to Demonstrate Quality and Value, for more information on Healthcare Effectiveness Data and Information Set and quality reporting.

Sports/Camp Physicals

CPT guidelines recommend that preventive medicine service codes (**99381–99395**) be reported when possible for physicals performed to determine participation eligibility. These codes most accurately describe the services performed in that they are preventive and age appropriate in nature and physicians offer counseling on topics such as appropriate levels of exercise or injury prevention. However, the need for these services often arises after the child has had a yearly preventive medicine service, thereby rendering this service non-covered by some health plans, which allow only 1 preventive service per year. In this case, the parent may be billed if the payer contract allows because the service is non-covered.

Office visit codes (**99212–99215**) may be used if a problem is discovered during the service. Outpatient consultation codes (**99241–99245**) might be considered if the coach or school nurse requested the physician's opinion of a suspected problem (ie, exercise cough associated with reduced performance in cold weather). The medical record must include documentation of the written or verbal request as well as a copy of the written report with the physician's opinion or advice that was sent back to the coach or school nurse. *ICD-10-CM* code **Z02.5** is reported for an encounter for examination for participation in sports. If the preparticipation physical evaluation is incorporated into the annual well health supervision visit, use code **Z00.121** or **Z00.129** in lieu of **Z02.5**. Any problems or conditions that are addressed during the course of the visit would also be reported.

When reporting sports or camp physicals for patients with Medicare or Medicaid managed care plans, check the plan's policy on payment for these services and instructions for coding and billing. Under some Medicaid plans, school and preparticipation physical evaluations may be covered even when the child has already had an annual preventive medicine service.

Immunizations

Vaccine services are reported using 2 families of *CPT* codes—one for the vaccine serum (the product) and one for the services associated with the administration of the vaccine. Exceptions to this fall under those patients receiving vaccines through the Vaccines for Children (VFC) program. See the Vaccines for Children Program section later in this chapter for more details on VFC coding.

Vaccines and Toxoids

> The administration of immune globulins (including palivizumab [Synagis]) is not reported using the immunization administration codes. See codes 96365–96368, 96372, 96374, and 96375. Medications, including birth control, are reported with 96372 (therapeutic, prophylactic, or diagnostic subcutaneous or intramuscular injection).

Codes **90476–90756** are used to report the vaccine or toxoid product only. They do not include the administration of a vaccine.
- **Appendix III**, Vaccine Products: Commonly Administered Pediatric Vaccines, provides a quick reference to codes, descriptors, and the number of vaccine components for each vaccine linked to the brand and manufacturer for each.
- The exact vaccine product administered needs to be reported to meet the requirements of immunization registries, vaccine distribution programs, and reporting systems (eg, Vaccine Adverse Event Reporting System), as well as for payment.

Chapter 9. Preventive Services

- Codes may be specific to the product manufacturer and brand, schedule (ie, number of doses or timing), chemical formulation, dosage, appropriate age guidelines, and/or route of administration.
- Codes for combination vaccines (eg, **90707**, measles, mumps, rubella, and varicella virus vaccine) are available, as are separate codes for single-component vaccines (eg, **90716**, varicella virus vaccine).
- It is not appropriate to code each component of a combination vaccine separately using separate vaccine product codes when a combination vaccine is administered. However, if a combination vaccine is commercially available but a physician elects to administer the component vaccines due to unavailability or other clinical reason, each vaccine product administered would be separately reported.

> The word *component* refers to an antigen in a vaccine that prevents disease(s) caused by 1 organism.

New Vaccines/Toxoids

The *CPT* Editorial Panel, in recognition of the public health interest in vaccine products, has chosen to publish new vaccine product codes prior to US Food and Drug Administration (FDA) approval. The American Medical Association (AMA) uses its *CPT* site (www.ama-assn.org/practice-management/cpt/category-i-vaccine-codes) to provide updates of *CPT* Editorial Panel actions on new vaccine products. Once approved by the *CPT* Editorial Panel, vaccine/toxoid product codes are typically made available for release on a semiannual basis (July 1 and January 1). As part of the electronic distribution, there is a 6-month implementation period from the initial release date (ie, codes released on January 1 are eligible for use on July 1; codes released on July 1 are eligible for use on January 1). Codes for products pending FDA approval are indicated with a lightning bolt symbol (⚡) and will be tracked by the AMA to monitor FDA approval status. The lightning bolt symbol will be removed once the FDA status changes to "approved." Refer to the AMA *CPT* site indicated earlier for the most up-to-date information on codes with this symbol. More rapid code release and implementation may occur when a government agency has identified an urgent need for a vaccine to address an emergent health issue and the FDA has granted that vaccine an expedited review process. In such cases, codes may be approved and released on an *immediate* (ie, outside the normal code consideration schedule) or *rapid* (ie, within the normal code consideration schedule but released shortly after approval with an implementation date within 3 months of release) basis.

Before administering any new vaccine product or an existing vaccine product with new recommendations, make certain the CDC, in the *Morbidity and Mortality Weekly Report,* or the AAP, in *Pediatrics,* has endorsed the use or recommendations of the vaccine. You may also want to verify with a patient's health plan that the vaccine is covered.

If a vaccine enters the market this year and is FDA approved, recommendations for use are published by the CDC or AAP, and no code exists for the specific vaccine, use code **90749** (unlisted vaccine/toxoid) and list the specific vaccine given.

National Drug Code

Table 9-2. National Drug Code Format Examples		
Product	**10-digit NDCs**	**11-digit NDCs (Added zero [0] is underscored.)**
RotaTeq 2-mL single-dose tube, package of 25	0006-4047-20 (4-4-2 format)	00006-4047-20[a] 00006-4047-01[b]
Fluzone Quadrivalent 0.50-mL prefilled single-dose syringe, package of 10	49281-420-50 (5-3-2 format)	49281-0420-50[a] 49281-0420-88[b]
Synagis 0.5-mL in 1 vial, single dose	60574-4114-1 (5-4-1 format)	60574-4114-01

Abbreviation: NDC, National Drug Code.

[a] Used when payer requires NDC from outer packaging.
[b] Used when payer requires NDC from unit-of-use (eg, single-dose vial).

Many payers, specifically Medicare, Medicaid, other government payers (eg, Tricare), and other private payers, require the use of the National Drug Code (NDC) when reporting vaccine product codes. The NDCs are universal product identifiers for medications, including vaccines. NDCs are found on outer packaging, product labels, and/or product inserts. This is discussed more fully in **Chapter 1**, The Basics of Coding.

NDCs are 10-digit, 3-segment numbers that identify the product, labeler, and trade package size. The Health Insurance Portability and Accountability Act of 1996 standards require an 11-digit code. **Table 9-2** shows how 10-digit codes are converted to the 11-digit format for reporting.

If you are not currently reporting vaccines with NDCs, be sure to coordinate the requirements with your billing software company. For more information on NDCs, visit www.fda.gov/Drugs/InformationOnDrugs/ucm142438.htm.

Immunization Administration

CPT codes **90460** and **90461** *or* **90471–90474** are reported *in addition to* vaccine/toxoid code(s) **90476–90756**.

Codes **90460** and **90461**

90460   Immunization administration through 18 years of age via any route of administration, with counseling by physician or other qualified health care professional; first or only component of each vaccine or toxoid administered

+90461   each additional vaccine or toxoid component administered
            (List separately in addition to code for primary procedure.)

When reporting codes **90460** and **90461**

- Physicians or QHPs must provide *face-to-face* counseling to the patient and/or family (patient aged 18 years or younger) at the time of the encounter for the administration of a vaccine. (See the Codes **90471–90474** section later in this chapter for immunization administration [IA] without physician counseling or to patients older than 18 years. Also see the Coding for Counseling When Immunizations Are Not Carried Out section later in this chapter.)
- *CPT* defines a physician or other QHP as follows:

    A *"physician or other qualified health care professional"* is an individual who by education, training, licensure/ regulation, facility credentialing (when applicable), and facility privileging (when applicable) performs a professional service within his/her scope of practice and independently reports that professional service. These professionals are distinct from "clinical staff."

- Clinical staff will not qualify to perform the counseling reported under codes **90460** and **90461**. While state scope of practice may allow certain clinical staff to perform the service, it will not qualify them to report these codes. In the absence of counseling by a physician or QHP, administration services by clinical staff are reported with codes **90471–90474**. *CPT* defines clinical staff as follows:

    A clinical staff member is a person who works under the supervision of a physician or other qualified health care professional and who is allowed by law, regulation, and facility policy to perform or assist in the performance of a specified professional service, but who does not individually report that professional service. Other policies may also affect who may report specific services.

- When a private payer contract does not allow QHPs to report services under their own name and National Provider Identifier (NPI), check with the payer to determine the eligibility of these professionals to report immunization counseling (**90460**, **90461**) and report under the name and number of the supervising physician.
- Documentation of immunization counseling should include a listing of all vaccine components with notation that counseling was provided for all listed components with authentication (electronic or written signature and date) by the physician or other QHP. Supply of the Vaccine Information Statement (VIS) without discussion of risks and benefits does not constitute counseling. Some payers require documentation of parent or caregiver questions or concerns that were addressed during counseling.
- Code **90460** is reported for the *first (or only) component of each vaccine administered* (whether single or combination) on a day of service and includes the related vaccine counseling.
- Code **90461** is only reported in conjunction with **90460** and is used to report the work of counseling for *each additional component(s) beyond the first* in a given combination vaccine. (See the Vaccines for Children Program section later in this chapter for reporting administration of vaccines containing multiple components to this program.)
- Combination vaccines are those vaccines that contain multiple vaccine components. Refer to **Appendix III**, Vaccine Products: Commonly Administered Pediatric Vaccines, for the number of components in the most commonly reported pediatric vaccines.
- The IA codes include the physician or other QHP's work of discussing risks and benefits of the vaccines, providing parents with a copy of the appropriate CDC VIS for each vaccine given, the cost of clinical staff time to record each vaccine component administered in the medical record and statewide vaccine registry, giving the vaccine, observing and addressing reactions or side effects, and cost of supplies (eg, syringe, needle, bandages).

Code **90460** is reported for each individual vaccine administered because every vaccine will have, at minimum, 1 vaccine component. For combination vaccines, code **90461** is additionally reported for counseling on each additional component. No modifier is typically required for reporting multiple units of the IA codes. Most payers advise reporting multiple units of the same service on a single line of the claim. However, individual payer guidance may vary. The AAP is also aware of the decreased RVUs for codes **90460** and **90461** and is working closely with the CMS to resolve this.

If a significant, separately identifiable E/M service (eg, office or other outpatient service, preventive medicine service) is performed, the appropriate E/M service code appended with modifier **25** should be reported in addition to the vaccine and toxoid administration codes. If vaccines are given during the course of a preventive medicine service and another E/M service, both E/M services will need modifier **25** if required by the payer. See also the Reporting a Preventive Medicine Visit With a Problem-Oriented Visit section later in this chapter.

Examples

➤ **A 15-year-old patient presents for the influenza vaccine from his physician.** The ordering physician discusses risks of the vaccine and the disease for which it provides protection. The parent/guardian is given the CDC VIS. The parent/guardian consents; the nurse prepares the vaccine. The nurse administers the vaccine by intranasal spray, charts the required information, and accesses and enters vaccine data into the statewide immunization registry. The patient is discharged home after the nurse confirms that there are no serious immediate reactions.

ICD-10-CM	CPT
Z23 (encounter for immunization)	**90672** (influenza virus vaccine, quad [LAIV], live, intranasal use) **90460**

Teaching Point: Because the physician personally performed the counseling, code **90460** is reported for this single-component vaccine. Code **90460** is appropriate regardless of the route of administration. No other services are reported because the purpose of the visit was for administration of the vaccine only.

➤ **An adolescent presents for immunizations.** After you counsel the patient, clinical staff administer meningococcal conjugate vaccine, serogroups A, C, W, Y, quadrivalent, diphtheria toxoid carrier (MenACWY-D), vaccine and a quadrivalent influenza vaccine at the same encounter.

Report code **90460** with 2 units (1 unit for the first component of each vaccine given). Code **90461** is not reported because each vaccine contains only 1 component (ie, protects against 1 disease). Link the vaccine and administration *CPT* codes to *ICD-10-CM* code **Z23** on health insurance claims.

➤ **A 4-month-old established patient receives the diphtheria, tetanus toxoids, acellular pertussis, inactivated poliovirus, and *Haemophilus influenzae* type b (DTaP-IPV/Hib) combination vaccine; rotavirus vaccine (RV5); and pneumococcal conjugate vaccine (PCV13) from her certified pediatric nurse practitioner (CPNP) at the time of her preventive medicine visit.** The CPNP discusses the risks of each vaccine component (eg, tetanus, pertussis) and the diseases for which each vaccine component provides protection. The parent/guardian is given the CDC VIS for all vaccine components and consents for each of the additional vaccine components. The nurse charts the required information and enters data into the statewide immunization registry for each vaccine component in addition to the vaccine administrations.

ICD-10-CM	CPT
Z00.129 (routine child examination without abnormal findings)	**99391 25** (preventive medicine visit; younger than 1 year)
Z00.129, Z23 (encounter for immunization)	**90698** (DTaP-IPV/Hib) **90680** (RV5) **90670** (PCV13) **90460** × 3 units for counseling for first component of each of 3 vaccines **90461** × 4 units for counseling for additional components (ie, tetanus, pertussis, IPV, Hib)

●=New code ▲=Revised code #=Re-sequenced code +=Add-on code

Teaching Point: Because the child is younger than 18 years and vaccine counseling was performed by the CPNP with her own NPI, codes **90460** and **90461** may be reported as appropriate. The CPNP reports code **90460** for each vaccine administered for the work of counseling for the first component of each vaccine administered (diphtheria, rotavirus, and pneumococcus). Code **90461** is reported in conjunction with **90460** for each additional component that is part of the combination vaccine DTaP-IPV/Hib. Payers who have adopted the Medicare National Correct Coding Initiative (NCCI) edits will require that modifier **25** be appended to code **99391** to signify that it was significant and separately identifiable from the IA. (For more information on NCCI edits, see **Chapter 2**, Modifiers and Coding Edits.) *ICD-10-CM* code **Z00.129** is reported first, followed by code **Z23**.

➤ **A patient receives the DTaP-IPV/Hib vaccine as a combination vaccine and an influenza vaccine.**

Report **90460** for each vaccine administered (2 units) and **90461** with 4 units for counseling related to additional components of the 5-component combination vaccine (DTaP-IPV/Hib). The DTaP-IPV/Hib vaccine product is reported with code **90698**. *Note:* While not as common, some physicians provide single-component vaccines versus combinations. Therefore, for this example, **90460** would be reported with 4 units for the first components of the 4 vaccine products and **90461** with 2 units for the additional components of the DTaP vaccine. Link the vaccine and administration *CPT* codes to *ICD-10-CM* code **Z23** on health insurance claims.

Codes 90471–90474

90471	Immunization administration (includes percutaneous, intradermal, subcutaneous, or intramuscular injections); one vaccine (single or combination vaccine/toxoid)
+90472	each additional vaccine (single or combination vaccine/toxoid)
	(List separately in addition to code for primary procedure.) (Use code **90472** in conjunction with **90460**, **90471**, or **90473**.)
90473	Immunization administration by intranasal or oral route; one vaccine (single or combination vaccine/toxoid)
+90474	each additional vaccine (single or combination vaccine/toxoid)
	(List separately in addition to code for primary procedure.) (Use code **90474** in conjunction with **90460**, **90471**, or **90473**.)

Codes **90471–90474** will be reported when criteria for reporting the 2 pediatric IA codes (**90460** and **90461**) have not been met. This occurs when either of the following are true:

- The physician or QHP does not counsel the patient or family or does not document that the counseling was personally performed.
- The patient is 19 years or older.

The CMS assigned 0.40 RVUs to codes **90460**, **90471**, and **90473** and 0.36 RVUs to codes **90461**, **90472**, and **90474** in 2020 (2021 RVUs were not established at time of publication).

- Appropriate reporting of codes **90460** and **90461** in lieu of codes **90471–90474** should result in higher payment based on reporting of multiple units of code **90461** for *each additional vaccine component* versus reporting of codes **90472** and **90474** for *each additional vaccine product.*
- Individual payers may or may not assign payment values based on the RVUs published by the CMS. (Administration of vaccines provided through the VFC program is paid differently. See more about the VFC program later in this chapter.)

When reporting codes **90471–90474**

- Codes **90471–90474** are reported for each vaccine administered, whether single or combination vaccines.
- *Only one* "first" IA code (**90460**, **90471**, or **90473**) may be reported on a calendar day.

The "first" IA code can be reported from either family or either route of administration (eg, when a patient receives an immunization via injection and a second one via intranasal route, IA services can be reported with codes **90471** and **90474** or with codes **90473** and **90472**).

- The Medicare NCCI edits pair code **90460** with codes **90471** and **90473**, not allowing codes from the pairs to be reported on the same day of service by the same physician or physician of the same group and specialty. If a physician personally performs counseling on one vaccine but not on another when given during the same encounter, IA will be reported using codes **90460** (and **90461** if appropriate) and either **90472** (IA, each additional vaccine via injection) or **90474** (IA, each additional vaccine via intranasal or oral route).

For more information on vaccine administration, please see the following examples and **Appendix III**, Vaccine Products: Commonly Administered Pediatric Vaccines:

Examples

➤ **A 4-year-old patient is seen by clinical staff per physician's order to follow up on impetigo and clearance to return to preschool.** The father also requests that his daughter receive influenza vaccination. An interval history and very brief examination are obtained and documented with assessment that the impetigo has resolved. The patient is noted to be in good health with no contraindications to the immunization per CDC guidelines. Next, the VIS and the antipyretic dosage for weight are reviewed with the father, who provides consent for the immunization. The influenza vaccine is administered, and the child is observed for immediate reactions prior to discharge.

ICD-10-CM	CPT	
Z09 (encounter for follow-up examination after completed treatment for conditions other than malignant neoplasm) **Z87.2** (personal history of diseases of the skin and subcutaneous tissue)	**99211 25** (E/M service)	
Z23 (encounter for immunization)	**90686** (influenza vaccine [IIV4], preservative free, 0.5 mL, intramuscular) **90471** (IA, first injection)	

Teaching Point: If the payer follows NCCI edits, *CPT* code **99211** will never be paid separately on the same date as vaccine administration (ie, **90471** or **90460**), even with modifier **25**. See "Coding Conundrum: Reporting Evaluation and Management Services With Immunization Administration" later in this chapter for more information on reporting code **99211** with IA.

➤ **A 5-year-old established patient presented 2 weeks ago for her 5-year check and vaccines.** At that appointment, her physician provided counseling for each recommended vaccine component and corresponding VISs. The patient's mother asked that the vaccines be split, so only the DTaP and IPV vaccines were given at that encounter. The patient returns today and sees a nurse for an immunization-only visit to get the measles-mumps-rubella (MMR) and varicella vaccines.

ICD-10-CM	CPT
Z23 (encounter for immunization)	**90707** (MMR, live) **90471** (IA, first injection) **90716** (varicella vaccine) **90472** (IA, subsequent injection)

Teaching Point: Counseling for all vaccines occurred at the last encounter and all VISs were handed out, so only administration occurred today. *CPT* codes **90460** and **90461** would be reported with the appropriate codes for DTaP and IPV vaccines that were administered during the previous encounter. However, services on this date did not include physician counseling. (See "Coding Conundrum: Vaccine Counseling on Day Different From Administration" later in this chapter.) Only report codes **90460** and **90461** when physician counseling is provided on the date of vaccine administration.

➤ **A 19-year-old established patient presents for college entrance examination.** In addition to providing a preventive medicine service, the physician counsels the patient on the need for meningococcal serogroup B (MenB-4C) immunization. The vaccine is administered, and a medical history and physical form provided by the college are completed.

ICD-10-CM	CPT
Z02.0 (encounter for examination for admission to educational institution)	**99395 25** (preventive medicine service, established patient, 18–39 years old)
Z23 (encounter for immunization)	**90620** (MenB-4C) **90471** (IA, first injection)

Teaching Point: Because the patient is older than 18 years, code **90460** cannot be reported even though the physician provided counseling for the vaccine provided. Code **Z02.0** is appropriate as the reason the patient presented for the encounter. Code **Z00.00** (encounter for general adult medical examination without abnormal findings) is not reported because *ICD-10-CM* excludes reporting of code **Z00.00** in conjunction with codes in category **Z02**. Code **Z00.00** is reported in lieu of **Z02** when the patient receives a routine age- and gender-appropriate preventive medicine E/M service.

Coding Conundrum: Vaccine Counseling on Day Different From Administration

Current Procedural Terminology states that codes **90460** and **90461** are reported when the physician or other qualified health care professional (QHP) provides face-to-face counseling to the patient and family during the administration of a vaccine. However, there are situations in which vaccine counseling is performed on a day different from the actual administration. For example, the physician or QHP might provide vaccine counseling during an encounter, but because the child is ill, the vaccines are deferred to a later date. Or the physician or QHP may counsel the patient and parent on all vaccines needed during the annual preventive medicine service visit, but the parent refuses multiple vaccines on the same day, and some of the vaccines are given over a series of encounters for vaccine administration only. How would a physician then report immunization administration (IA)?

Because these circumstances split the actual administration from vaccine counseling, codes **90460** and **90461** cannot be reported. In these situations, IA is reported using codes **90471–90474** on the day the vaccines are administered without physician counseling on the same date.

Coding for Counseling When Immunizations Are Not Carried Out

Pediatricians may counsel patients and caregivers on the need for immunization but decide immunization is contraindicated or not obtain consent to immunize.

> When immunization counseling takes place at the time of a preventive evaluation and management service (well-child visit) and does not result in administration, the counseling is not separately reported.

- When the purpose of the encounter is immunization counseling and immunizations are not administered, preventive medicine counseling codes (**99401–99404**) may be reported based on the time spent in face-to-face counseling with the patient and/or caregivers.
  — Codes for E/M services to address health problems (eg, **99202**) may be reported in addition to **99401–99404** when preventive counseling is provided at the same encounter. Append modifier **25** (significant, separately identifiable E/M service) to the problem-oriented code (eg, **99202 25**) when reporting both services at the same encounter.
  — Codes **99401–99404** were assigned 1.12, 1.85, 2.53, and 3.24 total non-facility RVUs, respectively, in the 2020 Medicare PFS.

99401	Preventive medicine counseling and/or risk-factor reduction intervention(s) provided to an individual (separate procedure); approximately 15 minutes
99402	approximately 30 minutes
99403	approximately 45 minutes
99404	approximately 60 minutes

Capturing the reason an immunization was not carried out begins with a code from *ICD-10-CM* category **Z28**, immunization not carried out, and under-immunization status.
- Under-immunization is reported with code **Z28.3**.
- Contraindications to immunization are captured with codes in subcategory **Z28.0-**.

Z28.01	Immunization not carried out because of acute illness of patient
Z28.02	Immunization not carried out because of chronic illness or condition of patient
Z28.03	Immunization not carried out because of immune compromised state of patient
Z28.04	Immunization not carried out because of patient allergy to vaccine or component
Z28.09	Immunization not carried out because of other contraindication

- Other codes in category **Z28** provide for reporting of immunization not carried out due to patient reasons, caregiver refusal, or other specified reason.

Z28.1	Immunization not carried out because of patient decision for reasons of belief or group pressure
Z28.20	Immunization not carried out because of patient decision for unspecified reason
Z28.21	Immunization not carried out because of patient refusal
Z28.29	Immunization not carried out because of patient decision for other reason

Chapter 9. Preventive Services

Z28.81   Immunization not carried out due to patient having had the disease
Z28.82   Immunization not carried out because of caregiver refusal
Z28.83   Immunization not carried out due to unavailability of vaccine

Examples

➤ **Parents of a 2-month-old established patient come to their physician's office to discuss immunizations.** To date, they have refused to have their infant immunized. Although the physician has discussed the need for vaccines during the infant's previous visits, the parents indicate they have further questions. The physician spends 25 minutes counseling the parents about current recommendations, safety and efficacy of vaccines, and their importance in preventing disease.

ICD-10-CM	CPT
Z71.89 (other specified counseling) **Z28.3** (personal history of under-immunization status) **Z28.82** (vaccination not carried out because of caregiver refusal)	**99402** (risk-factor reduction counseling)

➤ **An 11-year-old girl (new patient) presents to a pediatrician for a preventive medicine service.** In addition to the preventive E/M service with no abnormal findings, the physician discusses risks of the HPV vaccine and the disease for which it provides protection. The parent/guardian is given the CDC VIS. The parent/guardian consents; the nurse prepares to administer the vaccine. However, the patient then refuses to receive the immunization, and counseling by the nurse does not change her decision. The physician returns to the examination room and provides additional counseling, but the patient continues to refuse the vaccine. The patient's mother wishes to discuss the decision with the child's father and return on a later date. A follow-up appointment is scheduled.

ICD-10-CM	CPT	
Z00.129 **Z28.21** (immunization not carried out because of patient refusal)	**99383**	

Teaching Point: Because no vaccine was administered, no charge for the product or the administration would be reported. Written procedures for documentation and reporting of expired and wasted vaccine doses may be required for vaccines provided under the VFC program. When the patient returns for follow-up, the codes reported will depend on the outcome of the encounter. If the vaccine is administered after additional physician counseling at the same encounter, code **90460** would be reported in addition to the appropriate vaccine product code. If the patient returns for administration by clinical staff without additional counseling by a physician, code **90471** would be reported in lieu of **90460**. Additional counseling at the follow-up physician visit that does not result in immunization may be reported with a preventive medicine counseling code (**99401–99404**) based on the physician's face-to-face time with the patient.

Note that modifier **JW** (drug amount discarded/not administered to any patient) is not typically appropriate when no vaccine was administered to the patient. Modifier **JW** is used to report waste from a single-dose vial/package when the required patient dose is less than the available single-dose amount. Two claim lines report the amounts administered and wasted. Follow payer instructions for reporting wasted vaccines and use of modifier **JW**.

➤ **A 3-year-old girl (established patient) presents to a pediatrician with symptoms of vomiting and diarrhea.** The girl's mother notes that the child's cousins had the same illness about a week ago. She is concerned that the child is getting dehydrated. The pediatrician reviews the patient's history and after an examination diagnoses gastroenteritis with mild dehydration and provides education on caring for the child. The pediatrician also takes the opportunity to again counsel the mother about the need for immunization against MMR, which she has previously refused. Recent outbreaks and the safety of immunization are discussed for 10 minutes and the mother agrees to revisit the issue with her husband, who has been strongly opposed in the past. The pediatrician documents the separate time and context of the counseling.

ICD-10-CM	CPT
A08.4 (viral intestinal infection, unspecified)	**99213 25** (low-level medical decision-making [MDM]: 1 acute, uncomplicated illness; assessment requiring an independent observer; and low risk of morbidity from treatment)
Z28.3 (under-immunization status) **Z28.21** (immunization not carried out because of patient refusal)	**99401**

Teaching Point: The pediatrician's time of 10 minutes spent in preventive counseling supports reporting **99401** because the midpoint was passed (8 minutes are required for reporting a code assigned 15 minutes).

Vaccines for Children Program

The VFC program makes vaccines available to children and teens up to 19 years of age who meet any of the following criteria: are enrolled in the Medicaid program (depending on the state Medicaid Managed Care), do not have health insurance, have no coverage of immunizations under their health plan, or are American Indians or Alaska Natives. Vaccines are provided at no cost to the participating physician or patient, and payment is made only for administration of the vaccine.

If reporting the VFC vaccine with administration codes and not the product code, data for the vaccine products administered must be captured for registry and quality initiatives. This can be accomplished by entering the vaccine codes with a $0 charge (if your billing system allows) and appending modifier **SL** (state-supplied vaccine) to the vaccine code. However, follow individual payer rules for reporting.

Providers are encouraged to use code **90460** for administration of a vaccine under the VFC program unless otherwise directed by a state program. If code **90461** is used for a vaccine with multiple antigens or components, it should be given a $0 value for a child covered under the VFC program. This applies to Medicaid-enrolled VFC-entitled children as well as non–Medicaid-enrolled VFC-entitled children (ie, uninsured, underinsured, and American Indian or Alaska Native children not enrolled in Medicaid).

Please be aware that some state Medicaid programs do have reporting rules that differ from VFC. *Be sure to get this policy in writing from your state Medicaid program* and follow it to avoid denied payment. The AAP continues to advocate to the CMS to allow for recognition and payment for component-based vaccine counseling and administration (ie, code **90461**). Under the current statute, administration can only be paid "per vaccine" and not component.

Participants in the VFC program should be aware of program-specific guidance, including storage of VFC vaccine separate from privately purchased vaccines. For more information on the VFC program, visit www.cdc.gov/vaccines/programs/vfc/index.html.

See "FAQ: Immunization Administration" at www.aap.org/cfp (access code AAPCFP26) for more discussion of coding for IA.

Screening Tests and Procedures

Recommendations for age-appropriate screening services are outlined in the AAP/Bright Futures "Recommendations for Preventive Pediatric Health Care" (www.aap.org/periodicityschedule) or in your state's EPSDT plan.

When routine vision, developmental, and/or hearing screening services are performed in conjunction with a preventive medicine visit, the diagnosis code for a routine infant or child health check should be linked to the appropriate screening service.

Hearing Screening

92551	Screening test, pure tone, air only
92552	Pure tone audiometry (threshold); air only (full assessment)
#92558	Evoked otoacoustic emissions, screening (qualitative measurement of distortion product or transient evoked otoacoustic emissions), automated analysis
92567	Tympanometry (impedance testing)
92568	Acoustic reflex testing, threshold portion
92583	Select picture audiometry

●=New code ▲=Revised code #=Re-sequenced code +=Add-on code

Audiometric tests require the use of calibrated electronic equipment, recording of results, and a written report with interpretation (eg, chart of hertz and decibels with pass/fail result for each ear tested and overall pass/fail result). Services include testing of both ears. If the test is applied only to 1 ear, modifier **52** (reduced services) must be appended to the code.

> When hearing screening is performed in the physician office because of a failed screening in another setting (eg, school), report *International Classification of Diseases, 10th Revision, Clinical Modification* codes from category **Z01.11-**. Code **Z01.110** is reported for a normal screening result following a failed screening. Code **Z01.118** indicates a failed repeat screening. An additional code is reported to identify the abnormality found following the failed repeat screening.

- Code **92551** (screening test, pure tone, air only) is used when earphones are placed on the patient and the patient is asked to respond to tones of different pitches and intensities. This is a limited study.
- Code **92552** (full pure tone audiometric assessment; air only) is used when earphones are placed on the patient and the patient is asked to respond to tones of different pitches and intensities. The threshold, which is the lowest intensity of the tone that the patient can hear 50% of the time, is recorded for a number of frequencies.
- Code **92558** (evoked otoacoustic emissions [OAEs] screening) is used when a probe tip is placed in the ear canal to screen for normal hearing function. The probe tip emits a repeated clicking sound (transient evoked emissions) or 2 tones at 2 frequencies (distortion product emissions). The sounds pass through the tympanic membrane and middle ear to the inner ear. In the inner ear, the sound is picked up by the hair cells in the cochlea, which, in turn, bounce the sound back in low-intensity sound waves (OAEs). These OAEs are recorded and analyzed by computerized equipment and the results are automated.

> Medicaid plans may offer physician resources providing hearing screening/testing coverage information and documentation forms/requirements.

- Code **92583** (select picture audiometry) is typically used for younger children. The patient is asked to identify different pictures with the instructions given at different sound intensity levels.
- Other commonly performed procedures include codes **92567** (tympanometry [impedance testing]) and **92568** (acoustic reflex testing, threshold portion). However, both codes may have limited coverage; check with payers.
- Automated audiometry testing is reported with Category III codes **0208T–0212T**. Verify individual payer payment policy before providing these services.

Examples

➤ **George is a 16-year-old established patient presenting for a preventive service and clearance to participate in school sports.** A complete preventive E/M service (**99394**) is provided. George has not received a hearing screening since he was 13 years old, so pure tone, air-only screening audiometry is performed (**92551**). No abnormalities are found, and George receives clearance to participate in sports. The *ICD-10-CM* code reported for each of the services is **Z00.129** (encounter for routine child health examination without abnormal findings).

➤ **Sally is a 6-year-old who failed a hearing screening at school and is referred to her pediatrician for additional evaluation.** Sally's parents indicate no prior concerns about her hearing, and risk-factor assessment is negative. The pediatrician chooses to perform screening audiometry (**92551**), which produces typical results. The *ICD-10-CM* code reported is **Z01.110** (encounter for hearing examination following failed hearing screening). If the MDM or total physician time (not including time of testing) supports a separate office or other outpatient E/M service, this is separately reported (eg, **99212**).

Vision Screening

99173	Screening test of visual acuity, quantitative, bilateral
99174	Instrument-based ocular screening (eg, photoscreening, automated-refraction), bilateral; with remote analysis and report
99177	with on-site analysis

0333T   Visual evoked potential, screening of visual acuity, automated, with report
0469T   Retinal polarization scan, ocular screening with on-site automated results, bilateral

- Screening test of visual acuity (**99173**) must use graduated visual stimuli that allow a quantitative estimate of visual acuity (eg, Snellen chart).
  - Medical record documentation must include a measurement of acuity for both eyes, not just a pass or fail score.
  - Code **99173** is only reported when vision screening is performed in association with a preventive medicine visit. It is not reported when it is performed as part of an evaluation for an eye problem or condition (eg, examination to rule out vision problems in a patient presenting with problems with schoolwork) because the assessment of visual acuity is considered an integral part of the eye examination.
- Instrument-based ocular screening (**99174**, **99177**) is used to report screening for a variety of conditions, including esotropia, exotropia, isometropia, cataracts, ptosis, hyperopia, myopia, and others, that affect or have the potential to affect vision. These tests are especially useful for screening infants, preschool patients, and those older patients whose ability to participate in traditional acuity screening is limited or very time intensive.
  - Code **99177** specifies screening using an instrument that provides an on-site (ie, in-office) pass or fail result. The result should be documented.
  - Code **99174** specifies the use of a screening instrument that incorporates remote analysis and report (by a physician located elsewhere).
  - These screenings cannot be reported in conjunction with codes **92002–92700** (general ophthalmologic services), **99172** (visual function screening), or **99173** (screening test of visual acuity, quantitative) because ocular screening is inherent to these services. An AAP policy statement on instrument-based pediatric vision screening is available at http://pediatrics.aappublications.org/content/130/5/983.full.
- Vision screening performed using an automated visual evoked potential system is reported with code **0333T**. This code applies to automated screening using an instrument-based algorithm with a pass or fail result. A report of the result must be documented. Report code **95930** only for comprehensive visual evoked potential testing with physician interpretation and report.
- Retinal polarization scanning (**0469T**) is used to detect amblyopia due to strabismus and defocus. Similar to code **99177**, results of each scan are generated on-site.

Developmental Screening and Health Assessment

Standardized screening instruments (ie, validated tests that are administered and scored in a consistent or "standard" manner consistent with their validation) are used for screening and assessment purposes as reported by codes **96110** and **96127**. Health risk assessments that are patient focused (**96160**) are differentiated from those such as maternal depression screening that are caregiver focused (**96161**) for the benefit of the patient.

Developmental Screening

96110   Developmental screening with scoring and documentation, per standardized instrument

   Structured screening for developmental delay is a universal recommendation of the "Recommendations for Preventive Pediatric Health Care" at 18-month and 2-year visits for autism spectrum disorder (ASD)–specific screening and at 9-month, 18-month, and 2- or 2½-year visits for other developmental screening. When reporting these screenings, code **96110** represents developmental screening with scoring and documentation per standardized instrument. (*Note:* Screening results should be included in the patient medical record.)

   ICD-10-CM codes **Z13.40–Z13.49** (eg, **Z13.42**, screening for global developmental delays [milestones]) may be reported to indicate screening for developmental disability in children when the screening is performed with or without a well-child visit at the same encounter.

   Code **96110**

- Is reported only for standardized developmental screening instruments. It is not reported when the pediatrician conducts an informal survey or surveillance of development as part of a comprehensive preventive medicine service (which is considered part of the history and is not separately billed).
- Does not require interpretation and report (ie, includes scoring and documentation only).
- Is *not* reported for brief emotional or behavioral assessment; see code **96127**.
- May be reported for each standardized developmental screening instrument administered. Medicaid Medically Unlikely Edits (MUEs) allow reporting of 3 screening instruments per date of service. See claim form examples 1 and 2 for reporting options.

Example

➤ **An 18-month-old girl presents to her primary physician with a complaint of a cut on her thumb.** A pediatrician assesses a minor laceration of the child's right thumb (**S61.011A**), cleans the wound, and applies a bandage. The pediatrician notes that developmental and ASD screenings were not performed at a well-child visit 2 weeks ago because the child's grandmother, who brought her, was not comfortable completing the screenings. The mother is given a standardized screening instrument for developmental status and ASD by clinical staff, who explain their purpose and how they should be completed. The nursing assistant scores the completed forms and attaches them to the child's medical chart. The physician interprets and documents the normal results of the instruments. The child will return for a scheduled 2-year-old preventive service.

Code **96110** is reported with 2 units of service (see Claim Form Example 1 for Multiple Units of Service), or **96110** and **96110 59** are reported (see Claim Form Example 2 for Multiple Units of Service), depending on payer requirements.

Teaching Point: *ICD-10-CM* codes **Z13.41** (autism screening) and **Z13.42** (screening for delayed milestones) help identify the reason for 2 units of service. Proactive recommendations and delivery of preventive services support quality initiatives.

Claim Form Example 1 for Multiple Units of Service

21. Diagnosis or nature of illness or injury (Relate A–L to service line below 24E)   ICD Ind. 0
A. **S61.011A**   B. **Z13.41**   C. **Z13.42**   D.

24. A. Dates of service	B. Place of service	C. EMG	D. Procedures, services or supplies CPT/HCPCS	Modifier	E. Diagnosis Pointer	F. Charges	G. Days or units	H. EPSDT	I. ID Qual	J. Rendering Provider #
1/2/2021–1/2/2021	11		99213	25	A	$$$	1		NPI	123456789
1/2/2021–1/2/2021	11		96110		BC	$$$	2		NPI	123456789

Abbreviations: *CPT, Current Procedural Terminology*; EMG, emergency; EPSDT, Early and Periodic Screening, Diagnostic, and Treatment; HCPCS, Healthcare Common Procedure Coding System; *ICD, International Classification of Diseases*; NPI, National Provider Identifier.

Claim Form Example 2 for Multiple Units of Service

21. Diagnosis or nature of illness or injury (Relate A–L to service line below 24E)   ICD Ind. 0
A. **S61.011A**   B. **Z13.41**   C. **Z13.42**   D.

24. A. Dates of service	B. Place of service	C. EMG	D. Procedures, services or supplies CPT/HCPCS	Modifier	E. Diagnosis Pointer	F. Charges	G. Days or units	H. EPSDT	I. ID Qual	J. Rendering Provider #
1/2/2021–1/2/2021	11		99213	25	A	$$$	1		NPI	123456789
1/1/2021–1/2/2021	11		96110		B	$$$	1		NPI	123456789
1/1/2021–1/2/2021	11		96110	59	C	$$$	1		NPI	123456789

Abbreviations: *CPT, Current Procedural Terminology*; EMG, emergency; EPSDT, Early and Periodic Screening, Diagnostic, and Treatment; HCPCS, Healthcare Common Procedure Coding System; *ICD, International Classification of Diseases*; NPI, National Provider Identifier.

Emotional/Behavioral Assessment

96127   Brief emotional/behavioral assessment (eg, depression inventory, ADHD scale), with scoring and documentation, per standardized instrument

Code **96127**
- Is reported for standardized emotional/behavioral assessment instruments.
- Represents the practice expense of administering, scoring, and documenting each standardized instrument. No physician work value is included. Physician interpretation is included in a related E/M service.
- Is *not* reported in conjunction with preventive medicine counseling/risk-factor reduction intervention (**99401–99404**) or psychiatric or neurologic testing (**96130–96139** or **96146**).

- Can involve 2 or more separately reported completions of the same form (eg, attention-deficit/hyperactivity disorder [ADHD] rating scales by teacher and by parent). Note that MUEs limit reporting to 2 units per claim line. When reporting to payers adopting MUEs, additional units beyond the first 2 must be reported on a separate claim line with an NCCI modifier (eg, **59**, distinct procedural service). As always, documentation should support the appropriateness of the additional units of service.
- Can be reported for standardized depression instruments that are required under US Preventive Services Task Force (USPSTF) and Bright Futures recommendations (see AAP/Bright Futures "Recommendations for Preventive Pediatric Health Care" [periodicity schedule] insert).

Example

➤ **A 12-year-old boy is seen for an established patient well-child health supervision and sports physical encounter.** In addition to the preventive medicine service, the physician's staff administers and scores a standardized depression screening instrument. The physician reviews the score, documents that the screening result is negative for symptoms of depression, and completes the preventive medicine service. Clearance is given to participate in sports.

The preventive medicine service code (**99394**) would be reported in addition to code **96127**. The diagnosis codes reported are **Z00.129** (encounter for routine child health examination without abnormal findings) and **Z13.31** (encounter for screening for depression). Link **Z00.129** and **Z13.31** to the claim service line for code **96127**. Inclusion of codes may support claims-based data collection for quality measurement (ie, number of adolescent patients screened for depression). A code for the sports physical (**Z02.5**) is not reported because *ICD-10-CM* excludes reporting of codes in category **Z02** in conjunction with codes in category **Z00**.

When the physician performs further evaluation of positive screening results, leading to a diagnosis of depression, code the preventive service with abnormal findings (**Z00.121**) followed by the appropriate code for the diagnosed depression (eg, **F32.0**, major depressive disorder, single episode, mild). When appropriate, a significant and separately identifiable E/M service to evaluate and manage depression may be reported by appending modifier **25** to an office or other outpatient E/M code (eg, **99213 25**). Documentation should clearly support the MDM of the separate service or, if billing based on time, the physician's total time (not including the time spent providing the separately reported preventive medicine service) and a summary of the service provided (eg, education on the condition, questions answered, patient and/or caregiver concerns, management options discussed, plan of care).

Health Risk Assessment

96160   Administration of patient-focused health risk assessment (eg, health hazard appraisal) with scoring and documentation, per standardized instrument

96161   Administration of caregiver-focused health risk assessment (eg, depression inventory) for the benefit of the patient, with scoring and documentation, per standardized instrument

Code **96160** is reported for a patient-focused health risk assessment. This is differentiated from code **96161**, which is used to report a health risk assessment focused on a caregiver for the benefit of the patient (eg, maternal depression screening). For standardized health risk assessments that focus on social issues related to the patient and the family, report **96160**.

- Code **96160** is reported for administration (with scoring and documentation) of a standardized patient-focused health risk assessment instrument (eg, health hazard appraisal). Code **96160** cannot be used in conjunction with assessment and brief intervention for alcohol/substance abuse (**99408** and **99409**).

Check individual payer guidance to determine if and for what purposes code **96160** is included as a covered and payable service under the payer's policies (eg, some Medicaid plans pay for adolescent health questionnaires reported with **96160**).

- Code **96161** is reported for administration of a health risk assessment to a patient's caregiver. Examples are a postpartum depression inventory administered to the mother of a newborn and administration of a standardized caregiver strain instrument to parents of a child who is seriously injured or ill.
- Report 1 unit of **96160** or **96161** for each standardized instrument administered. Payer edits may limit the number of times codes **96160** and **96161** may be reported for an individual patient and/or on the same date of service. MUEs are set to 3 units for **96160** and 1 unit for **96161** per claim line. Append modifier **59** to the code for additional units on a second claim line.
- Sparse coverage for codes **96160** and specifically **96161** has been noted by the AAP, and advocacy efforts are being made.

Example

➤ **As part of a health supervision visit for a 4-month-old established patient, the physician directs clinical staff to administer a screening for postpartum depression.** Clinical staff explain the purpose of the instrument to the infant's mother. After the mother has completed the screening instrument, clinical staff score and document the result in the patient record. The physician completes the preventive medicine service. Anticipatory guidance that advises the mother that her screening indicates no current signs of postpartum depression is included, along with a list of symptoms that should prompt a call to her physician.

ICD-10-CM	CPT
Z00.129 (encounter for routine child health examination without abnormal findings)	**99391** (preventive medicine visit) **96161** (administration of caregiver-focused health risk assessment [eg, depression inventory] for the benefit of the patient, with scoring and documentation, per standardized instrument)

Teaching Point: Screening for postpartum depression is caregiver focused (sign/symptoms of depression in mother) but performed in this setting for the benefit of the infant. This service is reported as a service provided to the infant with code **96161**. Check payer policy on adoption of code **96161** versus a requirement to report as a service to the mother (ie, to mother's health plan) with code **96127** (brief emotional/behavioral assessment [eg, depression inventory, ADHD scale], with scoring and documentation, per standardized instrument). Many Medicaid plans provide separate payment for maternal depression screening at well-child visits, but specific reporting instructions may apply. Also, never report *ICD-10-CM* code **Z13.32** (encounter for maternal depression screen) on the baby's chart/bill. Vaccines and administration services would also be reported.

Avoid denials! National Correct Coding Initiative edits bundle codes **96160** and **96161** with code **96110** and with IA (**90460–90474**) services, but a modifier is allowed when each code represents a distinct service and is clinically appropriate. Append modifier **59** (distinct procedure) to the bundled code (second column of NCCI edits) when these services are reported on the same date to a payer that has adopted NCCI edits.

Prevention of Dental Caries

Application of Fluoride Varnish

99188   Application of topical fluoride varnish by a physician or other qualified health care professional

- Topical fluoride application by primary care physicians is a recommended preventive service for children from birth through 5 years of age (Grade B rating by the USPSTF). This service may be covered when provided alone or in conjunction with other services. Coverage is usually limited to once every 6 months.
- *ICD-10-CM* code **Z29.3** is reported to identify an encounter for prophylactic fluoride administration. When applicable, diagnosis of dental caries may be reported as a secondary diagnosis with codes in category **K02**. Encounter for prophylactic fluoride administration is reported separately from the encounter for routine child health examination (**Z00.121** or **Z00.129**) when both services are provided at the same encounter.

Example

➤ **A 4-year-old established patient undergoes a routine preventive medicine service without abnormal findings.** In addition, a medical assistant who has been qualified by a required online training and assessment program applies fluoride varnish to the child's teeth under supervision of the pediatrician, who remains in the office suite.

The pediatrician reports code **99392** (established patient routine child health examination, age 1–4) and **99188** (application of fluoride varnish). Diagnosis code **Z00.129** (routine child health examination without abnormal findings) is linked to code **99392**. Diagnosis code **Z29.3** is linked to code **99188**. Follow payer-specific guidelines on the qualifications of the provider who performs fluoride application and other payment policy.

●=New code   ▲=Revised code   #=Re-sequenced code   +=Add-on code

Chapter 9. Preventive Services

- Although code **99188** specifies application by a physician or QHP, payers may allow billing of services by trained clinical staff under direct physician supervision (incident to). Some Medicaid plans require training of clinical staff through specific programs and documentation of training and/or certification. It is important to identify the requirements of individual payers prior to providing this service and maintain documentation demonstrating all coverage requirements were met.

Counseling to Prevent Dental Caries

Some payers will provide coverage for oral evaluation and health risk assessment or other dental preventive services when provided on the same day as a preventive medicine visit; other payers will allow services only when they are provided at an encounter separate from a preventive medicine visit. It is important to know payer requirements for reporting.

Preventive counseling for oral health may be included as part of the preventive medicine service (**99381–99395**) or, if performed at a separate encounter, reported under the individual preventive medicine counseling service codes (**99401–99404**) or with an office or outpatient E/M service code (**99202–99215**). *ICD-10-CM* code **Z13.84** may be reported for an encounter for screening for dental disorders.

Other Codes for Prevention of Dental Caries

- *Code on Dental Procedures and Nomenclature* (*CDT®*) codes also exist for topical application of fluoride varnish and fluoride. In addition, *CDT* codes exist for nutrition counseling to prevent dental disease, oral hygiene instruction, and oral evaluations. However, acceptance of these codes by health plans may be limited to state Medicaid plans.
- For those carriers (particularly state Medicaid plans under EPSDT) that cover oral health care, some will require a modifier. These modifiers are payer specific and should only be used as directed by your state Medicaid agency or other private payer.
  SC Medically necessary service or supply
  EP Services provided as part of Medicaid EPSDT program
  U5 Medicaid Level of Care 5, as defined by each state

Screening Laboratory Tests

- A test performed in the office laboratory should be billed using the appropriate laboratory code and, if performed, the appropriate blood collection code (**36400–36416**).
- Codes **36415** (collection of venous blood by venipuncture) and **36416** (collection of capillary blood specimen [eg, finger, heel, ear stick]) are used for any age child when the physician is not needed to perform the procedure. Code **36416** is not payable by Medicare, as it is considered bundled, and many private payers follow this rule and bundle it as well.
- When a physician's skill is required to perform venipuncture (eg, access is too difficult for other staff to attain) *on a child younger than 3 years*, codes **36400–36406** are reported based on the anatomical site of the venipuncture. Report code **36400** when performed on a femoral or jugular vein, **36405** when on the scalp vein, or **36406** when another vein is accessed.
- When a physician's skill is required to perform venipuncture on a child 3 years or older, code **36410** (venipuncture, age 3 years and older, necessitating physician's skill, for diagnostic or therapeutic purposes [not to be used for routine venipuncture]) is reported.
- If the physician performs the venipuncture as a convenience or because staff is not trained in the procedure, code **36415** is reported because the physician's skill was not required.
- Although typically not required, some payers will require that modifier **25** be appended to the E/M code if a separate and significant E/M service is reported on the same day of service.
- Laboratories and physician offices performing waived tests may need to append modifier **QW** to the *CPT* code for Clinical Laboratory Improvement Amendments (CLIA)–waived procedures. The use of modifier **QW** is payer specific. To review the list of CLIA-waived procedures, go to http://cms.hhs.gov/Regulations-and-Guidance/Legislation/CLIA/Categorization_of_Tests.html.
- *ICD-10-CM* allows separate reporting of special screening examinations (codes in categories **Z11–Z13**) in addition to the codes for routine child health examinations when these codes provide additional information. A screening code is not necessary if the screening is inherent to a routine examination. Payer guidelines for reporting screening examinations may vary. When specific *ICD-10-CM* codes are required to support payment for a screening service, be sure to link the appropriate *ICD-10-CM* code to the claim line for the screening service.

●=New code ▲=Revised code #=Re-sequenced code +=Add-on code

A positive finding on a screening test does not change the test to a diagnostic test. When a screening test results in an abnormal finding that has been identified at the time of code assignment, list first the code for the screening or preventive service followed by a code for the abnormal finding. Failure to list the screening code first may affect the patient's out-of-pocket costs for preventive services. Please see Chapter 11 for information on coding for diagnostic tests in non-facility settings.

Anemia

85018 QW   Blood count; hemoglobin

Screening for anemia is reported with *ICD-10-CM* code **Z13.0**, encounter for screening for diseases of the blood and blood-forming organs and certain disorders involving the immune mechanism.

Lead Testing

83655 QW   Lead, quantitative analysis

- This test does not specify the specimen source or method of testing. Alternative tests sometimes (although now rarely) used for lead screening are **82135** (aminolevulinic acid, delta), **84202** (protoporphyrin, red blood cell count, quantitative), and **84203** (protoporphyrin, red blood cell count, screen).
- Some states provide lead testing at no cost to patients covered under the Medicaid EPSDT program. Check your state Medicaid requirements for reporting this service.
- Report *ICD-10-CM* code **Z13.88** (encounter for screening for disorder due to exposure to contaminants) when performing lead screening. Some payers require **Z77.011**, contact with and (suspected) exposure to lead, in lieu of **Z13.88**.

To meet the Healthcare Effectiveness Data and Information Set (HEDIS) measure for percentage of children who turned 2 years of age in a measurement year and who had 1 or more capillary or venous lead blood test(s) for lead poisoning by their second birthday, a laboratory report of lead screening test result, or a note indicating the date the test was performed and the result or finding must be documented. See Chapter 3 for more information on HEDIS measures.

Tuberculosis Skin Test (Mantoux)

86580   Tuberculosis, intradermal (includes administration)

- The tuberculosis (TB) skin test (Mantoux) using intradermal administration of purified protein derivative (PPD) is the recommended diagnostic skin test for TB. (This is not the BCG TB vaccine.)
- Code **99211** is the appropriate code to report when the patient returns for the reading of a PPD test. In the case of a positive test result, when the physician sees the patient and forms a further diagnostic or treatment plan, the complexity may lead to a higher-level code (ie, **99212–99215**). The appropriate *ICD-10-CM* code is **Z11.1** (encounter for screening for respiratory TB).
- There is not a separate administration code reported when the TB test is performed.

Dyslipidemia

80061 QW   Lipid panel (must include total serum cholesterol, lipoprotein by direct measurement high-density cholesterol [HDL], and triglycerides) *or*

82465 QW   Cholesterol, serum, total

83718 QW   Lipoprotein, direct measurement, high-density cholesterol (HDL cholesterol)

84478 QW   Triglycerides

The appropriate *ICD-10-CM* code for dyslipidemia screening is **Z13.220** (encounter for screening for lipoid disorders). A code for relevant family history may be reported (eg, **Z83.438**, family history of other disorder of lipoprotein metabolism and other lipidemia) in addition to **Z13.220**.

Sexually Transmitted Infection

86701 QW   Antibody; HIV-1

G0433 QW   Infectious agent antibody detection by enzyme-linked immunosorbent assay (ELISA) technique, HIV-1 and/or HIV-2, screening

- Screening laboratory tests for chlamydia, gonorrhea, and syphilis require more than waived testing laboratory certification. These tests include those described by the following codes:

86631	Antibody; chlamydia
86632	Antibody; chlamydia, IgM
86703	Antibody; HIV-1 and HIV-2; single assay
87081	Culture, presumptive, pathogenic organisms, screening only
87110	Culture, chlamydia, any source
87205	Smear, primary source with interpretation; Gram or Giemsa stain for bacteria, fungi, or cell types

- *ICD-10-CM* codes supporting screening laboratory tests are **Z11.8**, encounter for screening for other infectious and parasitic diseases (eg, chlamydia); **Z11.3**, encounter for screening for infections with a predominantly sexual mode of transmission (eg, syphilis and gonorrhea); and **Z11.4**, encounter for screening for HIV. Codes in category **Z72**, problems related to lifestyle, may also be required to support screening of a sexually active adolescent.

Preventive Care Provided Outside the Preventive Visit

Counseling and/or Risk-Factor Reduction

Codes **99401–99404**, **99411**, and **99412** are used to report risk-factor reduction services provided for the purpose of promoting health and preventing illness or injury in persons without a specific illness.

Preventive medicine service codes (**99381–99395**) include counseling, anticipatory guidance, and/or risk-factor reduction interventions that are provided at the time of the periodic comprehensive preventive medicine examination. *CPT* states to "refer to codes **99401**, **99402**, **99403**, **99404**, and **99411–99412** for reporting those counseling/anticipatory guidance/risk-factor reduction interventions that are provided at an encounter separate from the preventive medicine examination." Therefore, according to *CPT*, do not report **99401–99404**, **99411**, or **99412** in addition to **99381–99397**.

- Risk factor reduction services will vary with age and address issues such as diet, exercise, sexual activity, dental health, injury prevention, safe travel, and family problems.
- Services are reported based on time.
- Counseling, anticipatory guidance, and risk-factor reduction interventions provided at the time of an initial or periodic comprehensive preventive medicine examination are components of the periodic service and not separately reported.
- Risk-factor reduction may be reported separately with other E/M services.
  - Evaluation and management services (other than preventive medicine E/M services) reported on the same day must be separate and distinct.
  - Time spent in the provision of risk-factor reduction may not be used as a basis for the selection of the other E/M code.
- When reporting a distinct E/M service, append modifier **25** to the code for the distinct E/M service.

Preventive Medicine, Individual Counseling Codes

99401	Preventive medicine counseling and/or risk-factor reduction intervention(s) provided to an individual (separate procedure); approximately 15 minutes
99402	approximately 30 minutes
99403	approximately 45 minutes
99404	approximately 60 minutes

Report codes **99401–99404**

- Based on a physician's or other QHP's face-to-face time spent providing counseling.
- For a new or an established patient.
- When the medical record includes documentation of the total counseling time and a summary of the issues discussed. Time is met when the midpoint is passed (eg, 8 minutes of service required to report a 15-minute service).
- Cannot be reported in addition to a preventive medicine service (eg, **99393**) because preventive counseling is already taken into account.

Figure 9-2 lists the range of times included for codes **99401–99404** based on the midpoint rule.

Chapter 9. Preventive Services

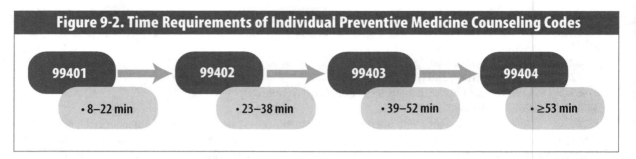

Figure 9-2. Time Requirements of Individual Preventive Medicine Counseling Codes

99401 • 8–22 min → 99402 • 23–38 min → 99403 • 39–52 min → 99404 • ≥53 min

See the Expectant Parent Counseling and Risk Reduction Intervention section later in this chapter for a discussion of counseling and risk-factor reduction intervention with expectant parents.

Examples

➤ **A physician provides counseling to parents of a child who is a picky eater and underweight.** The physician documents 20 minutes of face-to-face time spent with the parents discussing age-appropriate eating habits and assisting parents with a plan to encourage a healthy diet. Code **99401** (preventive medicine counseling and/or risk factor reduction intervention[s] provided to an individual [separate procedure]; approximately 15 minutes) is reported.

   Teaching Point: If the time of service had been 23 minutes or more, the midpoint between codes **99401** and **99402** (preventive medicine counseling; approximately 30 minutes) would be exceeded and code **99402** would be reported.

➤ **A mother requests counseling for her 14-year-old daughter who wishes to adopt a vegan diet.** The physician spends 30 minutes with the girl discussing why she wants to adopt a vegan diet (eg, avoid cruelty to animals), the importance of maintaining adequate nutrition, and a healthy approach to a vegan diet. A vitamin B_{12} supplement is also recommended.

ICD-10-CM	CPT
Z71.3 (dietary counseling and surveillance)	**99402** (risk-factor reduction counseling)

   Teaching Point: The physician's time of 30 minutes supports **99402**.

➤ **Parents of a 6-year-old request counseling for upcoming travel to Africa.** The pediatrician spends 25 minutes reviewing CDC recommendations for the areas of travel and counseling for potential health hazards for the child. Any recommended vaccines are administered, and the pediatrician recommends an appointment at a travel clinic for vaccines not available in the practice.

ICD-10-CM	CPT
Z71.84 (encounter for health counseling related to travel) **Z23** (encounter for immunization), if applicable	**99402** (risk-factor reduction counseling) Codes for vaccine products and administration

Expectant Parent Counseling and Risk Reduction Intervention

Codes **99401–99404** may be reported if a parent or family is seen by the physician to discuss a risk reduction intervention (ie, seeking advice to avoid a future problem or complication). If a family is referred by its obstetrician for an existing problem, the outpatient consultation should be reported using office-based consultation codes (**99241–99245**) or other appropriate E/M codes as directed by payer policy. (See **Chapter 7** for office and outpatient E/M services, **Chapter 8** for outpatient consultations, and **Chapter 16** for hospital E/M services.)

   ICD-10-CM code **Z76.81** (expectant parent[s] pre-birth pediatrician visit) would be reported for pre-birth counseling visits in addition to other *ICD-10-CM* codes as applicable. Family history codes may also be relevant for reporting the reason for pre-birth and/or preconception counseling (eg, **Z82.79**, family history of other congenital malformations, deformations, and chromosomal abnormalities).

When counseling and risk reduction interventions are provided to a mother or her fetus prior to delivery, report to the mother's insurance. Verification of the payer's benefit policy for these services is recommended prior to service; if non-covered, an advance beneficiary notice should be signed by the patient. An *advance beneficiary notice* or *waiver* is a written notice to the patient of noncoverage or potential out-of-pocket costs provided prior to delivery of a service. Verify payer requirements and applicable state regulations prior to using waivers in your practice. When used, a copy of the signed notice should be kept on file with the practice's billing records.

An encounter for a meet and greet is not considered a medically necessary service and will most likely not be covered. Check health plan contracts to determine if charging directly to the patient's caregiver is allowed and whether advance notification of noncoverage is required.

Preventive Medicine, Group Counseling Codes

99411   Preventive medicine counseling and/or risk factor reduction intervention(s) provided to individuals in a group setting (separate procedure); approximately 30 minutes

99412   approximately 60 minutes

Example

➤ **A group of 4 patients who have overweight attend a 30-minute session in the physician's office to discuss diet and exercise.** The physician conducts the counseling session.

ICD-10-CM	CPT
Z71.3 (dietary counseling and surveillance) **E66.3** (overweight) *Use additional code from category **Z68** to identify BMI.* **Z71.82** (exercise counseling)	**99411** (risk-factor reduction counseling, group)

    Teaching Point: Services are documented in each patient's medical record and are reported for each child. Services provided to a group of patients may not be reported as individual office E/M visits (**99202–99215**) because only face-to-face time spent counseling the individual patient may be reported based on time spent counseling and/or coordinating care when reporting office or other outpatient E/M visits.

    BMI codes in category **Z68** include

Z68.51   BMI <5th percentile
Z68.52   BMI 5th–<85th percentile
Z68.53   BMI 85th–95th percentile
Z68.54   BMI ≥95th percentile

Behavior Change Intervention

99406   Smoking and tobacco use cessation counseling visit; intermediate, >3 minutes up to 10 minutes
99407   intensive, >10 minutes
99408   Alcohol and/or substance (other than tobacco) abuse structured screening (eg, AUDIT, DAST), and brief intervention services; 15–30 minutes
99409   >30 minutes

    Behavior change interventions are for persons who have a behavior that is often considered an illness, such as tobacco use and addiction or substance use or misuse. Behavior change services may be reported when performed as part of the treatment of conditions related to or potentially exacerbated by the behavior or when performed to change the harmful behavior that has not yet resulted in illness.

● Behavior change intervention codes **99406–99409** are reported when
   — Services are provided by a physician or QHP for patients who have a behavior that is often considered an illness (eg, tobacco use and addiction, substance use or misuse).
   — Services involve specific validated interventions, including assessing readiness for and barriers to change, advising change in behavior, providing specific suggested actions and motivational counseling, and arranging for services and follow-up care.

     ●=New code   ▲=Revised code   #=Re-sequenced code   +=Add-on code

- Codes **99406–99409** include specific time requirements that must be met (eg, at least 15 minutes must be spent in counseling to support reporting of code **99408**).
- Do not separately report code **96160** for screening instruments used in conjunction with codes **99408** and **99409**.
- Medical record documentation supports the total time spent in the performance of the service, and a detail of the behavior change intervention is provided.
- Behavior change intervention services cannot be performed on a parent or guardian of a patient and reported under the patient's name.
- Behavior change interventions may be reported separately with preventive medicine or other E/M services.
  - Evaluation and management services reported on the same day must be separate and distinct.
  - Time spent in the provision of behavior change intervention may not be used as a basis for the selection of the other E/M code.
- When reporting a distinct E/M service, append modifier **25** to the code for the distinct E/M service (eg, **99213 25**).
- Code **99078** is reported when a physician counsels groups of patients with symptoms or an established illness. This service is reported for each participating child.

> See the Physician Group Education Services section in Chapter 11, Common Testing and Therapeutic Services in Office Settings, for an example of how code **99078** is used.

Examples

➤ **During an office visit for a 14-year-old new patient for an unrelated problem, it is learned that he has been smoking for 6 months but would like to quit.** The physician spends 10 minutes discussing specific methods to overcome barriers, pharmacological options, behavioral techniques, and nicotine replacement. The patient is referred to a community support group and a follow-up visit is scheduled in 2 weeks to provide additional encouragement and counseling as needed. Diagnosis is tobacco use.

ICD-10-CM	CPT
Use the code appropriate for problem addressed.	**99202–99205 25** (based on service performed and documented)
Z72.0 (tobacco use) **Z71.6** (tobacco abuse counseling)	**99406**

    Teaching Point: If only general advice and encouragement to stop smoking had been provided, it would be considered part of the new patient office visit. Counseling time must be documented. *ICD-10-CM* does not include a code for use of vaping products without a diagnosis of abuse or a vaping-related illness. Report **Z71.89** (other specified counseling) when counseling is focused on risks associated with vaping. See **F17.29-** for codes for nicotine dependence and vaping.

➤ **During a preventive medicine service for a 14-year-old established patient, it is learned that he frequently drinks beer and other alcoholic beverages.** The physician uses a structured screening tool to interview the patient about substance use. The result is positive, and the physician spends a total of 20 minutes interviewing the patient about substance use history and counseling the patient about risks associated with alcohol and drug use, not driving or riding with someone under the influence, and seeking an agreement to avoid future use.

ICD-10-CM	CPT
Z00.129 (routine child health examination without abnormal findings)	**99394 25** (preventive medicine visit)
Z71.89 (other specified counseling)	**99408**

Time of counseling should be specifically documented as beginning after conclusion of the preventive medicine service.

International Classification of Diseases, 10th Revision, Clinical Modification guidelines state that substance use codes (eg, **F10.99**, alcohol use, unspecified with unspecified alcohol-induced disorder) should only be assigned when the use is associated with a mental or behavioral disorder and such a relationship is documented by the provider.

Preventive Medicine Services Modifier

33   Preventive services

Modifier **33** is used to differentiate services provided as recommended preventive care when the service might also be provided for diagnostic indications. Some payers provide a listing of services for which modifier **33** is required when provided as a preventive service.

- The appropriate use of modifier **33** will reduce claim adjustments related to preventive services and corresponding payments to members.
- Modifier **33** should only be appended to codes represented in 1 or more of the following 4 categories:
  — Services rated A or B by the USPSTF
  — Immunizations for routine use in children, adolescents, and adults as recommended by ACIP
  — Preventive care and screenings for children as recommended by Bright Futures (AAP) and newborn testing (American College of Medical Genetics and Genomics)
  — Preventive care and screenings provided for women supported by HRSA

The US Preventive Services Task Force (USPSTF) grades A and B are defined as follows:

- **Grade A: The USPSTF recommends the service. There is high certainty that the net benefit is substantial.**
- **Grade B: The USPSTF recommends the service. There is high certainty that the net benefit is moderate or there is moderate certainty that the net benefit is moderate to substantial.**

Most health plans cover preventive services with grade A or B without cost to the patient (ie, no deductible, co-pay, or coinsurance).

- **DO *NOT* USE MODIFIER 33**
  — **When the *CPT* code(s) is identified as inherently preventive (eg, preventive medicine counseling)**
  — **When the service(s) is not indicated in the categories noted previously**
  — **With an insurance plan that continues to implement the cost-sharing policy on preventive medicine services (grandfathered health plan)**
- Check with your payers before fully implementing the use of modifier **33** to verify any variations in reporting requirements. Modifier **33** *is not used for benefit determination by some payers* and may be required by others only for services that may be either diagnostic/therapeutic or preventive.

Examples

➤ **A 3-year-old patient presents for her age-appropriate preventive medicine service.** An age-appropriate preventive medicine service is provided and documented. The child was recently seen by her dentist, who noted no damage to teeth and applied fluoride varnish to prevent caries. The child's mother notes concerns that she recently learned that her home may have a lead water service line. In addition to counseling the parents, the physician chooses to screen for lead.

ICD-10-CM	CPT
Z00.129	99392
Z00.129 Z13.88	83655 QW 33 (Lead, quantitative analysis)

Teaching Point: Append modifier **33** to code **83655** to indicate the preventive nature of the screening. In this case, the lead screening falls under Bright Futures recommendations for a 9-month-old. Note that the modifier does not have to be appended to code **99392** because that service is inherently preventive. Any immunization services provided are separately reported.

➤ **An 18-year-old is seen for an established patient office visit with request for immunization.** The patient's parents did not allow immunization after the patient was 7 years old and he would like to know if he may be immunized without their consent now that he has reached the age of majority in his state. The pediatrician discusses the parents' reasons for not immunizing and the patient's understanding of the risks and benefits of immunization and then counsels the patient about each vaccine/toxoid that will be administered on the date of service. Clinical staff administer and document the immunizations.

ICD-10-CM	CPT
Z23 (encounter for immunization) **Z28.3** (underimmunization status)	**90460 33** × the number of vaccine products administered **90461 33** × the number additional components in each combination vaccine Codes for each vaccine administered appended with modifier **33**

Teaching Point: Modifier **33** may be appended to the codes for the vaccine/toxoid products (eg, Tdap, meningococcal conjugate, and HPV products) and administration services to indicate the preventive nature of the immunization provided outside the typical immunization schedule.

Other Preventive Medicine Services

99429   Unlisted preventive medicine service

Code **99429** may be reported if these options are not suitable. If the unlisted code is used, most payers will require a copy of the progress notes filed with the claim.

Reporting a Preventive Medicine Visit With a Problem-Oriented Visit

When a problem or abnormality is addressed, *requires significant additional work* (eg, symptomatic atopic dermatitis, exercise-induced asthma, migraine headache, scoliosis), and is medically necessary, it may be reported using the office or other outpatient services codes (**99202–99205, 99212–99215**) in addition to the preventive medicine services code.

> Some payers have adopted policy that problem-oriented evaluation and management (E/M) services provided on the same date as a preventive medicine E/M service will be paid at 50% of the contractual amount agreed on under the health plan contract. When reporting to these payers, be sure to include all work related to the problem-oriented encounter in determining the level of service provided. Physicians should not reduce the level of service reported.

● The presence of a chronic condition(s) in and of itself does not change a preventive medicine visit to a problem-oriented visit; nor does it unilaterally support a separate problem-oriented E/M service (**99202–99205, 99212–99215**) with the well visit, unless it is significant and has been separately addressed.

● An insignificant problem or condition (eg, minor diaper rash, stable chronic problem, renewal of prescription medications) that does not require significant MDM or time cannot be reported as a separate E/M service.

   Although a separate E/M service is not reported when a minor problem or chronic condition requires less than significant additional work, the diagnosis code for the problem or chronic condition may be reported in addition to code **Z00.121** (routine child health examination with abnormal findings).

● It is important to make parents aware of any additional charges that may occur at the preventive medicine encounter. This includes, but is not limited to, a significant, separately identifiable E/M service.

— Some patients will be required to provide a co-payment for the non–preventive medicine visit code under the terms of their plan benefit even when there is no co-payment required for the preventive medicine visit. Legally, this co-payment cannot routinely be written off.

— The AAP has developed a template letter that can be used to outline what may not be covered under the no-cost-sharing preventive medicine services (www.aap.org/en-us/professional-resources/practice-transformation/getting-paid/Coding-at-the-AAP/Pages/Evaluation-and-Management.aspx).

Coding Conundrum: Reporting Evaluation and Management Services With Immunization Administration

Evaluation and management (E/M) services most often reported with the vaccine product and immunization administration (IA) include new and established patient preventive medicine visits (*Current Procedural Terminology* [*CPT*] codes **99381–99395**), problem-oriented visits (**99202–99215**), and preventive medicine counseling services (**99401–99404**).

If a patient is seen for the administration of a vaccine only, it is not appropriate to report an E/M visit if it is not medically necessary, significant, and separately identifiable. The E/M service must be clinically indicated.

Payers may require modifier **25** (significant, separately identifiable E/M service by the same physician on the same day of the procedure or other service) to be appended to the E/M code to distinguish it from the administration of the vaccine.

Do not report *CPT* code **99211** (established patient E/M, minimal level, not requiring physician presence) when the patient encounter is for vaccination only because Medicare Resource-Based Relative Value Scale (RBRVS) relative values for IA codes include administrative and clinical services (ie, greeting the patient, routine vital signs, obtaining a vaccine history, presenting the Vaccine Information Statement and responding to routine vaccine questions, preparation and administration of the vaccine, and documentation and observation of the patient following administration of the vaccine). However, if the service is medically necessary, significant, and separately identifiable, it may be reported with modifier **25** appended to the E/M code (**99211**). The medical record must clearly state the reason for the visit, brief history, physical examination, assessment and plan, and any other counseling or discussion items. The progress note must be signed with the physician's countersignature. For more information and clinical vignettes on the appropriate use of E/M services during IA, visit www.aap.org/cfp, access code AAPCFP26. Payers who do not follow the Medicare RBRVS may allow payment of code **99211** with IA. Know your payer guidelines, and if payment is allowed, make certain the guidelines are in writing and maintained in your office. Be aware that a co-payment may be required when the "nurse" visit is reported.

The same guidelines apply to physician visits (**99202–99215**).

When reporting both E/M services
- The documentation of the problem-oriented service must be distinct from that of the preventive service (even if included in the same encounter note) and clearly support the level of service reported.
- When the level of service is selected based on the physician's total time (on the date of the encounter) spent addressing the problem (not including any time spent providing the preventive service), the physician's total time spent addressing the problem must be distinctly documented in addition to documentation of the problem workup (eg, history of present illness, examination, records or test results reviewed), assessment, and plan.

    Documentation might indicate, "After completing the preventive service, I spent XX minutes evaluating and managing X condition."
- It is important to learn the payment policy of health plans commonly billed by your practice for billing of preventive and problem-oriented E/M services on the same date.
- Modifier **25** (significant, separately identifiable E/M service by the same physician on the same day of the procedure or other service) should be appended to the problem-oriented service code (eg, **99212**). If vaccines are given at the same encounter, append modifier **25** to the problem-oriented E/M service code and to the preventive medicine service code to avoid payer bundling edits that may allow payment only for IA.
- The AAP has developed an initial history questionnaire that promotes good documentation of preventive medicine services. Examples can be ordered from the AAP by calling 888/227-1770 or visiting https://shop.aap.org/product-list/?q=documentation%20forms. Additionally, some state Medicaid programs have developed documentation templates for preventive services delivered in their EPSDT program.
- *ICD-10-CM* well-care diagnosis codes (see code list earlier in this chapter in *ICD-10-CM* Codes for Preventive Care Visits) should be linked to the appropriate preventive medicine service code (**99381–99395**) and the sick care diagnosis code linked to the problem-oriented service code (**99202–99205, 99212–99215**).

In Claim Form Example 3, a patient received an established patient preventive service (**99393**) and a problem-oriented E/M service (**99212**) to address a plantar wart on the same date. The example shows diagnosis codes **Z00.121** and **B07.0** (plantar wart) listed in fields 21A and 21B. The A and B are diagnosis pointers used in column 24E to link the appropriate diagnosis codes to the procedure codes included on each service line. Note that diagnosis code **B07.0** (diagnosis pointer B) is linked to the preventive and problem-oriented services in column 24E. Modifier **25** is appended to code **99212** (field 24D under "Modifier") to indicate the significant, separately identifiable E/M service was provided in addition to the preventive medicine service (**99393**).

Claim Form Example 3: Preventive and Problem-Oriented Services

21. Diagnosis or nature of illness or injury (Relate A–L to service line below 24E)				ICD Ind. 0						
A. **Z00.121** B. **B07.0** C. D.										

24. A. Dates of service B. Place of service		C. EMG	D. Procedures, services or supplies CPT/HCPCS	Modifier	E. Diagnosis Pointer	F. Charges	G. Days or units	H. EPSDT	I. ID Qual	J. Rendering Provider #
1/2/2021– 1/2/2021	11		99393		AB	$$$	1		NPI	123456789
1/2/2021– 1/2/2021	11		99212	25	B	$$$	1		NPI	123456789

Abbreviations: *CPT, Current Procedural Terminology*; EMG, emergency; EPSDT, Early and Periodic Screening, Diagnostic, and Treatment; HCPCS, Healthcare Common Procedure Coding System; *ICD, International Classification of Diseases*; NPI, National Provider Identifier.

Examples

➤ **A 10-year-old boy receives a well-child (health supervision) visit.** This established patient also has previously diagnosed anxiety that is now exacerbated by health concerns of the grandmother who is his only caregiver. The grandmother notes she too is fearful about being too ill to care for her grandchild. Counseling with a licensed clinical social worker is recommended and arranged. The physician documents 20 minutes spent in counseling and coordinating care related to the patient's anxiety and the family's need for social support.

ICD-10-CM	CPT
Z00.121 (well-child check with abnormal findings) **F41.96** (anxiety) **Z63.79** (other stressful life events affecting family and household)	**99393** (preventive medicine visit)
F41.96 (anxiety) **Z63.79** (other stressful life events affecting family and household)	**99213 25** (office E/M service, total physician time 20–29 minutes)

Teaching Point: Documentation should clearly support the separate time of the problem-oriented E/M service, discussion topics, and plan of care for the problems addressed.

Codes for preventive counseling and risk-factor reduction intervention (eg, **99401**) are not appropriate for this example. Risk-factor reduction services are used for persons without a specific illness for which the counseling might otherwise be used as part of treatment. This patient has increased anxiety that prompts the counseling.

➤ **A 3-year-old boy with previously evaluated benign heart murmur is seen for a preventive medicine visit.** There are no new abnormal findings at the encounter.

ICD-10-CM	CPT
Z00.129 (well-child check without abnormal findings) **R01.0** (benign and innocent cardiac murmurs)	Preventive medicine visit **New Patient** **Established Patient** **99382** **99392**

Teaching Point: Because the benign heart murmur requires no additional workup or management, only the preventive medicine service is reported. The diagnosis code for the heart murmur may be reported as an additional diagnosis to the code for the well-child check but is not a finding of the well-child check.

See **Table 9-3** for additional illustration of coding for problem-oriented E/M services provided on the same date as preventive E/M services.

Coding Continuum Model: Problem-Oriented and Preventive Evaluation and Management on the Same Date

Table 9-3. Coding Continuum Model: Problem-Oriented and Preventive Evaluation and Management on the Same Date			
Code selection may be based on the complexity of medical decision-making or the total time spent by the physician or QHP solely devoted to the problem-oriented E/M on the date of the encounter.			
CPT Code Time Vignette (Appropriate preventive E/M service codes are also reported.)	**Medical Decision-making (2 of 3 elements required)**		
	Number and Complexity of Problems Addressed	**Amount and/or Complexity of Data Reviewed and Analyzed**	**Risk of Complications and/ or Morbidity or Mortality of Patient Management**
99212 (10–19 min) A 4-year-old presents today for a previously scheduled preventive service and follow-up visit for recurrent bilateral otitis media with effusion (**H65.196**) diagnosed 1 week ago, which is resolving.	Low Acute illness—resolving	Limited Assessment requiring an independent historian(s)	Minimal
99213 (20–29 min) A 4-year-old presents today for a previously scheduled preventive service and is found to have acute right otitis media with effusion (**H65.01**).	Low 1 acute, uncomplicated illness or injury	Limited Assessment requiring an independent historian(s)	Moderate Prescription of antibiotic
99214 (30–39 min) A 4-year-old presents today for a previously scheduled preventive service and follow-up visit for chronic bilateral otitis media with effusion (**H65.23**) diagnosed 1 week ago. On examination, eardrums are still inflamed, and the child complains of intermittent pain.	Moderate Chronic illness with exacerbation	Limited Hearing evaluation ordered Assessment requiring an independent historian(s)	Moderate Prescription of second-line antibiotic Consider/discuss tympanocentesis or referral to an allergist or otolaryngologist for tympanostomy.
99215 (40–54 min) A 4-year-old presents today for a previously scheduled preventive service and follow-up visit for chronic bilateral otitis media with effusion (**H65.23**) diagnosed 1 week ago. On examination, eardrums are still inflamed, and the child complains of intermittent pain.	40 minutes or more beyond (after) the time of the preventive medicine service is spent by the physician on the date of the encounter in evaluation of the otitis media, review of the number of previous infections and antibiotics used in treatment, shared decision-making with the parents, ordering of antibiotic including verifying inclusion in the patient's health plan formulary, ordering consultation with otolaryngology for evaluation and consideration of surgery and a hearing test, and documenting the problem-oriented service. (Documentation should specifically state time is separate from that spent providing the preventive medicine service and include details of the evaluation and counseling and/or coordination of care provided.)		
Abbreviations: *CPT, Current Procedural Terminology*; E/M, evaluation and management; QHP, qualified health care professional.			
Note regarding **99214** or **99215**: In many cases, a problem that requires these higher levels of E/M service may warrant delay of the preventive E/M service.			
Time-based E/M: Time is the total time spent in activities related to the problem-oriented E/M service by the physician or QHP on the date of the encounter. Do not include time of the preventive medicine service or time of other separately reported services.			

Chapter 9. Preventive Services

Resources

Bright Futures

AAP/Bright Futures "Recommendations for Preventive Pediatric Health Care" (also see insert) (www.aap.org/periodicityschedule)

Quality Measurement Information

US Department of Health and Human Services, Agency for Healthcare Research and Quality, National Guideline Clearinghouse (www.qualitymeasures.ahrq.gov)

CPT Category II codes (www.ama-assn.org/practice-management/cpt-category-ii-codes)

Physician Consortium for Performance Improvement (www.thepcpi.org)

Sports/Camp Physicals

"Sports and Camp Physicals" (June 2017 *AAP Pediatric Coding Newsletter*˚) (https://coding.solutions.aap.org/article.aspx?articleid=2629481)

"Preparing for Preparticipation Physical Evaluations" (July 2018 *AAP Pediatric Coding Newsletter*) (https://coding.solutions.aap.org/article.aspx?articleid=2685958)

Immunization and Vaccines

Appendix III, Vaccine Products: Commonly Administered Pediatric Vaccines

AMA Category I vaccine codes (www.ama-assn.org/practice-management/cpt/category-i-vaccine-codes)

CDC VFC program (www.cdc.gov/vaccines/programs/vfc/index.html)

Coding at the AAP vaccine coding (www.aap.org/en-us/professional-resources/practice-transformation/getting-paid/Coding-at-the-AAP/Pages/Vaccine-Coding.aspx)
>   Template Comment Letter for Members on Immunization Administration
>   Vaccine Counseling and Preventive Care Visits
>   Influenza Vaccines: Coding for the Current Season
>   Vaccine Coding Table
>   When Is It Appropriate to Report an E/M Service During Immunization Administration?
>
>   FAQ—Pediatric Immunization Administration Codes
>   CDC Vaccine Price List
>   New Versus Established Patient Status After Vaccine Only Encounter

AAP *Pediatric Vaccines: Coding Quick Reference Card 2021* (https://shop.aap.org/pediatric-vaccine-coding-quick-reference-chart-card-2021)

Laboratory Testing

CLIA-waived procedures list (http://cms.hhs.gov/Regulations-and-Guidance/Legislation/CLIA/Categorization_of_Tests.html)

National Drug Codes

US FDA NDC directory (www.fda.gov/drugs/drug-approvals-and-databases/national-drug-code-directory)

Oral Health Preventive Services

Oral Health Coding Fact Sheet for Primary Care Physicians (www.aap.org/en-us/Documents/coding_factsheet_oral_health.pdf)

AAP Section on Oral Health state-specific information (www.aap.org/en-us/about-the-aap/Committees-Councils-Sections/Oral-Health/Map/Pages/State-Information-and-Resources-Map.aspx)

Preventive Services: Patient/Payer Advocacy

Template letter to payers that deny code **99211** for evaluation of a TB skin test ("Coding Resources" at https://coding.aap.org; access code AAPCFP26)

"The Business Case for Pricing Vaccines" ("Coding Resources" at https://www.aap.org/en-us/Documents/practicet_businesscasepricingvacc.pdf; access code AAPCFP26)

What is Included in Preventive Medicine Encounters: Template Letter (www.aap.org/en-us/professional-resources/practice-transformation/getting-paid/Coding-at-the-AAP/Pages/Evaluation-and-Management.aspx)

Chapter 9. Preventive Services

Vision Screening

AAP Section on Ophthalmology and Committee on Practice and Ambulatory Medicine, American Academy of Ophthalmology, American Association for Pediatric Ophthalmology and Strabismus, and American Association of Certified Orthoptists "Instrument-Based Pediatric Vision Screening Policy Statement," *Pediatrics* (http://pediatrics.aappublications.org/content/130/5/983.full)

Test Your Knowledge!

1. **Which of the following may be an abnormal finding in a preventive medicine evaluation and management service?**
   a. Stable asthma requiring no evaluation and management
   b. A known congenital anomaly causing no new complaint
   c. New family history due to birth of a healthy sibling
   d. A new complaint of difficulty feeding or lack of appetite

2. **Which service is reported with code 90460?**
   a. Immunization of an 18-year-old patient with physician counseling
   b. Immunization administration on a date after the date of physician counseling
   c. Immunization of a 19-year-old patient
   d. Immunization with counseling provided by clinical staff

3. **How is provision of 2 developmental screening instruments at 1 encounter reported?**
   a. 96110 × 2 units
   b. Developmental screening is included in 99381 or 99391.
   c. 96110, 96110 59
   d. a or c

4. **Which code indicates a physician's skill is required for venipuncture on a 4-year-old?**
   a. 36400
   b. 36415
   c. 36410
   d. 36416

5. **Which of the following is true for behavior change intervention services (99406–99409)?**
   a. Codes 99406–99409 are reported for anticipatory tobacco abuse counseling.
   b. Codes 99406–99409 are reported for generalized counseling about diet and exercise.
   c. Codes 99406–99409 are subject to the midpoint rule for time of service.
   d. Codes 99406–99409 include specific time requirements that must be met.

Surgery, Infusion, and Sedation in the Outpatient Setting

Contents

Surgical Package Rules

Current Procedural Terminology (*CPT*®) surgical codes (**10004–69990**) are *packaged* or *global* codes. To understand documentation and coding of procedural services, it is necessary to know what is included in each service from a coding and payment perspective. *CPT* directs that each procedure code represents a "surgical package" of service components. These include

- Evaluation and management (E/M) services subsequent to the decision for surgery on the day before and/or day of surgery (including the history and physical examination)
- Local or topical anesthesia, including metacarpal, metatarsal, and/or digital block
- Immediate postoperative care
- Writing orders
- Evaluation of the patient in the recovery area
- Typical postoperative follow-up care

Using the *CPT* definition of the surgical package, relative value units (RVUs) are assigned to each procedure based on the typical preoperative, intraoperative, and postoperative physician work; practice expense (eg, procedure room, instruments, supplies, support staff); and professional liability. Payers that use RVUs to calculate payments will typically not pay separately for any components of the surgical package.

> The relative value units assigned to procedures include the typically used supplies under the practice expense component. Know your payer policies on this.

Medicare Surgical Package Definition

Most state Medicaid programs follow the Medicare definition of the surgical package. The Medicare definition differs from that of *CPT*.

- Medicare defines procedures as *minor* (procedures assigned a 0- or 10-day global period or endoscopies) or *major* (procedures assigned a 90-day global period). (**Table 10-1** includes global periods for common pediatric procedures.) *The day of surgery is day 0 (zero); the postoperative period begins the next day.*
- For minor procedures, the E/M visit on the date of the procedure is considered a routine part of the procedure *regardless of whether it is prior or subsequent to the decision for surgery.* In these cases, modifier **57** (decision for surgery) is not recognized.
- Medicare states an E/M code may be reported on the same day as a minor surgical procedure only when a significant, separately identifiable E/M service is performed with modifier **25** appended to the E/M code. *CPT* does not specifically include the initial E/M service prior to a minor procedure when the decision for surgery occurs at the visit.
- *CPT* also does not include care related to surgical complications in the surgical package. Medicare considers care related to complications following surgery to be included in the surgical package unless a return to the operating room is necessary.
- Global periods and minor or major surgery are not defined in *CPT*. Global periods are defined in the Medicare Physician Fee Schedule (MPFS). Although other payers can assign different global periods, most follow the MPFS.
- The RVUs and global period assigned to each service can be found in the current MPFS at www.cms.gov/medicare/medicare-fee-for-service-payment/physicianfeesched.

> Learn more about the Resource-Based Relative Value Scale in Chapter 4.

Most office and outpatient clinic procedures will have 0- or 10-day global periods. Exceptions are certain services such as care of fractures (discussed later in this chapter). The day of surgery is day 0 (zero); the postoperative period begins the next day.

Table 10-1. The Medicare Surgical Package			
Global Periods	**0-Day Global Surgeries**	**10-Day Global Surgeries**	**90-Day Global Surgeries**
Services before the date of surgery	Not included		All related services 1 day before surgery if after decision for surgery
Services on the date of procedure	E/M services typically included regardless of when decision for surgery is made		All related services except E/M services at which decision for surgery is made
Postoperative services	Typical postoperative care on the same date	All related care on date of service and 10 days following	All related care on date of service and 90 days following, including care for complications that does not require a return to the OR

Abbreviations: E/M, evaluation and management; OR, operating room.

Significant Evaluation and Management Service and Procedure

The Medicare Resource-Based Relative Value Scale is used by most private payers and Medicaid plans to determine RVUs and global periods for services. Under this payment methodology, procedural services include some preservice and post-service E/M by the performing physician. Payer edits, such as the National Correct Coding Initiative (NCCI) edits used by Medicare, Medicaid, and many other payers, also bundle E/M services with certain procedures.

For minor procedures, separate payment for a significant, separately identifiable E/M service is allowed when modifier **25** is appended to the E/M code. However, care should be taken to use modifier **25** only when documentation supports a significant and separately identifiable E/M service.

For major procedures (typically 90-day global period), modifier **57** may be appended when the decision for surgery or a procedure is made during the E/M service on the same date as the procedure. Documentation should clearly show E/M of the problem resulting in the initial decision to perform the related procedure.

Coding Conundrum: Procedure, or Evaluation and Management and Procedure?

The differences in the Centers for Medicare & Medicaid Services (CMS) and *Current Procedural Terminology* (*CPT*) surgical package guidelines may lead to confusion. Try to answer the following questions when determining if you should report a procedure alone or a procedure with an evaluation and management (E/M) service:

- Did you address a problem or condition prior to deciding to perform the procedure (above and beyond the usual preoperative care associated with the procedure) or a significant and separately identifiable problem? If yes, report an E/M service and procedure.
- Does the medical record documentation clearly support the performance of a medically necessary E/M service (required key components), the procedure (procedure note), the medical necessity for both, and the decision to perform the surgery? If yes, report an E/M service and procedure.
- Was the purpose of the visit for the procedure only? If yes, do not report an E/M service.
- Does the payer follow the *CPT* or CMS guidelines for reporting surgical procedures? If the focus of an E/M service is related to the procedure, the history and physical examination are part of preoperative service and only the surgical procedure should be reported.

Example

➤ **A physician sees a patient who returns for a previously planned incision in the lingual frenum.** On examination, the physician notes milia are present at the corners of the infant's mouth. The physician reexamines the frenum. Documentation includes notation of patient/caregiver consent, procedure, patient tolerance, outcome, and post-procedural examination finding (eg, breastfeeding without difficulty).

International Classification of Diseases, 10th Revision, Clinical Modification (ICD-10-CM)	*CPT*
Q38.1 (congenital ankyloglossia)	**41010** (incision in the lingual frenum to free the tongue)

Teaching Point: Although the physician noted milia, this does not support a significant and separately identifiable E/M service beyond the preservice/post-service work of the procedure that was provided or documented.

Reporting Postoperative Care

- Report *CPT* code **99024** (postoperative follow-up visit) for follow-up care provided during the global surgery period. No RVUs are assigned to **99024**, as the RVUs were included in the total value of the related procedure.
  - Reporting code **99024** allows a practice to track the number of visits performed during the postoperative period of specific procedures, calculate office overhead expenses (eg, supplies, staff, physician time) associated with the procedure, and potentially use the data to negotiate higher payment rates.
  - Payment for postoperative care is included as part of the procedure. Payers track the postoperative care provided.
  - If a physician is not providing or reporting the postoperative care typically performed for a procedure, payers may reduce payment for the surgical service.

> Payment of a surgical procedure may be reduced if the physician does not report code **99024**.

- When the physician who performed a procedure provides an unrelated E/M service during the postoperative period, modifier **24** (unrelated E/M service by the same physician during a postoperative period) should be appended to the E/M service code.
- When a physician *other than the surgeon* provides unrelated services to a patient during the postoperative period, the services are reported without a modifier. Despite the use of different National Provider Identifiers and diagnosis codes, some payers with assigned follow-up surgical periods will deny the service. The claim should be appealed for payment with a letter advising the payer that the service was unrelated to surgical care.

Example

➤ **A 4-year-old patient returns 8 days after removal of a foreign body from his right foot (10120 RT) with complaint of rhinorrhea and sore throat.** The physician diagnoses seasonal allergic rhinitis and acute pharyngitis. The physician also rechecks the wound on the right foot, which is healing as expected.

ICD-10-CM	CPT
J30.2 (other season allergic rhinitis) **J02.9** (acute pharyngitis, unspecified) **S90.851D** (superficial foreign body, right foot, subsequent encounter)	**99213 24**

    Teaching Point: Modifier **24** is reported to identify that the service provided was unrelated to the prior procedure. The medical decision-making (MDM) of the E/M service was low based on a low number and complexity of problems addressed (otitis media, pharyngitis), assessment requiring an independent historian, and minimal to low risk. The evaluation of the healing wound during the postoperative period is not included in determining the level of service for the encounter because it is included in postoperative care when provided during the 10-day global period.

> See Chapter 2 for more information on modifiers.

Supplies and Materials

99070   Supplies and materials provided by the physician over and above those usually included with the office visit or other services rendered

- Items such as elastic wraps, clavicle splints, or circumcision and suturing trays may be reported with this code. Remember that some supplies (eg, suturing trays, circumcision trays) may be included with the surgical procedure if the payer uses RVUs as its basis for payment.
- Only the supplies purchased in an office-based practice may be reported.

> If reporting code **99070**, identify the supplies or materials on the claim form and be prepared to submit an invoice.

- Some payers will require the use of Healthcare Common Procedure Coding System (HCPCS) codes. More specific HCPCS codes are available for a number of supplies (eg, codes **Q4001–Q4051** for cast and splint supplies). Use HCPCS codes when they are more specific.

For more information on Healthcare Common Procedure Coding System codes, see Chapter 1.

Reporting Terminated Procedures

When a procedure is started but cannot be completed due to extenuating circumstances, physicians should consider the individual situation, including the reason for termination of the procedure and the amount of work that was performed, when determining how to report the service rendered.

When a procedure was performed but not entirely successful (eg, portion of foreign body removed), it may be appropriate to report the procedure code that represents the work performed without modification.

- Only report reduced services (modifier **52**) or discontinued procedure (modifier **53**) when the service was significantly reduced from the typical service.
- If the work performed prior to discontinuation was insignificant, it may be appropriate to not report the procedure. If you choose to not report the procedure, consider whether the level of a related E/M service was increased due to the complexity of MDM associated with the attempted procedure, any complicating factors, and the revised management or treatment plan.

See an example of a discontinued service later in this chapter in the Removal of Impacted Cerumen section.

Common Pediatric Procedures

Minor Procedures That Do Not Have a Code

Some minor procedures are considered inherent to an E/M code or do not have separate *CPT* codes. However, any supplies used may be reported. The following procedures are included in an E/M service:

- Insertion or removal of an ear wick
- Removal of *nonimpacted* cerumen from the ear
- Nasal aspiration
- Nasogastric tube insertion without fluoroscopic guidance
- Removal of an umbilical clamp
- Removal of foreign bodies from skin that do not require an incision
- Puncture of abscess without aspiration
- Wound closure with adhesive strips only (eg, Steri-Strips, butterfly bandages)
- The use of fluorescein dye and a Wood lamp to examine for a corneal abrasion or foreign body of the eye

Common Procedure Values and Global Days

For other procedural services, verify separate reporting through your procedural coding reference. There is value in capturing the procedural services that are distinct from E/M services.

Example

➤ **A physician removes a foreign body from a child's nose.** If the MDM for the office visit supports code **99213** (level 3 established patient office E/M), the E/M service was assigned 2.11 total non-facility RVUs in 2020, whereas code **30300** (foreign body removal from nose) was assigned 5.40 non-facility RVUs in 2020.

Both services are reported only if a significant, separately identifiable E/M service, beyond the preservice work of the foreign body removal, is provided.

Table 10-2 details the number of global days for each of the commonly reported office procedures.

- Remember that when reporting any procedures containing 0, 10, or 90 global days, modifier **25** or **57** is required on any separately identifiable E/M service done on the same day (or, in some instances, the previous day prior to a planned major surgery).
- Those E/M services that are unrelated to the procedure that take place within the code's 10- or 90-day global period will require modifier **24**.

Table 10-2. Common Office Procedures and Global Days			
CPT Code	Description[a]	Global Period (d)	Total Non-facility RVUs (2020)
10060, 10061	Drainage of skin abscess	10	3.44, 5.97
10120, 10121	FB removal, SQ	10	4.31, 7.76
11200	Removal of skin tags	10	2.52
11760	Repair of nail bed	10	5.55
12001, 12011	Laceration repair, simple <2.5 cm	0	2.58, 3.15
12031, 12041, 12051	Laceration repair, intermediate <2.5 cm	10	7.17, 7.19, 7.73
16000, 16020	Burn care	0	2.09, 2.35
17110, 17111	Destruction benign lesions (eg, warts)	10	3.17, 3.72
17250	Chemical cautery	0	2.42
23500	Treatment of clavicle fracture	90	6.32
24640	Treatment elbow dislocation (nursemaid)	10	2.89
28190	FB removal, foot, subcutaneous (above fascia)	10	7.27
28490	Treatment big toe fracture (closed)	90	4.07
30300	Removal intranasal FB, office	10	5.40
30901	Nosebleed cautery/packing	0	4.09
41010	Incision in lingual frenulum	10	5.97
51701, 51702	Bladder catheterization	0	1.28, 1.74
54150	Circumcision	0	4.40

Abbreviations: CPT, Current Procedural Terminology; FB, foreign body; RVU, relative value unit; SQ, subcutaneous.

[a] Descriptors are abbreviated. Please see your 2021 coding reference for full descriptors and code selection.

Integumentary Procedures

Incision and Drainage

10060   Incision and drainage of abscess (eg, carbuncle, suppurative hidradenitis, cutaneous or subcutaneous abscess, cyst, furuncle, or paronychia); simple or single

10061   complicated or multiple

- The global period for codes **10060** and **10061** is 10 days.
- *CPT* does not provide differentiation between simple and complicated incision and drainage (I&D) and leaves code selection to the physician's judgment.
- The simple I&D procedure typically involves local anesthesia, an incision, expression of purulent drainage, obtaining a culture, irrigation, completely opening the cavity, and packing/dressing the wound.
- Complex I&D often typically involves a deeper incision, breakdown of multiple loculations, placement of a drain, and/or debridement of the cavity.
- The difference in RVUs for **10060** (3.44 total non-facility) and **10061** (5.97 total non-facility) indicates the significant additional work and practice expense associated with complicated or multiple I&D procedures.

Example

➤ **A 12-year-old presents with an abscess on his right lower leg.** The decision is made to perform I&D. The physician documents administration of local anesthetic, incision of skin above the abscess, and expression of purulent material. The wound was irrigated and packed. The patient will return in 3 days for reevaluation.

Code **10060** is reported for the procedure. All related visits (eg, follow-up visit to recheck the wound) within the 10 days following the date of surgery may be reported with code **99024** and no charge.

Removal of Skin Tags and Congenital Accessory Digits

11200   Removal of skin tags, multiple fibrocutaneous tags, any area; up to and including 15 lesions

Code **11200** is used to report the removal of a sixth digit from a newborn. It is equivalent to a skin tag and would not be assigned the code for an actual digit removal. The *ICD-10-CM* codes for accessory digits would be **Q69.0**, accessory fingers; **Q69.1**, accessory thumb; **Q69.2**, accessory toes; or **Q69.9**, unspecified. A 10-day global period applies under the MPFS.

Destruction of Benign Lesions (eg, Warts)

17110   Destruction (eg, laser surgery, electrosurgery, cryosurgery, chemosurgery, surgical curettement) of benign lesions other than skin tags or cutaneous vascular proliferative lesions; up to 14 lesions

17111   15 or more lesions

Report destruction of common or plantar warts, flat warts, or molluscum contagiosum with code **17110** or **17111** (with 1 unit of service), depending on the number of lesions removed. Do not report both **17110** and **17111** because they are mutually exclusive. Report *ICD-10-CM* using code **B08.1** for molluscum contagiosum, **B07.8** for common warts, or **B07.0** for plantar warts. A 10-day global period applies to both **17110** and **17111**.

Chemical Cauterization of Granulation Tissue

17250   Chemical cauterization of granulation tissue (ie, proud flesh)

Code **17250** is appropriately reported for cauterization of an umbilical granuloma. Do not report **17250** with removal or excision codes for the same lesion, for achieving wound hemostasis, or in conjunction with active wound care management. A 0-day global period applies.

Example

➤ **A 2-week-old presents for her well-baby check.** On examination, a moderate-sized umbilical granuloma is noted. The physician takes a very brief history and decides to cauterize. The routine well-baby check is completed in addition to cauterization of the umbilical granuloma.

ICD-10-CM	CPT
Z00.121 (encounter for routine child health examination with abnormal findings)	**99391 25**
P83.81 (umbilical granuloma)	**17250**

Teaching Point: Preservice work includes explanation of the procedure, obtaining informed consent, positioning and draping, preparing the site, and scrubbing in. Post-service work includes discussing follow-up care with parents and/or caregivers. Supplies and equipment, such as silver nitrate and an applicator, are included in the value assigned to the code when reporting to payers using RVUs. This service has a 0-day global period.

Laceration Repairs

12001–12018   Simple repair
12031–12057   Intermediate repair
13100–13160   Complex repair
● Categories of difficulty of wound repairs are described as
  — *Simple:* Superficial wound and/or subcutaneous wound requiring a simple single-layer closure or tissue adhesives. A 0-day global period applies.

— *Intermediate:* Includes the repair of wounds that, in addition to the requirements for simple repair, require layered closure of 1 or more of the deeper layers of subcutaneous tissue and superficial (non-muscle) fascia, in addition to skin (epidermal and dermal) closure. Intermediate repair includes limited undermining (defined as a distance less than the maximum width of the defect, measured perpendicular to the closure line, along at least 1 entire edge of the defect). Single-layer closure of heavily contaminated wounds that require extensive cleaning or removal of particulate matter also constitutes intermediate repair. A 10-day global period applies.

— *Complex:* Includes the repair of wounds that, in addition to the requirements for intermediate repair, require at least 1 of the following: exposure of bone, cartilage, tendon, or named neurovascular structure; debridement of wound edges (eg, traumatic lacerations or avulsions); extensive undermining (defined as distance equal to or greater than the maximum width of the defect, measured perpendicular to the closure line, along at least 1 entire edge of the defect); involvement of free margins of helical rim, vermilion border, or nostril rim; or placement of retention sutures. Necessary preparation includes creation of a limited defect for repairs or the debridement of complicated lacerations or avulsions. Complex repair does not include excision of benign (**11400–11446**) or malignant (**11600– 11646**) lesions, excisional preparation of a wound bed (**15002–15005**), or debridement of an open fracture or open dislocation. A 10-day global applies to most complex wound repairs. Late wound closure (**13160**) has a 90-day global period.

- Codes **12001–13160** are used to report wound closure using sutures, staples, or tissue adhesives (eg, Dermabond), singly or in combination with adhesive strips.
- Wound closure using adhesive strips (eg, Steri-Strips, butterfly bandages) only is considered inherent to the E/M service. However, the supplies (eg, Steri-Strips, butterfly bandages) may be reported separately using code **99070** (supplies and materials) or **A4450** (tape, non-waterproof, per 18 sq in). There are no specific HCPCS codes for Steri-Strips or butterfly bandages.
- Some payers may accept HCPCS code **G0168** (wound closure using tissue adhesive[s]) in lieu of simple repair codes (eg, **12001**, **12011**).
- Codes are reported based on the difficulty of the repair, measured length of the wound, and the location. To report wound repair, measure the length of the repaired wound(s) in centimeters.
  - If multiple wounds belong to the same category of difficulty and location, add the lengths and report with a single code.
  - If multiple wounds do not belong in the same category, report each repair separately with the more complicated repair reported as the primary procedure and the less complicated repair reported as the secondary procedure. Modifier **51** (multiple procedures) should be appended to the secondary code(s).
  - Simple ligation of vessels is considered as part of the wound closure.
- Wound debridement and/or cleaning and the provision of topical or injected local anesthesia are included in the wound repair code.
  - Debridement is considered a separate procedure only when gross contamination requires prolonged cleaning, excessive amounts of devitalized tissue are removed, or debridement is performed without immediate primary closure.
  - To report extensive tissue debridement, see codes **11042–11047** for selective debridement of subcutaneous, muscle, fascial tissues, and/or bone (includes debridement of dermis and epidermis when performed) or **97597** and **97598** for debridement of skin, epidermis, and/or dermis.

Know Your A, D, S Seventh Characters!

International Classification of Diseases, 10th Revision, Clinical Modification seventh characters A, D, and S define an encounter type for injuries and certain other diagnoses. Here are tips for remembering which character to use.

- A: active management of the initial injury or complications
- D: during healing of an injury that does not require active management (eg, routine follow-up, suture removal)
- S: scars and other sequela (effects of an injury) (Always report the sequela code before the injury code when the service is directed to the sequela.)

Seventh characters are also appended to codes for external cause of injury (eg, tripping).

Examples

➤ **A 10-year-old sustained a 1.5-cm laceration on his left knee requiring a simple (single layer) repair after a fall from playground equipment.**

ICD-10-CM	CPT
S81.012A (laceration without foreign body left knee, initial encounter) **W09.8XXA** (fall on or from other playground equipment, initial encounter) **Y92.838** (other recreation area)	**12001** (simple repair of superficial wounds of scalp, neck, axillae, external genitalia, trunk and/or extremities [including hands and feet]; 2.5 cm or less)

Teaching Point: Simple repair includes only the care on the date of the repair (0-day global period). Follow-up E/M visits are separately reported and do not require a modifier.

➤ **A 10-year-old fell from playground equipment and sustained a 1.5-cm laceration on his left knee and a 1.5-cm laceration on his left forearm. Each laceration required an intermediate repair.**

ICD-10-CM	CPT
S81.012A (laceration without foreign body left knee, initial encounter) **S51.812A** (laceration of left forearm without foreign body, initial encounter) **W09.8XXA** **Y92.838**	**12032** (intermediate repair, extremities, 2.6–7.5 cm)

Teaching Point: The measurement of both wounds (3 cm) is between 2.6 and 7.5 cm, both wounds are in the same family of anatomical sites, and both require the same level of repair. If the patient returns for wound follow-up within the 10 days following the date of repair, code **99024** (postoperative follow-up visit) is reported for the encounter because intermediate repair has a 10-day global period. There is no separate charge for care within the global period.

Suture Removal

The Medicare global surgery period for *CPT* codes **12001–12018** (simple repair of superficial wound) is 0 days, meaning payment includes the procedure or service plus any associated care provided on the same day of service. Therefore, practices may report a separate E/M service for removal of sutures placed in the office.

The Medicare global surgery period for intermediate (**12031–12057**) and complex (**13100–13153**) wound repairs is 10 days. Payment includes the procedure or service plus any associated follow-up care for a period of 10 days. Therefore, the charge for the procedure already includes suture removal by the same physician or a physician of the same group and specialty as part of the global surgical package.

When sutures are removed by another physician with a different tax identification number, an E/M office visit code may be reported for the suture removal. Some payers may allow reporting of HCPCS code **S0630**. Code **S0630** is for removal of sutures by a physician other than the physician who originally closed the wound. **S** codes are HCPCS Level II codes, designated by the Centers for Medicare & Medicaid Services and recognized by national BlueCross BlueShield payers, but coverage is on a payer-by-payer basis.

For aftercare of an injury, assign the acute injury code with the seventh character **D** (subsequent encounter). *ICD-10-CM* code **Z48.02** (encounter for removal of sutures) *is not reported* for removal of sutures placed to repair an injury.

Examples

➤ **An 8-year-old sustained a 0.5-cm laceration on her forehead.** The wound on her face requires a simple repair. She is seen in follow-up 7 days later. The wound is clean, and sutures are removed.

Visit	ICD-10-CM	CPT
Initial visit	**S01.81XA** (laceration without foreign body of other part of head, initial encounter)	**12011** (simple repair of the facial laceration 2.5 cm or less)
Follow-up visit	**S01.81XD** (laceration without foreign body of other part of head, subsequent encounter)	**99212** (problem-focused E/M visit, office or outpatient)

 Teaching Point: The seventh character **D** (ie, **S01.81XD**) is reported for encounters after the patient has received active treatment of the condition and is receiving routine care for the condition during the healing or recovery phase. Simple laceration repair has a 0-day global period, so any medically necessary follow-up care is separately reported.

➤ **A 3-year-old with 5 sutures placed in the emergency department presents at her pediatrician's office for suture removal.** The child is uncooperative and 2 clinical staff members are required to assist the pediatrician in removing the sutures. The physician's total time devoted to the patient's care on the date of service is 25 minutes.

ICD-10-CM	CPT
Appropriate code for injury with seventh character **D** (eg, **S51.812D**, laceration of left forearm without foreign body, subsequent encounter)	**S0630** (removal of sutures by a physician other than the physician who originally closed the wound), or **99213** (established patient E/M 20–29 minutes) based on the physician's total time

 Teaching Point: The 2021 office and other outpatient E/M codes may be reported based on the physician or other qualified health care professional's (QHP's) total time on the date of the encounter. Do not include time of clinical staff.

Other Repairs

Code **11760** (repair of nail bed) is reported when part or all of the nail plate is lifted and a laceration of the nail bed is repaired.

 Report code **40650** (repair of vermilion border of the lip) when a laceration of the full thickness of the lip and vermilion is repaired.

 Laceration repairs of the tongue (**41250–41252**) are reported based on size and location (eg, repair of laceration 2.5 cm or less, anterior two-thirds of the tongue is reported using code **41250**).

Burn Care

CPT code **16000** (initial treatment, first-degree burn, where no more than local treatment is required) is reported when initial treatment is performed for the symptomatic relief of a first-degree burn that is characterized by erythema and tenderness.

16020   Dressings and/or debridement of partial-thickness burns, initial or subsequent; small or less than 5% total body (eg, finger)

 Code **16020**

- Is used to report treatment of burns with dressings and/or debridement of small partial-thickness burns (second degree), whether initial or subsequent.
- An E/M visit with modifier **25** appended may be reported if a significant, separately identifiable E/M service is medically indicated, performed, and documented in addition to the burn care.

See Chapter 19 for coding of larger partial-thickness or full-thickness burns.

Chapter 10. Surgery, Infusion, and Sedation in the Outpatient Setting

Examples

➤ **A 9-year-old complaining of sunburn on her shoulders is seen by the physician.** There is redness and tenderness, but no blistering. Topical treatment is applied and an over-the-counter treatment for the first-degree burn is ordered.

ICD-10-CM	CPT
L55.0 (first-degree sunburn)	**16000** (first-degree burn requiring local treatment)

➤ **A 4-year-old is seen in the office after sustaining a burn on the first finger of her right hand from touching a hot pan.** The area is red and blistered. Following examination by the physician, the finger is treated with a topical cream and bandaged.

ICD-10-CM	CPT
T23.221A (second-degree burn of single finger, initial encounter) **X15.3XXA** (contact with other heat and hot saucepan or skillet, initial encounter)	**16020**

    Teaching Point: External cause of injury codes such as **X15.3XXA** are used to report the source, place, and/or intent of a burn injury. These codes are only required when state regulations mandate reporting cause of injury (typically applies to emergency department services). However, it is appropriate to report external cause of injury codes when the cause is known.

Negative Pressure Wound Therapy

97605   Negative pressure wound therapy (eg, vacuum assisted drainage collection), utilizing durable medical equipment (DME), including topical application(s), wound assessment, and instruction(s) for ongoing care, per session; total wound(s) surface area less than or equal to 50 square centimeters

97606   total wound(s) surface area greater than 50 square centimeters

97607   Negative pressure wound therapy (eg, vacuum assisted drainage collection), utilizing disposable, non-durable medical equipment, including provision of exudate management collection system, topical application(s), wound assessment, and instructions for ongoing care, per session; total wound(s) surface area less than or equal to 50 square centimeters

97608   total wound(s) surface area greater than 50 square centimeters

    Negative pressure wound therapy (NPWT), or vacuum-assisted closure in the management of traumatic and surgical wounds, has become commonly used by physicians in recent years.

    Codes **97605** and **97606** represent NPWT provided via a system that includes a *non-disposable* suction pump and drainage collection device.

    Codes **97607** and **97608** are used for NPWT that uses a *disposable* suction pump and collection system.

- Codes **97607** and **97608** are not reported in conjunction with codes **97605** and **97606**.
- Payer policies may limit coverage to care of specific types of wounds that require NPWT to improve granulation tissue formation and to certain types of NPWT equipment. Be sure to verify the coverage policy of the patient's health plan prior to provision of services.

    Negative pressure wound therapy

- Requires direct (one-on-one) physician or other QHP contact with the patient.
- May be initiated in a hospital or surgical center setting and continued in the home setting after discharge.
- Includes application of dressings.
- Is reported once for each session, which includes wound assessment and measurement and application of NPWT dressings and equipment.
- Is separately reported when performed in conjunction with surgical debridement (**11042–11047**).
- Documentation should include current wound assessment, including quantitative measurements of wound characteristics (eg, site, surface area, depth), any previous treatment regimens, debridement (when performed), prescribed length of treatment, dressing types and frequency of changes, and other concerns that affect healing.
- Encounters for ongoing NPWT may include documentation of progress of healing and changes in the wound, including measurement, amount of exudate, and presence of granulation or necrotic tissue.

    ●=New code ▲=Revised code #=Re-sequenced code +=Add-on code

- Supplies, including dressings, are reportable with HCPCS codes (eg, **A6550**, wound care set, for NPWT electrical pump, includes all supplies and accessories). Supplies for a disposable system are reported with code **A9272**, which also includes all dressings and accessories.

Removal of Foreign Bodies

Integumentary and Musculoskeletal Foreign Bodies

- Removal of a foreign body from within the subcutaneous tissues above the fascia is reported with a code from the integumentary system regardless of the site (eg, hand, foot).
- Musculoskeletal codes are reported when a foreign body is removed from *within the fascia, subfascial, or muscle*. Always check the *CPT* index to ensure you are reporting the most accurate code.
- Code **10120** (removal of a foreign body from subcutaneous tissue via simple incision) includes the removal of splinters or ticks when the physician has to "break open" or incise the skin to retrieve the splinter.
- Code **10121** is used to report the complicated removal of a foreign body by incision.
     Do not report codes **10120** or **10121** when a foreign body is removed using forceps alone with no incision. Instead, report an E/M service.

The physician determines whether the procedure is simple or complex, but the significant difference in physician work RVUs for the procedures may be used as an indicator of the difference—1.22 for **10120** versus 2.74 for **10121**. Clearly, a procedure described by code **10121** would involve double the time and effort of the simple procedure. *CPT* does not provide examples of simple versus complicated procedures.

- A complicated removal may require extended exploration and removal of multiple foreign bodies (eg, pieces of glass), use of imaging to help locate the foreign body, or removal that is complicated by the anatomical site of the foreign body (eg, area that is not easily seen) and will have a greater intensity of physician work.

The removal of an embedded earring requiring an incision would be reported with code **10120** or **10121**, depending on the complexity of the procedure required to remove it. If the earring is removed by wiggling it out or another method that does not require incision, this work is included in the E/M service.

- *Musculoskeletal foreign body:* Codes in the musculoskeletal system are not reported for removal of foreign bodies within the skin and subcutaneous fat. Examples of codes for removal of foreign bodies within the musculoskeletal system are
  - *Foot:* For foreign body removal *from within the fascia, subfascial, or muscle,* code **28190** is used to report the removal of a subcutaneous foreign body from the foot; code **28192** is used to report removal of a foreign body from the deep tissue of the foot.
  - *Upper arm or elbow:* Report removal of foreign bodies of the upper arm or elbow area from subcutaneous tissues within the fascia with **24200** or from deep, below the fascia, or in the muscle with **24201**.

Foreign Bodies of Other Body Sites

CPT includes codes for reporting removal of foreign bodies from many different body sites. **Table 10-3** summarizes foreign body removal services from areas other than skin or muscle.

Table 10-3. Codes for Removal of Foreign Bodies Other Than From Skin or Muscle

Site	Code(s)
Anal foreign body or fecal impaction	Use appropriate E/M code or **45999** (unlisted procedure, rectum) unless removed under anesthesia (**45915**, more than local anesthesia).
External auditory canal (For removal of impacted cerumen, see discussion later in this chapter.)	**69200** (removal foreign body from external auditory canal; without general anesthesia)
Eye	**65205** (removal of foreign body, external eye; conjunctival superficial) **65220** (removal of foreign body, external eye; corneal, without slit lamp)
Nose	**30300** (removal of intranasal foreign bodies when performed in the office) **30310** (removal of intranasal foreign bodies under general anesthesia)
Vagina	Use appropriate E/M code or **58999** (unlisted procedure, female genital system) unless removed under anesthesia (**57415**, more than local anesthesia).

Abbreviation: E/M, evaluation and management.

●=New code   ▲=Revised code   #=Re-sequenced code   +=Add-on code

Fracture and/or Dislocation Care

Casts/Strapping/Splints

- Codes for the application of casts, splints, or strapping (**29000–29590**) cannot be reported for the initial (first) application when fracture or dislocation care is reported because they are included as part of the global surgery package.
- May be reported when they are replacements for the initial application *or performed as part of the initial E/M visit and fracture care is not reported.*

  The following codes are commonly used when treating a fracture or dislocation:
- Application of splints
  — Short arm splint (forearm to hand): static (**29125**); dynamic (**29126**)
  — Finger splint: static (**29130**); dynamic (**29131**)
  — Short leg splint (calf to foot): **29515**
- Strapping
  — Shoulder: **29240**
  — Elbow or wrist: **29260**

Example

➤ **An established patient presents to an urgent care practice with an injury to the left wrist.** The patient states he tripped and fell while playing soccer with friends at a soccer field. After examination, a 3-view radiograph of the wrist is ordered and performed in the office. The physician interprets the radiograph, determines that the patient has a fracture of the left proximal scaphoid, and applies a short arm splint pending consultation with an orthopedist in 2 days.

ICD-10-CM	CPT
S62.035A (nondisplaced fracture of proximal third of navicular [scaphoid] bone of left wrist, initial encounter for closed fracture) **W01.0XXA** (fall on same level from slipping, tripping and stumbling without subsequent striking against object, initial encounter) **Y92.322** (soccer field as the place of occurrence of the external cause) **Y93.66** (activity, soccer) **Y99.8** (recreation or sport not for income or while a student)	**99212–99215 25** **29125** (application of short arm splint [forearm to hand]; static) **73110** (radiologic examination, wrist; complete, minimum of three views)

   Teaching Point: The physician reports splinting of the fracture because only the initial care and referral to an orthopedist were provided in lieu of restorative fracture care. An E/M service for evaluation of the extent of injury would be reported with modifier **25** appended to the E/M code. Payers must have accident information to determine if another party (eg, school, automobile, homeowner's insurance) is liable for a claim. Inclusion of codes for external cause of injury, although not required, may provide information that facilitates timely payment.

> When reporting codes for radiographs, documentation should include a report of the indication for the test, number of views, findings, and, when applicable, comparison to previous radiographs.
>
> - Do not report a charge for interpretation and report when reviewing images that have been previously interpreted (eg, by a radiologist).
> - The independent review of previously interpreted images is included in an evaluation and management service.

Supplies

- Supplies associated with fracture care may be billed with every application, including the initial casting, splinting, or strapping performed in association with the global surgery procedure code when the service is performed in the private office setting.
- HCPCS codes **A4580**, **A4590**, and **Q4001–Q4051** may be reported for cast supplies; codes **E1800–E1841** may be reported for splints. Check with your major payers and/or review their payment policies for reporting these supplies.

- HCPCS codes are accepted by many Medicaid and commercial payers and are very specific to the age of the patient and type of supply and/or material.
- A description of supplies may be required when reporting special supplies code **99070**.
- The following codes are commonly used:

99070	Supplies and materials (except spectacles)
A4565	Slings
A4570	Splint
L3650–L3678	Clavicle splints
Q4001–Q4051	Cast and splint supplies
S8450–S8452	Splint, prefabricated for finger, wrist, ankle, or elbow

Fracture and Dislocation Care Codes

Codes for fracture/dislocation care

- Are listed by anatomical location.
- Are provided (in most cases) for closed or open treatment, with or without manipulation, and with or without internal fixation.
- Most include a 90-day period of follow-up care under the Medicare global package.
- Include the initial casting, splinting, or strapping.
- Do not include radiographs or E/M to determine the extent of injury and treatment options.
- Fractures most commonly seen in a primary care pediatric practice include closed fractures (ie, skin is intact on presentation), and treatment is typically closed (ie, fracture site is not surgically opened) without manipulation (an exception is treatment of nursemaid elbow).
- *Clavicular fracture:* Report closed treatment without manipulation with code **23500**.
- *Nursemaid elbow:* Report closed treatment of radial head subluxation (nursemaid elbow) with manipulation with code **24640**. (This code has a 10-day global period.)
- *Radial fracture:* Report code **25500** for closed treatment of radial shaft fracture without manipulation and **25600** for closed treatment of distal radius fracture without manipulation.
- *Phalanx fracture:* Closed treatment of a proximal or middle phalanx, finger, or thumb (each) without manipulation is reported with code **26720**. Closed treatment of a distal phalangeal fracture (each) without manipulation is reported with code **26750**.
- *Great toe fracture:* Code **28490** is reported for the closed treatment of a fracture of the great toe, phalanx, or phalanges without manipulation.
- *Metatarsal fracture:* Report code **28470** for closed treatment of a metatarsal fracture without manipulation.
- *Lesser toe fracture:* Closed treatment of fracture, phalanx, or phalanges, other than great toe without manipulation, is coded with **28510**.
- When a patient presents for follow-up care after initial fracture care is provided in another setting (eg, emergency department, urgent care), it is necessary to determine if the provider of initial fracture care reported a code for fracture care with modifier **54** (surgical care only) or only reported casting/strapping for the initial care.
- If initial fracture care has been reported with modifier **54**, the physician providing continued fracture care reports the fracture care code with modifier **55** (postoperative care only) appended.

Ideally, documentation to support fracture care will include interpretation and report of radiographic findings, that appropriate stabilization or immobilization without neurovascular compromise was achieved, precautions, and instructions to return for follow-up care.

Tip: Unrelated services that are provided during the global surgery period by the same physician (or physician of the same group and specialty) may be reported. Modifier **24** would be appended to the unrelated E/M service.

Fractures not specified as displaced or non-displaced are reported with an *International Classification of Diseases, 10th Revision, Clinical Modification* code for a displaced fracture. Fractures not specified as open or closed are reported with a code for a closed fracture.

Chapter 10. Surgery, Infusion, and Sedation in the Outpatient Setting

●=New code ▲=Revised code #=Re-sequenced code +=Add-on code

Examples

➤ **An urgent care physician performs and documents a comprehensive evaluation on a child with multiple injuries, including a fracture of the shaft of the left clavicle and abrasions on the left upper arm and cheek, after a fall from the monkey bars.**

ICD-10-CM	CPT
S40.812A (abrasion upper arm, initial encounter) **S00.81XA** (abrasion face, initial encounter) **W09.8XXA** (fall from playground equipment, initial encounter)	**99202–99205 57**
S42.022A (displaced fracture shaft of clavicle, closed, initial encounter) **W09.8XXA**	**23500** (closed treatment clavicle fracture without manipulation)

Teaching Point: Because code **23500** is assigned a 90-day global period in the MPFS and is placed in the surgery section of *CPT*, many payers may require modifier **57** (decision for surgery) appended to the E/M code. Individual payers may have different policies.

➤ **A physician evaluates a 22-month-old girl (established patient) whose parents report that she will not move her left arm after falling on steps while holding her father's hand.** After obtaining history and physical examination to rule out other injuries, the physician diagnoses subluxation of the radial head that is reduced by manipulation. Reassessment after 10 minutes shows the child uses both arms now when presented with a balloon. The parents are counseled about potential for recurrent injury and avoidance. Follow-up will be at previously scheduled 2-year-old visit unless otherwise indicated.

ICD-10-CM	CPT
S53.032A (nursemaid's elbow, left, initial encounter) **W10.9XXA** (Fall [on] [from] unspecified stairs and steps)	**99213 25** (low-complexity MDM—acute uncomplicated injury with assessment requiring an independent historian and low risk of morbidity) **24640** (closed treatment of radial head subluxation in child, nursemaid elbow, with manipulation)

Teaching Point: The physician provided a significant and separately identifiable E/M service to evaluate extent of injury in addition to treatment of nursemaid elbow. Modifier **25** is required by most payers to indicate the E/M service was significant and separately identifiable from the preservice work of the minor procedure performed on the same date of service.

Ear, Nose, and Throat Procedures

Control of Nasal Hemorrhage

30901 Control nasal hemorrhage, anterior, simple (cautery or packing)
30903 Control nasal hemorrhage, anterior, complex (extensive cautery and/or packing) any method

- If performing cautery or packing on both sides, report **30901** with modifier **50**.
- If bleeding is controlled with manual pressure or placement of a nasal clamp (clip), only the appropriate level of E/M service is reported.

Example

➤ **A 7-year-old established patient presents with a facial injury sustained when he tripped and fell at school.** Part of his face hit the pavement, causing mild bruising on his nose and a significant nosebleed. The patient did not experience headache, vomiting, or loss of consciousness. Medical history was negative for a bleeding disorder, and family history was negative for a bleeding disorder within the family.

The patient had minimal abrasion and ecchymosis on the tip of the nose, with no pain on palpation over the bridge of the nose and cheeks. The septum was not deviated, and no hematoma was present. There was a moderate amount of crusted blood from the left naris, and small bleed medially of the left naris was visible. The remainder of the examination was normal. The decision was made to cauterize with silver nitrate and result of cautery was satisfactory.

ICD-10-CM	CPT
R04.0 (epistaxis) **S00.31XA** (abrasion of nose) **W01.0XXA** (fall on same level from slipping, tripping and stumbling without subsequent striking against object, initial encounter) **Y92.480** (sidewalk as the place of occurrence of the external cause) **Y93.01** (activity walking, marching, and hiking)	**99213 25** (MDM of low complexity—acute uncomplicated injury with low risk of morbidity from treatment) **30901**

Teaching Point: The physician provided a significant and separately identifiable E/M service to evaluate extent of injury in addition to treatment of the nosebleed. Only the 4 diagnosis codes may be linked to each procedure code on the claim. However, it is appropriate to include all diagnoses on the claim.

Removal of Impacted Cerumen

69209   Removal of impacted cerumen using irrigation/lavage, unilateral
69210   Removal of impacted cerumen requiring instrumentation, unilateral

> For cerumen removal that is not impacted, report the appropriate evaluation and management service code.

Modifier **25** should be appended to the significant, separately identifiable E/M service (eg, **99213**) provided on the same date as removal of impacted cerumen based on NCCI edits. Payers that use NCCI edits may deny the E/M service when submitted without modifier **25**.

Code **69209** is used to report removal of impacted cerumen by ear wash without direct visualization and instrumentation.

- *Do not report* **69209** for removal of cerumen that is not impacted.
- This code is intended to capture the practice expense associated with the service and is not valued to include physician work.
- Separately report any significant and separately identifiable E/M service provided by a physician or other QHP on the same date (modifier **25** may be appended to the E/M code when required by payers).
- For a bilateral procedure, report **69209** with modifier **50**.
- Do not report **69209** in conjunction with **69210** when performed on the same ear (modifiers **LT** and **RT** may be used to identify contralateral procedures).

Code **69210** is *only* reported when the physician, under direct visualization, removes impacted cerumen using, at a minimum, an otoscope and instruments such as wax curettes or by using an operating microscope and suction plus specific ear instruments (eg, cup forceps, right angles).

- Medical record documentation must support that the cerumen was impacted and removed by the physician and include a description of what equipment and method were used to perform the procedure.
- Report code **69210** with modifier **50** when bilateral procedures are performed.
- Removal of cerumen that is not impacted is included in an E/M code regardless of how it is removed.

Note: Medicare does not recognize modifier **50** when reported with code **69210** (impacted cerumen removal); therefore, those payers that follow Medicare payment policy will not recognize it and may deny the claim outright. Check with your payers.

Coding Conundrum: Unsuccessful Removal of Impacted Cerumen

If a physician or other qualified health care professional attempts to remove impacted cerumen but finds the impaction too hard for safe removal, what code is reported for the attempt? The answer depends on the individual situation, including the amount of work that was performed and whether another procedure was successful.

If the portion of the procedure completed required insignificant work and practice expense (eg, staff time), report only the services completed on that date (eg, evaluation and management).

If the patient is instructed to use softening drops and return later for removal, consider whether the effort and practice expense were sufficient to justify reporting the removal with reduced services modifier **52**.

If the procedure was discontinued after significant effort and practice expense due to extenuating circumstances or concerns that the procedure may threaten the patient's well-being, report the procedure code with modifier **53** (discontinued procedure).

If, after attempted removal by a physician is discontinued, softening drops are administered in the office and clinical staff perform removal of the impaction by lavage (**69209**), report only the completed procedure.

Examples

➤ **A physician orders removal of impacted cerumen from the right ear by lavage.** Clinical staff perform the lavage, removing the impacted cerumen. Because the child is uncooperative, the procedure takes 10 minutes.

ICD-10-CM	CPT
H92.01 (otalgia, right ear) **H61.21** (impacted cerumen, right ear)	**99202–99215 25** (Report if appropriate and use modifier **25** if required by payer.)
H61.21	**69209 RT** (**RT** indicates right ear.)

Teaching Point: This procedure was unilateral. If it were bilateral, modifier **50** would be appended to code **69209**. The anatomical modifier **RT** (right) is informational and typically does not affect payment. The extended time of service alone is not sufficient to support reporting increased procedural service (ie, modifier **22**).

➤ **Physician documents, "Impacted cerumen removed from both ears using an otoscope and curette," in a patient with complaint of decreased hearing.** Following the procedure, the patient's hearing is assessed as normal.

ICD-10-CM	CPT
H61.23 (impacted cerumen, bilateral)	**99202–99215 25** (Report if appropriate and use modifier **25** if required by payer.)
	69210 50 (bilateral removal of impacted cerumen using instrumentation)

Teaching Point: Unless a payer instructs otherwise, modifier **50** is appended to **69210** to indicate a bilateral procedure. An E/M service is reported only if significant and separately identifiable.

Digestive System Procedures

Incision in Lingual Frenulum

41010   Incision in the lingual frenum to free the tongue

Note that code **41115** (excision of lingual frenum) is not appropriate when an incisional release of tongue-tie is performed rather than excision (removal) of the frenum.

Example

➤ **A 14-day-old is seen for feeding difficulty caused by ankyloglossia.** The physician documents obtaining informed consent, positioning and restraining of the neonate, and gentle lifting of the tongue with a sterile, grooved retractor to expose the frenulum. The frenulum, adjacent to the ventral aspect of the tongue, is divided by 2 to 3 mm using sterile scissors. Afterward, the newborn is immediately returned to his mother for comfort and feeding. The latch appears improved. After feeding, the neonate is reevaluated with no evidence of complications. Code **41010** is reported for the procedure.

ICD-10-CM	CPT
Q38.1 (congenital ankyloglossia)	**41010**

Teaching Point: If a significant and separately identifiable E/M service was provided in addition to the preservice work of the procedure, modifier **25** would be appended to the appropriate E/M code. Any related visit within the 10 days following the procedure may be reported (with no charge) with code **99024**.

Gastrostomy Tube Replacement

43762   Replacement of gastrostomy tube, percutaneous, includes removal, when performed, without imaging or endoscopic guidance; not requiring revision of gastrostomy tract

43763   requiring revision of gastrostomy tract

- To report gastrostomy tube change without imaging or endoscopic guidance, see codes **43762** and **43763**.
- See codes **49450** and **43246** for placement with imaging or endoscopic guidance.
- A significant, separately identifiable E/M service on the same date may be reported with modifier **25** appended to the E/M code (eg, **99213 25**).
- An E/M service should not be reported when the encounter is solely for replacement of the gastrostomy tube.
- Codes **43762** and **43763** include the gastrostomy tube kit.

Genitourinary System Procedures

Urinary Catheterization

51701   Urinary catheterization, straight
51702   Urinary catheterization, temporary

- Code **51701** is reported when a non-indwelling bladder catheter (straight catheterization) is inserted (eg, for residual urine, for a urine culture collection).
- Code **51702** is reported when a temporary indwelling bladder catheter is inserted (ie, Foley).

> **Report code 51701 when you insert a urinary catheter to collect a clean-catch urine specimen, after which the catheter is removed.**

Lysis/Excision of Labial or Penile Adhesions

If lysis of labial or penile adhesions is performed by the application of manual pressure without the use of an instrument to cut the adhesions, it would be considered part of the E/M visit and not reported separately.

54450   Foreskin manipulation including lysis of preputial adhesions and stretching
54162   Lysis or excision of penile post-circumcision adhesions
56441   Lysis of labial adhesions

- Code **54450** does not require general anesthesia.
  - 1.98 RVUs and a 0-day global period are assigned when performed in a non-facility setting (eg, office).
  - This procedure is performed on the uncircumcised foreskin and the head of the penis. Adhesions are broken by stretching the foreskin back over the head of the penis onto the shaft or by inserting a clamp between the foreskin and the head of the penis and spreading the jaws of the clamp.

- Code **54162** is only reported when lysis is performed under general anesthesia or regional block, with an instrument, and under sterile conditions.
  - This code has an RVU of 7.39 when performed in a non-facility setting (eg, office) and a Medicare 10-day global surgery period.
  - If post-circumcision adhesions are manually broken during the postoperative period by the physician or physician of the same group and specialty who performed the procedure, it would be considered part of the global surgical package.
  - Report the service with *ICD-10-CM* code **N47.0**, adherent prepuce in a newborn, or **N47.5**, adhesions of prepuce and glans penis (patients older than 28 days).
- Code **56441** is performed by using a blunt instrument or scissors under general or local anesthesia.
  - The total RVUs for this procedure in a non-facility setting are 4.72.
  - This procedure also includes a Medicare 10-day global surgery period.
  - *ICD-10-CM* code **Q52.5** (fusion of labia) would be reported with *CPT* code **56441**.
  - When provided without anesthesia, modifier **52** may be appended to indicate reduced services. Payer guidance may vary in regard to use of modifier **52**.

Newborn Circumcision

When circumcisions are performed in the office

- If a payer does not base payment on a global surgical package, a supply code for the surgical tray can be reported with code **99070**. The description of the supply (circumcision tray) would need to be included on the claim form.
- Anesthetic creams (eutectic mixture of local anesthetics) are included in the circumcision code itself and should not be reported unless a third-party payer pays separately for topical anesthetic agents. In that case, they would be reported with code **99070**.

54150   Circumcision, using clamp or other device with regional dorsal penile or ring block

- If the circumcision using a clamp or other device is performed without dorsal penile or ring block, append modifier **52** (reduced services) to **54150**.
- 4.40 non-facility RVUs and a Medicare global period of 0 (zero) are assigned to code **54150**.
  - When an E/M service (eg, well-baby visit) is provided on the same date, append modifier **25** to the E/M code.
  - Link the appropriate *ICD-10-CM* code (eg, **Z00.110**, health check for newborn under 8 days old) to the E/M service and link *ICD-10-CM* code **Z41.2** (encounter for routine and ritual male circumcision) to the circumcision code.

54160   Circumcision, surgical excision other than clamp, device, or dorsal slit; neonate (28 days of age or less)

54161   older than 28 days

- Unlike code **54150**, Medicare has a global period of 10 days assigned to codes **54160** and **54161**. Services described by **54160** and **54161** are often provided in facility settings.

See Chapter 15 for information on reporting circumcision in a facility setting.

Hydration, Injections, and Infusions

Services included as inherent to an infusion or injection are the use of local anesthesia, starting the intravenous (IV) line, access to indwelling IV lines or a subcutaneous catheter or port, flushing lines at the conclusion of an infusion or between infusions, standard tubing, syringes and supplies, and preparation of chemotherapy agents.

- These codes are intended for reporting by the physician or other QHP in an office setting. They are not reported by a physician or other QHP when performed in a facility setting because the physician work associated with these procedures involves only affirmation of the treatment plan and direct supervision of the staff performing the services.
- If a significant, separately identifiable E/M service is performed, the appropriate code may be reported with modifier **25** appended. The diagnosis may be the same for the E/M service and codes **96360–96379**.

Documentation of medications administered in the outpatient pediatric practice should include

- **Order for medication**
- **Date and time of administration (include start/stop times for timed procedures)**
- **Medication, manufacturer, lot number, and expiration date**
- **Dose**
- **Route (eg, intramuscular) and site of administration (eg, left deltoid)**
- **Observations (eg, held by mother, no sign of adverse reaction after 5 minutes)**
- **Signature and credentials of individual administering medication**

Subcutaneous or Intramuscular Injection (Therapeutic, Prophylactic, and Diagnostic)

96372   Therapeutic, prophylactic, or diagnostic injection (specify substance or drug); subcutaneous or intramuscular

Report code **96372** for the administration of a diagnostic, prophylactic, or therapeutic (eg, antibiotic) subcutaneous or intramuscular (IM) injection. Do not report for the administration of a purified protein derivative test.

For administration of immunizations, see discussion of codes **90460, 90461**, and **90471–90474** in Chapter 9.

Examples

➤ **A 2-year-old established patient presents with moderate symptoms of croup that began last evening and worsened during the night.** After obtaining history and performing an examination, the physician recommends injection of dexamethasone sodium phosphate. A 7-mg dose of dexamethasone sodium phosphate is administered by IM injection. The child is observed for reaction and released to home with instructions and precautions.

ICD-10-CM	CPT
J05.0 (acute obstructive laryngitis [croup])	**99213 25** (established patient E/M with low MDM) **96372** (IM injection) **J1100** × 7 units (injection, dexamethasone sodium phosphate per 1 mg)

Teaching Point: The medication is reported with HCPCS code **J1100**, which indicates the unit of measure for reporting is 1 mg. Because 7 mg were administered, 7 units of service are reported. Also report the appropriate National Drug Code (NDC) and units.

See Chapter 1 for more information on National Drug Codes.

The E/M service included addressing an acute uncomplicated illness with prescription drug management, supporting code **99213**. (Although prescription drug management supports moderate MDM and code **99214**, neither the number and complexity of problems addressed nor the data to be reviewed and analyzed support this level. Two of 3 elements of MDM must meet the requirements for a level of MDM in 2021.) Modifier **25** must be appended to the E/M service code to indicate the significant, separately identifiable E/M service on the date of the injection for payers that use NCCI edits.

➤ **A 2-year-old girl presents with a fever (39.4°C [103.0°F]). Her mother states the girl has been tugging at her right ear for 2 days.** An expanded problem-focused history and examination are completed. When the doctor examines the ears, he notices that the right middle ear is very inflamed (pus is present) and the child is extremely uncomfortable. The child's mother states that it is very difficult to get her daughter to swallow medicine rather than spit it out. The doctor decides to administer a single injection of ceftriaxone sodium 600 mg to the child. The final diagnosis is right acute suppurative otitis media without rupture of eardrum. Medical decision-making is moderate.

Chapter 10. Surgery, Infusion, and Sedation in the Outpatient Setting

ICD-10-CM	CPT
H66.001 (acute suppurative otitis media without spontaneous rupture of ear drum, right ear)	**99213 25** (established patient level E/M with low MDM—acute uncomplicated problem with prescription drug management) **96372** (IM injection) **J0696** × 3 units (injection, ceftriaxone sodium, per 250 mg)

Teaching Point: The medication is reported with HCPCS code **J0696**, which indicates the unit of measure for reporting is 250 mg. Because 600 mg was administered, 3 units are reported per Medicare guidelines. However, if the payer accepts actual dosage, 2.4 units (2 units for the first two 250 mg of the medication and 0.4 units for the last 100 mg) would be reported rather than 3 units. Report also the appropriate NDC.

If the patient were scheduled for a series of injections of the same antibiotic over several days, report only the services rendered (eg, **96372** and **J0696**) each day (ie, do not report an E/M unless there is clinical indication for a significant and separately identifiable E/M service).

Modifier **25** must be appended to the E/M service code (**99213**) to indicate the significant, separately identifiable E/M service on the date of the injection for payers that use NCCI edits.

Hydration and Infusions

Hydration and infusion codes are reported based on the time when medication administration begins to the end of administration. Time must be documented.

When reporting multiple infusions on the same date, physicians select an initial service based on the service that is the primary reason for infusion services on that date.

Example

➤ **A patient receives infusion of a medication and a separate infusion of hydration fluid.** The physician determines whether the therapeutic infusion or the hydration was the primary service and selects the appropriate initial service code. The other service is reported with a code for sequential or subsequent administration.

Hydration

Codes **96360** (IV infusion, hydration; initial, 31 minutes to 1 hour) and **96361** (each additional hour)
- Are intended to report IV hydration infusion using prepackaged fluid and/or electrolyte solutions (eg, physiologic [normal] saline solution, D_5-0.45% physiologic saline solution with potassium).
- **96360** may be reported for hydration infusion lasting more than 31 minutes and up to 1 hour.
- **96361** is reported for each additional hour of hydration infusion and for a final interval of greater than 30 minutes beyond the last hour reported.

Code **96361** is reported if an IV hydration infusion is provided secondary or subsequent to a therapeutic, prophylactic, or diagnostic infusion and administered through the same IV access.
- Typically require direct physician supervision for purposes of consent, safety oversight, or supervision of staff with little special handling for preparation or disposal of materials.
- Do not typically require advanced training of staff because there usually is little risk involved and little patient monitoring required.
- Are reported based on the actual time over which the infusion is administered and do not include the time spent starting the IV and monitoring the patient after infusion.
- Medical record documentation must support the service reported.
- Are not reported when IV infusions are 30 minutes or less.
- Are not used to report infusion of drugs or other substances; nor are they reported when hydration is incidental to non-chemotherapeutic/diagnostic or chemotherapeutic services.

Intra-arterial and Intravenous Push Injections

96373   Therapeutic, prophylactic, or diagnostic injection (specify substance or drug); intra-arterial

96374   intravenous push, single or initial substance/drug

+96375   each additional sequential intravenous push of a new substance/drug (List separately in addition to **96365**, **96374**, **96409**, or **96413**)

- Each drug administered is reported separately with the appropriate infusion code.
- Report code **96373** for an initial intra-arterial injection and **96374** for an initial injection administered by IV push.
- Codes **96374** and **96375** are only used when the health care professional administering the substance or drug is in constant attendance during the administration *and* must observe the patient. The IV push must be less than 15 minutes.

> **Short infusions of less than 15 minutes are reported as a push (eg, 96374).**

- Sequential IV push of a new substance or drug is reported with add-on code **96375**.
- Code **96375** may be reported in addition to codes for IV infusion (**96365**), initial IV push (**96374**), or chemotherapy administration (**96409**, **96413**).
- Additional sequential IV push of the same substance or drug (**96376**) is not reported for services provided in the physician office (ie, is reported only by a facility).

Therapeutic, Prophylactic, and Diagnostic Infusions

96365   Intravenous infusion, for therapy, prophylaxis, or diagnosis (specify substance or drug); initial, up to 1 hour

+96366   each additional hour (List separately in addition to **96365** or **96367**.)

+96367   additional sequential infusion of a new drug/substance, up to 1 hour (List separately in addition to **96365**, **96374**, **96409**, **96413**.)

+96368   concurrent infusion (List separately in addition to **96365**, **96366**, or chemotherapy services **96413**, **96415**, or **96416**.)

Table 10-4 lists primary and additional IV infusion and IV push codes. See the table notes for additional instructions on reporting multiple services.

Codes **96365–96368**

- Are for infusions for the purpose of administering drugs or substances.
- Typically require direct physician supervision and special attention to prepare, calculate dose, and dispose of materials.
- If fluid infusions are used to administer the drug(s), they are considered incidental hydration and are not reported.
    Each drug administered is reported separately with the appropriate infusion code.
- Short infusions of less than 15 minutes are reported as a push (eg, **96374**).
- Only 1 initial service code (eg, **96365**) should be reported unless the protocol or patient condition requires that 2 separate IV sites must be used. A second IV site access is also reported using the initial service code with modifier **59** appended (eg, **96365**, **96365 59**).
- Subcutaneous infusion is reported with codes **96369–96371** (see **Table 10-4**).

Table 10-4. Primary and Additional Intravenous Infusion Codes[a]

For all services, you must specify the substance or drug administered.

Service (Select the primary reason for encounter irrespective of order of infusion services.)[b]	IV Infusion, for Therapy, Prophylaxis, or Diagnosis	Subcutaneous Infusion for Therapy or Prophylaxis[b]	Therapeutic, Prophylactic, or Diagnostic Injection IV Push
Initial service, up to 1 h	**96365** (16 min–1 h)	**96369** (16 min–1 h)	**96374** (IV push or infusion ≤15 min)
Each additional hour (>30 min) of *same substance or drug*	**+96366**[c] (List separately in addition to **96365**, **96367**)	**+96370** (Use **96370** in conjunction with **96369**.)	

Table 10-4 (*continued*)			
Service (Select the primary reason for encounter irrespective of order of infusion services.)[b]	**IV Infusion, for Therapy, Prophylaxis, or Diagnosis**	**Subcutaneous Infusion for Therapy or Prophylaxis**[b]	**Therapeutic, Prophylactic, or Diagnostic Injection IV Push**
Additional sequential infusion of *new substance or drug*	+96367[c]	+96371 (additional pump setup with new subcutaneous infusion site[s])	+96367
Sequential IV push of a *new substance/drug*	+96375		+96375
Concurrent infusion (Report only once per date of service.)	+96368		

Abbreviation: IV, intravenous.

[a] If IV infusion for hydration of longer than 30 minutes is provided in addition to a therapeutic infusion service (**96360**, **96365**, **96374**) through the same IV access, report +**96361** in addition to **96365** or **96374**.

[b] Includes pump setup and establishment of infusion site(s). Use **96369** and **96371** only once per encounter.

[c] Report **96367** only once per sequential infusion of same infusate mix. Report **96366** for each additional hour (includes final time unit of 31 minutes or more) beyond the first hour of the service reported with **96367**.

Coding Conundrum: Multiple and Concurrent Infusions or Injections

When administering multiple infusions, injections, or combinations, only 1 "initial" service code should be reported for a given date, unless protocol requires that 2 separate intravenous (IV) sites must be used.

- Do not report a second initial service on the same date due to an IV line requiring a restart, an IV rate not being able to be reached without 2 lines, or a need to access a port of a multi-lumen catheter.
- If an injection or infusion is of a subsequent or concurrent nature, even if it is the first such service within that group of services, a subsequent or concurrent code from the appropriate section should be reported. For example, the first IV push given subsequent to an initial 1-hour infusion is reported using a subsequent IV push code.

When services are performed in the physician's office, report as follows:

Initial Infusion

Report the code that best describes the key or primary reason for the service regardless of the order in which the infusions or injections occur. Only 1 initial service code (eg, **96365**) should be reported unless the protocol or patient condition requires using 2 separate IV sites. The difference in time and effort in providing this second IV site access is also reported using the initial service code with modifier **59**, distinct procedural service, appended (eg, **96365**, **96365 59**).

Sequential Infusion

This is an infusion or IV push of a new substance or drug following a primary or initial service. For example, if an IV push was performed through the same IV access subsequent to an IV infusion for therapy, the appropriate codes to report would be **96365** and **96375**. If an IV push was performed through a different IV access route, the services would be reported using codes **96365** and **96374**. Sequential infusions are reported only 1 time for the same infusate. However, if additional hours were required for the infusion, the appropriate "each additional hour" add-on code would be reported. Different infusates can be reported using the same code as the original sequential code. Hydration may not be reported concurrently with any other service. All sequential services require that there be a new substance or drug; only a facility may report a sequential IV push of the same drug using **96376**.

Concurrent Infusion

This is an infusion of a new substance or drug infused at the same time as another drug or substance. This is not time-based and is only reported once per day regardless of whether a new drug or substance is administered concurrently. Hydration may not be reported concurrently with any other service. A separate subsequent concurrent administration of another new drug or substance (the third substance or drug) is not reported.

Example

➤ **A 3-year-old established patient is seen with a complaint of vomiting and fever for the past 24 hours.** She has refused all food and liquids and last voided 12 hours prior to the visit. A detailed history and physical examination with moderate-level MDM are performed. Her diagnosis is bilateral acute suppurative otitis media and dehydration. Intravenous fluids are initiated with physiologic (normal) saline solution, and IV ceftriaxone (750 mg) is infused over 30 minutes for her otitis media. After 1 hour and 45 minutes of IV hydration, she urinates, begins tolerating liquids, and is released to home.

ICD-10-CM	CPT
E86.0 (dehydration) **H66.003** (acute suppurative otitis media without spontaneous rupture of ear drum, bilateral) **R11.10** (vomiting) **R50.9** (fever, unspecified)	**99214 25** (established patient office E/M) **96365** (IV infusion, for therapy) **96361** (IV infusion, hydration, each additional hour) **J0696** × 3 units (ceftriaxone sodium, per 250 mg) **J7030** (infusion, normal saline solution, 1,000 cc)

Teaching Point: Link the appropriate diagnosis code to each procedure (eg, code **H66.003** is linked to code **J0696**). If required by the payer, the medication and infusion solution may need to be reported with the NDC. The fluid used to administer ceftriaxone is not reported because it is considered incidental hydration.

Other Injection and Infusion Services

96523　　　　Irrigation of implanted venous access device for drug delivery systems

Code **96523** is used to report irrigation required for implanted venous access devices for drug delivery systems when services are provided on a separate day from the injection or infusion service. Do not report **96523** in conjunction with other services.

Chemotherapy and Other Highly Complex Drug/Biologic Agent Administration

Codes **96401–96549** are reported for chemotherapy administration. *CPT* defines *chemotherapy administration* as parenteral administration of non-radionuclide antineoplastic drugs, antineoplastic agents provided for treatment of non-cancer diagnoses and to substances such as certain monoclonal antibody agents, and other biologic response modifiers.

Example

➤ **A patient with severe persistent asthma is receiving injections of omalizumab 225 mg every 2 weeks.** The patient presents for administration of the medication. The medication is divided and injected at 2 different sites, as only 150 mg may be injected to a single site. The diagnosis code reported is **J45.50** (severe persistent asthma). Omalizumab injection is reported as a chemotherapy administration of monoclonal antibody (**96401**) with only 1 unit of service *unless prohibited by payer policy.* Omalizumab is provided in 150-mg single-use vials with an NDC of 50242-040-62. HCPCS code **J2357** (injection, omalizumab, 5 mg) is used to report the medication supplied by the physician practice. The following sample claim form illustrates reporting for this example:

Claim Form Sample National Drug Code

21. Diagnosis or nature of illness or injury (Relate A–L to service line below 24E) A. **J45.50** B. C. D.					ICD Ind. 0					
24. A. Dates of service	B. Place of service	C. EMG	D. Procedures, services or supplies CPT/HCPCS	Modifier	E. Diagnosis Pointer	F. Charges	G. Days or units	H. EPSDT	I. ID Qual	J. Rendering Provider #
1/1/2021–1/1/2021	**11**		**96401**		A	$$$	1		NPI	0123456789
N450242004062 UN2										
1/1/2021–1/1/2021	**11**		J2357		A	$$$	45		NPI	0123456789

Abbreviations: *CPT, Current Procedural Terminology*; EMG, emergency; EPSDT, Early and Periodic Screening, Diagnostic, and Treatment; HCPCS, Healthcare Common Procedure Coding System; *ICD, International Classification of Diseases*; NPI, National Provider Identifier.

Teaching Point: Check payer policies before reporting administration of omalizumab and other highly complex drug/biologic agents. *CPT* instructs that administration of certain monoclonal antibody agents may be reported with code **96401**. However, not all payers accept code **96401** for administration of omalizumab. Some payers limit reporting to code **96372** (subcutaneous or IM injection) and/or allow only 1 administration code despite requirements to administer by 2 or more separate injections.

The HCPCS codes and NDCs for the omalizumab are included on the claim with units based on the HCPCS code descriptor (225-mg dose/5-mg HCPCS unit = 45 units) and NDC quantity (payers may require NDC units per vial—UN2 or per gram—GR0.225) to identify the substance administered. Some payers allow reporting of the full amount of single-dose vials when only a portion of the medication is provided to a patient to account for drug waste. Report units for the full single-dose vial only as instructed by payer policy.

Moderate Sedation

Moderate sedation codes **99151–99153** and **99155–99157** are used for reporting moderate sedation when intraservice time is 10 minutes or more. **Table 10-5** contains sedation codes and descriptors.

Table 10-5. Moderate Sedation

Moderate sedation services provided by the same physician or other QHP performing the diagnostic or therapeutic service that the sedation supports, requiring the presence of an independent trained observer to assist in the monitoring of the patient's level of consciousness and physiological status;	Initial 15 min of Intraservice Time (Includes 10–22 min)	Each Additional 15 min of Intraservice Time[a]
patient younger than 5 years of age	**99151**	**+99153**
5 years or older	**99152**	**+99153**
Moderate sedation services provided by a physician other than the health care professional performing the diagnostic or therapeutic service that the sedation supports;	Initial 15 min of Intraservice Time (Includes 10–22 min)	Each Additional 15 min of Intraservice Time[a]
patient younger than 5 years	**99155**	**+99157**
5 years or older	**99156**	**+99157**

Abbreviation: QHP, qualified health care professional; +, designated add-on code.

[a] The *Current Procedural Terminology* midpoint rule applies. At least 8 minutes of time beyond the first or last full 15-minute period may be reported as an additional unit of service.

Moderate sedation is a drug-induced depression of consciousness.

● No interventions are required to maintain cardiovascular functions or a patent airway, and spontaneous ventilation is adequate.

● Moderate sedation codes are not used to report administration of medications for pain control, minimal sedation (anxiolysis), deep sedation, or monitored anesthesia care (**00100–01999**).

● Moderate sedation provided and reported by the same physician or QHP who is performing the diagnostic or therapeutic service requires the presence of an independent trained observer.

An *independent trained observer* is an individual qualified to monitor the patient during the procedure but who has no other duties (eg, assisting at surgery) during the procedure.

- Alternatively, a physician or QHP other than the person performing the diagnostic or therapeutic service may provide and report moderate sedation services.
- Codes **99151–99157** are distinguished by service provider, patient age, and time spent (see **Table 10-5**).

Codes **99151–99153** are reported when

- The administration of moderate sedation is provided by the physician who is simultaneously performing a procedure (eg, fracture reduction, vessel cutdown, central line placement, wound repair).
- An independent trained observer is present to assist the physician in the monitoring of the patient during the procedure or diagnostic service.

Codes **99155–99157** are reported when

- A second physician or QHP other than the health care professional performing the diagnostic or therapeutic services provides moderate sedation.

Codes **99153** and **99157** are reported for each additional 15 minutes of intraservice time. The midpoint between the end of the previous 15-minute period must be passed to report an additional unit of intraservice time (ie, intraservice time must continue for at least 8 minutes beyond the last full 15 minutes of intraservice time).

- Codes are selected based on intraservice time. Intraservice time
  - Begins with the administration of the sedating agent(s)
  - Ends when the procedure is completed, the patient is stable for recovery status, and the physician or other QHP providing the sedation ends personal continuous face-to-face time with the patient
  - Includes ordering and/or administering the initial and subsequent doses of sedating agents
  - Requires continuous face-to-face attendance of the physician or other QHP
  - Requires monitoring patient response to the sedating agents, including
    - Periodic assessment of the patient
    - Further administration of agent(s) as needed to maintain sedation
    - Monitoring of oxygen saturation, heart rate, and blood pressure
- Moderate sedation service of less than 10 minutes of intraservice time is not separately reported.
- Preservice work of moderate sedation services *is not separately reported* and is not included in intraservice time. Preservice work includes
  - Assessment of the patient's past medical and surgical history with particular emphasis on cardiovascular, pulmonary, airway, or neurologic conditions
  - Review of the patient's previous experiences with anesthesia and/or sedation
  - Family history of sedation complications
  - Summary of the patient's present medication list
  - Drug allergy and intolerance history
  - Focused physical examination of the patient, with emphasis on
    - Mouth, jaw, oropharynx, neck, and airway for Mallampati score assessment
    - Chest and lungs
    - Heart and circulation
    - Vital signs, including heart rate, respiratory rate, blood pressure, and oxygenation, with end-tidal carbon dioxide when indicated

> **Do not report a separate evaluation and management service for preservice or post-service work associated with moderate sedation.**

  - Review of any pre-sedation diagnostic tests
  - Completion of a pre-sedation assessment form (with American Society of Anesthesiologists physical status classification)
  - Patient informed consent
  - Immediate pre-sedation assessment prior to first sedating doses
  - Initiation of IV access and fluids to maintain patency
- Do not separately report or include the time of post-service work in the intraservice time. Post-service work of moderate sedation includes
  - Assessment of the patient's vital signs, level of consciousness, and neurologic, cardiovascular, and pulmonary stability in the post-sedation recovery period
  - Assessment of patient's readiness for discharge following the procedure

Chapter 10. Surgery, Infusion, and Sedation in the Outpatient Setting

— Preparation of documentation for sedation service

— Communication with family or caregiver about sedation service

● Oxygen saturation (**94760–94762**) cannot be reported separately.

> **Documentation of moderate sedation services must include all of the following:**
> - **The description of the procedure**
> - **Name and dosage(s) of the sedation agent(s)**
> - **Route of administration of the sedation agent(s) and who administered the agent (physician or independent observer)**
> - **The ongoing assessment of the child's level of consciousness and physiological status (eg, heart rate, oxygen saturation levels) during and after the procedure**
> - **The presence, name, and title of the independent observer or performing physician or other qualified health care professional**
> - **Total time from administration of the sedation agent(s) (start time) until the physician's face-to-face service is no longer required (end time)**

Examples

➤ **A 24-month-old requires a layered closure of a 2.5-cm laceration of the right knee in an urgent care setting.** Moderate sedation is required and is performed by the Pediatric Advanced Life Support–trained physician with an independent trained observer who has been trained in pediatric basic life support. The physician supervises the administration of the sedating agent and assesses the child until an effective, safe level of sedation is achieved and continues to assess the child's level of consciousness and physiological status while also performing the laceration repair. The procedure takes a total of 28 minutes from the time of administration of the agent until the physician completes the repair and determines the child is stable and face-to-face physician time is no longer required.

ICD-10-CM	CPT
S81.011A (laceration without foreign body, right knee, initial encounter) Codes for external cause, activity, and place of injury are reported when documented.	**12031** (intermediate repair of wound of extremities, 2.5 cm or less) **99151** (moderate [conscious] sedation, patient younger than 5 years, first 15 minutes) **+99153** (moderate [conscious] sedation, each additional 15 minutes of intraservice time)

Teaching Point: If a medically necessary, significant, and separately identifiable E/M service had also been performed, an E/M visit with modifier **25** appended could be reported. The agent itself should also be reported.

➤ **Same patient as previous example, except moderate sedation is performed by the Pediatric Advanced Life Support–trained physician while another physician performs the repair.** The procedure, from the time of administration of the agent until the repair is complete and the child is stable and no longer requires face-to-face physician time, takes a total of 28 minutes.

ICD-10-CM	CPT
S81.011A (laceration without foreign body, right knee, initial encounter) Codes for external cause, activity, and place of injury are reported when documented.	The physician repairing the wound reports **12031** (intermediate repair of wound of extremities, 2.5 cm or less)
	The physician performing moderate sedation reports **99155** (moderate [conscious] sedation, patient younger than 5 years, first 15 minutes) **+99157** (moderate [conscious] sedation, each additional 15 minutes of intraservice time)

Teaching Point: Each physician reports the service provided. The time of moderate sedation used in code selection is only the intraservice time.

Chapter 10. Surgery, Infusion, and Sedation in the Outpatient Setting

Resources

Global Periods and Relative Value Units

Medicare Physician Fee Schedule (www.cms.gov/medicare/medicare-fee-for-service-payment/physicianfeesched)

"The Surgical Package and Related Services" May 2018 *AAP Pediatric Coding Newsletter*" (https://coding.solutions.aap.org/article.aspx?articleid=2679119; subscription required)

Modifiers

"Modifier **25** and Minor Procedures" March 2018 *AAP Pediatric Coding Newsletter* (https://coding.solutions.aap.org/article.aspx?articleid=2673746; subscription required)

"Coding Challenge: Modifiers and Procedural Services (Online Exclusive)" May 2018 *AAP Pediatric Coding Newsletter* (https://coding.solutions.aap.org/article.aspx?articleid=2679120; subscription required)

Reduced or Discontinued Procedures

"Reporting Terminated Procedural Services" November 2014 *AAP Pediatric Coding Newsletter* (https://coding.solutions.aap.org/article.aspx?articleid=1921435; subscription required)

Suture Removal

"You Code It! Removal of Sutures" March 2018 *AAP Pediatric Coding Newsletter* (https://coding.solutions.aap.org/article.aspx?articleid=2673748; subscription required)

Test Your Knowledge!

1. **How is an unrelated evaluation and management (E/M) service provided during the global surgical period reported?**
   a. The appropriate E/M code appended with modifier **24**
   b. The appropriate E/M code appended with modifier **25**
   c. **99214**
   d. **99204**

2. **What global period is assigned to simple skin wound repair?**
   a. Zero (0) days
   b. 10 days
   c. 90 days
   d. The concept of global period does not apply to wound repairs.

3. **Layered closure of 1 or more of the deeper layers of subcutaneous tissue and superficial (non-muscle) fascia is what type of repair?**
   a. Complicated
   b. Simple
   c. Intermediate
   d. Complex

4. **Which codes describe infusion using prepackaged fluid and/or electrolyte solutions?**
   a. None; this service is included in a related E/M service.
   b. **96365, 96366**
   c. **96360, 96361**
   d. **96372**

5. **How many units of service are linked to code 96372 for an intramuscular injection of 7 mg of dexamethasone sodium phosphate?**
   a. 2
   b. 1
   c. 7
   d. 70

Common Non-facility Testing and Therapeutic Services

Chapter 11. Common Non-facility Testing and Therapeutic Services

Contents

●=New code ▲=Revised code #=Re-sequenced code +=Add-on code

This chapter includes discussion of codes for some of the most common tests and therapeutic services performed in physician offices and outpatient clinics.

Interpretation and Report

Many tests include recording of results and a report with interpretation. *Current Procedural Terminology* (*CPT*®) instructs
- *Results* are the technical component of a service. Testing leads to results; results lead to interpretation.
- *Reports* are the work product of the interpretation of test results.
- Certain procedures or services described in CPT involve a technical component (eg, tests), which produces results (eg, data, images, slides). For clinical use, some of these results require interpretation. Some *CPT* descriptors specifically require interpretation and reporting to report that code.

Pediatricians performing services that include an interpretation of results should become familiar with the types of reports typical for each test (eg, typical report produced for the interpretation of electrocardiogram [ECG] tracings). A report generated by an automated system is not typically sufficient to support reporting a service described as "with interpretation and report."

Professional and Technical Components

26   Professional component: When the physician or other qualified health care professional is reporting only the professional component of a service, append modifier **26** to the procedure code.

TC   Technical component: When reporting only the technical component of a service, append modifier **TC** to the procedure code.

Certain procedures (eg, ECGs, radiographs, surgical diagnostic tests, laboratory tests) include a professional and technical component. Modifiers are used to indicate that either the professional or technical component was performed, but not both.

> **When the physician owns the equipment and is performing the technical and professional services, a modifier should not be appended to the code.**

- The *professional component* includes the physician work (eg, interpretation of the test, written report).
- If a physician is performing a service or procedure with equipment owned by a facility or another entity and the codes are written as a global service, services are reported with modifier **26** (professional component).
- The *technical component* includes the costs associated with providing the service (eg, equipment, salaries of technical personnel, supplies, facility expense).
  CPT does not include a modifier for reporting the technical component. However, most payers recognize Healthcare Common Procedure Coding System (HCPCS) modifier **TC**. Facilities or an office providing use of its equipment would only report the same service using modifier **TC**.
- Some codes were developed to distinguish between the technical and professional components (eg, routine ECG codes **93000–93010**); however, many do not.

No modifier is appended when the code descriptor for the service identifies whether the professional, technical, or global service is being reported.

Examples

➤ **A pediatrician orders a 2-view chest radiograph on a child.** The child is sent to a neighboring physician's office (or outpatient department) for the radiograph (without interpretation). The films are then brought back to the office and the pediatrician interprets them and creates a report of the findings.
    Pediatrician: **71046 26** (radiologic examination, chest; 2 views)
    Neighboring physician's office: **71046 TC**

➤ **A pediatrician orders a 12-lead ECG on an adolescent patient.** The patient is sent to another office that has an ECG machine to perform the ECG. The tracings are taken back to the pediatrician for review and written interpretation and report.

Pediatrician: **93010** (routine ECG with at least 12 leads; interpretation and report only)

Other office: **93005** (routine ECG with at least 12 leads; tracing only, without interpretation and report)

Modifiers **26** and **TC** are not appended because the codes designate the professional and technical components.

Do not separately report review of another physician's interpretation and report or personal review of the tracing that has been interpreted by another physician. However, these activities contribute to the medical decision-making for any related evaluation and management (E/M) service.

When interpreting an ECG at a location remote from the site of the tracing, follow payer guidelines for reporting. The place of service for remote interpretation and report is typically the site where the technical component of the test was performed (eg, outpatient hospital). Payer guidelines may vary.

Supplies and Medications

Supplies and Materials

99070   Supplies and materials provided by the physician over and above those usually included with the office visit or other services rendered

The relative value units (RVUs) assigned to testing services include the value of supplies (eg, masks, tubing, gauze, needles) that are typically required for each service.

> If reporting code **99070**, identify the supplies or materials on the claim form and be prepared to submit an invoice.

- Supplies should be separately reported when a payer does not use a payment methodology based on the RVUs assigned to each code under the Medicare Physician Fee Schedule (MPFS). However, most payers today use a payment method based on RVUs and do not provide separate payment for supplies.
- Items such as elastic wraps, clavicle splints, or circumcision and suturing trays may be reported with this code. Remember that some supplies (eg, suturing trays, circumcision trays) may be included with the surgical procedure if the payer uses the Resource-Based Relative Value Scale as its basis for payment.
- Only the supplies purchased in an office-based practice may be reported.
- Some payers will require the use of HCPCS codes. HCPCS codes are available for a number of supplies (eg, codes **Q4001–Q4051** for cast and splint supplies). Use HCPCS codes when they are more specific than code **99070**.

Medications

Medications used in testing or treatment (eg, albuterol) are not included in the value of service and are separately reported using HCPCS codes (eg, **J7613**, albuterol, inhalation solution, US Food and Drug Administration [FDA]-approved final product, noncompounded, administered through durable medical equipment [DME], unit dose, 1 mg).

See **Table 11-1** for a list of the most commonly used HCPCS **J** codes.

- The practice must have incurred a cost for the medication reported.
- Most payers do not cover services reported with nonspecific codes.
- Check with payers to determine if they accept these HCPCS codes or if they require reporting with code **99070**.
- Drugs are listed with a base dosage. When the dosage exceeds the amount listed, report additional units for the total dosage administered.
- Some payers require use of the National Drug Code (NDC) instead of or in addition to **J** codes. The NDC should always be reported in addition to code **99070** or **J3490** (unclassified drug). You can find a list of NDCs at www.fda.gov/drugs/drug-approvals-and-databases/national-drug-code-directory.

> For more information on National Drug Codes, see Chapter 1.

Blood Sampling for Diagnostic Study

Collection of blood samples for testing (eg, venipuncture) in a physician practice is reported regardless of whether the laboratory test is performed in the office or at an outside facility.

Venipuncture

36400	Venipuncture, younger than age 3 years, necessitating the skill of a physician or other qualified health care professional, not to be used for routine venipuncture; femoral or jugular vein
36405	scalp vein
36406	other vein
36410	Venipuncture, age 3 years or older, necessitating the skill of a physician or other qualified health care professional (separate procedure), for diagnostic or therapeutic purposes (not to be used for routine venipuncture)
36415	Collection of venous blood by venipuncture
36416	Collection of capillary blood specimen (eg, finger, heel, ear stick)
36591	Collection of blood specimen from a completely implantable venous access device

Codes **36415** and **36416** are used for children of any age when the physician is not needed to perform the procedure. Code **36416** is considered bundled under the MPFS and, therefore, not separately payable. Some payers may follow this bundling practice.

- When a physician's skill is required to perform venipuncture (eg, access is too difficult for other staff to attain) on a child younger than 3 years, codes **36400–36406** are reported based on the anatomical site of the venipuncture as follows:
  - **36400** (femoral or jugular vein)
  - **36405** (scalp vein)
  - **36406** (another vein)
- When a physician's skill is required to perform venipuncture on a child 3 years and older, code **36410** is reported.

> If the physician performs the venipuncture as a convenience or because staff is not trained in the procedure, code 36415 is reported because the physician's skill was not required.

Although typically not required, some payers will require that modifier **25** be appended to the E/M code if an E/M service is reported on the same day of service.
- It is not appropriate to report *CPT* code **99211** (nurse visit) along with code **36415** if the nurse only collects the blood specimen and no medically necessary and separately identifiable E/M service is provided.
- Code **36591** (collection of blood specimen from a completely implantable venous access device) is reported only when in conjunction with a laboratory service.

> See Chapter 19 for discussion of arterial catheterization.

Arterial Puncture

36600	Arterial puncture, withdrawal of blood for diagnosis

Arterial puncture (eg, radial artery) with withdrawal of blood for diagnosis is reported with code **36600**.

> Specimen collection (eg, nasal or oral swab, collection of urine), other than blood sampling, is not separately reported.

Pathology and Laboratory Procedures

CPT laboratory codes may either be generic for a particular analyte that is independent of testing method or have a specific *CPT* code, depending on the method used for the particular analysis.
- A test performed in the office's laboratory should be billed using the appropriate laboratory code and, if performed, the appropriate blood collection code (**36400–36416**).
- Link the appropriate diagnosis code to the laboratory procedure and/or venipuncture and handling fee. The diagnosis must support the medical necessity or reason for the test or service.

●=New code ▲=Revised code #=Re-sequenced code +=Add-on code

Chapter 11. Common Non-facility Testing and Therapeutic Services

- If the *only service* provided is a urinalysis or obtaining a blood specimen, only the laboratory test and/or venipuncture or capillary stick is reported.
  - It is not appropriate to report a nurse visit (**99211**) in these cases.
  - If a medically necessary nursing E/M service is performed in compliance with payer guidelines (eg, incident to a physician's service) on the same date as venipuncture, append modifier **25** to code **99211**.
- Do not report any laboratory test that is *not performed* in the office (eg, thyroid, laboratory panels, phenylketonuria). Instead, report the appropriate blood-drawing code (**36415** or **36416**), when applicable, and handling fee code (**99000**).

     Exception: Follow state regulations and payer policies for physician billing of laboratory services performed by an outside laboratory. Generally, if the laboratory bills the pediatrician for the test, bill the patient using the appropriate laboratory analysis code with modifier **90** to indicate the procedure was performed in an outside laboratory.

Example

➤ **The physician orders a lead test and the nurse obtains the blood via venipuncture.** The specimen is sent to an outside laboratory for processing.

   Only the venipuncture (**36415**) and handling fee (**99000**) would be reported in addition to the E/M service and other procedures performed on that day.

Coronavirus (SARS-CoV-2) Testing

The coronavirus pandemic of 2019-2020 was occurring at the time this publication was written. Because the frequency at which we will see this virus is unclear, the codes for testing will be included until they are no longer needed. Related tests include those to detect the virus and those to detect antibodies to the virus as available at time of publication.

Coronavirus (SARS-CoV-2) Infection Testing

When multiple specimens are collected (eg, nasopharyngeal and oropharyngeal swabs), verify payer instructions for reporting separate assays on each specimen (eg, report **87635** and **87635 59**).

87635	Infectious agent detection by nucleic acid (DNA or RNA); severe acute respiratory syndrome coronavirus 2 (SARS-CoV-2) (Coronavirus disease [COVID-19]), amplified probe technique.
87426	Infectious agent antigen detection by immunoassay technique (eg, enzyme immunoassay [EIA], enzyme-linked immunosorbent assay [ELISA], immunochemiluminometric assay [IMCA]), qualitative or semi-quantitative, multiple-step method; severe acute respiratory syndrome coronavirus (eg, SARS-CoV, SARS-CoV-2 [COVID-19])

   See also HCPCS codes **U0001–U0004**, which may be used to identify tests developed by the Centers for Disease Control and Prevention and/or performed via high-throughput technologies.

Coronavirus (SARS-CoV-2) Antibody Testing

Testing for antibodies produced in response to COVID-19 infection may be performed in a single step (**86328**) or multistep (**86769**) method.

86328	Immunoassay for infectious agent antibody(ies), qualitative or semi-quantitative, single step method (eg, reagent strip); severe acute respiratory syndrome coronavirus 2 (SARS-CoV-2) (Coronavirus disease [COVID-19])

> **Code 86328 is reported with 1 unit per reagent strip regardless of the number of antibodies evaluated and reported.**

86769	Antibody; severe acute respiratory syndrome coronavirus 2 (SARS-CoV-2) (Coronavirus disease [COVID-19])

> **When 2 distinct analyses are performed (eg, IgG and IgM), report codes 86769 and 86769 59.**

Clinical Laboratory Improvement Amendments–Waived Tests

The Clinical Laboratory Improvement Amendments (CLIA) establish quality standards for all laboratory testing to ensure the accuracy, reliability, and timeliness of patient test results regardless of where the test was performed.

- A *laboratory* is defined as any facility that performs laboratory testing on specimens derived from humans for the purpose of providing information for the diagnosis, prevention, and treatment of disease or impairment or assessment of health.
- The term *CLIA waived* refers to simple laboratory examinations and procedures that have an insignificant risk of an erroneous result. One typical test that is CLIA waived is urinalysis without microscopy (**81002**). Other tests require higher levels of CLIA certification (eg, provider-performed microscopy).
  - Payers may require a practice's current CLIA certificate number on claims.
  - Some codes represent both CLIA-waived and higher complexity test systems.

> **Not Sure How a Test Is Categorized?**
>
> The Centers for Medicare & Medicaid Services list of Clinical Laboratory Improvement Amendments (CLIA)-waived tests (www.cms.gov/Regulations-and-Guidance/Legislation/CLIA/Categorization_of_Tests) includes codes, test names (product), manufacturers, and descriptions of use. See also the US Food and Drug Administration CLIA database at www.accessdata.fda.gov/scripts/cdrh/cfdocs/cfCLIA/results.cfm that includes tests of all categories by test system, manufacturer, or analyte.

- Laboratories and physician offices performing waived tests may need to append modifier **QW** to the *CPT* code for CLIA-waived procedures. The use of modifier **QW** is payer specific.

  Only a small number of CLIA-waived tests are exempt from the use of modifier **QW** (eg, **81002**, **81025**, **82272**). These are listed first on the Centers for Medicare & Medicaid Services list of waived tests referenced earlier in this chapter.

Laboratory Panel Coding

All laboratory test panels in *CPT* were specifically developed for coding purposes only and should not be interpreted as clinical parameters. (See codes **80047–80076** for a component listing of these panels.) For example, the lipid panel (**80061**) includes total cholesterol (**82465**), high-density lipoprotein cholesterol (**83718**), and triglycerides (**84478**). Any additional tests performed can be coded separately from the panel code. *Do not unbundle individual laboratory tests if a laboratory panel code is available.*

Direct Optical Observation

Direct optical observation is a testing platform that provides a result (ie, positive or negative) by producing a signal on the reaction chamber (eg, test strip with colored bands) that can be interpreted visually (eg, point-of-care influenza testing). (See codes **87804** [influenza], **87807** [respiratory syncytial virus], and **87880** [group A streptococcus].)

> Codes for direct optical observation may include instrument-assisted direct optical observation (eg, a reader device provides the result[s]). However, some codes specify instrument-assisted direct optical observation (eg, **80306**, presumptive drug testing).

Per *CPT,* when reporting tests using direct optical observation, the number of results (eg, 2 results—positive for influenza A and negative for influenza B) determines the units of service reported.

- Use code **87086** (culture, bacterial; quantitative colony count, urine) once per encounter for urine culture to determine the approximate number of bacteria present per milliliter of urine.
- Use of a commercial kit with defined media to identify isolates in a positive urine culture is reported with **87088** (culture, bacterial; quantitative colony count, urine with isolation and presumptive identification of each isolate).
- Code **81007** (urinalysis; bacteriuria screen, except by culture or dipstick) (CLIA waived) can be used for a bacteriuria screen by non-culture technique using a commercial kit. The type of commercial kit must be specified.
- Code **87070** (culture, bacterial; any other source except urine, blood, or stool) is reported for throat cultures.
- Use code **87045** to report culture, bacteria of the stool, aerobic, with isolation and preliminary examination (eg, Kligler [triple sugar] iron agar, lysine iron agar) for *Salmonella* and *Shigella* species. Additional pathogens are reported with code **87046** with 1 unit per plate.
- Culture, presumptive pathogenic organisms, screening only (**87081**), is reported for testing for a specific organism (eg, *Streptococcus*).
- Report services with the symptoms (eg, dysuria) or the confirmed diagnosis (eg, urinary tract infection).

Laboratory Tests Frequently Performed in the Office

Urinalysis

81000   Urinalysis, by dipstick or tablet reagent for bilirubin, glucose, hemoglobin, ketones, leukocytes, nitrite, pH, protein, specific gravity, urobilinogen, any number of these constituents; nonautomated, with microscopy

81001   as per **81000** with microscopy, but automated

81002   as per **81000** but without microscopy (CLIA waived)

81003   as per **81000** but without microscopy, automated (CLIA waived)

It is important to report the correct code for the urinalysis test performed.

- Code **81000** is reported when the results are shown as color changes for multiple analytes (eg, ketones, specific gravity) that are compared against a standardized chart (nonautomated) and when microscopy (in a second step, the urine is centrifuged and examined under microscope) is performed.
- Code **81002** is reported if the test results are obtained by the same method but a microscopic examination is not performed.
- Codes **81001** and **81003** are reported for urinalysis performed by a processor that reads the results (automated).

For urinalysis, infectious agent detection, semiquantitative analysis of volatile compounds, use code **81099**.

Urine Pregnancy Test

81025   Urine pregnancy test, by visual color comparison method (CLIA waived)

Report code **81025** with *International Classification of Diseases, 10th Revision, Clinical Modification* (*ICD-10-CM*) codes **Z32.00–Z32.02**, depending on the findings of the test (ie, unconfirmed result, positive result, or negative result).

Glucose Tests

82947   Glucose, quantitative, blood (without a reagent strip) (CLIA waived)

82948   blood, reagent strip

82951   Glucose tolerance test (GTT), 3 specimens (CLIA waived)

82952   each additional beyond 3 specimens (CLIA waived)

82962   Glucose, blood by glucose monitoring device(s) cleared by the FDA specifically for home use (CLIA waived)

83036   Hemoglobin; glycosylated (A_{1c}) (CLIA waived)

83037   Hemoglobin; glycosylated (A_{1c}) by device cleared by FDA for home use (CLIA waived)

Report code **83037** for in-office hemoglobin A_{1c} measurement using a device that is cleared by the FDA for home use. This test is not limited to use in a patient's home.

Code **82962** describes the method when whole blood is obtained (usually by finger-stick device) and assayed by glucose oxidase, hexokinase, or electrochemical methods and spectrophotometry using a small portable device designed for home blood glucose monitoring. The devices are also used in physician offices, during home visits, or in clinics.

Continuous glucose monitoring is reported with codes **95249–95251** (see discussion later in this chapter).

Hematology

85013   Spun microhematocrit (CLIA waived)

85018   Hemoglobin (CLIA waived)

85025–85027 Complete blood cell count, automated (**85025** is CLIA waived.)

88738   Hemoglobin (Hgb), quantitative, transcutaneous

If using a complete blood cell count (CBC) machine to perform only a hemoglobin test, follow these guidelines.

- If the CBC result is normal, only the hemoglobin may be reported because that was the medically necessary test ordered.
- If the CBC reveals an abnormality and it is addressed during the course of the visit, the CBC result may be reported. The abnormality would be linked to the procedure, and the medical record would need to include documentation for the ordering of the test and to support the medical necessity of the procedure.

Influenza—Point-of-Care Testing

| 87502 | Infectious agent detection by nucleic acid (DNA or RNA); influenza virus, for multiple types or sub-types, includes multiplex reverse transcription, when performed, and multiplex amplified probe technique, first 2 types or sub-types (CLIA waived) |
| 87804 | Infectious agent antigen detection by immunoassay with direct optical observation; influenza (CLIA waived) |

> Code **87502** describes a test that already takes into account the first 2 types or subtypes; therefore, do not report multiple units of code **87502** for the separate testing of influenza A and B.

- Code **87804** may be reported twice with modifier **59** appended to the second code when tests performed separately detect the influenza A and B antigen, providing 2 distinct results. This applies whether the test kit uses 1 or 2 analytic chambers to deliver 2 distinct results.
  - Check with payers; some do not recognize modifier **59** and may require reporting with 2 units of service and no modifier.
  - Some payers (eg, Medicaid plans) may limit units reported to the number of separate test kits used rather than following *CPT* instruction.

Lead Testing

| 83655 | Lead, quantitative analysis (CLIA waived) |

- This test does not specify the specimen source or the method of testing. Alternative tests sometimes (although rarely) used for lead screening are **82135** (aminolevulinic acid, delta), **84202** (protoporphyrin, red blood cell count, quantitative), and **84203** (protoporphyrin, red blood cell count, screen).
- Some states provide lead testing at no cost to patients covered under the Medicaid Early and Periodic Screening, Diagnostic, and Treatment program. Check your state Medicaid requirements for reporting this service.
- Report *ICD-10-CM* code **Z13.88** (encounter for screening for disorder due to exposure to contaminants) when performing lead screening. Some payers require **Z77.011**, contact with and (suspected) exposure to lead, in lieu of **Z13.88**.

> *International Classification of Diseases, 10th Revision, Clinical Modification* allows separate reporting of special screening examinations (codes in categories **Z11–Z13**) in addition to the codes for routine child health examinations (eg, **Z00.121, Z00.129**) when these codes provide additional information. A screening code is not necessary if the screening is inherent to a routine examination.

Mononucleosis—Heterophile Antibodies Screening

| 86308 | Heterophile antibodies; screening (CLIA waived) |

This code may be appropriate for rapid mononucleosis screening.

Papanicolaou Tests

- The laboratory performing the cytology and interpretation reports Papanicolaou (Pap) tests with codes **88141–88155**, **88164–88167**, or **88174** and **88175**.
- Obtaining a Pap test specimen is inherent to the physical examination performed during a preventive medicine visit or a problem-oriented office visit.
- Medicare does require reporting HCPCS code **Q0091** (screening Papanicolaou, obtaining, preparing, and conveyance of cervical and vaginal smear to laboratory) in addition to the E/M service for preventive medicine and problem-oriented office visits.
  - Some state Medicaid programs and commercial payers may also recognize obtaining a Pap test as a separate service.
  - Code **Q0091** cannot be reported when a patient must return for a repeat Pap test due to inadequate initial sampling.
  - If not reporting **Q0091**, a handling fee (**99000**) can be reported in addition to an E/M service if the Pap test was obtained and sent to a laboratory.
- The appropriate *ICD-10-CM* code to link to the E/M code or code **Q0091** is either **Z01.411** (encounter for gynecological examination [general] [routine] with abnormal findings) or **Z01.419** (encounter for gynecological examination [general] [routine] without abnormal findings).
- For screening cervical Pap test not part of a gynecologic examination, report *ICD-10-CM* code **Z12.4** (encounter for screening for malignant neoplasm of cervix).

- For high-risk patients, you may also report secondary diagnosis codes to indicate personal history of other medical treatment (**Z92.89**) or other contact with and (suspected) exposures hazardous to health (**Z77.9**).

Presumptive Drug Tests

#80305   Drug test(s), presumptive, any number of drug classes, any number of devices or procedures; capable of being read by direct optical observation only (eg, utilizing immunoassay [eg, dipsticks, cups, cards, or cartridges]); includes sample validation when performed, per date of service (CLIA waived)

#80306   read by instrument assisted direct optical observation (eg, utilizing immunoassay [eg, dipsticks, cups, cards, or cartridges]); includes sample validation when performed, per date of service

#80307   by instrument chemistry analyzers (eg, utilizing immunoassay [eg, EIA, ELISA, EMIT, FPIA, IA, KIMS, RIA]), chromatography (eg, GC, HPLC), and mass spectrometry either with or without chromatography (eg, DART, DESI, GC-MS, GC-MS/MS, LC-MS, LC-MS/MS, LDTD, MALDI, TOF); includes sample validation when performed, per date of service

- Presumptive drug class screening includes all drugs and drug classes performed by the respective methodology (eg, dipstick kit with direct optical observation) on a single date of service. Sample validation is included in presumptive drug screening service.
- Venipuncture to obtain samples for drug testing may be separately reportable with code **36415** (collection of venous blood by venipuncture).
- When testing is performed with a method using direct optical observation to determine the result, code **80305** is reported. Tests that have a waived status under CLIA may be reported with modifier **QW** (waived test).
- When a reader is used to determine the result of testing (eg, a dipstick is inserted into a machine that determines the final reading), code **80306** is reported.
- Testing that uses a chemistry analyzer or more effort than tests represented by codes **80305** and **80306** is reported with code **80307**.

Respiratory Syncytial Virus Test

87634   Infectious agent detection by nucleic acid (DNA or RNA); respiratory syncytial virus, amplified probe technique

87807   Infectious agent antigen detection by immunoassay with direct optical observation; respiratory syncytial virus (CLIA waived)

For assays that include respiratory syncytial virus with additional respiratory viruses, see **87631–87633**. Tests reported with codes **87631** and **87633** are CLIA waived. Append modifier **QW** if required.

Serum and Transcutaneous Bilirubin Testing

82247   Total bilirubin (CLIA waived)

82248   Direct bilirubin

88720   Transcutaneous total bilirubin

Streptococcal Test

87880   Infectious agent antigen detection by immunoassay with direct optical observation; streptococcus group A (CLIA waived)

87651   Infectious agent detection by nucleic acid (DNA or RNA); streptococcus, group A, amplified probe technique (CLIA waived)

87081   Culture, presumptive pathogenic organisms, screening only

87430   Enzyme immunoassay, qualitative, streptococcus group A

- Report the code based on the test method rather than on the site of specimen collection.
- Culture plates using sheep blood agar with bacitracin disks should be coded with **87081**.

Testing Stool for Occult Blood

82272   Blood, occult, by peroxidase activity (eg, guaiac), qualitative, feces, 1–3 simultaneous determinations, performed for other than colorectal neoplasm screening (CLIA waived)

- Code **82272** is reported when a single sample is obtained from a digital rectal examination or a multi-test card is returned from the patient and is tested for blood. Report **82272** with 1 unit when up to 3 cards are returned.

Tuberculosis Skin Test (Mantoux)

86580   Tuberculosis, intradermal

- This test is exempt from CLIA requirements.
- The tuberculosis (TB) skin test (Mantoux) using the intradermal administration of purified protein derivative (PPD) is the recommended diagnostic skin test for TB.
  — This is not the BCG TB vaccine.
  — The American Academy of Pediatrics (AAP) supports the use of the Mantoux test (TB, intradermal) for TB screening when appropriate
- A separate administration code *is not reported* when the PPD is placed.
- Code **99211** is the appropriate code to report the reading of a PPD test when that is the only reason for the encounter.

  The appropriate *ICD-10-CM* code is **Z11.1** (encounter for screening for respiratory TB). In the case of a positive test result when the physician sees the patient, the complexity may lead to a higher-level code.
- Because risk-based testing is recommended for pediatric patients, an E/M service to evaluate the need for testing may be indicated when testing is requested by a third party (eg, school, employer).
- If TB testing by cell-mediated immunity antigen response measurement, gamma interferon (**86480**) is ordered, and a specimen obtained, venipuncture (**36415**) may be separately reported.

Zika Virus Testing

86794   Zika virus, IgM
87662   Zika virus, amplified probe technique

- The amplified probe technique (**87662**) is used when potential exposure occurred 2 weeks or more prior to testing.
- The IgM test described by code **86794** is used when suspected patient exposure to the Zika virus was less than 2 weeks before testing.

Respiratory Tests and Treatments

Pulmonary Function Tests

National Correct Coding Initiative (NCCI) edits exist between office-based E/M services and all pulmonology services (**94010–94799**). Append modifier **25** to the E/M service code as appropriate when reporting a pulmonology service on the same claim.

> There is no code for peak flow analysis or oxygen administration. These services are considered part of the evaluation and management service and/or a component of pulmonary function testing.

- Codes include laboratory procedure(s) and interpretation of test results. If a separately identifiable E/M service is performed, the appropriate E/M service code may also be reported.
- When spirometry (**94010**) is performed before and after administration of a bronchodilator, report only code **94060** (bronchodilation responsiveness, spirometry as in **94010**, pre- and post-bronchodilator administration).
  — Code **94640** (nebulizer treatment) is inherent to (ie, included as part of) code **94060**.
  — Relative value units assigned to codes include typical supplies (eg, masks, tubing). Report codes for supplies only if the payer does not use an RVU payment methodology.
  — Medication is separately reported with the appropriate HCPCS code (eg, **J7613**, albuterol, inhalation solution, FDA-approved final product, noncompounded, administered through DME, unit dose, 1 mg).
- Measurement of vital capacity (**94150**) is a component of spirometry and is only reported when performed alone.
- Measurement of spirometric forced expiratory flows in an infant or child through 2 years of age is reported with code **94011**.
- Code **94012** is used to report measurement of bronchodilation spirometric forced expiratory flows (before and after bronchodilator) in an infant or child.
- Code **94013** is used to report measurement of lung volumes (eg, functional residual capacity, expiratory reserve volume, forced vital capacity) in an infant or child through 2 years of age.

> *Current Procedural Terminology* **guidelines allow reporting pulse oximetry (94760, 94761), but health plans using the Medicare Physician Fee Schedule will pay only if no other service is paid to the same physician on the same date (ie, some plans consider this an examination component similar to determining blood pressure).**

- Pulmonary stress testing (**94618**) includes measurement of heart rate, oximetry, and oxygen titration, when performed. If spirometry is performed prior to and following a pulmonary stress test, separately report 2 units of spirometry (**94010**).

Inhalation Treatment

94640   Pressurized or nonpressurized inhalation treatment for acute airway obstruction for therapeutic purposes and/or for diagnostic purposes such as sputum induction with an aerosol generator, nebulizer, metered dose inhaler (MDI) or intermittent positive pressure breathing (IPPB) device

94644   Continuous inhalation treatment with aerosol medication for acute airway obstruction; first hour (For services of less than 1 hour, use **94640**)

+94645   each additional hour (List separately in addition to code for primary procedure)

   Report **94640**
- When treatment such as aerosol generator, nebulizer, MDI, or IPPB device is administered.
- With modifier **76** (repeat procedure) with the number of units when more than 1 treatment is given on a date of service. Some payers require reporting with the number of units only and no modifier. Follow payer guidelines for reporting these services.
- When any treatment of less than 30 minutes is performed.

> *Current Procedural Terminology* **code 94060 includes spirometry and pre- and post-bronchodilation. Report only 94060 when 94010 and/or 94640 is a component of the 94060 service.**

   Current NCCI edit policy does not allow reporting code **94640** more than once per patient encounter. The AAP is working with NCCI edit staff to change this policy.
   Report codes **94644** and **94645** when
- A treatment lasts 31 minutes or longer.
- The total time spent in the provision of continuous inhalation treatments is documented in the medical record.

   Codes **94644** and **94645** are not reported by physicians when services are provided in a facility setting because no physician work value is assigned to these codes.

Nebulizer Demonstration or Evaluation

94664   Demonstration and/or evaluation of patient utilization of an aerosol generator, nebulizer, metered dose inhaler or IPPB device

- Code **94664** is reported only once per date of service.
- Report code **94664** (demonstration and/or evaluation of patient utilization of an aerosol generator, nebulizer, MDI, or IPPB device) when an initial or subsequent demonstration and/or evaluation is performed and documented.
- Physicians providing nebulizer instruction in conjunction with an E/M service may include the time of nebulizer instruction in the time of counseling and/or coordination of care or the total physician time on the date of an office E/M service (**99202–99205**, **99212–99215**) in lieu of reporting **94664**. No physician work is attributed to code **94664**.

   When the physician or nurse (of the same group and specialty) performs demonstration and/or evaluation of patient use of a device such as an MDI (**94664**) on the same day as a nebulizer treatment (**94640**), modifier **59** (distinct procedural service) should be appended to code **94664** to indicate to the payer that the services were separate and distinct and that both were clinically indicated.
- Per the Medicaid NCCI manual, the demonstration and/or evaluation described by code **94664** is included in code **94640** if the same device (eg, aerosol generator) is used for both services. The NCCI edits pair code **94664** with **94640** but allow an override of the edit with modifier **59** when both services are indicated (eg, treatment via nebulizer and teaching for MDI). However, some payers may not allow the use of modifier **59** in this instance if the 2 services did not occur at separate encounters. Check with your Medicaid payers.

Modifier **25** should be appended to an E/M service code reported on the same date to signify a separately identifiable service. All services must be documented in the medical record as significant, separately identifiable, and medically necessary.

Examples

➤ **A 6-year-old established patient with asthma arrives to the office in acute asthma exacerbation.** Pulse oximetry is performed and indicative of moderate asthma exacerbation. One nebulizer treatment is given via a small-volume nebulizer. Physical examination after first treatment shows decreased wheezing and work of breathing. Pulse oximetry is remeasured and normal. An asthma control test is completed, scored, and documented. An order is written for continuing treatments at home, evaluation and education in use of MDI, and return to the office as needed. The nurse documents her evaluation of use and education for home use of the MDI. Later the same day, the patient returns, again in acute exacerbation. A second nebulizer treatment is given by a small-volume nebulizer. Physical examination after the second treatment shows no improvement and the patient is borderline hypoxic on second pulse oxygen measurement. He is sent to the hospital to be admitted to observation by a hospitalist. Diagnosis is acute exacerbation of mild persistent asthma with hypoxemia.

ICD-10-CM	**J45.31** (mild persistent asthma with acute exacerbation) **R09.02** (hypoxemia)
CPT	**99214** or **99215 25** (office/outpatient E/M, established patient) **94640 76** × 2 units or **94640** × 2 (nebulizer treatments) **96160** (administration of asthma control test) **94664 59** (MDI demonstration) Medication (appropriate HCPCS code) **94761** (pulse oximetry, multiple determinations)

Teaching Point: Modifier **59** appended to **94664** indicates the MDI demonstration is reported in addition to nebulizer treatments provided via a different device. Physicians should also report any medications provided at the expense of the practice. HCPCS codes describe medications such as albuterol. (See HCPCS codes listed in **Table 11-1.**) The documented severity of the exacerbation in combination with a decision about hospital admission will support either **99214** (less than severe exacerbation) or **99215** (severe exacerbation).

Car Seat/Bed Testing

94780 Car seat/bed testing for airway integrity, for infants through 12 months of age, with continual clinical staff observation and continuous recording of pulse oximetry, heart rate and respiratory rate, with interpretation and report; 60 minutes

+94781 each additional full 30 minutes (List separately in addition to **94780**.)

To report codes **94780** and **94781**, the following conditions must be met:

- The patient must be an infant (12 months or younger). Reassessment after the patient is 29 days or older may be necessary.
- Continual clinical staff observation with continuous recording of pulse oximetry, heart rate, and respiratory rate is required.
- Vital signs and observations must be reviewed and interpreted and a written report generated by the physician.
- Codes are reported based on the total observation time spent and documented.
- If less than 60 minutes is spent in the procedure, code **94780** may not be reported.
- Each additional full 30 minutes (ie, not less than 90 minutes total) is reported with code **94781**.
- A significant, separately identifiable office or other outpatient E/M service [eg, **99213 25**]) may be reported on the same data as car seat/bed testing, when provided.

Table 11-1. Common Healthcare Common Procedure Coding System Codes

Inhalation Solution	Brand Name(s)[a]	J Code	Administration
Albuterol, inhalation solution, FDA-approved final product, noncompounded, administered through DME, concentrated form, 1 mg	Proventil, Ventolin	J7611	94640 or 94644 (for first hour)
Levalbuterol, inhalation solution, FDA-approved final product, noncompounded, administered through DME, concentrated form, 0.5 mg	Xopenex	J7612	94640 or 94644 (for first hour)
Albuterol, inhalation solution, FDA-approved final product, noncompounded, administered through DME, unit dose, 1 mg	AccuNeb, Proventil, Ventolin	J7613	94640 or 94644 (for first hour)
Levalbuterol, inhalation solution, FDA-approved final product, noncompounded, administered through DME, unit dose, 0.5 mg	Xopenex	J7614	94640 or 94644 (for first hour)
Levalbuterol, inhalation solution, compounded, administered through DME, unit dose, 0.5 mg	Levalbuterol hydrochloride	J7615	94640 or 94644 (for first hour)
Albuterol, up to 2.5 mg, and ipratropium bromide, up to 0.5 mg, FDA-approved final product, noncompounded, administered through DME	Albuterol, DuoNeb, ipratropium bromide	J7620	94640 or 94644 (for first hour)
Budesonide, inhalation solution, FDA-approved final product, noncompounded, administered through DME, unit dose form, up to 0.5 mg	Pulmicort	J7626	94640 or 94644 (for first hour)
Budesonide, inhalation solution, compounded product, administered through DME, unit dose form, up to 0.5 mg	Pulmicort Respules	J7627	94640 or 94644 (for first hour)
Injection	**Brand Name(s)[a]**	**J Code**	**Administration**
Epinephrine, 0.1 mg	Adrenalin chloride, Sus-Phrine	J0171	96372
Ampicillin, 500 mg	Omnipen-N, Totacillin-N	J0290	96372 (IM) (IV)[b]
Atropine sulfate, 0.01 mg	Atropen	J0461	96372
Penicillin G benzathine and penicillin G procaine, 100,000 units	Bicillin CR	J0558	96372
Penicillin G benzathine, 100,000 units	Bicillin L-A	J0561	96372
Ceftriaxone, per 250 mg	Rocephin	J0696	96372 (IM) (IV)[b]
Cefotaxime, per gram	Claforan	J0698	96372 (IM) (IV)[b]
Betamethasone acetate, 3 mg, and betamethasone sodium phosphate, 3 mg	Celestone Soluspan	J0702	96372
Dexamethasone acetate, 1 mg	Decadron-LA	J1094	96372
Dexamethasone sodium phosphate, 1 mg	Decadron	J1100	96372 (IM) (IV)[b]
Phenytoin sodium, per 50 mg	Dilantin	J1165	96374
Diphenhydramine hydrochloride, up to 50 mg	Benadryl	J1200	96372
Immunoglobulin, IM, 1 cc Immunoglobulin, IM, >10 cc	Gammar Gamastan	J1460 J1560	96372
Immunoglobulin, 500 mg	Gammar-IV	J1566	96374

Table 11-1 (*continued*)			
Injection (*continued*)	**Brand Name(s)**[a]	**J Code**	**Administration**
Gentamicin, up to 80 mg	Garamycin	**J1580**	**96372** (IM) (IV)[b]
Glucagon, per 1 mg	GlucaGen	**J1610**	**96374**
Heparin sodium (heparin lock flush), per 10 units	Hep-Lock	**J1642**	**96374**
Hydrocortisone sodium succinate, up to 100 mg	Solu-Cortef	**J1720**	**96374**
Promethazine hydrochloride, up to 50 mg	Phenergan	**J2550**	**96372**
Other	**Brand Name(s)**[a]	**J Code**	**Administration**
Prednisolone, oral, 5 mg	Delta-Cortef	**J7510**	None
Prednisone, immediate release or delayed release, oral, 1 mg	Rayos	**J7512**	None
Antiemetic drug, rectal/suppository, not otherwise specified	Phenergan	**J8498**	None
Dexamethasone, oral, 0.25 mg	Decadron	**J8540**	None

Abbreviations: DME, durable medical equipment; FDA, US Food and Drug Administration; IM, intramuscular; IV, intravenous.

[a] Brand names are furnished for identification purposes only. No endorsement of the manufacturers or products is implied.

[b] For IV administration codes, see **Table 10-4**.

The 2020 Healthcare Common Procedure Coding System codes were released subsequent to the publication of this book. Refer to www.aap.org/cfp for updates.

Example

➤ **A male neonate born at 34 weeks' gestation was released from the hospital 2 weeks ago with instructions to the parents to use only a car bed when transporting him until the pediatrician retests and determines that the neonate can safely ride in a car seat.** The newborn is seen in the outpatient clinic for a preventive medicine visit, and car seat testing is conducted for a period of 1 hour and 45 minutes. The physician reviews and interprets the nurse's records of pulse oximetry, heart and respiratory rates, and observations during the testing period. The interpretation is documented in a formal report and plan of care clearing the neonate to begin use of a rear-facing car seat. The plan of care is discussed with the parents, who also receive further instruction on appropriate use of the car seat.

ICD-10-CM	Codes for conditions of the newborn and **P07.37** (preterm newborn, gestational age 34 completed weeks)
CPT	**94780** (car seat/bed testing; first 60 minutes) **94781** (each additional full 30 minutes)

Teaching Point: In this scenario, a total of 105 minutes of testing was conducted. This would be reported with 1 unit of code **94780** for the initial 60 minutes of testing and 1 unit of code **94781** for the last 45 minutes (only 1 full period of 30 minutes beyond the first 60 minutes was performed). The 15 minutes beyond the last full 30-minute period are not separately reported. An associated preventive E/M service with modifier **25** would be separately reportable.

Pediatric Home Apnea Monitoring

94774   Pediatric home apnea monitoring event recording including respiratory rate, pattern and heart rate per 30-day period of time; includes monitor attachment, download of data, review, interpretation, and preparation of a report by a physician or other qualified health care professional

94777   review, interpretation and preparation of report only by a physician or other qualified health care professional

● Codes **94774** and **94777** are reported once per 30-day period.

- Codes **94774** and **94777** are reported by the physician.
  — Code **94774** (includes technical and professional services) is reported by the physician when he or she orders home monitoring, chooses the monitor limits, and arranges for a home health care provider to teach the parents about monitor use and response to alerts. It includes reviewing and interpreting downloaded data and preparation of the report.
  — Code **94777** is a professional service reported when the physician receives the downloaded information, reviews the patterns and periods of abnormal respiratory or heart rate, and summarizes, in a written report, the findings and recommendations for continuation or discontinuation of monitoring. This information is provided to the primary care physician and/or the family.
- Codes **94775** and **94776** are reported by the home health agency because there is no physician work involved.

> **See Chapter 20 for more information on pediatric home apnea monitoring.**

Home Ventilator Management

94005 Home ventilator management care plan oversight of a patient (patient not present) in home, domiciliary or rest home (eg, assisted living) requiring review of status, review of laboratories and other studies and revision of orders and respiratory care plan (as appropriate), within a calendar month, 30 minutes or more

- Services include determining ventilator settings, establishing a plan of care, and providing ongoing monitoring.
- Ventilator management includes all the E/M services (ie, physical examination, review of the medical record or diagnostic tests performed, counseling the patient and/or parents, coordinating care with other health care professionals, and documenting the medical record) performed by the physician responsible for providing the ventilation management.
- Code **94005** is used to report home ventilator management care plan oversight. It may only be reported when 30 or more minutes of care plan oversight is provided within a calendar month.

Allergy and Clinical Immunology

Allergy Testing

95004 Percutaneous tests (scratch, puncture, prick) with allergenic extracts, immediate type reaction, including test interpretation and report, specify number of tests

95017 Allergy testing, any combination of percutaneous (scratch, puncture, prick) and intracutaneous (intradermal), sequential and incremental, with venoms, immediate type reaction, including test interpretation and report, specify number of tests

95018 Allergy testing, any combination of percutaneous (scratch, puncture, prick) and intracutaneous (intradermal), sequential and incremental, with drugs or biologicals, immediate type reaction, including test interpretation and report, specify number of tests

95024 Intracutaneous (intradermal) tests with allergenic extracts, immediate type reaction, including test interpretation and report, specify number of tests

95027 Intracutaneous (intradermal) tests, sequential and incremental, with allergenic extracts for airborne allergens, immediate type reaction, including test interpretation and report, specify number of tests

95028 Intracutaneous (intradermal) tests with allergenic extracts, delayed type reaction, including reading, specify number of tests

- *CPT* codes for allergy testing are reported by type of test.
  — Percutaneous, immediate type reaction (**95004**)
  — Intracutaneous (intradermal) with immediate (**95024**, **95027**) or delayed type reaction (**95028**)
  — Any combination of percutaneous and intracutaneous, sequential and incremental tests with venoms (**95017**) or with drugs or biologicals (**95018**)
- Specification of the number of tests applied is required for accurate reporting of the units of service provided. Medicaid NCCI edits do not allow inclusion of positive or negative controls in the number of tests reported.
- Codes **95004**, **95017**, **95018**, **95024**, and **95027** include test interpretation and report. Code **95028** includes reading.

  An E/M service should not be reported for interpretation and report. However, if a significant, separately identifiable E/M service is performed and documented, it may be reported with modifier **25** appended to the appropriate E/M code.

●=New code   ▲=Revised code   #=Re-sequenced code   +=Add-on code

Chapter 11. Common Non-facility Testing and Therapeutic Services

Example

➤ **A patient with seasonal allergies undergoes percutaneous testing with 24 allergenic extracts.** A clinician administers the extracts per the physician's order and monitors the patient for signs of reaction. For each extract administered, the reaction (eg, size of wheal) or lack of reaction is noted. The physician interprets the test and creates a report of the findings.

The physician reports code **95004** with 24 units of service. If a significant E/M service is provided on the same date and is separately identifiable in the documentation from the preservice and post-service work of the testing (eg, interpretation and report), append modifier **25** to the code for the E/M service provided.

See "Allergy Skin Testing: Codes, Unit Counts, and Tips for Reporting" in the February 2020 *AAP Pediatric Coding Newsletter*™ for more information (https://coding.solutions.aap.org/article.aspx?articleid=2759685; subscription required).

- Patch and photo patch testing are reported with code **95044–95056**.
- Specific challenge testing (**95060–95079**) is coded according to target organ (eg, ophthalmic mucous membrane, nasal, inhalation bronchial challenges without pulmonary function testing, ingestion).
- Nasal cytology, a test for allergy-type cells (eosinophils) or infection-type cells (neutrophils) on a nasal scraping, is reported with code **89190**.
- Nitric oxide expired gas determination is reported with code **95012**. Nitric oxide determination by spectroscopy should be reported with code **94799**.

Allergen Immunotherapy

Codes for allergen immunotherapy are reported based on the service provided: preparation and provision of allergen extract only, administration only, or combined provision and administration.

An appropriate office or outpatient code may be reported with allergen immunotherapy codes. Modifier **25** is appended to the E/M service when it is performed and documented.

Preparation and Provision of Extract Only

95144	Professional services for the supervision of the preparation and provision of antigens for allergen immunotherapy, single-dose vials(s) (specify number of vials)
95145	Professional services for the supervision of the preparation and provision of antigens for allergy immunotherapy (specify number of doses); single stinging insect venom
95146	2 stinging insect venoms
95147	3 stinging insect venoms
95148	4 stinging insect venoms
95149	5 stinging insect venoms
95165	Professional services for the supervision of preparation and provision of antigens for allergen immunotherapy; single or multiple antigens (specify number of doses)
95170	Professional services for the supervision of preparation and provision of antigens for allergen immunotherapy; whole body extract of biting insect or other arthropod (specify number of doses)

- Codes **95144–95170** are used to report preparation and provision of antigens for allergen immunotherapy without administration of the allergenic extract.
  - Codes **95144–95170** describe the preparation of the antigen, the antigen extract itself, the physician's assessment and determination of the concentration and volume to use based on the patient's history and results of previous skin testing, and the prospective planned schedule of administration of the extract.
  - The number vials must be specified when reporting code **95144**.
  - Report codes **95145–95170** based on the *number of doses* (eg, preparation of 2 vials that will provide 20 doses of extract containing 4 insect venoms is reported with code **95148** and 20 units of service).
  - Services may be reported at the time the allergenic extract is prepared because injections occur on later dates (prospectively planned) or may not occur at all.
  - Administration of the allergenic extract is not included.
- Report **95146–95149** for preparation of extracts containing more than 1 single stinging venom (eg, code **95146** is reported for 2; code **95147** is reported for 3).

●=New code   ▲=Revised code   #=Re-sequenced code   +=Add-on code

National Correct Coding Initiative Immunotherapy Edits

The Medicaid National Correct Coding Initiative (NCCI) manual instructs that for purposes of reporting units of service (UOS) for antigen preparation (ie, *Current Procedural Terminology* codes 95145–95170), the physician reports "number of doses." The NCCI program defines a dose for reporting purposes as 1 mL. Thus, if a physician prepares a 10-mL vial of antigen, the physician may only report a maximum of 10 UOS for that vial even if the number of actual administered doses is greater than 10. Verify payer policies on units of service before reporting.

Administration of Extract Only

95115   Professional services for allergen immunotherapy not including provision of allergenic extracts; single injection

95117   2 or more injections

Either code **95115** or **95117** (not both) are used to report administration of the allergenic extract only. Report based on the number of injections when another health care professional (eg, the patient's allergist) has prepared and supplied the allergenic extract or when a physician (usually an allergist) administers the prospectively prepared extract (ie, prepared with the intent to administer on a planned schedule).

Example

➤ **The pediatrician administers 3 injections of allergen extract for a patient with allergic rhinitis due to pollen.** The extract was prepared and supplied by an allergist.

The pediatrician will report code **95117** with *ICD-10-CM* code **J30.1**.

Combined Provision of Allergenic Extract With Administration

Current Procedural Terminology (CPT) recommends codes 95120–95134 be reported only when specifically required by the payer. These codes are not assigned relative value units in the Medicare Physician Fee Schedule that many payers use as a basis for physician payment. The Centers for Medicare & Medicaid Services (CMS) Medicare program will only accept codes 95115, 95117, and 95144–95170 and will not allow payment for codes 95120–95134. State Medicaid and commercial payers may follow the CMS Medicare guidelines or may have their own established guidelines. Therefore, before reporting these services, research the reporting policies of your major payers.

See your *CPT* code manual or other code reference for full code descriptors for 95120–95134.

- Codes **95120–95134** are reported when the entire service of preparing, providing, and administering (injection) allergenic extract is performed at 1 patient encounter.
- Codes **95131–95134** are reported for extracts containing more than 1 single stinging insect venom.
- Codes **95115** and **95117** *cannot* be reported with codes **95120–95134**.
- Codes **95120** and **95125** are reported based on the number of injections administered (ie, a single injection or ≥2 injections).
- Codes **95130–95134** are reported per injection. Therefore, if 2 separate injections of 2 stinging insect venoms (eg, wasp and bee) are provided, code **95131** would be reported 2 times.
- For rapid desensitization per hour, see code **95180**.

Example

➤ **An allergist prepares a 10-dose vial of allergen extract and administers 1 dose at the time of the visit (allergenic extract was prepared with the intent to administer on a planned schedule).**

The allergist will report code **95165** with 10 units of service and **95115** with 1 unit of service and the specific diagnosis code. Allergic rhinitis due to pollen would be reported with *ICD-10-CM* code **J30.1** or, if due to food, code **J30.5**. Alternately, code **95120** would describe provision of allergenic extract and a single injection if required by a payer.

Epinephrine Auto-injector Administration

Administration of epinephrine via an epinephrine auto-injector in the office or other outpatient setting is reported with code **96372** (therapeutic, prophylactic, or diagnostic injection [specify substance or drug]; subcutaneous or intramuscular). Follow payer guidance for reporting an EpiPen kit furnished by the practice.

- Many payers require submission of code **J0171** (injection, adrenalin, epinephrine, 0.1 mg) with 1 unit for 1 injection.
- Other payers may require code **J3490** (unclassified drugs). Inclusion of the NDC provides additional information on the exact product.

Example

➤ **The patient has a reaction to the allergenic extract.** The physician injects epinephrine using an auto-injector device (eg, EpiPen Jr).

The injection using an auto-injection device would be reported as an intramuscular injection with code **96372**. Although code **J0171** is used to report provision of epinephrine, the auto-injector is not described by this code. Prior to claim submission, it is advisable to verify payer policy addressing submission of code **J0171** (epinephrine 0.01 mg) versus **J3490** (unspecified drug) with the product NDC to specify the exact product provided.

Immunoglobulins

> Note: This information does not apply to immunization services. See Chapter 9.

When reporting codes **90281–90399**, remember that they are only for the cost of the immunoglobulin and the appropriate separate administration code should also be reported (eg, **96372**, **96374**).

- A significant, separately identifiable E/M service performed during the same visit may also be billed if indicated.
- *ICD-10-CM* diagnosis codes to support immunoglobulin services include codes from categories **D80–D84** for certain disorders involving the immune mechanism or codes for specific conditions, such as mucocutaneous lymph node syndrome (**M30.3**).

Example

➤ **An infant with moderate pulmonary hypertension is seen for administration of the second of 5 monthly doses of palivizumab.** A nurse administers the immunoglobulin under direct physician supervision.

Code **96372** (intramuscular injection) is reported in addition to code **90378** (respiratory syncytial virus, monoclonal antibody, recombinant, for intramuscular use, 50 mg, each). The appropriate number of units reported for the dose given is 1 unit per 50 mg. The NDC for each vial should be included on claims for most payers.

> See Chapter 1 for more information on reporting National Drug Codes.

Hearing Screening and Other Audiological Function Testing Codes

(For central auditory function evaluation, see 92620, 92621.)

Audiometric tests require the use of calibrated electronic equipment, recording of results, and a written report with interpretation (eg, chart of hertz and decibels with pass/fail result for each ear tested and overall pass/fail result). Services include testing of both ears. If the test is applied to 1 ear only, modifier **52** (reduced services) must be appended to the code.

> Medicaid plans may offer physician resources providing hearing screening/testing coverage information and documentation forms/ requirements.

- Code **92551** (screening test, pure tone, air only) is used when earphones are placed on the patient and the patient is asked to respond to tones of different pitches and intensities. This is a limited study to identify the presence or absence of a potential hearing problem. Code **92551** is not used to report hearing screenings performed on newborns and infants.

> **Report hearing tests conducted following a failed hearing screening with *International Classification of Diseases, 10th Revision, Clinical Modification* code Z01.110 if results are normal. If findings are atypical, report code Z01.118 and a code to identify the abnormality.**

- Code **92552** (full pure tone audiometric assessment) is used when earphones are placed on the patient and the patient is asked to respond to tones of different pitches and intensities. The threshold, which is the lowest intensity of the tone that the patient can hear 50% of the time, is recorded for a number of frequencies.
- Air and bone thresholds (**92553**) may be obtained and compared to differentiate among conductive, sensorineural, or mixed hearing losses. Air and bone thresholds are obtained in a similar manner.

> **Automated audiometry testing is reported with Category III codes 0208T–0212T.**

- Code **92558** is reported for evoked otoacoustic emissions, screening (qualitative measurement of distortion product or transient evoked otoacoustic emissions), with automated analysis. This is used when the results are obtained automatically (ie, no interpretation and report is required). Coverage for this is typically limited to newborn screening, including follow-up newborn screening from a failed screen in the hospital and screening on younger children. Check with your payers, however.
- Code **92583** (select picture audiometry) is typically used for younger children. The patient is asked to identify different pictures with the instructions given at different intensity levels.
- Distortion product evoked otoacoustic emissions codes are reported based on the number of frequencies used. Code **92587** is used to report testing for confirmation of the presence or absence of a hearing disorder, 3 to 6 frequencies. Code **92588** is reported when a comprehensive (quantitative analysis of outer hair cell function by cochlear mapping) diagnostic evaluation with a minimum of 12 frequencies is performed. Interpretation and written report are required. Do not report these codes for automated analysis.
- Other commonly performed procedures include codes **92567** (tympanometry [impedance testing]) and **92568** (acoustic reflex testing, threshold portion). Code **92550** is reported when tympanometry and reflex threshold measurements are performed.
- Optical coherence tomography of the middle ear with interpretation and report is reported with Category III codes based on whether the service was unilateral (**0485T**) or bilateral (**0486T**). Be sure to verify payer policy prior to provision of services.
- Most audiological procedures are bundled with impacted cerumen removal services (**69209, 69210**) and, therefore, will not be separately payable. Report only the audiology test to payers that bundle impacted cerumen removal services.

Example

➤ **A 3-year-old with bilateral acute recurrent otitis media undergoes optical coherence tomography of the middle ears to evaluate the presence and purulence of effusion in the middle ears.** After sufficient images are collected and areas of interest identified, a printout of selected data is obtained and reviewed by the physician or other qualified health care professional (QHP), who creates a report of the findings. Diagnosis is bilateral acute recurrent otitis media with effusion.

ICD-10-CM	H66.006 (acute suppurative otitis media without spontaneous rupture of ear drum, recurrent, bilateral)
CPT	0486T (optical coherence tomography of middle ear, with interpretation and report; bilateral)

Teaching Point: If a unilateral procedure were performed, code **0485T** would be reported in lieu of **0486T**. Note that the printout produced in testing is not the physician or QHP interpretation and report but provides information for the interpretation and report.

Endocrinology Services

95250   Ambulatory continuous glucose monitoring of interstitial tissue fluid via a subcutaneous sensor for a minimum of 72 hours; physician or other qualified health care professional (office) provided equipment, sensor placement, hook-up, calibration of monitor, patient training, removal of sensor, and printout of record

#95249   patient-provided equipment, sensor placement, hookup, calibration of monitor, patient training, and printout of recording

95251   Ambulatory continuous glucose monitoring of interstitial tissue fluid via a subcutaneous sensor for a minimum of 72 hours; analysis, interpretation and report

- When ambulatory glucose monitoring using monitoring equipment is initiated and data are captured for a minimum of 72 hours, report either **95249** or **95250** based on the supplier of the equipment (patient or physician office).
- Physicians report code **95249** only if the patient brings the data receiver to the physician's or other QHP's office with the entire initial data collection procedure conducted in the office.
- Report code **95249** only once for the entire duration of time that a patient has a receiver even if the patient receives a new sensor and/or transmitter. If a patient receives a new or different model of receiver, code **95249** may be reported again when the entire initial data collection procedure is conducted in the office.
- Analysis, interpretation, and report (**95251**) may be performed without a face-to-face encounter on the same date of service. This service is reported only once per month.

Emotional/Behavioral Assessment

96127   Brief emotional/behavioral assessment (eg, depression inventory, attention-deficit/hyperactivity disorder [ADHD] scale), with scoring and documentation, per standardized instrument

Code **96127**

- Represents the practice expense of administering, scoring, and documenting each standardized instrument. No physician work value is included. Physician interpretation is included in a related E/M service.
- May be used for screening but also for assessment in monitoring treatment efficacy and to support clinical decision-making.
- Not reported in conjunction with **96105**, **96125**, and **99483**.
- Two separate completions (eg, by teacher and parent) of the same form may be separately reported (ie, 2 units of service). When reporting multiple units of service, it is advisable to learn if the payer has specific guidance for reporting the total number of units as a single line item or requires splitting to multiple claim lines. Medically Unlikely Edits may apply.

Example

➤ **The mother of an 8-year-old girl expresses concerns about the child daydreaming and not paying attention at school.** The parent version of a behavior assessment system for children is administered to the mother and scored for the physician's review. The physician recommends that an additional behavioral assessment be completed by the girl's teacher to confirm or rule out predominantly inattentive ADHD.

The appropriate E/M service code (preventive medicine visit, new or established patient office visit, or consultation) would be reported in addition to code **96127**. Because the physician did not diagnose ADHD, assign *ICD-10-CM* code **R41.840** for symptoms of attention and concentration deficit.

Please see

- **Chapter 14 for discussion of diagnostic testing of the central nervous system**
- **Chapter 9 for discussion of developmental screening, brief emotional and/or behavioral assessment, and health risk assessment as preventive services**
- **Chapter 2 for more information on Medically Unlikely Edits**

Radiology Services

The following general guidelines are for reporting radiology services:

- Report only the service provided. See the Professional and Technical Components section earlier in this chapter for appropriate reporting when the physician does not provide the global service.
- A signed written report of the physician's or QHP's interpretation of imaging is an integral part of the professional component of a radiologic service.
- A reference to *image* in *CPT* may refer to an image on film or in digital format. Images must contain anatomical information unique to the patient for which the imaging service is provided.

- Certain health plans, including Medicaid plans, may require use of modifier **FX** (x-ray taken using film) when reporting the technical component or global radiology service (ie, combined professional and technical components). Verify health plan requirements, as payment may be reduced for radiographs taken using film.

Several categories of codes for radiology services have been revised in recent years. The following sections highlight some of these changes. Please see your coding reference for a full listing of codes and reporting instructions.

Imaging Guidance

Many procedures include imaging guidance. When a code descriptor for a procedure or *CPT* instruction indicates that the procedure includes imaging guidance, do not separately report a code for supervision and interpretation of imaging (eg, radiography, fluoroscopy, ultrasonography, magnetic resonance imaging, computed tomography, nuclear medicine).

- Do not report imaging guidance when a non–imaging-guided tracking or localizing system (eg, radar, electromagnetic signals) is used.
- If you do not own or lease the equipment but are only reporting the professional service of interpreting the image and writing the report, refer to the modifier **26** discussion in the Professional and Technical Components section earlier in the chapter.

Abdominal Radiographs

74018	Radiologic examination, abdomen; 1 view
74019	2 views
74021	3 or more views
74022	Radiologic examination, complete acute abdomen series, including 2 or more views of the abdomen (eg, supine, erect, decubitus), and a single view chest

Report code **74022** when a series of radiographs are obtained to view the abdomen and chest as workup of acute abdominal illness or pain. An acute abdomen series includes 2 abdominal views and a single chest view.

Chest Radiographs

71045	Radiologic examination, chest; single view
71046	2 views
71047	3 views
71048	4 or more views

- The types of views (eg, frontal and lateral) obtained no longer affect coding of chest radiographs.
- Do not separately report a single-view chest radiograph when obtained in conjunction with an acute abdomen series (**74022**).

Hip Radiographs

73501	Radiologic examination, hip, unilateral, with pelvis when performed; 1 view
73502	2-3 views
73503	performed minimum of 4 views
73521	Radiologic examination, hips, bilateral, with pelvis when performed; 2 views
73522	3-4 views
73523	minimum of 5 views
73525	Radiologic examination, hip, arthrography, radiological supervision and interpretation
73592	Radiologic examination lower extremity, infant, minimum of 2 views

Codes **73501–73523** include radiograph of the pelvis when performed. Do not separately report a single-view radiograph of the pelvis (**72170**) when performed in conjunction with a radiograph of the hip.

Total Spine Radiographs

72081	Radiologic examination, spine, entire thoracic and lumbar, including skull, cervical and sacral spine if performed (eg, scoliosis evaluation); one view
72082	2 or 3 views
72083	4 or 5 views
72084	minimum of 6 views

Codes **72081–72084** describe imaging of the entire thoracic and lumbar spine and, when performed, the skull, cervical, and sacral spine.

Do not separately report codes for views of the individual spinal segments or skull when performed in conjunction with radiologic examination of the spine. Rather, select the code that represents the total number of views obtained.

Administrative Services and Supplies

Administrative Services

Codes in this section cover some of the administrative aspects of medical practice.

99071 Educational supplies, such as books, tapes, and pamphlets, for the patient's education at cost to physician or other qualified health care professional

99075 Medical testimony

99082 Unusual travel (eg, transportation and escort of patient)

Codes **99071–99082** are for administrative services.

- Code **99071** may be reported when the physician incurs costs for educational supplies and provides them to the patient at his or her cost.
- Code **99075** may be reported when a physician presents medical testimony before a court or other administrative body.
- None of these services are assigned Medicare RVUs.
- HCPCS code **S9981** (medical records copying fee, administrative) or **S9982** (medical record copying fee, per page) may be reported when it is appropriate to charge for copies of medical records. Commercial payers and some Medicaid programs may accept **S** codes.
  - State medical insurance departments or medical associations determine the amount a practice can charge for copying medical records. Be sure to know the state charge limitations and do not overcharge.
  - The Health Insurance Portability and Accountability Act of 1996 (HIPAA) regulations, where more stringent, will override state regulations. For information on charges to patients for copying health records, see www.hhs.gov/hipaa/for-professionals/privacy/guidance/access/index.html#newlyreleasedfaqs.

Physician Group Education Services

99078 Physician or other qualified health care professional qualified by education, training, licensure/regulation (when applicable), educational services rendered to patients in a group setting (eg, prenatal, obesity, or diabetic instructions)

Code **99078** is used to report physician educational services provided to established patients in group settings (eg, obesity or diabetes classes).

- There are no time requirements.
- Modifier **25** (significant, separately identifiable E/M service) should *not* be appended to the E/M service because **99078** is an adjunct service.
- Documentation in each medical record includes the education and training provided, follow-up for ongoing education, and total time of the education.
- Services are reported on each participating child.
- Payers may require that these services be reported differently.
- For preventive medicine and risk-factor reduction counseling to patients in a group setting, see codes **99411** and **99412**.

Resources

Allergy Testing

"Allergy Skin Testing: Codes, Unit Counts, and Tips for Reporting" February 2020 *AAP Pediatric Coding Newsletter* (https://coding.solutions.aap.org/article.aspx?articleid=2759685; subscription required)

CLIA Test Categorization

Waived test systems and analytes (www.accessdata.fda.gov/scripts/cdrh/cfdocs/cfClia/analyteswaived.cfm)

Centers for Medicare & Medicaid Services CLIA categorization (www.cms.hhs.gov/CLIA)

HIPAA Release of Patient Records

Individuals' Right under HIPAA to Access their Health Information: Questions and Answers About HIPAA's Access Right (45 CFR §164.524) (www.hhs.gov/hipaa/for-professionals/privacy/guidance/access/index.html#newlyreleasedfaqs)

National Drug Codes

US FDA NDC Directory (www.fda.gov/drugs/drug-approvals-and-databases/national-drug-code-directory)

Test Your Knowledge!

1. **Which of the following modifiers is used to indicate a physician provided only the professional component of a service?**
   a. **26**
   b. **TC**
   c. **25**
   d. No modifier is required.

2. **Which code is reported when venipuncture for a 6-year-old child requires a physician's skills?**
   a. **36400**
   b. **36410**
   c. **36415**
   d. **36416**

3. **Spirometry is performed before and after administration of a bronchodilator. What code is reported?**
   a. **94640**
   b. **94010**
   c. **94060**
   d. **94010** x 2

4. **What modifier is appended to the code for the audiometry service to indicate it was performed bilaterally?**
   a. **50**
   b. Report the code without a modifier x 2 units of service.
   c. **52**
   d. No modifier is required, as all audiological function testing services are bilateral.

5. **What is included in an acute abdomen series?**
   a. 2 abdominal views and a single chest view
   b. Any 3 views of the abdomen
   c. 1 view of the chest and abdomen
   d. 2 chest views and an abdominal view

Outpatient Management of Chronic and Complex Conditions

Contents

Outpatient Management of Chronic and Complex Conditions

Children with chronic and complex health care needs require greater levels and amounts of multidisciplinary medical, psychosocial, rehabilitation, and habilitation services than their same-aged peers. The child with special health care needs will require extra services, such as prolonged services and care management, with an increased frequency of evaluation and management (E/M) visits.

Codes have been developed with the aim of capturing the components of care that go beyond those included in pre-service, intraservice, and post-service values of the traditional face-to-face visit. This chapter provides an overview and examples of many of these services.

- Transitional care management (TCM) (**99495, 99496**) may be provided to help patients transition from a stay in a facility to their home environment without gaps in their care management.
- Chronic care management (CCM) (**99490, 99439, 99491**) and complex chronic care management (CCCM) (**99487, 99489**) are monthly services provided by a single physician to manage or coordinate services for all of a patient's health care needs.
- Care plan oversight (CPO) (**99339, 99340; 99374, 99375; 99377, 99378; 99379, 99380**) is another monthly service provided by a single physician in supervision of health care services typically delivered by qualified nonphysician health care professionals (QNHCPs) (eg, therapists), home health, or hospice services.
- Awareness of the codes for these services and the related coding instructions may offer additional opportunities for providing and/or coordinating comprehensive care for all children.
  - Codes and payment policy for many of these services continue to evolve.
  - Many restrictions to reporting care management services in conjunction with other non–face-to-face services have been reduced in 2021.
- Reporting these services and the diagnosis codes representing the patient's chronic and complex conditions can play an important role in demonstrating the higher quality, lower cost care that is a key element of emerging payment methodologies.

> See Chapter 4 for information on emerging payment methodologies such as value-based purchasing.

- Payers that have adopted value-based or enhanced payment initiatives, such as per-member, per-month payment models, may consider certain care management services bundled into the services for which the enhanced payment is made. However, practices may choose to assign codes for use in internal calculations of the cost to provide enhanced care in comparison to any enhanced payments.
- To take advantage of opportunities for providing and reporting services related to management of chronic conditions and complex health care needs, physicians must identify the services that their practice capabilities will support. For instance, provision of TCM services requires timely identification of patients who are discharged from an inpatient or observation stay so that contact may be made with the patient within 2 business days of facility discharge.
- Payers may also require specific electronic capabilities (eg, having an electronic health record [EHR] that meets specifications required by the Medicaid Promoting Interoperability Program and/or Merit-based Incentive Payment System [MIPS]).

To support billing and payment, standardized procedures are necessary for identifying the need for services and for documenting physician orders and delivery of services. Electronic systems may be used to identify patients whose records include specific diagnoses and/or services that may indicate the need for care management.

For more information on preparing your practice to care for patients with complex health care needs, see the American Academy of Pediatrics (AAP) policy statement, "Patient- and Family-Centered Care Coordination: A Framework for Integrating Care for Children and Youth Across Multiple Systems" (https://pediatrics.aappublications.org/content/133/5/e1451).

- This policy statement, coauthored by the AAP Council on Children With Disabilities and the Medical Home Implementation Project Advisory Committee, outlines the essential partnerships that are critical to this framework.
- To further augment and facilitate the recommendations in this policy statement, refer to the freely accessible Boston Children's Hospital Care Coordination Curriculum (www.pcpcc.org/resource/care-coordination-curriculum). This curriculum provides content that can be adapted to the needs of any entity (eg, a single practice, a network of practices, parent and family organizations, a statewide organization). By design, most of the content is universally relevant, but the curriculum is optimally used when it is adapted and customized to reflect local needs, assets, and cultures.

Preventive Services for Children With Chronic and Complex Health Care Needs

Like typical children, children with chronic and complex health care needs also should receive periodic preventive care visits. Preventive medicine evaluation and management (E/M) services may take longer for medically complex children. However, preventive E/M services are not reported based on time and prolonged service does not apply. Only report a separate E/M service on the date of a preventive E/M service when a problem is addressed that requires significant physician work (medical decision-making or time) and is separately identifiable in the documentation.

Please see Chapter 9 for more information on reporting preventive E/M services and separately reportable services on the same date. Services such as chronic care management do not prevent separate reporting of preventive services.

Tracking Time of Periodic Services

Some codes for care management services are reported only when a specific amount of time is spent providing the service during 1 calendar month. Services typically occur on multiple days within the month. *Each segment of time must be documented.*

Documentation and tracking of time for services that are reported on a periodic basis, such as time spent in CCM activities in a calendar month, require establishment of routine processes to prevent lost revenue due to not capturing all billable services. Practice and system capabilities vary. Potential tracking mechanisms include

- Electronic health record flow sheets designed to capture each activity and the related time throughout a period of service and provide a report of time per patient within each period of service.
- Stand-alone time-tracking software may also offer a solution for documenting time of service.
- Work-arounds in existing electronic systems, such as EHR templates for clinical staff appointments that are assigned pseudocodes to track time (see example that follows). Pseudocodes are never used on claims; instead, they provide a basis for tracking time-based services.
- Manual systems, such as spreadsheets, that are updated at the time of each activity.

Be sure to identify the reporting period of care management services. Transitional care management services (99495, 99496) are reported for a 30-day period beginning with the date of discharge from a facility setting. Other services are reported per calendar month of service, including all chronic care management, care plan oversight, psychiatric collaborative care management, and care management for behavioral health conditions.

Collaboration with system vendors, professional colleagues, and practice management consultants may be invaluable to successful delivery, documentation, and reporting of time-based services.

The following example illustrates one semiautomated method of using pseudocodes:

Example

➤ **A pediatrician is providing care management to a child with 2 or more chronic conditions.** The pediatrician's clinical staff spend 25 minutes over the course of a month in care management activities in support of the plan of care developed by the pediatrician. On the date of each activity, clinical staff document the nature of the activity as well as the start and stop times. They also select a pseudocode (COORD) and 1 unit of service for each minute spent providing a service. No charge is generated by entry of COORD. However, billing staff will generate a report of the patients for whom COORD was entered during a calendar month. For those patients who received care meeting the requirements of CCM or CCCM, the pediatrician reports the appropriate codes (ie, **99490, 99439, 99491, 99487, 99489**).

Coding for Management of Complex Medical Conditions

Management of complex medical conditions may be reported with multiple codes for individual services or codes that describe either a combination of face-to-face and non–face-to-face services (eg, TCM) or a period of non–face-to-face services reported with 1 or more codes based on time of service.

Many inclusion and exclusion rules are applied to the services discussed in this chapter.

- Certain niche services (eg, management of end-stage renal disease) may be considered components of or an alternative to comprehensive care management.
- The same time and activity is never used to support multiple codes (eg, time used to support reporting of an online digital E/M service code is not included in time of CCM).

> **More information on services that may be frequently provided as part of managing complex health conditions are found in the following chapters:**
>
> - **Chapter 8: services provided in a patient's home, group home, or nursing facility**
> - **Chapter 13: services by qualified nonphysician health care professionals**
> - **Chapter 14: behavioral and mental health services**
> - **Chapter 20: digital medicine services including remote patient monitoring services**

Care Management Services

Transitional Care Management Services

Transitional care management (**99495, 99496**) includes services provided to a new or an established patient whose medical and/or psychosocial problems require moderate- or high-complexity medical decision-making (MDM) during the transition from the following settings to the patient's home, domiciliary, rest home, or assisted living facility:

- Inpatient hospital including partial, acute, rehabilitation, and long-term acute stays
- Observation care
- Skilled nursing or nursing facility

Transitional care management commences on the date of discharge and continues for the next 29 days. There are no specific requirements for time spent in TCM services. However, TCM activities should be documented on the dates provided.

Moderate to high MDM is a requirement for TCM. Follow-up care that includes low-intensity services such as discussion of improving or normal laboratory results, which require only straightforward or low MDM, are not reported with codes for TCM.

Transitional care management includes a combination of patient care activities by a physician or other qualified health care professional (QHP) and clinical staff working under supervision of a physician or QHP. **Table 12-1** includes code descriptors and activities that may be provided as part of a TCM service.

The 2020 Medicare Physician Fee Schedule values for TCM services were 5.20 total non-facility relative value units (RVUs) for code **99495** and 6.87 RVUs for **99496**. Total non-facility RVUs include values for physician work, practice expense, and liability.

- This equated to $187.67 and $247.94, respectively, for providing TCM services over a 30-day period (calculated at $36.0896 per RVU). Figures for 2021 were not available at the time of publication.
- 2020 physician work RVUs assigned were 2.36 for **99495** and 3.10 for **99496**. Work RVUs are often used in salary calculations for employed physicians.

> **For more information on how relative value units affect payment, see Chapter 5.**

- Transitional care management services are not limited to the attending provider of the related facility stay (eg, hospitalist) or any specific specialty.
  - The individual reporting TCM provides or oversees the management and/or coordination of services necessary *for all* the patient's medical conditions, psychosocial needs, and activities of daily living.
  - Only 1 individual may report TCM for each qualifying patient within 30 days of discharge. Another TCM service may not be reported by the same individual or group for any subsequent discharge(s) within those 30 days.
  - Hospital or observation discharge services (ie, **99238, 99239,** or **99217**) may be reported by the same individual reporting TCM services. Discharge services do not qualify as the required face-to-face visit for TCM.
- The TCM services begin on the date of discharge (day 1 of 30-day period) and continue for the next 29 days.
- One face-to-face visit with the reporting physician or QHP is included in addition to non–face-to-face services performed by the physician/QHP and/or licensed clinical staff under the direction of the physician/QHP.

  Codes **99495** and **99496**
- Require initial patient contact, a face-to-face visit with the reporting physician or QHP, and medication reconciliation *within specified time frames.*

Table 12-1. Transitional Care Management at a Glance	
Patient Population	
New or established patients whose medical and/or psychosocial problems require moderate- or high-complexity MDM during a 30-day transition period beginning with date of discharge from a facility setting to the patient's home, domiciliary, rest home, or assisted living facility.	
99495 Transitional care management services with the following required elements: • Communication (direct contact, telephone, electronic) with the patient and/or caregiver within 2 business days of discharge • Medical decision-making of at least moderate complexity during the service period • Face-to-face visit, within 14 calendar days of discharge[a]	**99496** Transitional care management services with the following required elements: • Communication (direct contact, telephone, electronic) with the patient and/or caregiver within 2 business days of discharge • Medical decision-making of high complexity during the service period • Face-to-face visit, within 7 calendar days of discharge[a]
Non–face-to-face services provided by the physician or other QHP may include	
• Obtaining and reviewing the discharge information • Reviewing, ordering, or following up on pending diagnostic tests and treatments • Communication or education provided to family and/or other caregivers • Interaction with other QHPs who will assume/reassume care of the patient's system-specific problems • Scheduling assistance for necessary follow-up services • Arranging referrals and community resources as necessary	
Licensed clinical staff time (under the direction of the physician or other QHP) may include face-to-face and non–face-to-face time spent	
• Communicating with the patient and/or family or other caregivers about aspects of care and with other agencies and community services utilized by the patient • Patient and/or family/caregiver education to support self-management, independent living, and activities of daily living • Assessment and support for adherence to treatment plan and medication management • Facilitating access to care and other services needed by the patient and/or family, including identification of community and health resources	
Abbreviations: MDM, medical decision-making; QHP, qualified health care professional. [a] Medication reconciliation and management must occur no later than the date of the face-to-face visit.	

To provide direct patient contact within 2 business days of discharge and to schedule appointments within 7 or 14 days, practices must have a process for receiving notification of observation and inpatient hospital discharges. Failure to make contact within 2 business days of discharge or to provide a face-to-face visit within 14 days of discharge eliminates the possibility of reporting transitional care management services.

- Medication management must occur *no later than* the date of the face-to-face visit.
  - *Medication reconciliation* refers to the process of avoiding inadvertent inconsistencies across transitions in care by reviewing the patient's complete medication regimen at the time of admission, transfer, and discharge and comparing it with the regimen being considered for the new setting of care.
  - Clinical staff may perform and document medication reconciliation under general supervision of the physician or QHP.
- Code selection is based on the level of MDM and the date of the first face-to-face visit, as shown in **Table 12-2**. Note that all 3 components (communication within 2 business days, type of MDM, and timing of face-to-face visit) must be met to report TCM services, although only the MDM and time of the face-to-face visit differentiate code selection.

Table 12-2. Levels of Transitional Care Management		
Type of Medical Decision-making	**Face-to-face Visit Within 7 Days**	**Face-to-face Visit Within 8 to 14 Days**
Moderate complexity	99495	99495
High complexity	99496	99495

- The first face-to-face visit is included in the TCM service and is not reported separately.
- Additional face-to-face E/M services (eg, **99212–99215**) during the 30-day TCM period but provided on dates subsequent to that of the first included face-to-face visit may be separately reported.

- The TCM services cannot be reported when provided during a postoperative portion of the global period of a service reported by the same physician or other physician of the same specialty and same group practice. For example, a surgeon would not report TCM during a postoperative period, but a primary pediatrician may report TCM when managing all of the patient's medical conditions following hospital discharge. Transitional care management is not reported for postoperative care alone.
- Documentation includes the timing of the initial post-discharge communication with the patient or caregivers, date of the face-to-face visit, and complexity of MDM over the 30-day service period. *Medical decision-making is defined by the E/M service guidelines.*
- Follow payer guidelines for reporting. The Centers for Medicare & Medicaid Services (CMS) allows reporting of TCM services once the included face-to-face visit has been completed (ie, prior to the end of the service period). Other payers may not allow billing until the complete service period has elapsed.

Examples

To help illustrate the use of codes for management of complex medical conditions, examples in this chapter will focus on one patient, Isadora (Izzy) Doe, who has cystic fibrosis with failure to thrive and developmental delay.

➤ **Izzy, a child with cystic fibrosis, is discharged from the hospital after an admission for recurrent *Pseudomonas aeruginosa* infection.** Two days after discharge, the physician speaks with Izzy's mother. Clinical staff assess adherence with the treatment plan and educate the parents on management of the child. The child is seen by the physician in follow-up 10 days after discharge. The pediatrician and clinical staff monitor and coordinate the child's ongoing treatment through the 29th day following discharge. The MDM is highly complex.

Code **99495** is reported. Although the MDM is highly complex, this service did not meet the requirements for code **99496** because the face-to-face visit did not occur within 7 days of discharge. Diagnosis codes may include **E84.0** (cystic fibrosis with pulmonary manifestations), **B96.5** (*Pseudomonas* as the cause of diseases classified elsewhere), and, if pneumonia is current, **J15.1** (pneumonia due to *Pseudomonas*).

➤ **Izzy, a child with cystic fibrosis, is discharged from the hospital after an admission for recurrent *Pseudomonas aeruginosa* infection.** Two days after discharge, the physician speaks with Izzy's mother. Clinical staff assess adherence with the treatment plan and educate the parents on management of the child. The child is seen by the physician in follow-up 5 days after discharge. The pediatrician and clinical staff monitor and coordinate the child's ongoing treatment through the 29th day following discharge. The MDM is highly complex.

Code **99496** is reported. Diagnoses are as noted in the previous example.

Chronic Care Management (CCM) Services

Chronic care management services are management and support services that are provided by physicians or QHPs or by clinical staff under the direction of a physician or QHP to individuals with 2 or more chronic conditions who reside at home or in a domiciliary, rest home, or assisted living facility.

Single Disease Management

The Centers for Medicare & Medicaid Services (CMS) added coverage of comprehensive care management services for a single high-risk disease (principal care management) effective January 1, 2020. The CMS implemented Healthcare Common Procedure Coding System codes **G2064** and **G2065** for reporting these services. Subscribers to the *AAP Pediatric Coding Newsletter*™ can find information on principal care management in the April 2020 article, "2020 Medicare Rule Changes: A Preview of *CPT* Changes?" (https://coding.solutions.aap.org/article.aspx?articleid=2763376).

The appropriate CCM code(s) is reported once per calendar month by only 1 individual who has assumed the management role for all the patient's care. This may be a primary pediatrician or a subspecialist, but only the 1 individual may report CCM services in a calendar month. Face-to-face E/M services may be separately reported by the same individual during the same calendar month.

Chronic care management

- Includes provision or oversight of the management and/or coordination of services, as needed, for all the patient's medical conditions, psychosocial needs, and activities of daily living.

- Requires creation, implementation, monitoring, and revision (as needed) of a comprehensive care plan for all the patient's health problems (discussed later in this chapter).
- Cannot be reported if performed within the postoperative portion of the global period of a surgery or procedure reported by the same physician or a physician of the same specialty and same group practice.
- Cannot be reported for any post-discharge CCM services within 30 days of discharge *if reporting* code **99495** or **99496** (TCM services).
  - When care management resumes after a discharge in a new month, start a new period or report TCM services (**99495**, **99496**) as appropriate.
  - If discharge occurs in the same month, continue the reporting period or report TCM services.

Example

➤ **Izzy is discharged on April 15, 2021. Transitional care management is provided through a period ending on May 14, 2021.** Only the time spent in CCM services provided from May 15, 2021, through May 31, 2021, may be considered for that calendar month per *Current Procedural Terminology* (*CPT*®).

Individual payers may adopt Medicare policy that allows reporting of both TCM and CCM during the same time period as long as each service is unique. Report overlapping services only when specifically allowed in payer policy.

Chronic Care Management Required Practice Capabilities

A practice providing CCM services must have all of the following specific capabilities:
- Use of an EHR system that allows care providers timely access to clinical information.
- Use of a medical record form and format that are standardized within the practice.
- Identification of patients who require care management using a standardized methodology (see description later in this chapter).
- Adoption of an internal care management process to provide care management services in a timely manner following identification of need for these services.
- Ability to provide access to care providers or clinical staff 24 hours a day, 7 days a week, including providing patients and caregivers with a means to make contact with health care professionals in the practice to address urgent needs, regardless of the time of day or day of the week.
- Ability to provide continuity of care through scheduling of the patient's successive routine appointments with a designated member of the care team.
- Provision of timely access and management for necessary follow-up when a patient is discharged from the emergency department or hospital.
- Patient and caregiver engagement and education.
- The individual reporting CCM oversees activities of the care team.
- All care team members providing services are clinically integrated.

Adopting a standardized methodology to identify patients who may qualify for CCM services may involve developing checklists or processes for identifying characteristics of patients with complex health care needs (eg, any patient with chronic or episodic conditions that are expected to last at least 12 months and increase the risk of morbidity and mortality, acute exacerbation or decompensation, or functional decline may require CCM services). Examples of such characteristics (*examples only; not a practice guideline*) include
- Number of chronic conditions
- Number of visits for nonroutine care in the past year
- Number of days the child did not attend school due to the health condition
- Emergency department visits or hospitalizations in the past 6 months
- Number of current medications or medications prescribed or revised in the last 6 months
- Number of physicians and other providers (eg, home health care provider, nutritionist)
- Lack of resources (eg, housing, health plan coverage, access to care in community)
- Assistance required for activities of daily living
- Other psychosocial considerations (eg, language barriers, multiple family members with complex care needs)

Activities of CCM

Services include all face-to-face and non–face-to-face clinical staff time spent in CCM activities. Time spent in other reported clinical staff services (eg, time of prolonged clinical staff service [**99415**, **99416**]) may not be included to meet requirements for reporting CCM.

●=New code ▲=Revised code #=Re-sequenced code +=Add-on code

Care management activities include

- Face-to-face and non–face-to-face time spent communicating with and engaging the patient and/or family, caregivers, other professionals, community services, and agencies
- Developing, revising, documenting, communicating, and implementing a comprehensive care plan
- Collecting health outcomes data and registry documentation
- Teaching patient and/or family/caregiver to support patient self-management, independent living, and activities of daily living
- Identifying community and health resources
- Facilitating access to care and other services needed by the patient and/or family
- Management of care transitions not reported as part of TCM (**99495**, **99496**)
- Ongoing review of patient status, including review of laboratory and other studies not reported as part of an E/M service
- Assessment and support for adherence to the care plan

Chronic care management codes were developed to align with Medicare coverage of CCM. The CMS has specific coverage criteria that may be adopted by Medicaid and private health plans, including 2 points of consideration for physicians.

1. Practices providing CCM services must have certain capabilities, including use of an EHR.
   — Health plans may adopt the CMS requirement for use of an EHR that meets certification requirements of the Medicaid Promoting Interoperability Program and/or MIPS in place on December 31 of the prior year.
2. Chronic care management activities are provided by clinical staff under the supervision of the physician or QHP reporting CCM services. Check with payers for the level of supervision required.
   — The CMS has allowed an exception to the Medicare requirement for direct supervision (ie, physician presence in the office suite when staff perform activities) for CCM services, allowing staff to perform CCM activities under the physician's or QHP's general supervision (ie, available as needed by phone) as long as all other incident-to requirements are met.

> **See Chapter 13 for information on incident-to requirements.**

Development of a Plan of Care

A plan of care must be developed or revised *and a copy provided to each patient* receiving CCM services.

- A comprehensive plan of care for health problems is based on a physical, mental, cognitive, social, functional, and environmental evaluation. It is intended to provide a simple and concise overview of the patient and be a useful resource for patients, caregivers, and providers. See **Figure 12-1** for an example of a plan of care.
- Creation, monitoring, or revision of a plan of care must be documented. Plans created by other entities (eg, home health agencies) cannot be substituted for a care plan established by the individual reporting CCM services.

Defining a Plan of Care

Current Procedural Terminology defines a *care plan* or *plan of care* as required for chronic care management and complex chronic care management services as

- Based on a physical, mental, cognitive, social, functional, and environmental assessment
- Comprehensive for all health problems
- A typical plan of care is not limited to, but may include
  — Problem list
  — Expected outcome and prognosis
  — Measurable treatment goals
  — Cognitive assessment
  — Functional assessment
  — Symptom management
  — Planned interventions
  — Medical management
  — Environmental evaluation
  — Caregiver assessment
  — Interaction and coordination with outside resources and other health care professionals and providers
  — Summary of advance directives

These elements are intended to be a guide for creating a meaningful plan of care rather than a strict set of requirements. They should be utilized only as appropriate for the individual.

The plan should be updated periodically based on status or goals changes. The entire care plan should be reviewed at least annually.

Chapter 12. Outpatient Management of Chronic and Complex Conditions

Codes for CCM and Complex CCM

Chronic care management includes multiple levels of complexity with codes describing each. **Table 12-3** provides code descriptors for CCM (**99490**, **99439**, **99491**) and CCCM (**99487**, **99489**) services.

● Only 1 type of CCM service is reported per calendar month.
— **99487** and **99491** or **99490** are not reported for the same month.
— **99490** and **99491** are not reported for the same month.

Table 12-3. Chronic Care Management Services
A comprehensive care plan must be developed, revised, or monitored and shared with the patient/caregivers for each type of CCM service.
Patient Population for All CCM Services Patients have multiple (≥2) chronic or episodic conditions expected to last ≥12 months, or until the death of the patient, that place the patient at significant risk of death, acute exacerbation/decompensation, or functional decline.
99490 Chronic care management services by clinical staff **Work Required** ● ≥20 minutes of clinical staff activity directed by a physician/QHP, per calendar month ● May include <30 minutes personally spent by a pediatrician or QHP in CCM services as long as ≥20 minutes are spent within a calendar month (including time of clinical staff) **99439** each additional 20 minutes of clinical staff time directed by a physician or QHP, per calendar month (List separately in addition to **99490**) ● Report up to 2 units of **99439** in a calendar month in addition to **99490** ● May combine time spent by a physician/QHP in addition to time of clinical staff
#99491 Chronic care management services by physician **Work Required** ● ≥30 minutes of time personally spent by a physician or QHP, per calendar month
99487 Complex chronic care management services by clinical staff/physician/QHP **Work Required** ● Moderate- or high-complexity medical decision-making ● ≥60 minutes of clinical staff activity directed by a physician or other QHP, per calendar month (may include time spent personally by a physician or other QHP) **+99489** ● each additional 30 minutes per calendar month (List separately in addition to **99487**)
Abbreviation: CCM, chronic care management; QHP, qualified health care professional.

The significant difference in work and practice expense required for delivery of CCCM services is reflected in the 2020 total non-facility RVUs assigned to codes **99490** (1.17), **99491** (2.33), **99487** (2.56), and **99489** (1.24).

● These codes are reported in any calendar month when the time requirements are met.
    Only time spent by clinical staff employed directly by or under contract with the reporting professional's practice is included.
● For **99491**, only count the time personally performed by the physician or other QHP. Time spent by clinical staff is not counted toward the time to support **99491**.
● More than 1 clinical staff member may spend time in CCM activities on a single date. Count all time that is not overlapping, but do not count the same period more than once.
    If multiple clinical staff members meet about 1 patient, count the time for only 1 staff member (eg, 3 staff members spend 5 minutes discussing a patient; the total time of the CCM activity is 5 minutes).
● Time, activities (eg, patient education), and identification of the individual conducting each activity must be documented. Visit www.aap.org/cfp (access code AAPCFP26) for an example of a worksheet for tracking CCM service times.
● Do not count any time of the clinical staff on the day of an initiating visit (eg, the creation of the care plan, initial explanation to patient and/or caregiver, obtaining consent).

> The midpoint rule commonly applied for coding based on time does not apply to chronic care management or complex chronic care management services (99487, 99489, 99490, 99439, 99491).

Figure 12-1. Example Plan of Care

This plan of care has been written by A Great Pediatric Practice to help us work with you to be as healthy as possible. This plan will allow you to share with us what is important to you and will let you know what to expect from us.

We will keep a copy of this plan and make changes as necessary. We will share this with other people who take care of you (for example, other doctors or therapists), as needed, to help them take care of you. You can also share this with others, such as family members, who help you take care of yourself.

Date	01/15/2021	Primary pediatrician	Dr Joe	Page 1 of 2

About Me

Name	Isadora Doe	I like to be called	Izzy	Date of birth	12/25/2014
Primary caregivers	Jenny Doe—mother; James Doe—father; Ellen Wright—mother's aunt				
Preferred contact information	Jenny Doe—MamaJ@hotmail.net, James Doe—DaddyJ@hotmail.net Ellen Wright—555/555-5555				
Secondary contact information	Jenny Doe—555/555-4444, James Doe—555/555-5554				
Preferred pharmacy	Family Drug Store	Preferred hospital		Children's Hospital-Main	

Who Do I Call When I Need Care or Have Questions?

My care coordinator	Bonnie Wood, LPN; 555/444-3333, ext 22; bwood@GreatPeds.care

Important Health Information

I am allergic to	No known allergies
I have difficulty with	Airway clearance techniques, gaining weight, infections, keeping up with schoolwork
Equipment I need (for example, wheelchair)	Percussion vest, aerosol generator
Community assistance	Mother reports no food or housing insecurity.

My Health Concerns (include concerns from patient and caregiver perspectives)

Concerns	What I can expect for each concern
Cystic fibrosis	Coordinated care with pulmonologist and respiratory therapist
Failure to thrive	Continue high calorie diet and consultation with nutritionist

My Health Goals

Goals	Plans of action
Cystic fibrosis: Maintain lung function and infections.	Continue daily percussion therapy, medications, and quarterly visits to Cystic Fibrosis Clinic.
Failure to thrive: Increase growth rate to achieve goal of 10th–≥50th percentile for age.	Continue enzyme and nutrition therapy; monitor weight and height.

My Planned Care

Specialty care	Cystic Fibrosis Clinic visit quarterly or as needed
Preventive care	Next preventive visit 06/12/2021
Scheduled follow-up visit	02/25/2021 8:00 am Call for urgent appointment as needed.
Nutrition therapy	ABC Home Care biweekly appointments
Respiratory therapy	ABC Home Care weekly appointments for 1 month
School counselor	Coordinates IEP changes, available at 555/555-5555
Other: School nurse is available only 2 days a week. Alert teacher of any changes to nutrition therapy. School requires physician signature annually on chronic illness form due to potential for missed school.	
Notes:	
Patient signature	
Parent signature	
Care coordinator signature	

- When provided during the same calendar month, behavioral or psychiatric collaborative care management (PCCM) services (**99484**, **99492–99494**) may be separately reported. Do not count the same minutes of time (eg, 1:00–1:15 pm) toward CCM and behavioral or PCCM services.
- If the physician personally performs clinical staff activities, his or her time may be counted toward the required clinical staff time to meet the elements of codes **99487**, **99489**, **99490**, and **99439**. If a physician or QHP personally performs at least 30 minutes of CCM services, see code **99491**.

When CCM services are provided to a patient *with moderate to high MDM and the reporting physician or QHP has personally spent 30 minutes or more in CCM activities,* consider whether the requirements for code **99487** (ie, ≥60 minutes and moderate to high MDM) have been met based on the combined time of the physician or QHP and clinical staff.

See examples for each level of CCM in **Table 12-4**.

Table 12-4. Chronic Care Management Coding Examples

The patient in each example is Izzy, who has cystic fibrosis and failure to thrive due to exocrine pancreatic insufficiency and has just completed a 30-day period of TCM. *ICD-10-CM* diagnosis codes may include **E84.0** (cystic fibrosis with pulmonary manifestations), **B96.5** (*Pseudomonas* as the cause of diseases classified elsewhere), **E84.8** (cystic fibrosis with other manifestations), **K86** (exocrine pancreatic insufficiency), and **R62.51** (failure to thrive), in addition to codes for any other conditions addressed.

Example	Code Assignment
Izzy is receiving CCM services. Time began the day after the 30-day period of TCM was completed. Clinical staff spend 65 minutes in the remainder of the calendar month implementing the care plan and responding to questions and concerns. MDM is moderate.	Code **99487** (CCCM of at least 60 minutes with moderate to high MDM) is reported by supervising physician Dr Joe. *Tip:* No time spent during the TCM period is counted toward the time of CCCM or CCM.
Izzy is receiving continued CCM services. During the calendar month, MDM included the decision to start tube feeding to address worsening feeding problems. A total of 95 minutes of combined physician and clinical staff time was spent in CCM activities for Izzy in the calendar month.	Dr Joe reports code **99487** for the first 60 minutes and **99489** (CCCM, each additional 30 minutes) for the additional 35 minutes. One unit of **99489** is reported for each full 30 minutes after the first 60 minutes of CCM in a calendar month.
Izzy is receiving continuing CCM services. Dr Joe spends 40 minutes revising Izzy's plan of care. Clinical staff also spent 15 minutes in CCM activities during the calendar month.	Dr Joe reports **99491** (CCM, personally performed by a physician or QHP, at least 30 minutes in the calendar month). Only Dr Joe's time is counted toward **99491**.
Izzy is receiving CCM services for cystic fibrosis with exocrine pancreatic insufficiency with attention to a gastrostomy and supervision of enteral nutrition. Dr Joe's clinical staff spend 20 minutes in CCM activities. Dr Joe also personally spends 10 minutes in CCM activities.	Dr Joe reports **99490** (CCM with at least 20 minutes of clinical staff time). Dr Joe and the clinical staff's combined time is counted toward **99490**. *Tip:* Dr Joe did not personally spend 30 minutes in CCM activities to support **99491**.
Izzy is receiving continued CCM services. Dr Joe personally spends 10 minutes in CCM activities in addition to 30 minutes spent by clinical staff.	**99490**, **99439** × 1 (CCM of at least 20 minutes and at least 20 minutes beyond the first 20 minutes in a calendar month) are reported for 40 minutes combined time of Dr Joe and clinical staff.

Abbreviations: CCM, chronic care management; CCCM, complex chronic care management; *ICD-10-CM, International Classification of Diseases, 10th Revision, Clinical Modification;* MDM, medical decision-making; QHP, qualified health care professional; TCM, transitional care management.

Care Plan Oversight Services

Care plan oversight is recurrent physician or QHP supervision of a complex patient or a patient who requires multidisciplinary care and ongoing physician or QHP involvement. Transitional care management or CCM/CCCM services would not be reported in conjunction with CPO services. (See the "Coding Conundrum: Chronic Care Management or Care Plan Oversight?" box later in this chapter to compare CPO with CCM services.) Care plan oversight services are not face-to-face and reflect the complexity and time required to supervise the care of the patient. The codes are reported separately from E/M office visits.

Medicare requires the use of Level II Healthcare Common Procedure Coding System codes for CPO services provided to patients under the care of a home health agency (**G0181**) or hospice (**G0182**). To report these **G** codes, Medicare requires a minimum of 30 minutes of physician supervision per calendar month. Because some state Medicaid programs may follow suit, check with your payer to learn its requirements for reporting these services.

Table 12-5 provides a comparison of CPO services, including patient population, work included, and services not separately reported. (Work included and services not separately reported are the same for all CPO services).

Care plan oversight services
- Are reported only by the individual (ie, physician/QHP) who has the predominant supervisory role in the care of the patient or is the sole provider of the services.
- A face-to-face service with the patient must have been provided by the physician prior to assuming CPO. The CMS requires a face-to-face visit within 6 months prior to CPO services.
- Include
  — Regular development and/or revision of care plans
  — Review of subsequent reports of the patient's status
  — Review of related laboratory or other diagnostic studies
  — Communication (including telephone calls) for purposes of assessment or care decisions with health care professionals, family members, surrogate decision-makers (eg, legal guardians), and/or key caregivers involved in the patient's care
  — Integration of new information into the medical treatment plan or adjustment of medical therapy
  — Team conferences
  — Prolonged E/M service before and/or after direct patient care when the same time is attributed to CPO
- Are reported once per month based on the amount of time spent by the physician during that calendar month.

Table 12-5. Care Plan Oversight Service Codes at a Glance

Patient Population

Patients receiving CPO require complex and multidisciplinary care modalities involving regular physician development and/or revision of care plans. The patient is not present at the time of service.

Individual physician supervision of a patient *in home, domiciliary, or rest home or assisted living facility (not under the care of a home health or hospice agency)* **99339** 15–29 min **99340** ≥30 min	Supervision of patient *under care of home health agency in home, domiciliary, or equivalent environment* **99374** 15–29 min **99375** ≥30 min
Supervision of *hospice patient* **99377** 15–29 min **99378** ≥30 min	Supervision of a *nursing facility patient* **99379** 15–29 min **99380** ≥30 min

Work Included in CPO Services

- At least 15 minutes by physician in regular development and/or revision of care plans
- Review of subsequent reports of the patient's status and related laboratory or other diagnostic studies
- Communication (including telephone calls) for assessment or care decisions with individuals (eg, family, caregivers, health care professionals) involved in patient's care
- Integration of new information into the medical treatment plan or adjustment of medical therapy

May Be Separately Reported When the Time of Each Service Is Distinct and Nonoverlapping

98966–98968, 99441–99443 Telephone services
98970–98972, 99421–99423 Online digital services
99358, 99359 Prolonged E/M service before and/or after direct patient care

May Not Be Reported in the Same Calendar Month as CPO

94005 Home ventilator management care plan oversight
99091 Collection and interpretation of physiologic data
99487–99491 Care management services

Abbreviations: CPO, care plan oversight; E/M, evaluation and management.

Chapter 12. Outpatient Management of Chronic and Complex Conditions

Coding Conundrum: Chronic Care Management or Care Plan Oversight?

Chronic care management (CCM) personally performed by a physician or other qualified health care professional (QHP) (**99491**) is similar to care plan oversight (CPO) for patients in their home setting, under care of home health or hospice, or residing in a nursing facility (**99339, 99340; 99374, 99375; 99377–99380**). Which should be reported for a physician's or QHP's services?

There are differences in code selection, as shown in this box. Additionally, practices reporting CCM must meet certain qualifications (eg, provides access to care providers or clinical staff 24 hours a day, 7 days a week, including providing patients and caregivers with a means to make contact with health care professionals in the practice to address urgent needs, regardless of the time of day or day of the week). Specific practice qualifications are not required for CPO.

Service	CPO	CCM Personally Performed by the Physician or QHP
Codes and total RVUs (non-facility)	**Codes requiring 15 minutes** **99339**: 2.19 **99374, 99377**, and **99379**: 1.98	Requires at least 30 minutes in a month **99491** 2.33
	Codes requiring 30 minutes **99340**: 3.05 **99375, 99378, 99380**: 2.96	
Level of physician/QHP involvement	Must personally perform services	Must personally perform services
Number of chronic conditions	≥1	≥2
Care plan work	Regular development and/or revision	Comprehensive care plan established, implemented, revised, or monitored

Abbreviations: CCM, chronic care management; CPO, care plan oversight; QHP, qualified health care professional; RVU, relative value unit.

Unlike nonphysician chronic care management and transitional care management services, time included in care plan oversight is only that of the physician or other qualified health care professional and not that of clinical staff.

- Includes cumulative time beginning on the first day of the calendar month and ending the last day of the calendar month.
- Are reported based on the patient's location or status (eg, home, hospice) and the total time spent by the physician within a calendar month. Less than 15 minutes' cumulative time within a calendar month cannot be reported.
- Are reported separately from other office or other outpatient, hospital, home, nursing facility, or domiciliary E/M services.
- Do not require specific practice capabilities as are defined for CCM services.
- Require recurrent supervision of therapy. Provision of very low-intensity or infrequent supervision services is considered part of the pre- and post-encounter work for home, office/outpatient, hospital, and nursing facility or domiciliary visit codes.

Example

➤ **A physician reviews a final report from a home health nurse on a patient who no longer requires home health after the first week of the calendar month.** These low-intensity services would be included in related E/M services and are not reported as CPO services.

Time spent on the following activities may not be considered CPO:
- Travel time to or from the facility or place of domicile
- Services furnished by clinical staff (ancillary or incident-to staff)
- Very low-intensity or infrequent supervision services included in the pre- and post-encounter work for an E/M service
- Interpretation of laboratory or other diagnostic studies associated with a face-to-face E/M service
- Informal consultations with health professionals not involved in the patient's care
- Routine postoperative care provided during the global surgery period of a procedure

- Time spent on telephone calls or online digital E/M or in medical team conferences if they are separately reported with codes **99441–99443**, **99421–99423**, or **99367**

A CPO billing worksheet can be used to track time of CPO services based on documentation in the patient's medical record and used to support billing when time in a calendar month supports reporting a CPO service. A template is found online at www.aap.org/cfp (access code AAPCFP26). See the "Care Plan Oversight Encounter Worksheet" box for an example of a completed CPO log. Electronic time-tracking software may be used in lieu of a worksheet.

Care Plan Oversight Encounter Worksheet

Physician: Dr Joe   Patient Name: Izzy Doe   Month: February 2021
Supporting documentation is found in patient's medical record.

Date of Service	Documented Service	Start Time	End Time	Total Minutes	Monthly Subtotal
02/04/2021	Review of diet log and weights with patient's mother	12:00 pm	12:06 pm	6	6
02/04/2021	Discussion with Dr Endocrine	12:15 pm	12:21 pm	6	12
02/15/2021	Review of laboratory results and discussion with Mrs Doe	5:15 pm	5:25 pm	10	22
02/16/2021	Discussion with Dr Pulmonary	5:30 pm	5:45 pm	15	37

Time Requirements per Calendar Month	Patient in Home, Domiciliary, or Rest Home (eg, assisted living facility)	Patient Under the Care of a Home Health Care Agency	Hospice Patient	Nursing Facility Patient
15–29 min	**99339**	**99374**	**99377**	**99379**
≥30 min	**99340**	**99375**	**99378**	**99380**
≥30 min Medicare code		**G0181**	**G0182**	

Code Supported: **99340**

See www.aap.org/cfp for an online version of this worksheet (access code AAPCFP26).

Medical Team Conferences

Medical team conference codes are used to report participation by a minimum of 3 physicians and/or QHPs or QNHCPs of different specialties in conferences to coordinate or manage care and services for established patients with chronic or multiple health conditions (eg, child who is ventilator dependent with developmental delays, seizures, and gastrostomy tube dependence for nutrition).

Table 12-6 provides an overview of the patient population, code descriptors, and services not separately reported with medical team conference services.

Medical team conferences require

- *Face-to-face participation* by a minimum of 3 physicians and/or QHPs or QNHCPs from different subspecialties or disciplines (eg, speech-language pathologists, dietitians, social workers), with or without the presence of the patient, family member(s), community agencies, surrogate decision-maker(s) (eg, legal guardian), and/or caregiver(s).
  — Participation by telephone is not reported.
  — Verify payer policies for participation via interactive audiovisual communication (telemedicine). Participation in team conferences via telemedicine *has not yet been added* to the lists of services reported with modifier **95** or the Medicare list of services approved for provision via telehealth.
- Active involvement in the development, revision, coordination, and implementation of health care services needed by the patient by each participant.
- Face-to-face evaluations and/or treatments within the previous 60 days, by the participant, that are separate from any team conference.
- Only 1 individual from the same specialty may report codes **99366–99368** for the same encounter. However, physicians of different specialties may each report their participation in a team conference.

Chapter 12. Outpatient Management of Chronic and Complex Conditions

- Medical record documentation supporting the reporting physician's or QHP's contributed information and subsequent treatment recommendations and the time spent from the beginning of the review of an individual patient until the conclusion of the review.
- Medical team conferences may not be reported if the facility or organization is contractually obligated to provide the service, they are informal meetings or simple conversations between physicians and other QHPs and QNHCPs, or less than 30 minutes of conference time is spent in the team conferences.

   Codes differentiate provider (physician vs other health care professional) and between face-to-face and non–face-to-face (patient and/or family is not present) patient team conference services.

- *CPT* instructs that physicians *or other QHPs* who may report E/M services should report their participation in a team conference with the patient and/or family present using E/M codes (based on key components [MDM only for office and other outpatient E/M services] or time, when appropriate per the instructions for the E/M service provided).

Table 12-6. Medical Team Conference Services

Patient Population

Established patients with chronic and multiple health conditions or with congenital anomalies (eg, cleft lip and palate, craniofacial abnormalities)

Physician or Qualified Health Care Professional Service

99367   Medical team conference with interdisciplinary team of health care professionals, patient and/or family not present, 30 minutes or more; participation by physician

(Physicians report other evaluation and management codes when patient or caregivers attend conference.)

Nonphysician Service

99366 Medical team conference with interdisciplinary team of health care professionals, face-to-face with patient and/or family, 30 minutes or more; participation by nonphysician qualified health care professional

99368 Medical team conference with interdisciplinary team of health care professionals, patient and/or family not present, 30 minutes or more; participation by nonphysician qualified health care professional

Work Required

- At least 30 minutes of face-to-face services from different specialties or disciplines
- Performed face-to-face evaluations or treatments of the patient, independent of any team conference, within the previous 60 days
- Presentation of findings and recommendations
- Formulation of a care plan and subsequent review/proofing of the plan

Do not report during the service time of

99487–99491 Chronic care management services

Examples

For each of the following examples, a team meets to discuss the care of Izzy, a child with cystic fibrosis with pulmonary manifestations (**E84.0**), exocrine pancreatic insufficiency (**E84.8**, **K86**), and failure to thrive (**R62.51**). Each participant in the conference has completed his or her evaluation of the patient within 60 days prior to the conference.

➤ **A primary care pediatrician, endocrinologist, pulmonologist, and medical nutrition therapist participate in discussion and planning, including changes to Izzy's respiratory therapy and medications, potential side effects of treatment, and option of enteral feeding.** The conference lasts 60 minutes.

CPT

99367   Each participating physician (if they are different specialties and/or from different practices [ie, separate tax identification numbers])

99368   Each QNHCP (eg, medical nutrition therapist)

   Physicians who provide a face-to-face visit (eg, consultation, **99241–99245**) on the same date as a *medical team conference without the patient/family present* should report codes for the individual services provided. A payer may require modifier **25** (significant, separately identifiable E/M service) on the code for the face-to-face visit.

➤ **A primary care pediatrician, endocrinologist, pulmonologist, and medical nutrition therapist participate in discussion and planning with Izzy's parents present.** The conference lasts 60 minutes. No other E/M services are provided by the physicians on this date.

CPT

99366	Each nonphysician QHP (eg, medical nutrition therapist)
99202–99499	Each participating physician (if they are different specialties and/or from different practices [ie, separate tax identification numbers]) reports an E/M service based on the place of service and applicable time-based coding instructions.

Physicians who provide a face-to-face visit on the same date as a medical team conference *with the patient/family present* should report the appropriate E/M code for the site of the visit and may also report an appropriate prolonged service code (eg, **99354**, **99355**, or, if in conjunction with an office or other outpatient code, **99417**) for time extending beyond the parameters designated by the E/M code and to the minimum time of the appropriate prolonged service code.

- If licensed QHPs (including clinical nurse specialists and clinical nurse practitioners) participated in a conference without direct physician supervision, they may report the service (**99367**) if it is within the state's scope of practice and they use their own National Provider Identifier. State Medicaid and commercial payers may follow these Medicare requirements or have their own specific rules.
- Code **99367** is the only code that may be reported by a physician, and it can only be reported when the patient and/or family is not present at the team conference.
- When the physician participates in a medical team conference with the patient and/or family present, the appropriate-level E/M code for the setting (eg, inpatient hospital) will be reported based on the place of service and documented level of service.
- Time reported for medical team conferences may not be used in the determination of time for CPO (**99339**, **99340**; **99374–99380**), CCM services (**99487–99491**), prolonged services (**99354–99359**), psychotherapy (**90832–90853**), or any E/M service.

Advance Care Planning

99497	Advance care planning including the explanation and discussion of advance directives such as standard forms (with completion of such forms, when performed), by the physician or other qualified health care professional; first 30 minutes, face-to-face with the patient, family member(s) and/or surrogate
+99498	each additional 30 minutes (List separately in addition to code for primary procedure)

Advance care planning includes

- A face-to-face service by a physician or QHP to a patient, family member, or surrogate spent in counseling and discussion of advance directives
- Completion of forms, when applicable (eg, Health Care Proxy, Durable Power of Attorney for Health Care, Living Will, and Medical Orders for Life-Sustaining Treatment)

> Active management of problems is not included in advance care planning. Other evaluation and management (E/M) services provided on the same date as advance care planning may be separately reported *with the exceptions of* hourly critical care services (99291, 99292), inpatient neonatal and pediatric critical care (99468, 99469; 99471–99476), and initial and continuing intensive care services (99477–99480). Append modifier 25 to the E/M code for active management of problems.

Because the *CPT* prefatory language and code descriptors for advance care planning do not include other instruction on the time required for reporting, these services may be reported based on general *CPT* instruction to report when the midpoint is passed (eg, 1 unit of **99498** may be reported for services of 46–75 minutes).

- Do not report code **99497** for less than 16 minutes of physician face-to-face time. Exceptions may apply for payers with policy requiring that the time be met or exceeded.

Advance care planning services may be considered bundled to enhanced payment methodologies (eg, patient-centered medical home receiving per-member, per-month care coordination fees) and not separately paid. However, *CPT* requires reporting of the code that is specific to the service provided regardless of payment policy. Advance care planning services should not be reported as another service (eg, office visit) in an effort to avoid denial as a bundled service.

Relative value units assigned for a non-facility site of service are 2.41 for **99497** and 2.11 for **99498** ($86.98 versus $76.15, respectively, when paid at the 2020 Medicare conversion factor of $36.0896 per RVU).

CPT instructs that codes reported should accurately describe the service rendered and physicians should not report a code that merely approximates the service provided, so it would be inappropriate to report another service that may have higher RVUs and payment values.

However, when a payer does not recognize advance care planning codes or the main reason for an encounter is other than advance care planning, consultation codes **99241–99245** or other E/M service codes (eg, **99212–99215**) may be appropriately reported.

Example

➤ **A child and his parents, who have learned at a recent visit that the child's prognosis is poor, return for advance care planning.** The physician spends 50 minutes face-to-face with the patient and parents, assesses their understanding of the diagnosis, and confirms and documents the desire to limit lifesaving measures and decisions about palliative care. A plan of care is developed and documented, and an appointment with the supportive care team at the hospital is scheduled.

CPT

99497	Advance care planning, initial 30 minutes
99498 × 1	each additional 30 minutes

The physician's face-to-face time of 50 minutes spent providing the advance care planning supports reporting **99497** with 1 unit of **99498** for the final 20 minutes of service.

Prolonged Services Without Direct Patient Contact

Prolonged services without direct patient contact (**99358**, **99359**) are reported when a physician or QHP provides prolonged service that does not involve face-to-face care.

Guidelines for reporting non-direct prolonged services include

- Prolonged service before and/or after direct patient care does not include time spent by clinical staff.
- Service must be related to another service conducted by a face-to-face physician or other QHP.
  - Prolonged service must relate to a service or patient where direct (face-to-face) patient care has occurred or will occur and to ongoing patient management.
  - The primary service may be an E/M service (with or without an assigned time), a procedure, or other face-to-face service.
- The place of service does not affect reporting.
- May be reported on a different date than the related primary service. *CPT* does not specify a time frame (eg, within 1 week of related service) for provision of prolonged service before and/or after direct patient care.
- Cannot be reported for time spent in provision of and reported with codes for
  - Care plan oversight services (**99339, 99340; 99374–99380**)
  - Chronic care management (**99487, 99489, 99490, 99439, 99491**)
  - Medical team conferences (**99366–99368**)
  - Online medical evaluations (**99421–99423**)
  - Interprofessional telephone/internet/EHR consultations (**99446–99452**)
  - Anticoagulant management for a patient taking warfarin (**93792, 93793**)
- For time of prolonged service on the date of an office or other outpatient E/M service (**99205** or **99215**), see code **99417**.
- Time is met when the midpoint is passed.
  - Less than 30 minutes' total duration on a given date cannot be reported.
  - Less than 15 minutes beyond the first hour or beyond the final 30 minutes is not reported separately. Use code **99359** to report the final 15 to 30 minutes of prolonged service on a given date. **Table 12-7** breaks down the time requirements.

Example

➤ **A physician requested and received medical records from the former physician of a child with cystic fibrosis with exocrine pancreatic insufficiency requiring enteral feeding via gastrostomy.** On a day before the date of the initial consultation service, the physician spends 35 minutes reviewing and summarizing the medical records and documents his time in the medical record. The physician reports

Table 12-7. Non–face-to-face Prolonged Services at a Glance	
99358 Prolonged evaluation and management service before and/or after direct patient care; first hour **+99359** each additional 30 minutes (Use in conjunction with code **99358**.)	
Prolonged service must be related to another service provided by the same individual.	
Total Duration of Prolonged Service Without Direct Face-to-face Contact	**Code(s) and Units of Service Reported**
<30 min	Not separately reported
30–74 min	**99358** × 1
75–104 min	**99358** × 1 and **99359** × 1
≥105 min	**99358** × 1 and **99359** × 2

CPT
99358 (prolonged physician services without direct patient contact; 30–74 minutes)

International Classification of Diseases, 10th Revision, Clinical Modification
E84.8, **K86** (cystic fibrosis and exocrine pancreatic insufficiency)
Z93.1 (gastrostomy status)

See Chapter 7 for prolonged service on the same date as an office or other outpatient E/M service reported with 99202–99205 or 99212–99215 and for discussion of prolonged clinical staff services.

See chapters 8 and 16 for discussion of face-to-face prolonged services.

Related Services Discussed in Other Chapters

Psychiatric Collaborative Care Management Services

Psychiatric collaborative care management services are provided to patients who have a new or existing psychiatric disorder that requires a behavioral health assessment; care plan implementation, revision, or monitoring; and provision of brief interventions. These services involve the efforts of a team of 3 health care professionals: a treating physician or QHP, a behavioral health care manager, and a psychiatric consultant. The treating physician or QHP reports codes **99492–99494** when all requirements for reporting are met. Evaluation and management and other services may be reported separately by the same physician or QHP during the same calendar month.

Please see Chapter 14 for information on reporting psychiatric collaborative care management services and general behavioral health integration care management services.

General Behavioral Health Integration Care Management

Code **99484** was created for reporting provision of behavioral health integration care management services by other than the PCCM model. The services are performed by clinical staff for a patient with a behavioral health condition (including substance use) that requires care management services (face-to-face or non–face-to-face) of 20 or more minutes in a calendar month. The service must be initiated and supervised by a physician or QHP who may report E/M services (ie, is not reported by QNHCPs whose scope of practice does not include E/M services under state regulations or when not allowed by payer policy). A documented treatment plan is required as well as all activities specified in the code descriptor.

Online Digital Evaluation and Management Services

An online digital medical evaluation (**99421–99423**) is a non–face-to-face E/M service by a physician or other QHP who may report E/M services to a patient using internet resources in response to a patient's online inquiry.

This is in contrast with telemedicine services, which represent interactive audio and video telecommunications systems that permit real-time communication between the physician, at the distant site, and the patient, at the originating site.

Codes **98970–98972** are used by a QNHCP to report an online assessment and management service. The reporting guidelines for codes **98970–98972** are the same as those required for online services provided by the physician or QHP.

> **Please see Chapter 20 for more information about online digital medical services.**

Remote Physiologic Monitoring

#▲**99457**   Remote physiologic monitoring treatment management services, 20 minutes or more of clinical staff/physician/other qualified health care professional time in a calendar month requiring interactive communication with the patient/caregiver during the month

#+●**99458**   each additional 20 minutes

Code **99457** is reported for time spent managing care when the results from a monitoring device(s) are used for treatment management services. This code requires 20 or more minutes of time spent using the results of physiologic monitoring to manage a patient under a specific treatment plan. When the time of service extends a full 20 minutes beyond the first 20 minutes, report code **99458** in addition to **99457**.

> **Please see Chapter 20 for more information on remote physiologic monitoring services and on interprofessional consultations.**

Telephone Evaluation and Management Services

Telephone services (**99441–99443**) are non–face-to-face E/M services provided at the request of a patient or caregiver by a physician or other QHP who may report E/M services to a patient using the telephone.

Codes **98966–98968** are used to report telephone assessment and management services by health care professionals who may not report E/M services (eg, occupational therapists, speech-language pathologists).

> **Please see Chapter 8 for more details on telephone services codes.**

Interprofessional Telephone/Internet Consultations

Patients with chronic conditions may often require collaboration between their primary pediatrician and a subspecialist.

A consultation request by a patient's attending or primary physician or QHP soliciting opinion and/or treatment advice *by telephone, internet, or EHR* from a physician with specialty expertise (consultant) is reported by the consultant with interprofessional consultation codes **99446–99449** or **99451**. These consultations do not require face-to-face contact with the patient by the consultant.

The physician requesting the consultation may report code **99452** when 16 to 30 minutes is spent preparing for the referral and/or communicating with the consultant in a service day. Alternatively, prolonged service codes may be reported by the requesting individual when supported by the time of service.

After-hours and Special Services

Codes **99050–99060** are used to report services that are provided after hours or on an emergency basis and are an adjunct to the basic E/M service provided.

> **Please see Chapter 7 for more details on after-hours and special services codes.**

Reporting a Combination of Complex Medical Management Services

Services such as CCM and TCM offer a means of reporting many activities of care management with 1 or 2 codes that describe the complexity and period of care. However, these codes do not always apply (eg, patient does not meet criteria) or a payer does not provide benefits for care management services. In these cases, it may be necessary to report a combination of codes for non–face-to-face services provided to a child with complex health care needs. These may include CPO, online or telephone E/M services, prolonged services, and team conference services.

➤ Each of these services has been discussed, at least briefly, in this chapter. **Table 12-8** provides examples of services provided in a calendar month in the care of a child requiring complex medical management services.

Teaching Point: If all services are allowed by Izzy's health plan, Dr Bill would be paid approximately $289.44 for providing non-face-to-face services in this example in addition to the $123.43 paid for the preventive medicine visit.

Code **99340**, which requires 30 minutes of physician time, is supported by the 52 minutes Dr Bill spent on January 5 and 6, which were not included in other reported services. This service is valued at about $110.07 (when calculated at the 2020 Medicare conversion factor of 36.0896×3.05 total non-facility RVUs).

In this vignette, the practice is not reporting CCM services even though the time requirements were met. Dr Bill and his clinical staff spent 67 minutes in CCM services, **99490** and **99439** $\times$ 2 ($118.01, 3.27 combined RVUs $\times$ 36.0896) but instead reports code **99340**, which does not require the practice capabilities or multiple chronic conditions of CCM. A physician whose practice meets the required capabilities for CCM, and whose patient also meets the requirements for CCM, could report **99490** and **99439** in lieu of **99340**, potentially increasing payment by about $8.

Dr Bill's 52 minutes could also be reported with **99491** (CCM time personally spent by a physician) but that service is valued at about $84.09 (2.33 RVUs $\times$ 36.0896).

Code **99442** is applicable for the phone call initiated by the patient's mother on January 16, and this time is not included in the time of CPO (or CCM, when reported).

Dr Bill also reports **99452** (1.04 total non-facility RVUs, $37.53) for his participation in the interprofessional consultation on January 24 addressing changes to Izzy's care plan. This service is not paid under the Medicare Physician Fee Schedule, and other payers may also deny coverage.

Table 12-8. A Combination of Services Provided in Complex Medical Management

The patient in this example is Izzy, who just moved to a new town. These services represent Izzy's first encounter and related care with Dr Bill, a general pediatrician who will be Izzy's primary care physician. Diagnoses are **E84.8**, **K86** (cystic fibrosis with exocrine pancreatic insufficiency), **Z93.1** (gastrostomy status), **Z00.129** (routine child health check without abnormal findings), and **Z71.89** (other specified counseling).

Date and Service	Codes Reported	RVUs/Average Payment[a]
January 3 Dr Bill reviews Izzy's medical records, spending 30 minutes at noon and another 20 minutes after regular office hours to complete the review and document his findings. The total time spent is documented.	*ICD-10-CM* **E84.8, K86, Z93.1** *CPT* **99358** (prolonged E/M service before and/or after direct patient care; first hour)	3.15, $113.68
January 5 Dr Bill sees Izzy and provides and documents a preventive medicine visit. No new or exacerbated problems are addressed. During the visit, Izzy's mother relates that the child's new school has requested updated medical information, especially as related to routine and emergency care.	*ICD-10-CM* **Z00.129, E84.8, K86, Z93.1** *CPT* **99383** (preventive medicine visit, 5–11 years of age, new patient)	3.42, $123.43
January 5 Dr Bill spends 40 minutes developing a care plan and seeking input from a cystic fibrosis clinic 175 miles away whose physicians will also be caring for Izzy. Time spent is documented in the medical record. Dr Bill's clinical staff coordinates with Izzy's mother to schedule Izzy's first appointment at the cystic fibrosis clinic. Total time spent is 15 minutes.	*ICD-10-CM* **E84.8, K86** *CPT* Only Dr Bill's time (40 minutes) is counted toward the time of CPO. (See Teaching Point for more information.)	N/A; included in CPO total
January 6 Dr Bill spends an additional 12 minutes on a call with the patient's mother to discuss the care plan. All services and the time spent are documented in the medical record.	*ICD-10-CM* **E84.8, K86** *CPT* 12 minutes are counted toward CPO.	N/A; included in CPO total

	Table 12-8 (*continued*)	
Date and Service	**Codes Reported**	**RVUs/Average Payment**[a]
January 16 Izzy's mother calls Dr Bill with concerns that her child is not receiving appropriate accommodations at her new school. Dr Bill spends 15 minutes on the telephone with the mother and suggests a conference with the school nurse and administrator. The physician documents the time spent on the telephone call, the history, and issues discussed.	*ICD-10-CM* **Z71.89, E84.8, K86** *CPT* **99442** (telephone E/M service; 11–20 minutes of medical discussion)	0.78, $28.15
January 24 Dr Bill spends 35 minutes in an internet consultation with a specialist at Izzy's cystic fibrosis clinic discussing recommended changes to Izzy's plan of care. Izzy and her mother are not present.	*ICD-10-CM* **E84.8, K86** *CPT* **99452** (interprofessional referral service[s], 30 minutes)	1.04, $37.53
January 31 Dr Bill's total time spent in CPO (on January 5 and 6) is totaled and a claim is submitted.	*ICD-10-CM* **E84.8, K86** *CPT* **99340** (CPO, patient at home, ≥30 minutes) Total CPO time in the calendar month was 52 minutes.	3.05, $110.07
	Totals	**Totals** 11.44, $412.87

Abbreviations: CPO, care plan oversight; CPT, *Current Procedural Terminology*; E/M, evaluation and management; ICD-10-CM, *International Classification of Diseases, 10th Revision, Clinical Modification*; N/A, not applicable; RVU, relative value unit.

[a] 2020 total non-facility RVUs multiplied by 2020 conversion factor $36.0896. The 2021 RVUs and conversion factor were not available at time of publication.

- Be sure to review payer guidance on reporting of these services, as National Correct Coding Initiative edits or other payment policy may require appending modifiers to indicate distinct periods were spent in the provision of each service. For instance, prolonged E/M service is bundled to CPO, but a modifier may be appended to indicate distinct services within the same reporting period. Guidance for reporting and coverage may vary.
- Practices with the capabilities required for reporting CCM services in lieu of CPO may still report the CPO codes when the service provided and nature of the patient presentation support reporting CPO services. Physicians must determine the appropriate code selection based on the practice capabilities, services rendered, and nature of the patient presentation.

Resources

Care Plan Oversight

Care Plan Oversight Encounter Worksheet (www.aap.org/cfp, access code AAPCFP26)

Chronic Care Management

"Chronic Care Management 2021," October 2020 *AAP Pediatric Coding Newsletter*™ (http://coding.aap.org; subscription required)

"Chronic Care Management: Documenting a Plan of Care," December 2019 *AAP Pediatric Coding Newsletter* (https://coding.solutions.aap.org/article.aspx?articleid=2756867; subscription required)

"Chronic Care Management Documentation and Tracking Examples," December 2019 *AAP Pediatric Coding Newsletter* (https://coding.solutions.aap.org/article.aspx?articleid=2756869; subscription required)
CCM Tracking Worksheet (www.aap.org/cfp, access code AAPCFP26)

Patient- and Family-Centered Care Coordination

AAP policy statement, "Patient- and Family-Centered Care Coordination: A Framework for Integrating Care for Children and Youth Across Multiple Systems" (https://pediatrics.aappublications.org/content/133/5/e1451)

Boston Children's Hospital Care Coordination Curriculum (www.pcpcc.org/resource/care-coordination-curriculum)

Principal Care Management

"2020 Medicare Rule Changes: A Preview of *CPT* Changes?" April 2020 *AAP Pediatric Coding Newsletter* (https://coding.solutions.aap.org/article.aspx?articleid=2763376; subscription required)

Transitional Care Management

"Transitional Care Management: Revisiting the Basics," July 2017 *AAP Pediatric Coding Newsletter* (https://coding.solutions.aap.org/article.aspx?articleid=2634452; subscription required)

Test Your Knowledge!

1. **Which of the following is required for transitional care management (TCM)?**
   a. The patient was discharged to home, domiciliary, rest home, or assisted living facility.
   b. Medication reconciliation is required.
   c. An interactive contact within 2 business days of discharge
   d. All of the above

2. **Which is required for chronic care management (CCM) services reported with code 99490?**
   a. All patients receiving CCM services must be provided a copy of their plan of care.
   b. At least 30 minutes of clinical staff time spent in CCM activities must be documented.
   c. Physicians must personally spend 20 minutes performing CCM activities.
   d. The patient must have at least 3 chronic conditions.

3. **Which of the following is always true of TCM (99495)?**
   a. A face-to-face visit must occur within 30 days of patient discharge.
   b. At least moderate-complexity medical decision-making is required.
   c. Physicians and clinical staff must spend 20 minutes providing TCM services.
   d. Transitional care management services begin on the date of the first face-to-face visit after discharge.

4. **Which of the following is an example of time used to support care plan oversight?**
   a. Time of a face-to-face visit
   b. Time spent by clinical staff
   c. Physician time integrating new information into the patient's care plan
   d. Time of phone calls reported with codes 99441–99443

5. **Which codes correctly report 90 minutes of physician prolonged service before or after a related face-to-face service?**
   a. Only 99358
   b. 99358 × 1, 99359 × 1
   c. 99359 × 2
   d. 99358 × 1, 99359 × 2

Chapter 12. Outpatient Management of Chronic and Complex Conditions

CHAPTER 13

Qualified Nonphysician Health Care Professional Services

Contents

In their quest to provide comprehensive and high-quality care to patients, pediatric physicians are including more qualified nonphysician health care professionals (QNHCPs) (eg, nutritionists) in their practices and using clinical staff to their full potential.

This chapter focuses on services that are provided by health care professionals other than physicians and other qualified health care professionals (QHPs), such as nurse practitioners and physician assistants (who often practice and report services much as physicians do).

Terminology

> Throughout the *Current Procedural Terminology*® code set, the use of terms such as *physician, qualified health care professional,* or *individual* is not intended to indicate that other entities may not report the service. In selected instances, specific instructions may define a service as limited to professionals or other entities (eg, hospital, home health agency).

To help differentiate, the following definitions will apply in discussions and examples in this chapter:

- **Qualified health care professional (QHP):** Advanced practice providers, such as advanced practice nurses, clinical nurse specialists, and physician assistants, whose scope of practice includes evaluation and management (E/M) services beyond minimal services incident to a physician (ie, **99211**).
- **Qualified nonphysician health care professional (QNHCP):** A broad category of health care professionals who typically would not independently prescribe and manage, whose professional services are typically performed under the order and supervision of a physician or QHP, and whose scope of practice does not include E/M services beyond **99211**. Sometimes they are able to bill under their own National Provider Identifier (NPI). This category includes providers such as clinical psychologists, licensed counselors, dietitians/nutritionists, health educators, and lactation consultants, among others.
- **Clinical staff member** (as defined by *Current Procedural Terminology* [*CPT*]): A health care team member who works under the supervision of a physician or other QHP and who is allowed by law, regulation, and facility policy to perform or assist in the performance of a specific professional service but *does not individually report that professional service.* These include, but are not limited to, registered nurses (RNs), licensed practical nurses (LPNs), and medical assistants (MAs).

    CPT references *clinical staff member* mostly in the context of staff who provide components of physician or QHP services, such as obtaining patient history, and services that are always billed by a supervising physician or QHP (eg, nurse visit, medication administration), as discussed in the Incident-to Requirements: Supervision of Nonphysician Health Care Professionals section later in this chapter.

> Staff who perform *only administrative functions,* such as receptionist, scheduling, billing, dictation, or scribing, are not clinical staff for coding purposes.

Including Qualified Nonphysician Health Care Professionals in Your Practice

Services by QNHCPs, provided under a physician's or QHP's order within a physician group practice, can be an integral part of providing a full scope of care in the medical home.

- Billing and coding must align not only with coding guidelines but also state scope of practice (see the Scope of Practice Laws section later in this chapter) and individual payer policies on credentialing, contracting, and billing for services of the specific QNHCP.
- *Before including QNHCPs within your group practice,* it is important to seek expert advice on related state regulations for scope of practice and supervision requirements, enrollment and payment policies of the group's most common payers, and best practices in employment and/or contractual agreements.
- The number of services that may be provided can be estimated based on current patient diagnoses or history of referral for services. Reports from electronic health records or billing software may be used in this estimation (eg, report of the number of unique patient accounts containing a diagnosis indicating mental or behavioral health conditions).

When physicians choose to arrange for services provided within their practice by QNHCPs who are not employed or contracted with their group practice, additional counsel should be obtained to avoid conflict with anti-kickback and/or self-referral regulations.

Chapter 13. Qualified Nonphysician Health Care Professional Services

Payment for QNHCP services begins with negotiating and contracting with payers for coverage and payment of services as described by *CPT* and/or Healthcare Common Procedure Coding System (HCPCS) codes. (A list of HCPCS codes that may be used to report nonphysician education services is included in the Healthcare Common Procedure Coding System Codes section later in this chapter.)

● Payers may pay separately for these services when your practice can demonstrate the overall cost savings (eg, decrease in physician or emergency department visits, decreased hospital care) that may be achieved through expanded care in the physician practice.

> **For more on quality and performance measurement, see Chapter 3.**

● If payers do not agree to directly compensate for individual services, consider opportunities for shared savings and other revenue that may be realized when QNHCP services support quality improvement initiatives (eg, per-member, per-month compensation for meeting certain quality measures) and redirection of physician and QHP time to services that are restricted to or best delivered within their scope of practice.

Physicians should be especially aware of each payer's policy addressing use of E/M codes for services provided by QNHCPs or clinical staff. Medicare and payers that adopt Medicare policy do not allow reporting of E/M services provided by QNHCPs or clinical staff other than **99211** (E/M visit not requiring physician face-to-face service) and other services that specifically indicate work of clinical staff under physician supervision (eg, transitional care management [TCM] or chronic care management [CCM]).

Example

➤ *CPT* **describes codes 99401–99404 as representing services provided face-to-face by a physician or other QHP for the purpose of promoting health and preventing illness or injury. However, some payers directly instruct that codes such as 99401 may be reported for specific services by specific clinical staff or by QNHCPs such as medical nutritionists or certified lactation consultants.** See the Breastfeeding Support/Lactation Services section later in this chapter for an example of payer policy that includes reporting of codes **99401–99404** for lactation counseling by an RN.

Always keep a printed or electronic copy of payer guidance that conflicts with *CPT* or standard billing practices.

> **For more information on chronic care management and transitional care management, see Chapter 12.**

Scope of Practice Laws

Scope of practice is a term used by state licensing boards for various professions to define the procedures, actions, and processes that are permitted for a licensed individual. Scope of practice may also address the delegation of health care activities to unlicensed individuals who the delegating physician or other QHP/QNHCP has ascertained has the education, training, and/or certification necessary to safely perform the activity. Additional limitations on scope of practice of QNHCPs and on delegation to clinical staff may come from Medicaid programs, health care systems, or health care professional membership organizations.

Physicians, RNs, clinical nurse practitioners, physician assistants, LPNs, physical therapists, and licensed nutritionists are among some of the professions for which scope of practice laws are defined. Some states limit the autonomous practice of advanced practice professionals and require these QHPs to have written collaboration agreements and require general or direct supervision by a physician. Prescribing authority may also be limited. Verify your state's requirements for all clinicians and appropriate inclusions in any collaboration/supervision agreements.

Every state has laws and regulations that describe the requirements of education and training for health care professionals. However, some states do not have different scope of practice laws for every level of professional (eg, LPN). Health systems, government payers, and health care professional membership organizations may also define or limit the scope of practice or delegation to QNHCPs and clinical staff.

Scope of practice should be taken into consideration when delegating directly or through standing orders (eg, physician writes order that recommended screening instruments will be completed for all patients presenting for well-baby/well-child [health supervision] examinations).

While scope of practice provides guidance on what services may be performed by QNHCPs and clinical staff, certain codes also limit who can report specific services. For instance, nurses are allowed to counsel for and administer immunizations, but administration codes **90460** and **90461** are only reported when a physician or QHP has provided immunization counseling. Likewise, E/M services are reported only by a physician or QHP, although QNHCPs and clinical staff may perform tasks included in the service (eg, activities of CCM).

National Provider Identifier

The NPI is a unique identification number for covered health care professionals. The NPI is required on administrative and financial transactions under the Health Insurance Portability and Accountability Act of 1996 (HIPAA) administrative simplification provisions.

- Anyone who directly provides health care services (eg, physical therapist, nutritionist, audiologist) can apply for and receive an NPI.
- Usually only those who will bill for services and/or order services or prescription drugs will need an NPI.
- The NPI is included on medical claims to indicate who ordered, provided, or supervised the provision of services.

Incident-to Requirements: Supervision of Nonphysician Health Care Professionals

When physicians or other QHPs bill under their NPI for services performed by clinical staff or QNHCPs, an incident-to policy may apply. For those payers that align with Medicare policy, see detailed requirements online at https://aap.org/cfp, access code AAPCFP26 ("Medicare Requirements for Incident-to Services by Nonphysician Professionals and Clinical Staff"). See also Chapter 12, section 30.6, of the *Medicare Claims Processing Manual* and Chapter 15, section 60, of the *Medicare Benefit Policy Manual* at http://cms.gov/manuals (select "Internet-Only Manuals (IOMs)"). Check with your payers and obtain a copy of their specific policies for reporting services provided by clinical staff and/or QNHCPs incident to a physician's service.

> **Incident-to provisions apply only in the office or other outpatient setting.**

- The Centers for Medicare & Medicaid Services defines *incident to* as "services incident to the service of a physician or other professional permitted by statute to bill for services incident to their services when those services meet all of the requirements applicable to the benefit."
  — Incident-to services are always provided as a continuation of a physician's services and do not address new problems (eg, a nursing visit performed at patient or caregiver request and not based on a physician's recommendation is not an incident-to service).
  — A supervising physician or QHP must be present *in the office suite* and available to assist, as needed, at the time of service.
  — A treatment plan or order must be documented by a physician or QHP prior to provision of services by a QNHCP or clinical staff provision of services billed incident to a physician or QHP.
  — The individual providing the incident-to service must be an employee (direct or leased) or working under contract with the physician practice (ie, paid as a practice expense).
- Although certain QHPs and QNHCPs otherwise may bill for their services under their own NPI when they provide medically necessary services (within their state's scope of practice), the incident-to provision allows for reporting under the name and NPI of a supervising physician when the requirements of incident-to billing are met.
  — Payment for QHPs and QNHCPs billing under the incident-to provision may be 100% of the physician payment versus 85% when reporting under the QHP's and QNHCP's individual NPI.

> **While Medicare and many other payers reduce payment to 85% of the Physician Fee Schedule amount when a qualified health care professional provides a service outside of the incident-to requirements (eg, new patient visit), this is not the case for all payers.**

  — Payers may not allow reporting of a certain service as incident to a physician's service (eg, psychotherapy) when the service is not included under the contract between the payer and physician.
- Nonphysician providers without their own NPIs must report services incident to a physician and must meet all incident-to requirements, including physician presence in the office suite and continuation of a physician's previously established plan of care.

- Medicare makes an exception by not requiring the physician's presence in the office suite for CCM, TCM, and behavioral health integration activities by clinical staff. Private payers may also allow inclusion of time spent by clinical staff without direct supervision when reporting these services.

Examples

➤ **A patient returns as directed by a pediatrician for a dressing change on a previously treated partial-thickness burn.** The physician is in the office suite at the time of service. An MA removes the dressing, washes the burn, and applies a new dressing. The MA instructs the patient to return to the practice for a scheduled follow-up visit in 2 days. Code **99211** (established patient E/M not requiring a physician's presence) is reported for this encounter.

➤ **An MA, as allowed under state scope of practice laws, administers an intranasal influenza vaccine that was ordered and directly supervised by the physician who documented counseling provided to the patient and/or caregivers.** Codes for the vaccine and administration (**90460**, **90672**) would be reported under the physician's NPI. If a pediatric nurse practitioner had ordered the treatment, the service would be reported under that practitioner's NPI.

Documentation Requirements and Tips When Reporting Incident-to Services

- Physicians and QHPs must document their order for a service or treatment (eg, injection) that will be performed as incident to or document their plan for a follow-up visit in the treatment plan (eg, follow-up visit in 1 week for weight check).
- To demonstrate compliant incident-to billing, QNHCPs and clinical staff providing services in continuation of a physician's plan of care *should, ideally, reference the date of the physician order for the service.* This may be documented in the chief complaint for the encounter (eg, "Patient is seen today per Dr Green's 1/2/2021 order for dressing change to left arm wound in 3 days").
- Documentation of incident-to services should fully describe the services provided, including date of service, assessment, concerns noted and addressed, details of care provided (eg, wound cleansed and new bandage applied), and education and/or instructions for home care and follow-up.
  - Inclusion of the supervising physician's name also supports that incident-to requirements were met.
  - Medical record documentation must reflect the identity, including credentials and legible signature of the person providing the service.

For Medicare purposes, the physician or QHP billing the service is not required to sign documentation prepared by the clinical staff. Other payer and state regulations may require physician authentication. Documentation might be as simple as "service performed/provided under the direct supervision of Dr X." When applicable, the supervising physician's signature must be legible.

Healthcare Common Procedure Coding System Codes

HCPCS Level II codes may be reported when the narrative differs from the *CPT* code for the service. What follows is a small sample of HCPCS codes and modifiers that may be used for services by QNHCPs. Payer guidance for reporting HCPCS or *CPT* codes may vary.

Note that HCPCS codes may include the term *nonphysician provider* (NPP) rather than QNHCP or QHP. These codes are only reported when services are provided by NPPs unless otherwise instructed by a payer. It is advisable to retain copies of a payer's written policies and guidance for reporting HCPCS codes.

G0108	Diabetes outpatient self-management training services, individual, per 30 minutes
G0109	Diabetes outpatient self-management training services, group session (2 or more), per 30 minutes
S0315	Disease management program; initial assessment and initiation of the program
S0316	Disease management program, follow-up/reassessment
S0317	Disease management program; per diem
S0320	Telephone calls by a registered nurse to a disease management program member for monitoring purposes; per month
S9441	Asthma education, NPP; per session
S9443	Lactation classes, NPP, per session
S9445	Patient education, not otherwise classified, NPP, individual, per session
S9446	group, per session

S9449	Weight management classes, NPP, per session
S9451	Exercise class, NPP, per session
S9452	Nutrition class, NPP, per session
S9454	Stress management class, NPP, per session
S9455	Diabetic management program, group session
S9460	nurse visit
S9465	dietitian visit
S9470	Nutritional counseling, dietitian visit

Payers may also instruct certain QNHCPs to report services by appending a HCPCS modifier to the *CPT* or HCPCS code for services provided.

AE	Registered dietitian
AH	Clinical psychologist
AJ	Clinical social worker
HA	Child/adolescent program
HN	Bachelor's degree level
HO	Master's degree level (eg, licensed master social worker)
HP	Doctoral level
HQ	Group setting
UN	Two patients served
UP	Three patients served
UQ	Four patients served
UR	Five patients served
US	Six or more patients served

Nonphysician Services

Nonphysician Evaluation and Management Services

Nursing Visit

| 99211 | Office or other outpatient visit for the evaluation and management of an established patient, that may not require the presence of a physician or other qualified health care professional. Usually, the presenting problem(s) are minimal. |

When clinical staff and/or QNHCPs who do not independently report E/M services provide an E/M service that is not described by another procedure code, code **99211** is reported.

Report **99211** when
- Services meet the incident-to requirements of the payer.
- Problems addressed have previously been addressed by ordering physician or QHP and services are a continuation of care.
- The service is provided based on physician orders and within scope of practice and license.
- The service is rendered face-to-face with the patient/caregiver.

Never report **99211** when
- Another procedure code describes the service provided (eg, **36415**, venipuncture).
- The physician performs a face-to-face E/M service on the same date.
- The patient is new or the problem has not been addressed by a physician.

Examples

➤ **A physician orders counseling about diet and exercise by a nurse in the practice for a 16-year-old patient who has obesity with borderline hypertension (follow-up visit not on same day as physician visit).** The follow-up visit is conducted by an RN who documents the patient's weight, body mass index (BMI), and blood pressure. The nurse spends 10 minutes face-to-face with the patient going over dietary guidelines, demonstrating proper portion sizes, and encouraging him to continue an exercise routine and healthier diet.

The RN is not a registered dietitian or licensed medical nutritionist who may report medical nutrition therapy. This service was provided in continuation of the physician's plan of care and under direct (in-office) physician supervision. Code **99211** is reported. Most payers will deny code **99211** when reported on the same date as a physician's E/M service (**99202–99205, 99212–99215**).

➤ **A physician orders education and training on proper use of a metered-dose inhaler (MDI) for a patient seen in the emergency department and treated for new-onset asthma.** A respiratory therapist who provides asthma education part time in the physician's office sees the patient. The patient presents with an MDI and spacer. The therapist demonstrates proper use and evaluates the patient's use of the MDI. The patient is instructed to keep a follow-up appointment with the ordering physician in 10 days.

    94664   Demonstration and/or evaluation of patient utilization of an aerosol generator, nebulizer, metered dose inhaler or IPPB device

This service is not reported with code **99211** because code **94664** describes the service performed.

➤ **Clinical staff assess the site of a previously administered tuberculosis skin test per a physician's instruction.** The negative result is documented by the clinician who authenticates the record.

If the clinician found a positive or questionable reaction requiring E/M by a supervising physician or other QHP, only the E/M service (eg, **99213**) would be reported.

Education and Training for Patient Self-management

98960   Education and training for patient self-management by a qualified, nonphysician health care professional using a standardized curriculum, face-to-face with the patient (could include caregiver/family) each 30 minutes; individual patient

98961   2–4 patients

98962   5–8 patients

Report codes **98960–98962** when

- The purpose of these services is to teach the patient and caregivers how to self-manage the illness or disease or delay disease comorbidities in conjunction with the patient's professional health care team.
- A physician prescribes the services and a standardized curriculum is used. A standardized curriculum is one that is consistent with guidelines or standards established or recognized by a physician or QNHCP society, association, or other appropriate source (eg, curriculum established or endorsed by the American Academy of Pediatrics).
- Qualifications of the QNHCPs and the content of the program are consistent with guidelines or standards established or recognized by a physician or QNHCP society, association, or other appropriate source.
  - These codes apply to diabetic and asthma self-management training—important categories of patient self-management education and training. Such training can be provided by nurse educators or other clinicians who have received special education and/or certification from accreditation societies or state licensing panels.
  - These services could be reported by the supervising physician when the services are rendered by the appropriately certified professional and acknowledged by the payer via the payer contract or published guidance.
- Education and training services are provided to patients with an established illness or disease.
- When a standardized curriculum is not used in the provision of health behavior assessment and intervention, see codes **96156, 96158, 96159**, and **96164–96171**.

> **Qualifications of the qualified nonphysician health care professionals (QNHCPs) and the content of patient self-management education (98960–98962) must be consistent with guidelines or standards established or recognized by a physician or QNHCP society, association, or other appropriate source.**

Code selection is based on the general *CPT* instruction for reporting services based on time. Time is met when the midpoint is passed (ie, report code **98960** for 16 or more minutes of face-to-face time and with units of service for each additional full 30 minutes and the last 16–30 minutes).

Example

➤ **A 14-year-old patient was recently diagnosed with type 1 diabetes and is referred to the diabetes educator for continued training under an approved curriculum.** The certified nurse educator assesses what the patient and caregivers have learned since diagnosis and uses a standardized curriculum to provide additional education. The total documented time of service is 30 minutes.

Code **98960** is reported for the 30 minutes of service. If the time of service extended 16 to 30 minutes beyond the first 30 minutes, an additional unit would be reported.

The content, type, duration, and patient response to the training must be documented in the medical record.

The payer contract will determine if services are reported under the name of the asthma educator, supervising physician, or QHP. If the payer credentials educators, report under the name and NPI of the educator. If the payer does not credential educators, follow payer guidance for reporting. HCPCS modifiers and/or codes may be required to indicate the service was provided by a QNHCP.

Genetic Counseling Services

96040   Medical genetics and genetic counseling services, each 30 minutes face-to-face with patient/family

- Trained genetic counselors provide services that may include obtaining a structured family genetic history, pedigree construction, analysis for genetic risk assessment, and counseling of the patient and family.
- Only face-to-face time with the patient or caregiver is used in determining the units of service reported. Do not report genetic counseling of 15 minutes or less. Report code **96040** with units of service for the first and each additional 30 minutes and the last 16 to 30 minutes.
- Services may be provided during one or more sessions and may include review of medical data and family information, face-to-face interviews, and counseling services.
- For genetic counseling and education on genetic risks by a QNHCP to a group, see codes **98961** and **98962**.
- Genetic counseling by physicians and other QHPs who may report E/M services are reported with the appropriate E/M service code.

Health Behavior Assessments/Interventions

Codes **96156**, **96158**, **96159**, and **96164–96171** describe services to identify and address psychological, behavioral, emotional, cognitive, and interpersonal factors important to the assessment, treatment, or management of physical health problems.

> **Health behavior assessment and intervention services are provided to patients whose primary diagnosis is physical in nature. The assessment and interventions focus on factors complicating medical conditions and treatments.**

Physicians and other QHPs who may report E/M services (eg, **99214**, **99401–99412**) may not report codes **96156**, **96158**, **96159**, and **96164–96171**.

- Health behavior assessment/reassessment and/or intervention may be reported by psychologists, clinical social workers, licensed therapists, and other QNHCPs within their scope of practice and training.
  - It is important to verify health plan credentialing policies for these individuals to determine if services should be reported by the individual provider or under the name of a supervising physician or other QHP.
  - A practice might also include a master's level social worker under direction of a physician and/or licensed clinical social worker (LCSW) if state regulations/scope of practice allow inclusion of these QNHCPs who may be gaining clinical experience necessary to become an LCSW.
- Check payer guidelines for any required referral or prior authorization for services.

Health Behavior Assessment/Reassessment

96156   Health behavior assessment, or re-assessment (ie, health-focused clinical interview, behavioral observations, clinical decision making)

Health behavior assessment includes face-to-face evaluation of the patient's responses to disease, illness or injury, outlook, coping strategies, motivation, and adherence to medical treatment. Assessment is conducted through health-focused clinical interviews, observation, and clinical decision-making.

Face-to-face health behavior assessment and reassessment services are reported with code **96156**.

- Do not report adaptive behavior assessment or intervention (**97151–97158, 0362T, 0373T**) or psychiatric services (**90785–90899**) in conjunction with **96156**. Report only the predominant service when these services are provided on the same date.

> **See Chapter 14 for information on reporting adaptive behavior and psychiatric services.**

- When an E/M service is provided on the same date as health behavior assessment or reassessment (**96156**), the services are separately reported only if provided by different individuals (ie, a physician who can report E/M services and an QNHCP who does not report E/M services).

Example

➤ **A 15-year-old girl is undergoing maintenance chemotherapy. The patient is referred to an LCSW for health behavior assessment due to clinical indications that the patient is not adhering to her therapy regimen.** The social worker reviews the patient's medical records and the patient is assessed using a standardized questionnaire. The patient's parents are also interviewed.

Documentation includes the results of the assessment, recommended services to be provided, and coordination of feedback to interdisciplinary team members and family. The social worker facilitates treatment planning and follow-up care with the team members and family.

Code **96156** would be reported with the *International Classification of Diseases, 10th Revision, Clinical Modification* (*ICD-10-CM*) code appropriate to the reason for chemotherapy and, when applicable, underdosing of medication (codes in categories **T36–T50** with final character **6**) and a code for patient's noncompliance with medical treatment and regimen (**Z91.1-**).

Health Behavior Intervention

Health behavior interventions are used to report services that include promotion of functional improvement, minimizing psychological and/or psychosocial barriers to recovery, and management of and improved coping with medical conditions. Patient/family engagement and involvement are promoted.

Interventions may be provided to individual patients, a group of 2 or more patients, and/or a family with or without the patient present. Codes for each are shown in **Table 13-1**.

Table 13-1. Health Behavior Intervention Code Assignment	
Service Provided to	**Codes**
1 patient	**96158** Health behavior intervention, individual, face-to-face; initial 30 minutes **+96159** each additional 15 minutes (List separately in addition to code **96158**)
≥2 patients	**#96164** Health behavior intervention, group (2 or more patients), face-to-face; initial 30 minutes **#+96165** each additional 15 minutes (List separately in addition to code **96164**)
Family with patient present	**#96167** Health behavior intervention, family (with the patient present), face-to-face; initial 30 minutes **+96168** each additional 15 minutes (List separately in addition to code **96167**)
Family without patient present	**#96170** Health behavior intervention, family (without the patient present), face-to-face; initial 30 minutes **#+96171** each additional 15 minutes (List separately in addition to code **96170**)

Apply the following instruction for codes **96158, 96159,** and **96164–96171**:
- A standardized curriculum is not required.
- Codes **96158, 96164, 96167,** and **96170** are not reported for less than 16 minutes of service.
- The total time must be documented in the medical record.
  - Time is met when the midpoint is passed unless payer policy directs otherwise.
  - Codes for initial 30 minutes are reported only for 16 or more minutes.
  - Codes for each additional 15 minutes are reported only for 8 or more minutes beyond the last unit of service.
- Physicians and other QHPs who may report E/M services are instructed to report E/M (eg, **99214**) or preventive service E/M codes (eg, **99401–99404**) in lieu of health behavior intervention.

- The first-listed diagnosis should be the medical condition for which the patient may benefit from assessment and intervention focused on helping the patient better manage his or her health condition.
- Payers may deny claims if the first or only diagnosis is a psychiatric condition.

  Codes **96158**, **96159**, and **96164–96171** *are not* reported

- With psychiatric codes (**90785–90899**) when provided on the same day. Only the primary service is reported (ie, either **96158**, **96159**, and **96164–96171**, or **90785–90899**).
- With an E/M code (eg, **99202–99215**, **99401–99412**) on the same day when both services are provided by the same individual.
  — Verify health plan policy to determine if both services will be paid when reported by the same or different individuals on the same date.
  — Where health behavior intervention is reported under the name of a supervising physician, modifiers may be required to designate provision of services by a QHP (eg, **AJ**, clinical social worker).
  — Modifier **25** (significant and separately identifiable E/M service) may be appended to the E/M code when reported on the same date as a health behavior assessment or intervention.
- In conjunction with adaptive behavior assessment or treatment (**97151–97158**; **0362T**, **0373T**). Report only the predominant service.

Examples

➤ **A 15-year-old girl is undergoing maintenance chemotherapy and has undergone health and behavior assessment due to noncompliance with her chemotherapy regimen.** Based on the assessment conducted at a previous encounter, a QHP (eg, psychologist) works with the girl and her parents to facilitate family communication and provide education about the importance of compliance and family support of the maintenance chemotherapy. Documentation includes describing the patient's status, family involvement, and progress toward and/or modification of treatment goals based on patient progress or other confounding factors. Sixty minutes of face-to-face time with the patient and family is also documented. Feedback is provided to the pediatrician and other health care professionals. Follow-up care is coordinated.

Code **96167** is reported with 1 unit of service for the first 30 minutes of service. Code **96168** is reported with 2 units of service for the last 30 minutes of service.

➤ **A 15-year-old girl is undergoing maintenance chemotherapy and has undergone health and behavior assessment due to noncompliance with her chemotherapy regimen.** Based on the assessment conducted at a previous encounter, a psychologist works with the girl's parents (the patient is not present) to facilitate family communication and provide education about the patient's resistance to chemotherapy, engage and mobilize family support and problem-solving for treatment adherence, and clarify family roles and caregiver responsibilities. Documentation includes describing the patient's status, family involvement, and progress toward and/or modification of treatment goals based on patient progress or other confounding factors. Feedback is provided to the patient's pediatrician and other health care professionals. Follow-up care is coordinated. A total of 55 minutes spent face-to-face with the parents is also documented.

Code **96170** is reported with 1 unit of service for the first 30 minutes of service, and code **96171** is reported with 2 units of service for the last 25 minutes of service (1 unit for the full 15-minute period and 1 unit for the final 10 minutes [because the midpoint of 8 minutes beyond the last full period was passed]).

Breastfeeding Support/Lactation Services

Under the Patient Protection and Affordable Care Act (PPACA), most health insurance plans must provide coverage of breastfeeding support, counseling, and equipment to mothers for the duration of breastfeeding. These services are not subject to a deductible, co-pay, or coinsurance. However, many plans lack straightforward advice to patients or health care professionals on coverage and reporting requirements, and some plans provide no opportunity for lactation consultants to become in-network providers.

> Pediatricians may report preventive medicine counseling (eg, 99401) for lactation counseling in the absence of problems (typically billed to mother's health plan). When providing services related to feeding problems or maternal issues, report evaluation and management codes by site of service for these services (eg, office visit).

Lactation consultation services do not have a specific *CPT* code, and billing is a source of confusion for many providers. Less-specific codes are often used to report these services. Options for reporting services by QNHCPs may include

| S9443 | Lactation classes, nonphysician provider, per session |

Code **S9443** is the code most specific to lactation services. This code is included in some health plan policies for preventive medicine services. However, it is not paid under many health plan contracts.

S9445	Patient education, not otherwise classified, nonphysician provider, individual, per session
S9446	Patient education, not otherwise classified, nonphysician provider, group, per session
98960	Education and training for patient self-management by a qualified, nonphysician health care professional using a standardized curriculum, face-to-face with the patient (could include caregiver/family), each 30 minutes; individual patient
99401	Preventive medicine counseling and/or risk-factor reduction intervention(s) provided to an individual (separate procedure); approximately 15 minutes

Key considerations for reporting lactation services include

- Unless the newborn or infant has been diagnosed with a feeding problem, the mother is typically the patient and claims are filed to her health benefit plan.
- Practices must verify coverage and reporting instructions for each payer prior to service. Examples of coding instructions for lactation counseling from payers include
  - No cost share for supervision of lactation for women when billed to the mother's health plan by a physician with the appropriate E/M code and **Z39.1** (encounter for care and examination of lactating mother) billed in the principal diagnosis position.
  - Education and assistance with lactation, breast and nipple care, and breastfeeding are included in postpartum care and may not be separately billed per the policy of 1 Medicaid plan.
  - Lactation counseling is covered with no cost sharing when provided by lactation consultants or nursing staff employed by a credentialed physician or by a physician assistant or certified RN practitioner when under the supervision of a credentialed physician. (Lactation consultants are not credentialed and cannot receive direct payment for their services.) Bill the mother's plan using the appropriate procedure codes (**99401**, **99402**, and **99403**) and the appropriate diagnosis code (**Z39.1**). Counseling by the physician is integral to the examination of the newborn.
- Although included as a covered preventive service under the PPACA, breastfeeding services are often considered by payers to be included in E/M services provided to the mother by a physician or other QHP.
- Payer policies may not allow separate payment for lactation counseling on the same date as an E/M service.
- Challenges might be encountered in states where licensure is not yet enacted for lactation support professionals. Hurdles include credentialing and coverage by payers who cover only services provided by licensed health care professionals, although services provided incident to a physician or QHP may be allowed.
- When a medical condition (eg, feeding problem) was previously diagnosed by the physician on an earlier date, a QNHCP may see the mother and patient to identify the psychological, behavioral, emotional, cognitive, and social factors important to the prevention, treatment, or management of physical health problems. Behavioral health assessment and intervention codes **96156**; **96158** and **96159**; and **96164–96171** may be reportable for these services. Again, payer policy drives the provision (who may provide) of and payment for these services.
- *CPT* describes codes **99401–99404** as services provided face-to-face by a physician or other QHP for the purpose of promoting health and preventing illness or injury. When payer policy instructs to report these codes for services by a QNHCP (eg, lactation consultant), a written copy of the payer policy should be kept on file.
- Lactation counseling provided by a QNHCP in conjunction with a physician's or QHP's E/M service, although not always separately reported, may reduce the physician's time spent on history taking, counseling, and education. This may also support quality initiatives.

ICD-10-CM code **Z39.1** is reported for an encounter for care and examination of a lactating mother.

Medical Nutrition Assessments

| 97802 | Medical nutrition therapy; initial assessment and intervention, individual, face-to-face with the patient, each 15 minutes |

97803	Reassessment and intervention, individual, face-to-face with the patient, each 15 minutes
97804	group (2 or more individuals), each 30 minutes

Medical nutrition therapy is one of the services for which *CPT* instruction excludes reporting by a physician or QHP who may report E/M services.

- Many states restrict the provision of medical nutrition therapy to certain QNHCPs (eg, registered dietitian, licensed medical nutritionist). Practices providing medical nutrition therapy services should be aware of state licensing and scope of practice regulations as well as health plan credentialing policies.
- Coverage may also be limited to patients with certain conditions (eg, diabetes, kidney disease) and a limited number of units of service or visits per year.
- Payers that follow Medicare policy on reporting of E/M services will not accept codes **99202–99205**, **99212–99215**, or **99217–99499** performed by QNHCPs. (*Note:* **99211** is reportable by QNHCPs and clinical staff. Payers may adopt Medicare incident-to policy requirements.)
- Codes are reported when provided by a QNHCP who may report medical nutrition therapy services under his or her individual state's scope of practice.
- When medical nutrition therapy is provided as a preventive service, modifier **33** may be appended to codes **97802–97804**.

> **For more on modifier 33, see chapters 2 and 9.**

- Services are reported based on time. Per *CPT* instruction, a unit of time is met when the midpoint is passed.
  - Report code **97802** or **97803** with 1 unit for 8 to 22 minutes of service. An additional unit may be reported for each subsequent 15 minutes and the last 8 to 22 minutes of service.
  - Certain payers may require that the time in the code descriptor (eg, 15 minutes) be met or exceeded for each unit of service reported.
- Time must be documented.
- HCPCS codes may be required by certain payers when providing reassessment and subsequent intervention due to a change in diagnosis, medical condition, or treatment.

G0270	Medical nutrition therapy; reassessment and subsequent intervention(s) following second referral in same year for change in diagnosis, medical condition, or treatment regimen (including additional hours needed for renal disease); individual, face-to-face with the patient, each 15 minutes
G0271	group (2 or more individuals), each 30 minutes

Documentation of services should include the physician or QHP order for services, information on the medical need for services, medical nutrition therapy evaluation and plan for intervention, time, correspondence with the referring provider, date of service, and name, credentials, and signature of the provider of the medical nutrition therapy.

Examples

➤ **A 14-year-old girl was seen by her physician for a health supervision visit 1 week ago.** Her BMI was at the 90th percentile, her blood pressure was at upper limit of normal, and results of cholesterol screening indicated hypercholesterolemia. The patient was referred to the practice's registered dietitian for assessment and counseling on a diet to reduce the risk of cardiovascular and endocrine disorders. The dietitian meets with the child and her parents and spends 30 minutes discussing risk factors and developing a plan with goals to decrease weight, cholesterol, and blood pressure.

ICD-10-CM	CPT
Z71.3 (dietary counseling and surveillance) **E78.00** (pure hypercholesterolemia) **Z68.53** (BMI pediatric, 85th percentile to less than 95th percentile for age)	If payer allows billing under registered dietitian's NPI **97802** × 2 (medical nutrition therapy, initial assessment and intervention, individual, face-to-face with the patient, each 15 minutes) If payer requires billing under the NPI of the supervising physician **97802 AE** × 2 (medical nutrition therapy as above by a registered dietitian)

   ●=New code   ▲=Revised code   #=Re-sequenced code   +=Add-on code

Chapter 13. Qualified Nonphysician Health Care Professional Services

Teaching Point: Some Medicaid plans and/or private payers may require that medical nutrition therapy in the physician practice be provided under a physician's order and general supervision. Services are reported as if provided by the physician, but modifier **AE** indicates the service was provided by a registered dietitian.

➤ **A 12-year-old girl has become a vegetarian.** The patient's laboratory test results have shown iron deficiency, and she is referred by her pediatrician to a nurse practitioner in the same practice for consultation on a vegetarian diet that meets the patient's nutritional requirements. The nurse practitioner spends 15 minutes prior to the visit reviewing the patient's history and collecting resources for dietary education and planning. At the visit, the nurse practitioner spends 30 minutes with the patient and her parents learning the patient's reasons for choosing a vegetarian diet, assessing the patient's current diet, and counseling on the importance of a plant-based diet that is balanced to provide adequate nutrition. A plan is developed to encourage food choices that support adequate nutrition, and a follow-up visit is scheduled in 2 weeks. The nurse practitioner spends another 5 minutes documenting the encounter.

ICD-10-CM	CPT
Z71.3 (dietary counseling and surveillance) **E61.1** (iron deficiency)	**99215** (40–54 minutes total time)

Teaching Point: The nurse practitioner is qualified to provide an E/M service to manage the patient's iron deficiency. The office E/M service code is selected based on either medical decision-making or total physician time on the date of the encounter. The nurse practitioner's total time was 50 minutes, supporting **99215**. If the nurse practitioner is working under the physician's supervision in the office suite, the service may be reported by the physician and potentially paid at a higher Physician Fee Schedule rate.

Medical Team Conferences

99366   Medical team conference with interdisciplinary team of health care professionals, face-to-face with patient and/or family, 30 minutes or more; participation by nonphysician qualified health care professional

99368   Medical team conference with interdisciplinary team of health care professionals, patient and/or family not present, 30 minutes or more; participation by nonphysician qualified health care professional

Medical team conference codes are used to report participation by a minimum of 3 health care professionals (including physicians, QHPs, and QNHCPs) of different specialties in conferences to coordinate or manage care and services for established patients with chronic or multiple health conditions (eg, a child who is ventilator dependent with developmental delays, seizures, and a gastrostomy tube for nutrition).

- Codes differentiate provider (physician or QHP vs QNHCP) and between face-to-face and non–face-to-face (patient and/or family is not present) team conference services.
- If QHPs (including clinical nurse specialists and clinical nurse practitioners) participated in the conference without direct physician supervision, they may report team conference participation *without the patient or caregiver present* as if provided by a physician (**99367**) if it is within the state's scope of practice and they use their own NPI.
- State Medicaid and commercial payers may follow these Medicare requirements or have their own specific rules.
- Medical team conferences may not be reported when
  - The facility or organization is contractually obligated to provide the service or if they are informal meetings or simple conversations between physicians and QNHCPs (eg, therapists).
  - Less than 30 minutes of conference time is spent in a team conference.
- One unit of service is reported for each conference of 30 minutes or more.
- Medicare assigns a bundled (B) status to team conference services in the Medicare Physician Fee Schedule and does not allow separate payment for participation in medical team conferences. Payment policies may vary among Medicaid and private health plans.

  Medical team conferences require
- Face-to-face participation by a minimum of 3 health care professionals (any combination of QNHCPs, physicians, and/ or QHPs) from different subspecialties or disciplines (eg, speech-language pathologists, dietitians, social workers), with or without the presence of the patient, family member(s), community agencies, surrogate decision-maker(s) (eg, legal guardian), and/or caregiver(s).
- Active involvement in the development, revision, coordination, and implementation of health care services needed by the patient by each participant.

- That the participant has provided a face-to-face evaluations and/or treatment to the patient, separate from any team conference, within the previous 60 days.
- Only one individual from the same specialty may report codes **99366–99368** for the same encounter.
- Medical record documentation must support the reporting individual's participation, the time spent from the beginning of the review of an individual patient until the conclusion of the review, and the contributed information and subsequent treatment recommendations.

Examples

➤ **A care team meets to discuss the care plans for a 4-year-old girl with history of congenital heart disease, cerebrovascular accident with residual paraplegia, and developmental delays.** As the child nears entry to kindergarten, the pediatrician has requested input to the child's Individualized Education Plan and ongoing health care plan from all health care professionals. The pediatrician, cardiologist, physiatrist, occupational and physical therapists, speech-language pathologist, home care coordinator, and social worker attend the conference to discuss the child's current medical status, prognosis for the short and long term, and necessary accommodations for her education. The conference lasts 60 minutes. The patient and family are not present for the conference.

Qualified nonphysician health care professionals report participation using code **99368** when the patient/caregivers are not present. Assign appropriate *ICD-10-CM* codes for the specified developmental delays (codes in categories **F80–F88**) and other health concerns addressed.

> Physicians may report code 99367 when participating in a conference without the patient/parents present. *Current Procedural Terminology* allows reporting of code 99368 by nonphysician qualified health care professionals. However, reporting an evaluation and management code for participation when the patient or caregivers are present may be beneficial when allowed or required by individual payer policy. See Chapter 12 for information on physician participation in team conferences.

➤ **A patient with cerebral palsy requires coordination with multiple health care professionals (eg, physical and occupational therapists, neurologist, pediatrician).** Each participant in the conference has completed his or her evaluation of the patient within 60 days prior to the conference, and a team conference of 40 minutes is held to assess the current plan of care and therapy. The patient's family is present at this conference.

Code **99366** would be reported by the physical and occupational therapists. Physicians present at the conference would report an E/M code that best describes their services on this date (eg, office or other outpatient E/M service based on face-to-face time with the family spent in counseling and/or coordination of care).

Medication Therapy Management Services

99605	Medication therapy management service(s) provided by a pharmacist, individual, face-to-face with patient, with assessment and intervention if provided; initial 15 minutes, new patient
99606	initial 15 minutes, established patient
+99607	each additional 15 minutes (List separately in addition to **99605** or **99606**)

Medication therapy management services

- Are provided only by a pharmacist face-to-face with the patient or caregiver and usually in relation to complex medication regimens or medication adherence in conditions such as asthma and diabetes.
- Are provided on request of the patient or caregiver, prescribing physician, other QHPs, or prescription drug benefit plan (not reported for routine dispensing-related activities).
- Are reported with codes selected based on whether the patient is new or established and the pharmacist's face-to-face time with the patient.
- Include review of pertinent patient history (not limited to drug history).
- Include documentation of review of the pertinent patient history, medication profile (prescription and nonprescription), and recommendations for improving health outcomes and treatment compliance.
- *New patients* are those who have received no face-to-face service from the pharmacist or another pharmacist of the same clinic or pharmacy within 3 years prior to the current date of service.

- Unless otherwise specified by the payer policy, time is met when the midpoint is passed.
  — Report codes **99605** and **99606** for the first 8 to 22 minutes of face-to-face time with the patient.
  — When time exceeds 22 minutes, code **99607** may be reported for subsequent 15-minute periods and the last 8 to 22 minutes.
- Under the Medicare program, pharmacists may also provide services incident to a physician or QHP and report E/M services with code **99211** when allowed under the scope of practice as defined by state licensure.

Online Medical Assessment

98970 Qualified nonphysician health care professional online digital assessment and management service, for an established patient, for up to seven days, cumulative time during the 7 days; 5-10 minutes

98971 11-20 minutes

98972 21 or more minutes

   An online electronic medical assessment (**98970–98972**) is a non–face-to-face assessment and management service by an QNHCP to an established patient using internet resources in response to a patient's online inquiry.

> Online digital evaluation and management (E/M) services by a physician or other qualified health care professional (who may report E/M services) is reported with codes 99421–99423. See Chapter 20 for more information on online digital health care services.

- *Online assessment and management* refers to use of technology such as secure email and other asynchronous digital communication.

   This contrasts with *telemedicine services,* which represent interactive audio and video telecommunications systems that permit real-time communication between the QNHCP at the distant site and the patient at the originating site.
- Before providing online medical services, understand local and state laws, ensure that communications will be HIPAA compliant (eg, conducted through secure patient portal), establish written guidelines and procedures, educate payers and negotiate for payment, and educate patients.
- Codes **98970–98972** are time-based codes used by a QNHCP to report an online assessment and management service.
- One code and 1 unit of service are reported for the sum of communications pertaining to the online encounter during a 7-day period.
- The 7-day service period begins with the initial, personal QNHCP review of the patient-generated inquiry.
- All time spent addressing the presenting problem and any additional problems (including new unrelated problems addressed by online electronic communications) during the service period is cumulative and reported as one service.
- Online assessment and management includes
  — Review of the initial inquiry
  — Review of patient records or data pertinent to assessment of the patient's problem
  — Personal QNHCP interaction with clinical staff focused on the patient's problem
  — Development of management plans
  — Timely reply to the patient/caregiver's request for online service
  — Permanent record of the service (hard copy or electronic)
  — All related communications during a 7-day episode of care (eg, ordering laboratory or other testing, prescriptions, related phone calls)
  — Cumulative time of QNHCPs in the same group that are involved in the online digital E/M service
- Online digital assessment services (**98970–98972**) are *not* reported
  — For services of less than 5 minutes' cumulative time.
  — For new patient inquiries (although new problems may be addressed for established patients).
  — For electronic communication of test results, scheduling of appointments, or other communication that does not include assessment and management.
  — If the online digital inquiry occurs within the postoperative period of a previously completed procedure.
  — If the patient generates an online digital inquiry within 7 days of a previous treatment or E/M service and both services relate to the same problem.
  — If a separately reported assessment service occurs within 7 days of the initial online digital inquiry.
  — When care plan oversight (**99339–99340; 99374, 99375; 99377–99380**), CCM (**99487, 99489–99491**), TCM (**99495, 99496**), or collection of physiologic data (**99091**) are provided in the same period, do not count the time of communications related to these services toward the time of online digital medical services.

Example

➤ **The parents of a 17-year-old boy who is restricted from driving due to seizures contact the child's social worker due to increased behavioral issues since his younger brother started driving 2 weeks ago.** The social worker responds to the request and emails are exchanged to further clarify the nature of the problem and provide management options. The boy will be reevaluated at a regularly scheduled face-to-face appointment in 2 weeks. The cumulative time of the communications is 15 minutes.

The social worker reports code **98971**. If the patient had been seen within the past 7 days or scheduled for an appointment within the 7-day period, this service would not be separately reported.

Telephone Calls

98966   Telephone assessment and management services provided by a qualified nonphysician health care professional to an established patient, parent, or guardian not originating from related assessment and management service provided within the previous 7 days nor leading to an assessment and management service or procedure within the next 24 hours or soonest available appointment; 5–10 minutes of medical discussion

98967   11–20 minutes of medical discussion

98968   21–30 minutes of medical discussion

Codes **98966–98968** are used to report telephone assessment and management services by QNHCPs. Those QHPs who may independently provide and report E/M services report codes **99441–99443**.

Report codes **98966–98968** when

- The patient or caregiver initiates a call that is not in follow up to a service by the same QNHCP within the past 7 days.
- Five minutes or more is spent in assessment and management services (*time must be documented*).
- No decision to see the patient within 24 hours or at the next available appointment is made during the telephone service.

Services Not Reported as Telephone Assessment and Management

Most telephone services provided by clinical staff (eg, MA relaying physician instructions) are included in the practice expense value assigned to physician services and not separately reported.

Do not report telephone assessment and management services that

- Are related to a service provided by the QNHCP within the past 7 days, regardless of whether the service was planned or prompted by patient or caregiver concern.
- Result in an appointment within the next 24 hours or next available appointment. When telephone assessment and management results in scheduling the patient for an appointment within 24 hours or at the next available appointment, the service is considered preservice work to the face-to-face encounter.
- Are within a global period of another service.

> Telephone services by clinical staff may contribute to time of chronic care management (CCM) or transitional care management (TCM) when the services meet the description of the clinical staff activities included in CCM or TCM.

Example

➤ **The parents of a patient with autism spectrum disorder and failure to thrive contact their child's registered dietitian for advice because the patient refuses to eat more than a few bites at mealtime.** It has been 3 weeks since the dietitian provided education on meeting the child's nutritional needs and introducing new foods due to the child's refusal of many textures. The dietitian spends 18 minutes on the phone with the parents discussing concerns and techniques for encouraging the child to eat more at mealtime.

The dietitian reports code **98967** based on the time spent addressing the parents' concerns. This service would not be reported if the call were provided within 7 days of a previous service by the same provider or if the call resulted in an appointment within 24 hours or at the next available face-to-face appointment.

Chapter 13. Qualified Nonphysician Health Care Professional Services

Psychiatric Evaluation and Psychotherapy Without Evaluation and Management

+**90785**	Interactive complexity (List separately in addition to the code for primary procedure)
90791	Psychiatric diagnostic evaluation
90832	Psychotherapy, 30 minutes with patient and/or family member
90834	45 minutes with patient and/or family member
90837	60 minutes with patient and/or family member
90839	Psychotherapy for crisis; first 60 minutes
+**90840**	each additional 30 minutes (List separately in addition to code **90839**)
90846	Family psychotherapy (without the patient present), 50 minutes
90847	Family psychotherapy (conjoint psychotherapy) (with patient present), 50 minutes
90849	Multiple-family group psychotherapy
90853	Group psychotherapy (other than of a multiple-family group)
+**90863**	Pharmacologic management, including prescription and review of medication, when performed with psychotherapy services (List separately in addition to **90832**, **90834**, **90837**.)

> See Chapter 14 for information on codes for psychological and neuropsychological testing.

Mental and behavioral health services may be covered through a plan and provider network separate from other health care services. Qualified nonphysician health care professionals may be required to apply for network participation and sign contracts separate from those held by the practices with health benefit plans.

- The scope of services may also be limited by payer policies allowing specific licensed providers, such as licensed clinical psychologists, to report certain services, while other QNHCPs (eg, LCSWs) may report a smaller scope of services.
- Verify coverage and billing options prior to provision of services.

A payer may apply bundling edits that do not allow separate payment for mental and behavioral health services and E/M services provided in the same practice on the same date.

- Follow payer instructions for reporting services such as psychotherapy by a QNHCP under the name and NPI of a supervising physician and E/M services by the physician on the same date (typically applies only when both services are reported under a health benefit plan).

> Healthcare Common Procedure Coding System modifiers identifying the type of provider (eg, **AJ**, clinical social worker) may be necessary to override edits that bundle evaluation and management and mental or behavioral health services on the same date.

See the Healthcare Common Procedure Coding System Codes section earlier in this chapter for HCPCS modifiers or your current HCPCS coding reference for additional modifiers.
- Psychiatric diagnostic evaluation or reevaluation (**90791**) is reported once per day.
  Do not report psychotherapy codes (**90832–90840**) on the same date of service as **90791**.
- Psychotherapy times are for face-to-face services with a patient and/or family member.
  The patient must be present for all or some of the service except when reporting family psychotherapy without the patient present (**90846**). This allows for the participation of others in the psychotherapy session for the patient as long as the patient remains the focus of the intervention. The patient must be present for a significant portion of the session.
- Psychiatric services may be reported "with interactive complexity" (**90785**) when at least 1 of the following conditions is present:
  — The need to manage maladaptive communication (related to, eg, high anxiety, high reactivity, repeated questions, disagreement) among participants that complicates delivery of care
  — Caregiver emotions or behavior that interferes with the caregiver's understanding and ability to assist in the implementation of the treatment plan
  — Evidence or disclosure of a sentinel event and mandated report to a third party (eg, abuse or neglect with report to state agency) with initiation of discussion of the sentinel event and/or report with patient and other visit participants
  — Use of play equipment, other physical devices, interpreter, or translator to communicate with the patient to overcome barriers to therapeutic or diagnostic interaction between the physician or other QHP and a patient who
    - Is not fluent in the same language as the physician or other QHP

- Has not developed, or has lost, the expressive language communication skills to explain his or her symptoms and response to treatment or the receptive communication skills to understand the physician or other QHP if he or she were to use typical language for communication
- Family psychotherapy (**90846**, **90847**), which uses family psychotherapy techniques to benefit the patient (eg, attempting to improve family communication or alter family interactions that negatively affect the patient; encouraging interactions to improve family functioning) is different from psychotherapy (**90832–90840**).
  - Family psychotherapy includes sessions with the entire family as well as sessions that may not include the patient.
  - Do not report family psychotherapy of 25 minutes or less.
- In reporting, choose the code closest to the actual time (**Table 13-2**). Do not report psychotherapy of less than 16 minutes' duration.
- Do not report psychotherapy for crisis (**90839**, **90840**) for service of less than 30 minutes or on the same date as other psychiatry services (**90785–90899**).
- Code **90863** was created for medication management when provided on the same day as psychotherapy by QHPs who may not report E/M codes (ie, psychologists licensed to prescribe).
  - **90863** is an add-on code and may only be reported in addition to one of the stand-alone psychotherapy codes (ie, **90832**, **90834**, **90837**).
  - Time spent providing medication management is not included in the time spent in psychotherapy.
- Prolonged services in the outpatient setting (**99354**, **99355**) or inpatient or observation setting (**99356**, **99357**) may be reported in addition to the psychotherapy service code **90837** when 90 minutes or longer of face-to-face time with the patient and/or family member is spent performing psychotherapy services that are not performed with an E/M service. Prolonged service may also be reported for 80 or more minutes of family psychotherapy.
- Do not report psychotherapy codes in conjunction with codes for adaptive behavior assessment or treatment services (**97151–97158, 0362T, 0373T**).

Table 13-2. Reporting Psychotherapy Services

Duration of Psychotherapy	CPT Codes
<16 min	Do not report.
16–37 min	**90832**
38–52 min	**90834**
53–89 min	**90837**

Abbreviation: *CPT, Current Procedural Terminology.*

Example

➤ **A clinical psychologist provides psychotherapy to a 16-year-old with a diagnosis of acute post-traumatic stress disorder.** An interval history and objective information are obtained. The patient's mental status is reexamined, and trauma-focused cognitive-behavioral therapy is continued from a previous session. The face-to-face time of the encounter is 40 minutes.

ICD-10-CM	CPT
F43.11 (acute posttraumatic stress disorder)	**90834** (psychotherapy, 45 minutes with patient and/or family member)

Code **90834** is reported based on *CPT* instruction to choose the code closest to the actual time.

See Chapter 14 for information on behavioral/mental health care services provided by qualified nonphysician health care professionals and/or clinical staff under supervision of a reporting physician.

Home Health Procedures/Services

99501	Home visit for postnatal assessment and follow-up care
99502	Home visit for newborn care and assessment
99503	Home visit for respiratory therapy care (eg, bronchodilator, oxygen therapy, respiratory assessment, apnea evaluation)
99504	Home visit for mechanical ventilation care
99505	Home visit for stoma care and maintenance including colostomy and cystostomy
99506	Home visit for intramuscular injections
99507	Home visit for care and maintenance of catheter(s) (eg, urinary, drainage, and enteral)
99509	Home visit for assistance with activities of daily living and personal care
99510	Home visit for individual, family, or marriage counseling
99511	Home visit for fecal impaction management and enema administration
99512	Home visit for hemodialysis
99600	Unlisted home visit service or procedure

Codes **99500–99600** are

- Typically reported for skilled nursing services ordered by a physician or QHP and are medically necessary services provided to a housebound patient. *Exception:* A nursing visit to a mother and newborn may be covered when provided within a specified period following hospital discharge (verify payer policy for coverage).
- Used to report services provided in a patient's residence (including assisted living apartments, group homes, nontraditional private homes, custodial care facilities, or schools).

> **Physicians and other qualified health care professionals providing evaluation and management services in a patient's home report code 99341–99350.**

- Not reported if another code more accurately describes the service provided (eg, report home medical nutrition therapy with **97802–97804** rather than **99509**).

Coverage of home health procedures or services by QHPs who are authorized to use E/M home visit codes (**99341–99350**) may also be reported with codes **99500–99600** if both services are performed and the patient's condition requires a significant, separately identifiable service. Modifier **25** would be appended to codes **99341–99350**.

Resource

Incident-to Billing

Medicare Claims Processing Manual Chapter 12, section 30.6, and *Medicare Benefit Policy Manual* Chapter 15, section 60 (http://cms.gov/manuals; select "Internet-Only Manuals (IOMs)")

Chapter 13. Qualified Nonphysician Health Care Professional Services

Test Your Knowledge!

1. **Which of the following terms describes the procedures, actions, and processes that are permitted for a licensed individual?**
   a. Incident to
   b. Qualified nonphysician health care professional
   c. Clinical staff
   d. Scope of practice

2. **Which of the following meets Medicare incident-to billing requirements?**
   a. A physician is available by phone when clinical staff provide a service.
   b. A nurse practitioner provides an evaluation and management (E/M) service to a new patient.
   c. Clinical staff administer an injection under direct supervision of the ordering physician.
   d. A nurse practitioner provides an E/M service to address a new problem.

3. **Which of the following is appropriately reported with code 99211?**
   a. A medical assistant phones a parent to advise of a normal test result.
   b. A nurse administers an injection of medication as ordered by a physician.
   c. A medical assistant performs a weight check on a child as ordered by the child's physician.
   d. All of the above

4. **When is a service addressing breastfeeding billable to the newborn's or infant's health plan?**
   a. When the mother has no health insurance
   b. Never
   c. Always
   d. When a newborn's or infant's feeding problem is evaluated

5. **Which Healthcare Common Procedure Coding System modifier indicates a service was provided by a registered dietitian?**
   a. **RD**
   b. **MN**
   c. **AE**
   d. **AJ**

●=New code ▲=Revised code #=Re-sequenced code +=Add-on code

Mental and Behavioral Health Services

Contents

Chapter 14. Mental and Behavioral Health Services

Physicians and Other Mental/Behavioral Health Providers

This chapter focuses on services that are provided to diagnose, manage, or treat mental and behavioral health conditions. Mental and behavioral health services may be covered through a provider network separate from other health care services. Physicians providing these services personally and/or through nonphysician staff within their practice must be aware of the coverage and payment policies of local and regional health plans and determine how these policies affect delivery and payment of services.

Services included in this chapter may be provided by

- Physicians and other qualified health care professionals (QHPs) and qualified nonphysician health care professionals (QNHCPs), including licensed clinical psychologists and licensed clinical social workers
- Allied health care professionals (AHPs), such as technicians and developmental specialists, who provide services ordered by and under the general supervision of physicians and QHPs
- Clinical staff working under direct physician supervision

Identifying which providers are included under terms such as "physician or other qualified health care professional" or "qualified, nonphysicians health care professional" is of particular importance for correct reporting of nonphysician provider services. These terms are used in *Current Procedural Terminology* (*CPT*®) and/or payer instruction.

Current Procedural Terminology Provider Definitions

Current Procedural Terminology (*CPT*) provides the following definitions of providers:

- **Physician or other qualified health care professional:** an individual who is qualified by education, training, licensure/regulation (when applicable), and facility privileging (when applicable) who performs a professional service within his or her scope of practice and independently reports that professional service
- **Clinical staff member:** a person who works under the supervision of a physician or other qualified health care professional and who is allowed by law, regulation, and facility policy to perform or assist in the performance of a specific professional service but does not individually report that professional service

Throughout the *CPT* code set, the use of terms such as "physician," "qualified health care professional," or "individual" is not intended to indicate that other entities may not report the service. In selected instances, specific instructions may define a service as limited to professionals or other entities (eg, hospital, home health agency).

In *CPT, clinical staff member* is primarily used in the context of staff who provide components of physician or QHP services, such as transitional care management and chronic care management (CCM), as well as services that are always billed under incident-to guidelines (eg, nurse visit, medication administration).

See Chapter 13 for more information on state scope of practice and billing and coding for services of nonphysician providers.

The *CPT* definition of *physician or other QHP* is used in relation to services such as evaluation and management (E/M) (**99202–99499**), which are typically within the scope of practice of physicians and advanced practice professionals but not of other QHPs and QNHCPs, whose scope of practice may be limited to specific specialized services. For example, a clinical social worker may be limited to reporting psychotherapy provided without an E/M service.

Including Nonphysician Providers in Your Practice

Services such as behavioral health assessment by a licensed social worker or licensed psychologist may be provided within a general pediatric group practice and can be an integral part of providing a full scope of care in the medical home. However, billing and coding of these services must align not only with coding guidelines but also state scope of practice and individual payer policies on credentialing, contracting, and billing for services of the specific QNHCP.

Payment and Coverage Issues for Mental/Behavioral Health Services

Behavioral health services may be covered through a plan and provider network separate from other health care services. When arranging for or providing behavioral health services, it is very important to explore the patient's health plan policy options.

- Failure to credential and, when applicable, contract with behavioral health plans may lead to unpaid or underpaid charges.

●=New code ▲=Revised code #=Re-sequenced code +=Add-on code

Chapter 14. Mental and Behavioral Health Services

- Payer policies may allow specific licensed professionals, such as licensed clinical psychologists and licensed clinical social workers, to directly provide and report certain services. Other QNHCPs (eg, licensed master social workers) may be limited to providing services under direct supervision and reporting in the name of the participating health care professional (eg, licensed clinical psychologist or psychiatrist).
- General pediatricians and other QHPs may be ineligible to participate in the behavioral health plan network and limited to reporting E/M services to the health plan based on time.

The American Academy of Pediatrics (AAP) Council on Early Childhood, Committee on Psychosocial Aspects of Child and Family Health, and Section on Developmental and Behavioral Pediatrics included the following information about coverage of treatment of emotional and behavioral health problems in the policy statement, "Addressing Early Childhood Emotional and Behavioral Problems" (https://pediatrics.aappublications.org/content/138/6/e20163023):

American Academy of Pediatrics Policy Statement

"Without adequate payment for screening and assessment by primary care providers and management by specialty providers with expertise in early childhood mental health, treatment of very young children with emotional and behavioral problems will likely remain inaccessible for many children. Given existing knowledge regarding the importance of early childhood brain development on lifelong health, adequate payment for early childhood preventive services will benefit not only the patients but society as well and should be supported. Mental health carve-outs should be eliminated because they provide a significant barrier to access to mental health care for children. Additional steps toward equal access to mental health and physical health care include efficient prior authorization processes; adequate panels of early childhood mental health providers; payment to all providers, including primary care providers, for mental health diagnoses; sustainable payment for co-located mental health providers and care coordination; payment for evidence-based approaches focused on parents; and payment for the necessary collection of information from children's many caregivers and for same-day services. Advocacy for true mental health parity must continue."

Integration of psychiatric and/or developmental/behavioral health care professionals into the primary care practice may also require an understanding of health plan payment policies. Payer edits may not allow separate payment for mental and behavioral health services when E/M services are provided in the same practice on the same date. Verify coverage and billing options prior to provision of services.

Learn more about payer edits in Chapter 2 and about American Academy of Pediatrics payer advocacy in Chapter 4.

- Payers often place limitations on the diagnoses that may be paid under a patient's health benefits versus a separate behavioral health benefit.
  - Pediatricians may be required to report codes for symptoms rather than diagnosed conditions (eg, sadness in lieu of depression). This conflicts with *International Classification of Diseases, 10th Revision, Clinical Modification (ICD-10-CM)* guidelines.
  - *ICD-10-CM* guidelines instruct, "Codes that describe symptoms and signs, as opposed to diagnoses, are acceptable for reporting purposes when a related definitive diagnosis has not been established (confirmed) by the provider."
  - Adherence to these guidelines when assigning *ICD-10-CM* diagnosis codes is required under the Health Insurance Portability and Accountability Act of 1996. Payers are required to accept codes reported in compliance with the official guidelines for code selection and reporting.
  - When payers deny claims appropriately reported with codes **F01–F99** (mental, behavioral and neurodevelopmental disorders), pediatricians may report the issue using the AAP online Hassle Factor Form (www.aap.org/en-us/professional-resources/practice-transformation/getting-paid/Pages/Hassle-Factor-Form-Concerns-with-Payers.aspx) or seek the assistance of an AAP pediatric council (www.aap.org/en-us/professional-resources/practice-transformation/getting-paid/Pages/aap-pediatric-councils.aspx).
- Healthcare Common Procedure Coding System (HCPCS) modifiers identifying the type of health care professional (eg, **AJ**, clinical social worker) may be necessary to override edits that bundle E/M services provided by a physician/QHP and mental/behavioral health services provided by a QNHCP on the same date.
- Relevant HCPCS modifiers include

AH	Clinical psychologist
AJ	Clinical social worker
AM	Physician, team member service
HA	Child/adolescent program
HN	Bachelor's degree level
HO	Master's degree level

HP	Doctoral level
HQ	Group setting
TL	Early intervention/individualized family service plan (IFSP)
UN	Two patients served
UP	Three patients served
UQ	Four patients served
UR	Five patients served
US	Six or more patients served

Reporting Codes F01–F99

Diagnosis of behavioral and mental health conditions is typically based on the criteria set forth in the *Diagnostic and Statistical Manual of Mental Disorders,* 5th Edition (*DSM-5*) classification system.

● Often, a simple crosswalk from the *DSM-5* diagnosis to the *ICD-10-CM* code supporting the diagnosis can be made. However, the classifications are not always equivalent.

DSM-5 does not differentiate Asperger syndrome from autism spectrum disorder (ASD). *ICD-10-CM* provides a specific code for Asperger syndrome (**F84.5**) in addition to codes for autistic disorder (**F84.0**) and other pervasive developmental disorders (eg, Rett syndrome, **F84.2**).

● It is important that documentation clearly reflects a diagnostic statement separate from the assignment of an *ICD-10-CM* code as required by official guidance for *ICD-10-CM*.

  — This statement should include the findings supporting the diagnosis (eg, observations made during the appointment, history, standardized rating scale results, pertinent physical examination findings).

> *International Classification of Diseases, 10th Revision, Clinical Modification* codes for behavioral and emotional disorders with onset usually occurring in childhood and adolescence (F90–F98) may be reported for patients of any age. Disorders in this category typically have onset during childhood but may continue throughout life and not be diagnosed until adulthood.

  — Failure to document the information supporting the diagnostic statement could affect the patient's access to care and the physician's payment for services provided.

● *ICD-10-CM* includes codes for specifying how an accident or injury happened (eg, unintentional or accidental; intentional, such as suicide or assault).

  — Management of patients who have sustained injury or illness (eg, poisoning) due to intentional self-harm are reported with codes signifying the intent (eg, **T52.92XA**, toxic effect of unspecified organic solvent, intentional self-harm, initial encounter).

  — If the intent of the cause of an injury or other condition is unknown or unspecified, code the intent as accidental intent. All transport accident categories assume accidental intent.

  — External cause codes for events of undetermined intent are only for use if the documentation in the record specifies that the intent cannot be determined at the encounter (eg, suspected abuse under investigation).

Current Procedural Terminology Add-on Codes

Many mental and behavioral health services are described by a combination of a base code with add-on codes representing extended services. Add-on codes (marked with a + before the code) are always performed in addition to a primary procedure and are never reported as a stand-alone service. Add-on codes describe additional intraservice work and are not valued to include preservice and post-service work like most other codes.

Central Nervous System Assessments/Tests

The following codes are used to report the services provided during testing of central nervous system functions. Central nervous system assessments include, but are not limited to, memory, language, visual/motor responses, and abstract reasoning/problem-solving abilities. The mode of completion can be by a person (eg, paper and pencil) or via automated means. The administration of these tests will generate material that will be interpreted and formulated into a report by a physician or other QHP or an automated result.

●=New code   ▲=Revised code   #=Re-sequenced code   +=Add-on code

> Standardized instruments are used in the performance of central nervous system assessment/testing services. *Standardized instruments are validated tests administered and scored in the consistent or "standard" manner performed during their validation.* Informal checklists created by a physician or electronic health record developer are not considered standardized instruments.

Claims for testing are typically reported after the final date of testing services, with the appropriate codes for each date of service reported on the single claim. However, payer instructions may vary, and some require reporting with only the date on which testing services are completed (see example in discussion of **96112** and **96113** in the next section).

Central nervous system assessments and tests are not reported in conjunction with adaptive behavior treatment (**97151–97158, 0362T, 0373T**).

Developmental Testing

96112   Developmental test administration (including assessment of fine and/or gross motor, language, cognitive level, social, memory and/or executive functions by standardized developmental instruments when performed), by physician or other qualified health care professional, with interpretation and report; first hour

+96113   each additional 30 minutes (List separately in addition to code for primary procedure)

Developmental testing services, which include interpretation and report, are described by codes **96112** and **96113**.

> Developmental screening services are described by code 96110. Developmental screening using an objective standardized instrument, including scoring and documentation, is typically done by clinical staff. Interpretation and counseling on the score are included in the related E/M service.

Codes **96112** and **96113**

- Allow reporting of developmental testing in which the child is observed doing standardized tasks that are then scored, with interpretation and report.
- Include assessment of motor, language, social, and/or cognitive function by standardized developmental instruments (eg, scales of infant and toddler development) and include objective assessments as well.
- Billing time includes both face-to-face time spent in testing and time of interpretation and report.
  - Although not specifically stated in the code descriptor, interpretation and report is included as intraservice work in the assignment of work relative value units for these services.
  - Payer policies may vary on reporting of time spent in interpretation and report. Check the policies of individual health plans when reporting.
- Code selection is based on time spent per hour by the physician or QHP.
  - The midpoint rule applies to developmental testing; time is met when the midpoint is passed.
  - The first hour of service (**96112**) may be reported for 31 minutes or more.
  - Report 1 unit of code **96113** for time of at least 16 minutes beyond the first hour or beyond the last 30-minute period of service.
- If a developmental instrument does not meet the criteria of being an objective instrument with the subjective element and does not take a minimum of 31 minutes to complete including interpretation and report, refer to code **96110** instead.

Do not report **96110** if also reporting code **96112** or **96113** on the same day for the same patient.

Examples

➤ **A 5-year-old boy previously diagnosed with ASD but not enrolled in early intervention due to family circumstances presents for extended developmental testing after he could not be successfully assessed for kindergarten entry.** Developmental tests are administered, with total testing time on this date of 75 minutes. The child returns and spends a total of 60 minutes to complete testing 1 week later. After testing is completed, the developmental pediatrician spends another 60 minutes on the same date interpreting the test results and 60 minutes formulating a report of the findings and recommendations. Code **96112** is reported for the 75 minutes of service on the first date. Because the midpoint between 60 and 90 minutes (76 minutes) was not passed, **96113** is not reported. On the second date of service, codes **96112** (first 60 minutes of testing) and **96113** with 4 units of service (2 hours interpreting the testing results and developing the report) are reported. On the final date of service (ie, the day of the feedback session), submit 1 claim for all cumulative services detailed *by separate dates of service.*

Teaching Point: Some payers may require the entire service be reported on a single claim and single date of service. For these payers, report code **96112** (for the 60 minutes of testing on the first day) and 6 units of **96113** (for the remaining 195 minutes) on the date of the second session. Remember, the midpoint must be passed for the additional units to be billed. In this case, the remaining time was only 15 minutes.

➤ **A 10-year-old established patient has shown a progressive pattern of academic struggles since the first grade.** He says the fourth-grade work is "too hard." His parents wonder if he is "lazy" or if he may not be "smart enough." His school psychologist says there is no reason for her to do any psychoeducational testing. The physician administers a Kaufman Brief Intelligence Test, 2nd Edition, and a Wide Range Achievement Test, 4th Edition, to briefly assess overall cognitive level and academic achievement levels. The tests are scored and interpreted. A concise written report is created for the parents to take to the school psychologist. Total time devoted to face-to-face testing, interpretation, and report was 110 minutes.

Code **96112** is reported for the first hour of testing, and code **96113** is reported with 2 units of service for the additional 50 minutes of service (1 unit for the first 30 minutes after the first hour and another unit for the final 20 minutes).

Neuropsychological and Psychological Testing

Neuropsychological and psychological testing evaluation services typically include integration of patient data with other sources of clinical data, interpretation, clinical decision-making, treatment planning, and report.
- Interactive feedback, conveying the implications of psychological or neuropsychological test findings and diagnostic formulation, is included when performed.
- Testing by a physician or QHP is separately reportable as an evaluation service on the same or a different date.
- Testing codes differentiate tests administered by a physician or other QHP, by a technician, or via an electronic platform.

Neurobehavioral Status Examination

★**96116**   Neurobehavioral status examination (clinical assessment of thinking, reasoning and judgment [eg, acquired knowledge, attention, language, memory, planning and problem solving, and visual spatial abilities]), by physician or other qualified health care professional, both face-to-face time with the patient and time interpreting test results and preparing the report; first hour

+**96121**   each additional hour

> Mini-mental status examination performed by a physician would be included as part of the central nervous system physical examination of an evaluation and management service and not separately reportable.

- Documentation of these services includes scoring, informal observation of behavior during the testing, and interpretation and report. It should include the date and time spent in testing, time of interpretation and report, reason for the test, and titles of all instruments used.
- Neurobehavioral status examination is reported based on the time of face-to-face testing and includes time interpreting test results and preparing a report.
- The unit of time is 60 minutes and time is met when the midpoint is passed (ie, at least 31 minutes of time is required for the first or last unit of service).

Example

➤ **An 8-year-old boy, previously diagnosed with attention-deficit/hyperactivity disorder (ADHD), predominantly inattentive type, is being evaluated for gradual problems with remembering directions, organizing his school materials and his room at home, and other behavior concerns.** The physician performs a neurobehavioral status examination, which involves clinical assessments and observations for impairments in acquired knowledge, attention, learning, and memory. The results indicate the need for further standardized language, memory, and intelligence testing. The total time for testing, scoring, and report writing is 3½ hours.

This service is reported with codes **96116** (neurobehavioral status examination) and **96121** with 2 units for the additional 2½ hours of testing, scoring, and report writing. The diagnosis code would be *ICD-10-CM* code **F90.0** (ADHD, predominantly inattentive type). Additional *ICD-10-CM* codes may be assigned for specific developmental disorders diagnosed following testing (eg, **F81.2**, mathematics disorder).

Psychological and Neuropsychological Testing Services

Codes for psychological and neuropsychological testing differentiate test administration by physicians and QHPs, technicians, or automated systems. A combination of testing evaluation and test administration and scoring services is typically reported on a single claim.

The tests selected, test administration, and method of testing and scoring are the same regardless of whether the testing is performed by a physician, QHP, or technician.

Testing Evaluation Services by a Physician or Other Qualified Health Care Professional With Interpretation and Report

96130	*Psychological* testing evaluation services by physician or other qualified health care professional, including integration of patient data, interpretation of standardized test results and clinical data, clinical decision making, treatment planning and report, and interactive feedback to the patient, family member(s) or caregiver(s), when performed; first hour
+96131	each additional hour (List separately in addition to code for primary procedure)
96132	*Neuropsychological* testing evaluation services by physician or other qualified health care professional, including integration of patient data, interpretation of standardized test results and clinical data, clinical decision making, treatment planning and report, and interactive feedback to the patient, family member(s) or caregiver(s), when performed; first hour
+96133	each additional hour (List separately in addition to code for primary procedure)

- These services follow standard *CPT* time definitions (ie, a minimum of 31 minutes must be provided to report a 1-hour unit of service). The time reported in codes **96130–96133** is the face-to-face time with the patient and the time spent integrating and interpreting data.
- *Time spent in test administration and scoring is not included in time used to support codes 96130–96133.* Separately report psychological/neuropsychological test administration and scoring services (**96136–96139**) on the same or different days (ie, each service is separately reported on the same claim). Report the total time of evaluation and testing services at the completion of the entire episode of evaluation on a single claim with each date of service listed separately.

> Time of 30 minutes or less would not be reported with codes **96132** and **96133**.

- Documentation of these services includes scoring, observation of behavior, and interpretation and report. It should include the date and time spent in testing and the time spent integrating and interpreting data, reason for the testing, and titles of all instruments used.

> The time reported in codes **96130–96133** is the face-to-face time with the patient and the time spent integrating and interpreting data. Time spent in face-to-face testing and in integration and interpretation of data must be documented to support the time used in code selection. An itemization of time for each activity is preferable.

Example

➤ **An adolescent patient with history of brain surgery is referred for neuropsychological evaluation due to difficulties with memory and reading.** A physician spends 2 hours reviewing the patient's medical records, interpreting data from tests administered and scored on an earlier date by a technician, and creating a report (copied to the referring physician) of the diagnosis and recommendations for treatment. Another 40 minutes was spent providing interactive feedback to the patient and caregivers.

Code **96132** and 2 units of **96133** are reported for 2 hours and 40 minutes spent in data interpretation, interactive feedback, and report writing. If the physician also personally administered and scored tests, codes **96136** and **96137** would also be reported based on the time of testing and scoring. Test administration and scoring by a technician would be reported separately with codes **96138** and **96139** based on the time of service (see discussion of codes **96138** and **96139** in the Technician-Administered Testing section later in this chapter).

Teaching Point: Report code **96133** with 1 unit of service in addition to **96132** for time of 91 to 150 minutes. Time of 151 minutes or more supports additional units of service for code **96133** (include 1 unit for 31–59 minutes beyond the last full hour).

Testing Administration Services

Test administration and scoring services are selected based on time of service. The midpoint rule applies. Separate codes are reported based on whether testing and scoring are personally performed by a physician or QHP or are performed by a technician.

> At least 2 distinct tests must be administered and scored to report codes **96136–96139**. Do not separately count subtests in a multifaceted test (eg, Wechsler Preschool and Primary Scale of Intelligence is 1 test with 14 subtests). Code **96127** (brief emotional/behavioral assessment with scoring and documentation, per standardized instrument) may be reported for administration and scoring of a single standardized test.

Table 14-1. Calculating Units of Service for Time of Test Administration and Scoring

Total time of administration and scoring	16–45 min	46–75 min	76–105 min	>106 min (each 30 min or last 16 min beyond the final full 30-min period)
Performed by a physician/QHP	**96136** (1 unit)	**96136** and **96137** (1 unit each)	**96136** (1 unit) and **96137** (2 units)	**96136** (1 unit) and units of **96137** for each 30 min or the last 16 min beyond the final full 30-min period
Performed by a technician	**96138** (1 unit)	**96138** and **96139** (1 unit each)	**96138** (1 unit) and **96139** (2 units)	**96138** (1 unit) and units of **96139** for each 30 min or the last 16 min beyond the final full 30-min period

Abbreviation: QHP, qualified health care professional.

Physician or Qualified Health Care Professional Administration and Scoring

96136 Psychological or neuropsychological test administration and scoring by physician or other qualified health care professional, two or more tests, any method; first 30 minutes

+96137 each additional 30 minutes after first 30 minutes (List separately in addition to code for primary procedure)

- Services include administration of a series of tests, recording of behavioral observations made during testing, scoring, and transcription of scores to a data summary sheet.
- Codes are selected based on time of testing and scoring. Time is met when the midpoint is passed (ie, a minimum of 16 minutes for 30-minute codes). Refer to **Table 14-1** for more details.
- *Do not include* time spent in integration of patient data or interpretation of test results in the time reported with codes **96136** and **96137**. This time is included with psychological and neuropsychological test evaluation services (**96130–96133**).
- Psychological or neuropsychological test administration *using a single test/instrument,* with interpretation and report by a physician or QHP, is reported with code **96127** (brief emotional/behavioral assessment [eg, depression inventory, ADHD scale], with scoring and documentation, per standardized instrument).

Examples

➤ **A physician spends 50 minutes administering tests, recording observations, scoring, and transcribing results to a data summary sheet.** Codes **96136** and **96137** are reported with 1 unit of service each.

Teaching Point: Because the time of service exceeded 16 minutes beyond the first 30 minutes, code **96137** is reported in addition to **96136**.

➤ **An adolescent whose family reports psychotic behavior is referred for psychological testing evaluation.** The patient undergoes physician-administered psychological testing to evaluate emotionality, intellectual abilities, personality, and psychopathology and to make a mental health diagnosis and treatment recommendations as applicable. The total time of face-to-face testing is 45 minutes. The physician's total time of evaluation and data integration and interpretation is 75 minutes. Codes **96136** and **96130** are reported.

   Teaching Point: Test administration and scoring time of 45 minutes is reported with code **96136**. Seventy-five minutes of physician testing evaluation service is reported with code **96130**.

Technician-Administered Testing

Testing and administration services performed by a technician are reported with codes **96138** and **96139**.

96138   Psychological or neuropsychological test administration and scoring by technician, two or more tests, any method; first 30 minutes

+96139   each additional 30 minutes (List separately in addition to code for primary procedure)

● Codes **96138** and **96139** do not include the work of a physician or QHP. These codes are valued for practice expense and medical liability only.

● Evaluation services by the physician or QHP are reported with codes **96130–96133** whether provided on the same or a different date. Do not include time for evaluation services (eg, integration of patient data or interpretation of test results in the time of technician-administered testing) in time of test administration and scoring.

Example

➤ **An adolescent patient is referred for neuropsychological testing.** A technician spends 40 minutes administering and scoring tests. The technician also notes any behavioral observations. Code **96138** is reported with 1 unit of service.

   Teaching Point: When a physician or QHP provides evaluation services, including integration and interpretation of data from tests administered by a technician, on the same or different date, see codes **96132** and **96133** for those services.

Automated Testing and Result

When a single test instrument is completed by the patient via an electronic platform without physician, QHP, or technician administration and scoring, report code **96146**.

96146   Psychological or neuropsychological test administration, with single automated, standardized instrument via electronic platform, with automated result only

● Code **96146** does not include scoring by a health care professional or interpretation and report. Results are generated via the electronic platform.

● If a test is administered by a physician, QHP, or technician, do not report **96146**. For brief emotional/behavioral assessment, see code **96127**.

Example

➤ **A child who is recovering from a concussion is provided a single computerized test for post-concussion symptoms.** The patient completes the test and the automated result is included in the patient's medical record.

   Code **96146** is reported in addition to the code representing the physician's related E/M service (eg, **99213**).

Adaptive Behavior Assessment and Treatment Services

Adaptive behavior services address
● Deficient adaptive behaviors, such as impaired social, communication, or self-care skills
● Maladaptive behaviors, such as repetitive and stereotype behaviors
● Behaviors that risk physical harm to the patient, others, and/or property

   Codes for adaptive behavior services are a combination of Category I and Category III (emerging technology) *CPT* codes. Adaptive behavior services may be delivered by a physician or QHP, behavioral analyst, and/or licensed psychologist working with assistant behavior analysts or technicians.

It is important to verify health plan policies for coverage and payment of adaptive behavior services, including any required provider qualifications (eg, certification, licensure) prior to provision of services.

- Most states mandate coverage of adaptive behavior services for patients diagnosed with ASD. Some states require that behavior analysts providing ASD-related assessment and/or treatment be certified by the Behavior Analyst Certification Board as a Board-Certified Behavior Analyst.
- In the discussion of adaptive behavior services, the QHP includes behavior analysts and licensed psychologists who can independently report these services.

See your procedure coding reference (eg, *CPT* coding manual) for specific instructions for reporting these services.

The general rule that time is met when the midpoint is passed applies because *CPT* doesn't include category-specific instructions on the time of service for adaptive behavior services (eg, at least 8 minutes of service is required to support a service specified as 15 minutes).

Healthcare Common Procedure Coding System Codes for Adaptive Behavior Assessment and Treatment Services

Some payers (eg, Medicaid plans) have required HCPCS codes in lieu of *CPT* codes for certain adaptive behavior assessment and treatment services. Examples of HCPCS codes used in health plan policies for adaptive behavior services include

H0025	Behavioral health prevention education service (delivery of services with target population to affect knowledge, attitude and/or behavior)
H0031	Mental health assessment by nonphysician
H0032	Mental health service plan development by nonphysician
H2014	Skills training, per 15 minutes
H2019	Therapeutic behavioral services, per 15 minutes
H2027	Psychoeducational service, per 15 minutes
S5108	Home care training to home care client, per 15 minutes
S5111	Home care training, family; per session

HCPCS codes are often interpreted and used differently by individual health plans. It is important to verify each payer's policy for coverage and payment of adaptive behavior services and to submit codes that comply with each payer's policy.

See **Chapter 1** for more information on HCPCS codes.

Adaptive Behavior Assessment

#97151	Behavior identification assessment, administered by a physician or other qualified health care professional, each 15 minutes of the physician's or other qualified health care professional's time face-to-face with patient and/or guardian(s)/caregiver(s) administering assessments and discussing findings and recommendations, and non-face-to-face analyzing past data, scoring/interpreting the assessment, and preparing the report/treatment plan
#97152	Behavior identification supporting assessment, administered by one technician under the direction of a physician or other qualified health care professional, face-to-face with the patient, each 15 minutes
0362T	Behavior identification supporting assessment, each 15 minutes of technicians' time face-to-face with a patient, requiring the following components:

- administration by the physician or other qualified health care professional who is on site;
- with the assistance of two or more technicians;
- for a patient who exhibits destructive behavior;
- completion in an environment that is customized to the patient's behavior

Behavior identification assessment (**97151**) is conducted by a physician or other QHP and may include

- Analysis of pertinent past data (including medical diagnosis)
- A detailed behavioral history
- Patient observation
- Administration of standardized and/or non-standardized instruments and procedures
- Functional behavior assessment
- Functional analysis
- Guardian/caregiver interview to identify and describe deficient adaptive behaviors, maladaptive behaviors, and other impaired functioning secondary to deficient adaptive or maladaptive behaviors

If the physician or other QHP personally performs the technician activities, his or her time engaged in these activities should be included as part of the required technician time to meet the components of the code.

●=New code   ▲=Revised code   #=Re-sequenced code   +=Add-on code

- Codes **97151**, **97152**, and **0362T** may be repeated on the same or different days until the behavior identification assessment (**97151**) and, if necessary, supporting assessment(s) (**97152**, **0362T**) are complete.
- Code **97152** is reported for assessment by a technician. The reporting physician or QHP is not required to be on-site during the assessment. See code **0362T** when multiple technicians and a customized assessment environment are required due to destructive behavior(s) of the patient.
- Code **0362T** represents testing of a patient who demonstrates destructive behavior (ie, maladaptive behaviors associated with a high risk of medical consequences or property damage) and requires multiple technicians and an environment customized to the patient and behavior. The reporting physician or QHP is required to be on-site (ie, immediately available and interruptible to provide assistance and direction throughout the performance of the procedure). The reporting physician or QHP is not required to be in the room during testing.
- Only count the time of 1 technician when 2 or more technicians are present. Code **0362T** is reported based on a single technician's face-to-face time with the patient and not the combined time of multiple technicians (eg, 1 hour with 3 technicians equals 1 hour of service) despite the expectation that more than 1 technician will be needed.

Examples

➤ **A 3-year-old boy with symptoms of ASD presents for assessment.** The physician/QHP spends 1 hour face-to-face with the patient and/or guardian(s)/caregiver(s) administering assessments and discussing findings and recommendations and 38 minutes of non–face-to-face time analyzing past data, scoring/interpreting the assessment, and preparing the report/treatment plan. The total time of service is 1 hour, 38 minutes. Code **97151** is reported with 7 units (1 for each full 15 minutes of service and 1 for the last 8 minutes).

    Teaching Point: If fewer than 8 minutes past the last full 15 minutes of service were provided, only the number of 15-minute periods of service would be reported (eg, 1 hour, 37 minutes equals 6 units).

➤ **An additional assessment of the 3-year-old from the previous example is required to assess behavior that interferes with acquisition of adaptive skills.** A technician, under the physician's or QHP's direction, observes and records occurrence of the patient's deficient adaptive and maladaptive behaviors and the surrounding environmental events several times in a variety of situations. The physician/QHP reviews and analyzes data from those observations. The face-to-face time of the technician is 1 hour.

    Code **97152** is reported with 4 units of service.

➤ **An 11-year-old boy with ASD requires evaluation due to increased self-injury and aggression toward others.** A team of technicians conducts the assessment session in a room that is devoid of any objects that might cause injury. A physician/QHP is on-site and immediately available throughout the session. The technicians implement functional analysis as directed by the physician/QHP and record data. Graphed data are reviewed and analyzed by the physician/QHP to identify the environmental events in whose presence the level of behavior was highest and lowest. The technicians spend a total of 90 minutes face-to-face with the patient during the assessment.

    Code **0362T** is reported with 6 units of service.

Adaptive Behavior Treatment

Adaptive behavior treatment services address specific treatment targets and goals based on results of previous assessments and include ongoing assessment and adjustment of treatment protocols, targets, and goals. Codes describe services to the individual patient, groups of patients, families, and an individual patient who exhibits destructive behavior.

    Codes for adaptive behavior treatment specify services provided by protocol (**97153**, **97154**) or with protocol modification (**97155**, **97158**, **0373T**). Behavior treatment with protocol modification requires adjustments be *made in real time* rather than for a subsequent service.

Adaptive Behavior Treatment by Protocol

#97153   Adaptive behavior treatment by protocol, administered by technician under the direction of a physician or other qualified health care professional, face-to-face with one patient; each 15 minutes

#97154   Group adaptive behavior treatment by protocol, administered by technician under the direction of a physician or other qualified health care professional, face-to-face with two or more patients, each 15 minutes

- Adaptive behavior treatment by protocol to a single patient (**97153**) and group adaptive behavior treatment by protocol (**97154**) are administered by a technician under the direction of a physician/QHP, using a treatment protocol *designed in advance* by the physician or other QHP, who may or may not provide direction during the treatment.
  — The service described by code **97153** is face-to-face with only 1 patient.
  — Code **97154** is reported for services delivered face-to-face with 2 or more patients but not more than 8 patients.
- Codes **97153** and **97154** do not include protocol modification.
- If the physician/QHP personally performs the technician activities, his or her time spent engaged in these activities should be reported as technician time. The physician is not required to be on site during the provision of these services.

Examples

➤ **A 4-year-old girl presents with deficits in language and social skills and emotional outbursts in response to small changes in routines or when preferred items are unavailable.** A QHP directs a technician in the implementation of treatment protocols and data collection procedures. The technician conducts a treatment session in the family home with multiple planned opportunities for the patient to practice target skills. The QHP reviews the technician's recorded and graphed data to assess the child's progress and determine if any treatment protocol needs adjustment. The technician spends 1 hour at the patient's home with face-to-face time of the treatment session lasting 50 minutes. Code **97153** is reported with 3 units of service.

  Teaching Point: Only the technician's face-to-face time with the patient is used to determine the units of service. This service may also be conducted in a community setting (eg, playground, store).

➤ **Peer social skills training in a small group is recommended for a 7-year-old girl with deficits in social skills.** A technician conducts the group session using treatment protocols and data collection procedures as previously designed by a QHP. The QHP reviews the technician's recorded and graphed data to assess the child's progress and determine if treatment protocols need adjustment. The total face-to-face time of the session is 60 minutes. Code **97154** is reported with 4 units.

Adaptive Behavior Treatment With Protocol Modification

#**97155**	Adaptive behavior treatment with protocol modification administered by physician or other qualified health care professional, which may include simultaneous direction of technician, face-to-face with one patient, each 15 minutes
#**97158**	Group adaptive behavior treatment with protocol modification, administered by physician or other qualified health care professional, face-to-face with multiple patients, each 15 minutes
0373T	Adaptive behavior treatment with protocol modification, each 15 minutes of technicians' time face-to-face with a patient, requiring the following components:

- administration by the physician or other qualified health care professional who is on site;
- with the assistance of two or more technicians;
- for a patient who exhibits destructive behavior;
- completion in an environment that is customized to the patient's behavior.

- Adaptive behavior treatment with protocol modification (**97155**) is administered by a physician/QHP *face-to-face with a single patient.*
  — The physician/QHP resolves 1 or more problems with the protocol and may simultaneously direct a technician in administering the modified protocol *while the patient is present.*
  — Physician/QHP direction to the technician without the patient present is not reported separately.
- Group adaptive behavior treatment with protocol modification (**97158**) is reported when a physician/QHP provides *face-to-face* protocol modification services with up to 8 patients in a group. The physician/QHP monitors the needs of individual patients and adjusts treatment techniques during the group sessions, as needed.
- Adaptive behavior treatment with protocol modification (**0373T**) is reported for services to a patient who presents with 1 or more destructive behavior(s).
  — The service time is based on a single technician's face-to-face time with the patient and not the combined time of multiple technicians.
  — The physician/QHP must be on site and immediately available during the service described by code **0373T**.

●=New code ▲=Revised code #=Re-sequenced code +=Add-on code

Chapter 14. Mental and Behavioral Health Services

Examples

➤ **A 5-year-old boy previously showed steady improvements in language and social skills at home as a result of one-to-one intensive applied behavior analysis intervention, but skill development seems to have recently reached a plateau.** A QHP modifies the previously used written protocols to incorporate procedures designed to build the child's language and social skills into daily home routines (eg, play, dressing, mealtimes). The QHP demonstrates the procedures to the technician and directs the technician to implement the protocols with the child. The QHP then observes and provides feedback as the technician implements the procedures with the child. The technician's face-to-face time with the patient is 45 minutes. Code **97155** is reported with 3 units of service.

   Teaching Point: Time spent by the technician and QHP without the patient present is not included in the time of service.

➤ **A 13-year-old girl is reported to be isolated from peers due to poor social skills and odd behavior.** The child attends a group treatment session that focuses on peer social skills. A QHP begins the group session by asking each patient to briefly describe 2 of their recent social encounters with peers, one that went well and one that did not. The information is used to develop a group activity in which each patient has the opportunity to practice the skills she or he used in the encounters that went well and to problem-solve the interactions that did not go well. The QHP helps each patient identify social cues that were interpreted correctly and incorrectly and what she or he could have done differently. The QHP also provides prompts and feedback individualized to each patient's skills. The QHP ends the session by summarizing the discussion. The total time of the session was 70 minutes, including a 10-minute break (ie, 60 minutes of group session). Code **97158** is reported with 4 units of service.

   Teaching Point: Only the QHP's face-to-face time spent providing the service is reported.

➤ **A 16-year-old boy has had 2 surgeries to relieve esophageal blockages due to pica involving repeated ingestion of small metal objects (eg, paper clips, pushpins).** The patient's pica behavior has not responded to previous treatment. The QHP supervising the patient's treatment plan has previously developed written protocols for reducing the patient's pica. A technician carefully inspects the room before the session to make sure there are no potential pica items on the floor. Two technicians are present, with one presenting the patient with a series of trials in which the patient is presented with a food item and a nonhazardous item that resembles a pica item. The second technician prompts the patient to choose the food item and blocks attempts to choose the pica item. The patient's response to each trial is recorded. The QHP is on site and available to assist as needed. The total session lasts 40 minutes. Code **0373T** is reported with 3 units.

   Teaching Point: Although 2 technicians were present, time is counted only once. The midpoint rule allows reporting a unit of service for the final 10 minutes of service.

Family Adaptive Behavior Treatment Guidance

Family adaptive behavior treatment guidance (**97156**) and multiple-family group adaptive behavior treatment guidance (**97157**) are administered by a physician or QHP face-to-face with guardian(s)/caregiver(s) and involve identifying potential treatment targets and training guardian(s)/caregiver(s) to implement treatment protocols designed to address deficient adaptive or maladaptive behaviors.

#97156   Family adaptive behavior treatment guidance, administered by physician or other qualified health care professional (with or without the patient present), face-to-face with guardian(s)/caregiver(s), each 15 minutes

#97157   Multiple-family group adaptive behavior treatment guidance, administered by physician or other qualified health care professional (without the patient present), face-to-face with multiple sets of guardians/caregivers, each 15 minutes

● Family adaptive behavior treatment guidance (**97156**) provided to the caregiver(s) of one patient may be performed with or without the patient present.

   Adaptive behavior treatment where the parent(s) or guardian(s) are present but not part of the therapy would not qualify as family adaptive behavior treatment.

● Family adaptive behavior treatment guidance provided to the caregiver(s) of multiple patients (**97157**) is performed without the patients present. The group must be no larger than the caregiver(s) of 8 patients.

Examples

➤ **The parents of a 6-year-old boy seek training on procedures for helping the child communicate using picture cards during typical family routines (a skill he previously developed in adaptive behavior treatment therapy sessions with technicians).** A physician/QHP trains the parents. The service includes reviewing the written treatment and data collection protocols with the parents, demonstrating how to implement the cards in role-plays and with the child, and having the parents implement the protocols with the child while the provider observes and provides feedback. The time of service is 1 hour.

Code **97156** is reported with 4 units of service.

➤ **The parents of a 3-year-old boy who has pervasive hyperactivity and no functional play, social, or communication skills seek training on how to manage his hyperactive and disruptive behavior and help him develop appropriate play, social, and communication skills.** The parents attend a group session (without the patient) led by a physician who asks each set of parents to identify 1 skill to be increased or 1 problem behavior to be decreased in their own child. The physician describes how behavior analytic principles and procedures could be applied to the behavior identified by the parents of this 3-year-old patient. The physician demonstrates a procedure (eg, prompting the child to speak instead of whining when he wants something; not giving him preferred items when he whines). The parents then role-play, implementing that procedure. Other group participants and the physician provide feedback and make constructive suggestions. That process is repeated for skills/behaviors identified by other sets of parents. The group session ends with the physician summarizing the main points, answering questions, and giving each set of parents a homework assignment to practice the skills they worked on during the session. The session lasts 110 minutes. Code **97157** is reported with 7 units.

Teaching Point: The last 5 minutes are not reported because the midpoint of 8 minutes beyond the last full 15-minute period (105 minutes) was not passed.

Habilitative and Rehabilitative Modifiers

Adaptive behavior services may be either habilitative or rehabilitative. *Habilitative* services are those provided to help an individual learn skills not yet developed and to keep and/or improve those skills. *Rehabilitative* services help a patient keep, get back, or improve skills that have been lost or limited due to illness, injury, and/or disability. Because the Patient Protection and Affordable Care Act provides that certain health plans must provide equal coverage for habilitative and rehabilitative services and count each type of service separately, it may be necessary to indicate that a service is habilitative or rehabilitative. Modifiers **96** (habilitative services) and **97** (rehabilitative services) are appended to procedure codes to designate the nature of a service. Modifiers **96** and **97** may not be adopted for use by all payers or may have limited utility. Verify payer policies for these modifiers when providing habilitative and rehabilitative services.

See Chapter 2 for more information on modifiers **96** and **97**.

Health and Behavior Assessments/Interventions

Health and behavior assessment and intervention procedures (**96156**, **96158**, **96159**, and **96164–96171**) are used to identify and address psychosocial, behavioral, emotional, cognitive, and interpersonal factors important to the assessment, treatment, or management of physical health problems.

The patient's primary diagnosis is physical in nature, and the focus of the assessment and interventions is on factors complicating medical conditions and treatments. These codes describe assessments and interventions to improve the patient's health and well-being using psychological and/or psychosocial interventions designed to ameliorate specific disease-related problems.

These services do not represent preventive medicine counseling and risk factor reduction interventions.

● Physicians and QHPs who can provide and report E/M services do not report **96156**, **96158**, **96159**, or **96164–96171**. Evaluation and management codes including preventive medicine services are reported instead.

● When an E/M service is provided by a physician or QHP on the same date that an AHP provides health and behavior assessment/intervention, each service is separately reported by the individual providing the service. The same provider cannot report both services.

●=New code   ▲=Revised code   #=Re-sequenced code   +=Add-on code

- May be reported by psychologists, clinical social workers, licensed therapists, and other AHPs within their scope of practice who have specialty or subspecialty training in health and behavior assessment or intervention procedures.
- Are not reported with psychiatric codes (**90785–90899**) when provided on the same day. Only the primary service is reported (ie, **96156, 96158, 96159,** and **96164–96171** or **90785–90899**).
- Are not reported with adaptive behavior assessment or treatment (**97151–97158, 0362T, 0373T**).
- Are not used in conjunction with a primary diagnosis of mental disorder. (Payers may deny claims when a diagnosis code indicating mental disorder is included for these services.)

Health Behavior Assessment

96156   Health behavior assessment, or re-assessment (ie, health-focused clinical interview, behavioral observations, clinical decision making)

Health behavior assessment includes evaluation of the patient's responses to disease, illness or injury, outlook, coping strategies, motivation, and adherence to medical treatment. Assessment is conducted through health-focused clinical interviews, observation, and clinical decision-making.

Code **96156** is not reported based on time. Report only 1 unit of service.

Example

➤ **A 16-year-old boy has juvenile myoclonic epilepsy.** He has recently had seizures, is suspected of not taking his medication, and has not been completing schoolwork. The boy's parents are concerned that he is not coping well with the limitations that epilepsy has required (eg, not starting to drive). The patient is assessed using standardized questionnaires. The child's parents are also interviewed.

Code **96156** would be reported with, for example, *ICD-10-CM* code **G40.B09**, juvenile myoclonic epilepsy, not intractable, without status epilepticus.

Health Behavior Intervention

Table 14-2. Health Behavior Intervention Codes		
Health Behavior Intervention Provided to	**Initial Code**	**Add-on Code**
Individual, face-to-face;	**96158** initial 16–30 min	**+96159** each additional 15 min (List separately in addition to code **96158**)
Group (2 or more patients), face-to-face;	**#96164** initial 16–30 min	**#+96165** each additional 15 min (List separately in addition to code **96164**)
Family (with the patient present), face-to-face;	**#96167** initial 16–30 min	**#+96168** each additional 15 min (List separately in addition to code **96167**)
Family (without the patient present), face-to-face;	**#96170** initial 16–30 min	**#+96171** each additional 15 min (List separately in addition to code **96170**)

Codes **96158, 96159,** and **96164–96171**
- Are time-based services requiring documentation of the time spent face-to-face with the patient(s) and/or family.
- Do not report **96158, 96164, 96167,** or **96170** for less than 16 minutes of service.
- Include promotion of functional improvement, minimizing psychological and/or psychosocial barriers to recovery, and management of and improved coping with medical conditions.
- Emphasize active patient/family engagement and involvement. These interventions may be provided individually, to a group (≥2 patients), and/or to the family, with or without the patient present.

Refer to **Table 14-2** for a breakdown of the health and behavior intervention codes.

Examples

➤ **Health and behavior intervention is provided to a 12-year-old girl undergoing treatment for persistent attention and concentration deficits following a traumatic brain injury.** Results from a health and behavior assessment are used to develop a plan for coping and complying with her physician's treatment plan in her daily activities. Thirty minutes is spent with the patient discussing the behavior and suggested coping skills.

Code **96158** with 1 unit of service would be reported with, for example, *ICD-10-CM* codes **R41.840**, attention and concentration deficit, and **S06.301S**, unspecified focal traumatic brain injury with loss of consciousness of 30 minutes or less, sequela.

➤ **Three patients with sickle cell anemia and identified needs for better treatment adherence take part in a group intervention.** Based on assessments conducted at previous encounters, the clinical psychologist works with the patients to gain understanding and acceptance of their physician's care plan, addresses barriers to compliance, and helps each patient develop goals for better compliance. A total of 55 minutes is spent face-to-face with the group of patients.

Code **96164** (1 unit for first 30 minutes) and **96165** with 2 units of service (1 full 15-minute period and 1 unit for the last 10 minutes because the midpoint of 8 minutes beyond the last full period was passed). *ICD-10-CM* codes appropriate to each patient's condition (eg, **D57.1**, sickle-cell disease without crisis) are reported.

Psychiatric Services

Psychiatric services include diagnostic services, psychotherapy, and other services to an individual, a family, or a group. Comprehensive services may be provided by a multidisciplinary team (eg, a psychiatrist, developmental-behavioral pediatrician, nurse practitioner, psychologist, clinical social worker, and/or clinical counselor).

However, in many parts of the country, children's mental and behavioral health professionals are not available. General pediatricians must often take on management of minor mental health problems and, when possible, consult with a mental/behavioral health professional at a distant location or arrange for services via telemedicine services. (See the Payment and Coverage Issues for Mental/Behavioral Health Services section earlier in this chapter for important considerations for general pediatricians providing psychiatric services.)

An emerging method of delivering mental health services is *psychiatric collaborative care management* (PCCM), in which care is directed by a primary care pediatrician or QHP and provided in collaboration with a psychiatric consultant. See the Psychiatric Collaborative Care Management Services section later in this chapter for more information.

Interactive Complexity

+90785 Interactive complexity

Psychiatric services to children may include interactive complexity. According to *CPT,* psychiatric procedures may be reported "with interactive complexity" when at least one of the following is present:

- The need to manage maladaptive communication (related to, eg, high anxiety, high reactivity, repeated questions, disagreement) among participants that complicates delivery of care
- Caregiver emotions or behavior interfering with the caregiver's understanding and ability to assist in the implementation of the treatment plan
- Evidence or disclosure of a sentinel event and mandated report to third party (eg, abuse or neglect with report to state agency) with initiation of discussion of the sentinel event and/or report with the patient and other visit participants
- Use of play equipment, other physical devices, interpreter, or translator to communicate with the patient to overcome barriers to therapeutic or diagnostic interaction between the physician or other QHP and a patient who either
  — Is not fluent in the same language as the physician or other QHP
  — Has not developed, or has lost, either the expressive language communication skills to explain his or her symptoms and response to treatment or the receptive communication skills to understand the physician or other QHP if he or she were to use typical language for communication

Add-on code **90785** is reported when interactive complexity complicates delivery of psychiatric services, including diagnostic psychiatric evaluation (**90791, 90792**), psychotherapy (**90832, 90834, 90837**), psychotherapy when performed with an E/M service (**90833, 90836, 90838**), and group psychotherapy (**90853**).

- Interactive complexity indicates an *increased complexity of work* as opposed to an extended duration of services.
- Interactive complexity is not billed in conjunction with psychotherapy for crisis (**90839, 90840**).

- Interactive complexity applies only to the psychiatric portion of a service including both psychiatric and E/M components. Code **90785** is never reported alone and is not reported in conjunction with E/M services alone.
- Do not report code **90785** in conjunction with adaptive behavior treatment (**97153–97158**; **0373T**).

Examples

➤ **A 10-year-old patient undergoes psychiatric evaluation.** The child is accompanied by separated parents, reporting the child has recently demonstrated significant anxiety when leaving either or both parents. The child's teachers report that the child appears to feign illness and seek reasons to contact a parent during the school day. The parents are extremely anxious and repeatedly ask questions about the treatment process. Each parent continually challenges the other's observations of the patient.

Codes **90791** (psychiatric diagnostic evaluation) and **90785** (interactive complexity) are reported.

➤ **A 6-year-old girl is seen for psychotherapy.** The child was placed in foster care following hospitalization for head injuries sustained due to physical abuse and neglect by her mother and the mother's boyfriend. The service includes the psychologist's review of the child's medical record and telephone interviews with the child's social worker and teacher. The mother refuses a request for interview. The psychologist interviews the foster mother, who expresses concerns that the child is grieving the loss of contact with 2 half-siblings who are in their father's custody and is fearful of making emotional connections with her foster parents. The psychologist uses play to gain trust and evaluate the child. The psychologist and foster mother agree on a treatment plan and then discuss the plan with the child in terms she can understand. Following the service, the psychologist provides a report to the patient's social worker.

Codes **90791** (psychiatric diagnostic evaluation) and **90785** (interactive complexity) are reported.

Psychiatric Diagnostic Evaluation

90791   Psychiatric diagnostic evaluation
90792   Psychiatric diagnostic evaluation with medical services

Psychiatric diagnostic evaluation (**90791**) and psychiatric diagnostic evaluation with medical services (**90792**) include an integrated biopsychosocial assessment, including history, mental status, and recommendations. When medical services (ie, medical assessments and physical examination other than mental status, when indicated) are included, code **90792** is reported.

- Psychiatric diagnostic evaluation or reevaluation (**90791**, **90792**) is reported once per day. Do not report psychotherapy codes (**90832–90839**) on the same date of service as **90791** or **90792**.
- The same individual may not separately report E/M services on the same date as psychiatric diagnostic evaluation.
- Report code **90785** for interactive complexity in addition to code **90791** or **90792**, when applicable.

Health plans may not cover mental health consultation, testing, or evaluation that is performed to assess custody, visitation, or parental rights.

- **Verify health plan contractual obligations prior to providing services that may lack medical necessity and determine if a waiver of liability must be signed by the patient(s) prior to beginning the service.**
- **A waiver of liability (similar to Medicare's advance beneficiary notice) is the patient's agreement to pay out of pocket for services not covered by his or her health plan.**
- **Modifier GA (waiver of liability statement issued as required by payer policy, individual case) may be appended to the code reported to indicate the waiver is on file.**

When services are requested for purposes that a health plan may not consider medically necessary, failure to obtain the responsible party's signature on a waiver of liability _prior to the service_ may release the patient from the obligation to pay based on contractual agreement between the provider and health plan.

Examples

➤ **A 14-year-old girl is referred by her primary care pediatrician for evaluation and treatment of depression with suicidal ideation.** The psychologist obtains information on the presenting problem and situation. A statement of need and expectations is documented. Current symptoms and behaviors are documented. The patient has no history of previous psychiatric treatment. The patient denies previous substance use treatment and current use of alcohol or drugs. Her current medication regimen of fluoxetine 10 mg once a day is documented. She has no current medical problems and is not allergic to any medications. The patient's family and social status (current and historical), school status/functioning, and resources are obtained and documented. A diagnosis of moderate major depressive disorder, single episode, and parent-child relationship problem is documented.

   Code **90791** is reported in conjunction with *ICD-10-CM* codes **F32.1** (major depressive disorder, single episode, moderate) and **Z63.8**, other specified problems related to primary support group.

➤ **A 15-year-old girl was admitted through the emergency department (ED) following a suicide attempt.** The girl is evaluated by a psychiatrist for admission to inpatient psychiatric care. The psychiatrist performs a psychiatric diagnostic evaluation of this patient, who previously attempted suicide at age 13 years and has a history of recurrent major depressive disorder. The patient also expresses fear that she may be pregnant and has been exposed to a sexually transmitted infection. Medical history includes nausea with vomiting for the last week and last menstrual period 6 weeks ago. Laboratory tests are ordered to rule out pregnancy and/or infection, and consultation with a gynecologist is ordered. Diagnoses are severe major depressive disorder without psychosis (**F33.2**), nausea with vomiting (**R11**), and pregnancy test, unconfirmed (**Z72.40**).

   Code **90792** is reported for combined psychiatric and medical evaluations.

➤ **A 17-year-old girl wishes to be evaluated for purposes of determining her ability to accept responsibility for herself.** The girl is seeking emancipation from her mother, who is currently living with an abusive boyfriend and will not allow her to move in with her aunt while finishing high school. An attorney has advised obtaining a psychological evaluation to support the girl's claims that she is psychologically prepared to take this action. The girl's health plan considers this service not medically necessary but allows for patient payment when a waiver of liability is obtained prior to the service. She agrees to sign the waiver and pay for the service. An evaluation is completed, and a report of the evaluation is provided to the girl and her attorney.

   The service is reported to the health plan with modifier **GA** (waiver of liability statement issued as required by payer policy, individual case) appended to code **90791**.

Psychotherapy

CPT defines *psychotherapy* as the treatment of mental illness and behavioral disturbances in which the physician or QHP, through definitive therapeutic communications, attempts to alleviate the emotional disturbances, reverse or change maladaptive patterns of behavior, and encourage personality growth and development.

Progress notes for psychotherapy services should include

- **Start and stop times of psychotherapy**
- **Service type**
- **Diagnosis**
- **Interval history (eg, increase/decrease in symptoms, current risk factors)**
- **Names and scores of standardized rating scales used in monitoring progress**
- **Therapeutic interventions (eg, type of therapy, medications)**
- **Summary of goals and progress**
- **An updated treatment plan**
- **Date and signature of performing provider**

These elements should be documented in the progress note in the patient record rather than the protected psychotherapy notes. Protected psychotherapy notes *are not disclosed* for purposes of receiving or supporting accurate payment.

- Services include ongoing assessment and adjustment of psychotherapeutic interventions and may include involvement of informants in the treatment process.
- Codes differentiate psychotherapy services to individuals (with and without E/M services), an individual family or groups of families, and groups of patients. Codes for each are provided in the following discussions.
- Separate codes (**90839, 90840**) are reported for psychotherapy for crisis (see the Psychotherapy for Crisis section later in this chapter).

  Pertinent instructions for coding for all psychotherapy services are
- Psychotherapy times are for face-to-face services with a patient and/or family member. The patient must be present for all or some of the service except when reporting family psychotherapy without the patient present (**90846**). This allows for the participation of others in the psychotherapy session for the patient as long as the patient remains the focus of the intervention. Documentation must support that the patient was present for a significant portion of the session.
- For psychotherapy with biofeedback, see codes **90875** and **90876** (see Psychotherapy With Biofeedback section later in this chapter).
- Psychotherapy differs from family psychotherapy (**90846, 90847**). Family psychotherapy uses techniques to benefit the patient (eg, attempting to improve family communication or alter family interactions that negatively affect the patient; encouraging interactions to improve family functioning). Family psychotherapy includes sessions with the entire family as well as sessions that may not include the patient.
- In reporting, choose the code closest to the actual time (**Table 14-3**). Do not report psychotherapy of less than 16 minutes' duration.
- Do not report psychotherapy codes in conjunction with codes for adaptive behavior assessment or treatment services (**97153–97158, 0362T, 0373T**).
- Psychotherapy of more than 45 minutes is often considered unusual and may require health plan precertification.

Table 14-3. Reporting Psychotherapy Services	
Duration of Psychotherapy	*CPT* **Codes**
<16 min	Do not report.
16–37 min	**90832, 90833**
38–52 min	**90834, 90836**
53–89 min	**90837, 90838**
≥26 min	**90846, 90847**
Abbreviation: *CPT, Current Procedural Terminology.*	

Psychotherapy With Evaluation and Management

+**90833**   Psychotherapy, 30 minutes with patient when performed with an evaluation and management service
+**90836**   45 minutes with patient when performed with an evaluation and management service
+**90838**   60 minutes with patient when performed with an evaluation and management service

Psychiatrists and other physicians who provide a combination of psychotherapy and E/M services (eg, **99213**) on the same date may report an E/M code and an add-on code for psychotherapy (**90833, 90836, 90838**).

- To report both E/M and psychotherapy, the 2 services must be significant and separately identifiable.
- Time may not be used as the basis of E/M code selection. Evaluation and management code selection must be based on the level of key components of history, examination, and medical decision-making (MDM), *or MDM alone in the case of office and other outpatient E/M services,* when reported in conjunction with psychotherapy.
- Prolonged services *may not* be reported when psychotherapy with E/M (**90833, 90836, 90838**) is reported.

Example

➤ **An 8-year-old boy presents for psychotherapy.** The psychiatrist provides psychotherapy services with face-to-face time of 40 minutes and also provides an E/M service to reevaluate the effectiveness and patient reaction to current medications. The office E/M service includes low-complexity MDM based on the low number and complexity of problems (1 stable chronic illness) with moderate risk of morbidity of prescription drug management. Codes reported are **99213** and **90836**.

The 40 minutes of time is only the face-to-face time of psychotherapy services and does not include the time of the E/M service. Because the midpoint between 30 and 45 minutes was passed, code **90836** (45 minutes) is reported in lieu of **90833** (30 minutes). No modifier is required (eg, modifier **25**) because the add-on codes were assigned values that took into account the overlapping practice expense of the 2 services (eg, same clinical staff and examination room).

Psychotherapy Without Evaluation and Management

90832	Psychotherapy, 30 minutes with patient and/or family member
90834	45 minutes with patient and/or family member
90837	60 minutes with patient and/or family member
+90863	Pharmacologic management, including prescription and review of medication, when performed with psychotherapy services

When psychotherapy is provided without an E/M service on the same date, codes **90832**, **90834**, and **90837** are reported based on the face-to-face time of service.

● To accommodate reporting of pharmacologic management by psychologists who have prescribing privileges but who cannot provide E/M services, add-on code **90863** is reported in addition to the appropriate code for psychotherapy without E/M.

Only a psychologist with prescribing authority may provide pharmacologic management. Other QHPs may provide psychotherapy but must collaborate with a physician or advance practice professional who provides pharmacologic management.

● Physicians and QHPs providing pharmacologic management report the service with an E/M code.

● Prolonged services in the outpatient setting (**99354**, **99355**) or inpatient or observation setting (**99356**, **99357**) may be reported in addition to the psychotherapy service code **90837** when 90 minutes or longer of face-to-face time with the patient and/or family member is spent performing psychotherapy services, *which are not performed with an E/M service.*

● Code **90863** is an add-on code and may only be reported in addition to one of the stand-alone psychotherapy codes (ie, **90832**, **90834**, **90837**). Time spent providing medication management is not included in the time spent in psychotherapy.

Example

➤ **An 8-year-old boy presents for psychotherapy.** The licensed clinical psychologist (whose state scope of practice includes prescribing authority) provides psychotherapy services with face-to-face time of 40 minutes and also provides a pharmacologic management service to reevaluate the effectiveness and patient reaction to current medications. Codes reported are **90834** and **90863**.

Psychotherapy With Biofeedback

90875	Individual psychophysiological therapy incorporating biofeedback training by any modality (face-to-face with the patient), with psychotherapy (eg, insight oriented, behavior modifying or supportive psychotherapy); 30 minutes
90876	45 minutes

When psychotherapy incorporates biofeedback training, code **90875** or **90876** is reported based on the face-to-face time of the combined services. Do not separately report codes for psychotherapy (**90832–90838**) or biofeedback training (**90901**).

Example

➤ **A child with chronic pain is provided psychotherapy and biofeedback training to help her cope with and control her pain.** The face-to-face time of service is 45 minutes.

Code **90876** is reported for the combined services. Were biofeedback training provided on a date when no psychotherapy was provided, code **90901** would be reported. Time of service is not a factor in reporting code **90901**.

Psychotherapy for Crisis

90839   Psychotherapy for crisis; first 60 minutes
+90840   each additional 30 minutes (List separately in addition to code **90839**)

Psychotherapy for crisis is provided on an urgent basis to a patient requiring mobilization of resources to defuse a crisis and restore safety. It also incorporates implementation of psychotherapeutic interventions to minimize the potential for psychological trauma.

- This includes assessment and history of a crisis state, a mental status examination, and a disposition.
- The presenting problem is typically life-threatening or complex and requires immediate attention to a patient in high distress.
- Codes **90839** and **90840** are reported based on the total face-to-face time the physician or QHP spends with the patient and/or family providing psychotherapy for crisis on a single date of service. Time is cumulative for all psychotherapy for crisis on the same date even if time is not continuous.
  — Code **90839** is reported for the first 30 to 74 minutes of psychotherapy for crisis on a single date of service. For psychotherapy for crisis with face-to-face time of less than 30 minutes' duration, report individual psychotherapy codes (**90832** or **90833**).
  — Add code **90840** for each additional block of time (each 30 minutes beyond the first 74 minutes and once for up to 30 minutes of the last full 30-minute period).
- Do not report psychotherapy for crisis (**90839**, **90840**) for service of less than 30 minutes or on the same date as other psychiatry services (**90785–90899**).

Example

➤ **Parents of a 16-year-old established patient with depression and history of substance use phone his psychologist's office requesting an immediate appointment because the patient has phoned his mother at work saying he planned to kill himself.** The patient's grandfather has arrived at the patient's home to find the patient distraught and prepared to follow through with self-harm. The psychologist is consulted and speaks to the mother to determine the nature of the crisis. The parents agree to evaluation and possible inpatient admission. The psychologist meets the family in the ED of the hospital, examines the patient, obtains agreement for inpatient treatment, and makes arrangements for admission. The total face-to-face time of the encounter is 45 minutes.

Code **90839** is reported. Although the code descriptor states "first hour," the instructions for reporting psychotherapy for crisis instruct that code **90839** is reported for the first 30 to 74 minutes of face-to-face service.

Family and Group Psychotherapy

90846   Family psychotherapy (without the patient present), 50 minutes
90847   Family psychotherapy (conjoint psychotherapy) (with patient present), 50 minutes
90849   Multiple-family group psychotherapy

While family members may act as informants during individual psychotherapy, psychotherapy using family psychotherapy techniques is reported with codes **90846** and **90847** based on whether the patient is present for the service.

- Psychotherapy to a group of individual patients includes discussion of individual and/or group dynamics. Processes may include interpersonal interactions, support, emotional catharsis, and reminiscing.
- The focus of family psychotherapy is on family dynamics and/or subsystems within the family (eg, parents, siblings) and on improving the patient's functioning by working with the patient in the context of the family.
- Do not report family psychotherapy for services of fewer than 26 minutes.
- Prolonged service may also be reported in conjunction with code **90847** (family psychotherapy, 50 minutes) when 80 minutes or longer of face-to-face time with the patient and family are spent performing psychotherapy.

- Codes for individual psychotherapy (**90832–90838**) may be reported on the same day as family psychotherapy codes **90846** and **90847** when the services are separate and distinct. Append modifier **59** (distinct procedural service) to the group psychotherapy code when both services are reported on the same date.
- When multiple families participate in family psychotherapy at the same session, code **90849** is reported once for each family.

90853   Group psychotherapy (other than of a multiple-family group)

- Report code **90853** with 1 unit of service for each group member. Documentation should support the individual patient's involvement in the group session, the duration of the session, and issues that were presented.
- No time is assigned to code **90853**. This service is reported with 1 unit of service regardless of the time of service.

Other Psychiatric Services

The following services are often bundled under payer contracts (ie, considered components of other services) or non-covered. However, check plan benefits, especially for Medicaid patients, as there may be circumstances in which these services are separate benefits. Plan-specific modifiers are often required when coverage of the following services is a health plan benefit:

90882   Environmental intervention for medical management purposes on a psychiatric patient's behalf with agencies, employers, or institutions

90885   Psychiatric evaluation of hospital records, other psychiatric reports, psychometric and/or projective tests, and other accumulated data for medical diagnostic purposes

90887   Interpretation or explanation of results of psychiatric, other medical examinations and procedures, or other accumulated data to family or other responsible persons, or advising them how to assist patient

     Do not report code **90887** in conjunction with adaptive behavior services (**97151–97158**, **0362T**, **0373T**).

90889   Preparation of report of patient's psychiatric status, history, treatment, or progress (other than for legal or consultative purposes) for other individuals, agencies, or insurance carriers

     Code **90889** should not be reported in conjunction with psychological or developmental testing, as the codes for these services include time for report writing.

Evaluation and Treatment of Substance Use

The initial evaluation of a child for alcohol and/or substance use is often in the context of an E/M service. When more than 50% of the physician/QHP time with the patient is spent in counseling and/or coordinating care, E/M codes are selected based on the total face-to-face time of the service in a non-facility setting or total unit/floor time in a facility setting (eg, ED, hospital unit). Office E/M services (**99202–99205**, **99212–99215**) may be reported for the physician or other QHP's total time on the date of service, as described in **Chapter 7**.

ICD-10-CM Coding for Use, Abuse, and Dependence

The guidelines for *ICD-10-CM* offer specific guidance for reporting diagnoses of mental and behavioral disorders due to psychoactive substance use.

- Code **Z71.41** is reported as the first-listed code when an encounter is primarily focused on alcohol abuse counseling and surveillance. An additional code for alcohol abuse or dependence (**F10.-**) is additionally reported.
- Code **Z71.51** is reported as the first-listed code when an encounter is primarily for drug abuse counseling and surveillance of drug abuser. Codes for drug abuse or dependence (**F11–F16**, **F18**, or **F19**) are reported in addition to code **Z71.51**.
- The codes for psychoactive substance *use* disorders (**F10.9-**, **F11.9-**, **F12.9-**, **F13.9-**, **F14.9-**, **F15.9-**, **F16.9-**) are to be used only when the psychoactive substance use is associated with a physical, mental, or behavioral disorder and such a relationship is documented by the provider. Note that codes for inhalant use (**F18.9-**) and polysubstance or indiscriminate drug use (**F19.9-**) are not included in this instruction.
- New guidance was added for vaping or electronic nicotine delivery systems. Specifically, for vaping of nicotine, assign code **F17.29-**, nicotine dependence, other tobacco products. Electronic nicotine delivery systems are noncombustible tobacco products.
- Subcategories of codes for mental and behavioral disorders due to psychoactive substance use indicate *use* and *abuse* of and *dependence* on various psychoactive substances. These categories do not include abuse of nonpsychoactive substances such as antacids, laxatives, or steroids that are reported with category **F55**. Each subcategory offers a spectrum of use, abuse, and dependence with extended information such as *with intoxication, with withdrawal,* and *with delusions.*

- When documentation refers to use of, abuse of, and dependence on the same substance (eg, alcohol, opioid, cannabis), only 1 code should be assigned to identify the pattern of use based on the following hierarchy:
  — If both use and abuse are documented, assign only the code for abuse.
  — If both abuse and dependence are documented, assign only the code for dependence.
  — If use, abuse, and dependence are all documented, assign only the code for dependence.
  — If both use and dependence are documented, assign only the code for dependence.
- Selection of codes for mental and behavioral disorders due to psychoactive substance use for substance abuse or dependence in remission (categories **F10–F19** with **-.11**, **-.21**) requires the provider's clinical judgment. The appropriate codes for in remission are assigned only on the basis of provider documentation unless otherwise instructed by the classification.
- Mild substance use disorders in early or sustained remission are classified to the appropriate codes for substance abuse in remission, and moderate or severe substance use disorders in early or sustained remission are classified to the appropriate codes for substance dependence in remission.

Management/Treatment of Alcohol and Substance Use Disorders

Coding for management/treatment of alcohol and substance use disorders is largely payer driven. Psychotherapy codes may be applicable, or E/M codes may be selected based on time of counseling and/or coordination for ongoing counseling on alcohol and/or substance use disorders. However, many health plans and Medicaid programs require use of HCPCS codes for reporting assessments and management/treatment of alcohol and/or substance use disorders.

Examples of HCPCS codes include

H0001	Alcohol and/or drug assessment
H0005	Alcohol and/or drug services; group counseling by a clinician
H0007	Alcohol and/or drug services; crisis intervention (outpatient)
H0014	Alcohol and/or drug services; ambulatory detoxification
H0016	Alcohol and/or drug services; medical/somatic (medical intervention in ambulatory setting)
H0022	Alcohol and/or drug intervention service (planned facilitation)
H0047	Alcohol and/or other drug abuse services, not otherwise specified
T1006	Alcohol and/or substance abuse services, family/couple counseling
T1007	Alcohol and/or substance abuse services, treatment plan development and/or modification

Individual health and Medicaid plans may have different definitions for the services reported with HCPCS codes. Prior authorization of services is often required.

General behavioral health integration (GBHI) care management services (**99484**) may also be provided for substance use disorders; see the General Behavioral Health Integration Care Management section later in this chapter for a discussion.

Alcohol and/or Substance Use Screening/Testing

> Codes for findings of drugs and other substances not normally found in blood (**R78.-**) are not reported in conjunction with codes for substance use (**F10–F19**).

Presumptive Drug Class Screening

Presumptive drug class screening is typically used to identify possible use or nonuse of a drug or drug class. These tests are often used to verify compliance with treatment, identify undisclosed drug use, and monitor for relapse in patients with known use or dependence.

Urine is often the specimen used for testing in outpatient settings. *ICD-10-CM* codes for use or dependence (**F10–F19**) or counseling (eg, **Z71.51**) are often sufficient to support the need for testing. However, payer policies may vary, so it is advisable to verify each plan's policy and any coding requirements.

When the specimen used for alcohol/drug testing is blood, report *ICD-10-CM* code **Z02.83** (encounter for blood-alcohol and blood-drug test). When blood test findings are positive in a patient not diagnosed with substance use (**F10–F19**), report codes from category **R78.-** (findings of drugs and other substances, not normally found in blood) in addition to code **Z02.83**.

When findings of blood alcohol testing are positive, codes in category **Y90.-** are used to report the alcohol level. Codes in category **Y90** are reported secondary to codes for associated alcohol-related disorders. See **Table 14-4** for a listing of related codes in categories **R78** and **Y90**.

Table 14-4. *International Classification of Diseases, 10th Revision, Clinical Modification* **Abnormal Finding Drug Blood Test**	
R78.0	Finding of alcohol in blood (Use additional external cause code [**Y90.-**] for detail regarding alcohol level.)
R78.1	Finding of opiate drug in blood
R78.2	Finding of cocaine in blood
R78.3	Finding of hallucinogen in blood
R78.4	Finding of other drugs of addictive potential in blood
R78.5	Finding of other psychotropic drug in blood
R78.6	Finding of steroid agent in blood
R78.89	Finding of other specified substances, not normally found in blood
R78.9	Finding of unspecified substance, not normally found in blood
ICD-10-CM **Evidence of Alcohol Involvement Determined by Blood Alcohol Level**[a]	
Y90.0	Blood alcohol level of <20 mg/100 mL
Y90.1	Blood alcohol level of 20–39 mg/100 mL
Y90.2	Blood alcohol level of 40–59 mg/100 mL
Y90.3	Blood alcohol level of 60–79 mg/100 mL
Y90.4	Blood alcohol level of 80–99 mg/100 mL
Y90.5	Blood alcohol level of 100–119 mg/100 mL
Y90.6	Blood alcohol level of 120–199 mg/100 mL
Y90.7	Blood alcohol level of 200–239 mg/100 mL
Y90.8	Blood alcohol level of ≥240 mg/100 mL
Y90.9	Presence of alcohol in blood, level not specified

Abbreviation: *ICD-10-CM, International Classification of Diseases, 10th Revision, Clinical Modification.*

[a] Code first any associated alcohol-related disorders (**F10**).

Presumptive drug class screening includes all drugs and drug classes performed by the respective methodology (eg, dipstick kit with direct optical observation) on a single date of service. Sample validation is included in presumptive drug screening service. Venipuncture to obtain samples for drug testing may be separately reportable with code **36415** (collection of venous blood by venipuncture).

When testing is performed with a method using direct optical observation to determine the result, code **80305** is reported. Tests that have a waived status under the Clinical Laboratory Improvement Amendments may be reported with modifier **QW** (waived test).

80305   Drug test(s), presumptive, any number of drug classes, any number of devices or procedures; capable of being read by direct optical observation only (eg, utilizing immunoassay [eg, dipsticks, cups, cards, or cartridges]), includes sample validation when performed, per date of service

When a reader is used to determine the result of testing (eg, a dipstick is inserted into a machine that determines the final reading), code **80306** is reported.

80306   read by instrument assisted direct optical observation (eg, utilizing immunoassay [eg, dipsticks, cups, cards, or cartridges]), includes sample validation when performed, per date of service

Testing that uses a chemistry analyzer or more effort than tests represented by codes **80305** and **80306** is reported with code **80307**.

International Classification of Diseases, 10th Revision, Clinical Modification code **F40.231** (fear of injections and transfusions) may be used for patients who have a phobia of needles.

80307   by instrument chemistry analyzers (eg, utilizing immunoassay [eg, EIA, ELISA, EMIT, FPIA, IA, KIMS, RIA]), chromatography (eg, GC, HPLC), and mass spectrometry either with or without chromatography, (eg, DART, DESI, GC-MS, GC-MS/MS, LC-MS, LC-MS/MS, LDTD, MALDI, TOF); includes sample validation when performed, per date of service

Some plans require use of HCPCS codes for reporting alcohol/drug screening or testing. Code **H0048** allows for reporting of the collection and handling of specimens other than blood for alcohol and/or drug testing. Code **H0003** is used to report the analysis of a screening test for alcohol and/or drugs.

H0003   Alcohol and/or drug screening; laboratory analysis of specimens for presence of alcohol and/or drugs

H0048   Alcohol and/or other drug testing: collection and handling only, specimens other than blood

Examples

➤ **A psychologist is consulted by an ED physician to evaluate and recommend treatment options for an intoxicated 17-year-old patient who presented with a scalp laceration.** Although not notably intoxicated at the encounter, the patient admits to alcohol dependence since age 14 years and intoxication on arrival to the ED. His blood alcohol level on admission was 22 mg/100 mL. The psychologist recommends treatment for alcoholism through a local community health center. The documented diagnosis is alcohol dependence with intoxication.

   ICD-10-CM codes reported are **F10.229** (alcohol dependence with intoxication, unspecified) and **Y90.1** (blood alcohol level of 20–39 mg/100 mL).

➤ **A patient who is dependent on cannabis is seen in follow-up.** A urine sample is tested for the presence of drugs and the result is negative. The patient's diagnosis is cannabis dependence, in remission.

   Codes **Z02.83** (encounter for blood-alcohol and blood-drug test) and **F12.21** (cannabis dependence, in remission) are reported.

Definitive Drug Testing

When necessary to identify specific drugs or metabolites, a definitive drug test may be ordered. Definitive drug identification methods identify individual drugs and distinguish between structural isomers but not necessarily stereoisomers. Definitive drug tests are reported with codes **80320–80373** based on drug classes (eg, alcohol[s] or non-opioid analgesics) as identified in the Definitive Drug Classes Listing in the Pathology and Laboratory section of *CPT* references.

Behavioral Health Integration

Behavioral health integration includes PCCM and GBHI. These services are differentiated by the required elements of service. Psychiatric collaborative care management services (**99492–99494**) include a defined team of health care professionals providing care using a specific care method. General behavioral health integration (**99484**) services do not include specific types of providers or a specified method of delivery.

Psychiatric Collaborative Care Management Services

99492   Initial psychiatric collaborative care management, first 70 minutes in the first calendar month of behavioral health care manager activities, in consultation with a psychiatric consultant, and directed by the treating physician or other qualified health care professional, with the following required elements:
- outreach to and engagement in treatment of a patient directed by the treating physician or other qualified health care professional;
- initial assessment of the patient, including administration of validated rating scales, with the development of an individualized treatment plan;
- review by the psychiatric consultant with modifications of the plan if recommended;
- entering patient in a registry and tracking patient follow-up and progress using the registry, with appropriate documentation, and participation in weekly caseload consultation with the psychiatric consultant; and
- provision of brief interventions using evidence-based techniques such as behavioral activation, motivational interviewing, and other focused treatment strategies.

99493   Subsequent psychiatric collaborative care management, first 60 minutes in a subsequent month of behavioral health care manager activities, in consultation with a psychiatric consultant, and directed by the treating physician or other qualified health care professional, with the following required elements:
- tracking patient follow-up and progress using the registry, with appropriate documentation;
- participation in weekly caseload consultation with the psychiatric consultant;
- ongoing collaboration with and coordination of the patient's mental health care with the treating physician or other qualified health care professional and any other treating mental health providers;
- additional review of progress and recommendations for changes in treatment, as indicated, including medications, based on recommendations provided by the psychiatric consultant;

- provision of brief interventions using evidence-based techniques such as behavioral activation, motivational interviewing, and other focused treatment strategies;
- monitoring of patient outcomes using validated rating scales; and
- relapse prevention planning with patients as they achieve remission of symptoms and/or other treatment goals and are prepared for discharge from active treatment.

+99494   Initial or subsequent psychiatric collaborative care management, each additional 30 minutes in a calendar month of behavioral health care manager activities, in consultation with a psychiatric consultant, and directed by the treating physician or other qualified health care professional (List separately in addition to code for primary procedure)

       (Use **99494** in conjunction with **99492**, **99493**)

Psychiatric collaborative care management includes use of validated rating scales in monitoring patient outcomes. Do not separately report use of standardized rating scales (eg, **96127**).

Psychiatric collaborative care management services are reported by a supervising physician or QHP for services by a behavioral health care manager (BHM) working under the supervision of the reporting physician or QHP. Psychiatric collaborative care management services are provided to patients who have a new or existing psychiatric disorder that requires a behavioral health assessment; care plan implementation, revision, or monitoring; and provision of brief interventions. The treating physician or QHP reports codes **99492–99494** when all requirements for reporting are met. Evaluation and management and other services may be reported separately by the same physician or QHP during the same calendar month.

Each team member's role is defined in *CPT* as follows:

- The treating physician or QHP
  - Directs the BHM and continues to oversee the patient's care, including prescribing medications, providing treatments for medical conditions, and making referrals to specialty care when needed.
  - Engages the services of the psychiatric consultant who does not directly bill for PCCM services (ie, the treating physician's or QHP's practice contracts with the psychiatric consultant for this component of the PCCM service).
  - Acts in a supervisory role to the BHM (may be a direct employee or contractual employee but should represent a practice expense like other clinical staff and QNHCPs).
  - May personally perform behavioral health care management activities. When those activities are not used to meet criteria for a separately reported service (eg, office E/M), his or her time may be counted toward the required time for PCCM.
  - Is ultimately responsible for delivery, documentation, and billing of PCCM services in compliance with *CPT* and payer policies.
- The BHM is a QNHCP or clinical staff member with master- or doctoral-level education *or* specialized training in behavioral health who provides behavioral health care management services under the treating physician's or QHP's supervision and in consultation with a psychiatric consultant. The BHM provides the following services, as needed:
  - Assessment of needs including the administration of validated rating scales.
  - Development of a care plan.
  - Provision of brief face-to-face and non–face-to-face interventions.
  - Ongoing collaboration with the treating physician or QHP.
  - Consultation with the psychiatric consultant at least weekly (typically non–face-to-face).
  - Maintenance of a registry.
  - May also provide and report other services (within BHM's scope of practice) in the same calendar month as PCCM. These may include psychiatric diagnosis, psychotherapy, smoking and tobacco use cessation counseling (**99406**, **99407**), and alcohol and/or substance use structured screening and brief intervention services (**99408**, **99409**).
- The psychiatric consultant is a medical professional trained in psychiatry or behavioral health *and qualified to prescribe a full range of medications.* The psychiatric consultant typically does not see the patient or prescribe medications, except in rare circumstances. The psychiatric consultant advises and makes recommendations to the treating physician or QHP (typically via consultation with the BHM). The psychiatric consultant's services include recommending the following services, as needed:
  - Psychiatric and other medical differential diagnosis.
  - Treatment strategies addressing appropriate therapies.
  - Medication management.
  - Medical management of complications associated with treatment of psychiatric disorders.
  - Referral for specialty services.
  - The psychiatric consultant may directly provide and separately report E/M or psychiatric services, such as psychiatric evaluation (**90791**, **90792**), to a patient within a calendar month when the same patient receives PCCM services.

Chapter 14. Mental and Behavioral Health Services

Reporting requirements for PCCM services include

- Time of service is met when the midpoint is passed. Documentation must support provision of PCCM services for the required time.

    When service time does not meet the midpoint (ie, 36 minutes for **99492**, 31 minutes for **99493**, 16 minutes beyond last full period for **99494**), do no report PCCM.

- Services are provided for an episode of care defined as beginning when the treating physician or QHP directs the patient to the BHM and ending with
    - The attainment of targeted treatment goals, which typically results in the discontinuation of care management services and continuation of usual follow-up with the treating physician or other QHP
    - Failure to attain targeted treatment goals culminating in referral to a psychiatric care provider for ongoing treatment
    - Lack of continued engagement with no PCCM services provided over a consecutive 6-month calendar period (break in episode)

- A new episode of care starts after a break in episode of 6 calendar months or more.

- Medical necessity of PCCM services may be supported by documentation such as
    - A newly diagnosed condition
    - A patient's need for help engaging in treatment
    - A patient who has not responded to standard care delivered in a nonpsychiatric setting or who requires further assessment and engagement prior to consideration of referral to a psychiatric care setting

        These are typical patient scenarios. Other reasons for services may support medical necessity.

- Documentation of the patient's behavioral health conditions, psychosocial needs, and other factors influencing patient care may help support the necessity of services when health plans implement specific coverage criteria and/or prior authorization for PCCM services.

    Psychiatric collaborative care management services do not require establishment of a care plan for *all* the patient's health care needs. The services are directed to behavioral health needs. Patients may or may not have comorbid conditions that affect treatment and management.

- Psychiatric collaborative care management services may be reported in the same month as CCM services (**99487**, **99489–99491**) when the requirements for each service are met without overlap.

- Provision of PCCM services may support quality initiatives such as use of an electronic clinical data system to track care and administration of a validated rating scale (eg, depression screening instrument) during a 4-month period for patients diagnosed with major depression or dysthymia.

Example

➤ **A pediatrician orders PCCM services for a 15-year-old patient diagnosed with moderate depression, single episode.** A licensed clinical psychologist acting as the BHM discusses PCCM services with the patient and perform an initial assessment. Standardized assessment instruments are used in the assessment and a treatment plan including psychotherapy is agreed on. Later, the BHM enters the patient information into a registry that will be used to track medication compliance and progress. At a regularly scheduled conference call between the BHM and a consulting psychiatrist the patient's assessment is reviewed and the treatment plan approved. The supervising pediatrician is also consulted and approves the treatment plan. The BHM, whose scope of practice includes psychotherapy, provides 3 separately reportable individual psychotherapy sessions within the calendar month in addition to PCCM services. During the calendar month, the BHM documents 60 minutes of time spent in PCCM services.

ICD-10-CM	CPT
F32.1 (major depressive disorder, single episode, moderate)	**99492** (initial month PCCM service, first 70 minutes)
	90832, **90834**, or **90837** (psychotherapy without E/M based on time of service; 30, 45, or 60 minutes)

Teaching Point: Time of service for PCCM services is met when the midpoint is passed. In this example, the 60 minutes spent by the BHM supports reporting of code **99492**, which includes the first 70 minutes of PCCM services in the initial month of service.

Psychotherapy services may be reported on a separate claim prior to fulfilling the time requirement for PCCM. No time spent in provision of psychotherapy may be attributed to the time of PCCM services. If psychotherapy services were not within the scope of practice for the BHM, the patient might be referred to another provider (eg, the consulting psychiatrist), who would report the services rendered.

General Behavioral Health Integration Care Management

#99484   Care management services for behavioral health conditions, at least 20 minutes of clinical staff time, directed by a physician or other qualified health care professional, per calendar month, with the following required elements:
- Initial assessment or follow-up monitoring, including the use of applicable validated rating scales;
- Behavioral health care planning in relation to behavioral/psychiatric health problems, including revision for patients who are not progressing or whose status changes;
- Facilitating and coordinating treatment such as psychotherapy, pharmacotherapy, counseling and/or psychiatric consultation; and
- Continuity of care with a designated member of the care team

General behavioral health integration care management (**99484**) is reported by a physician or QHP for supervision of clinical staff who provide at least 20 minutes of GBHI services within a calendar month to a patient with a behavioral health condition (includes substance use). A treatment plan must be documented and address the patient's behavioral health condition(s), but a comprehensive health care plan is not required. General behavioral health integration is an outpatient service.

Clinical staff providing GBHI services are not required to have qualifications that would permit them to separately report services (eg, psychotherapy), but, if qualified and they perform such services, they may report such services separately. The time of the separately reported service is not used to support reporting **99484**.

Services must be provided under general physician supervision and in accordance with the licensing and scope of practice requirements of the state where services are provided. The individual supervising and reporting GBHI care management services must be able to report E/M services.

All the required elements of service listed in the code descriptor must be provided and documented.

Example

➤ **A 15-year-old presents to the primary care pediatrician with vague complaints of stomachaches, fatigue, excessive sleep, and atypically poor grades.** The primary care physician diagnoses the patient with a behavioral health disorder and recommends that the patient receive behavioral health care management as part of the treatment plan. Clinical staff provide behavioral health care planning and coordination of care with a psychologist in another practice as directed by the pediatrician. At least 20 minutes of clinical staff time is documented for contact with the patient and psychologist throughout the calendar month to assess progress using standardized rating scales and coordinating care, including facilitating access to community resources, as needed.

If clinical staff time of fewer than 20 minutes is documented in a calendar month, code **99484** is not reported. Code **99484** does not include requirements for a BHM or collaboration with a psychiatrist.

- *Use of validated rating scales is required and is not separately reported* (ie, do not report code **96127** for rating scales administered during the period of behavioral health care management services).
- Time may be face-to-face but more typically may be non–face-to-face. Clinical staff must be available to provide face-to-face services to the patient when requested.
- Evaluation and management and/or psychiatric services may be reported on the same date or in the same calendar month as GBHI services when performed, but these services cannot be used to support reporting of GBHI (ie, time of separately reported services is not counted toward the time of GBHI services).
- General behavioral health integration (**99484**) may be reported in the same month as CCM services (**99487, 99489–99491**) when the requirements for each service are met without overlap.
- The reporting individual may personally provide GBHI services and combine the time of service with that of clinical staff to support reporting code **99484**. However, the time of services that are separately reported (eg, 15 minutes spent providing an E/M service reported with code **99213**) cannot be included in the time supporting **99484**.
- General behavioral health integration (**99484**) and PCCM (**99492–99494**) may not be reported by the same provider in the same month.

- Clinical staff time spent coordinating care with the ED may be reported using **99484**, but time spent while the patient is an inpatient or is admitted to observation status may not be reported using **99484**.

Resources

AAP Policy Statement

"Addressing Early Childhood Emotional and Behavioral Problems" (https://pediatrics.aappublications.org/content/138/6/e20163023)

Payment/Denial Advocacy

AAP Hassle Factor Form (www.aap.org/en-us/professional-resources/practice-transformation/getting-paid/Pages/Hassle-Factor-Form-Concerns-with-Payers.aspx; AAP members only)

AAP Pediatric Councils (www.aap.org/en-us/professional-resources/practice-transformation/getting-paid/Pages/aap-pediatric-councils.aspx)

Test Your Knowledge!

1. **Which of the following is true of billing for mental and behavioral health services?**
   a. A qualified nonphysician health care professional may directly provide and report any mental or behavioral health service.
   b. Health plans always pay for both evaluation and management and mental health services provided in the same group practice on the same date.
   c. All payers deny medical claims appropriately reported with codes **F01–F99**.
   d. Services may be covered under a provider network separate from other health services.

2. **What *Current Procedural Terminology* codes are reported for 125 minutes of time spent in developmental testing with interpretation and report?**
   a. **96112** × 2
   b. **96112, 96113** (1 unit each)
   c. **96112, 96113** × 2
   d. **96112, 96113** × 3

3. **True or false? A physician who administers a single neuropsychological test that has multiple subtests may report code 96136 and, when applicable, 96137.**
   a. True
   b. False

4. **Which is true of code 97155 but not 0373T?**
   a. A physician or other qualified health care professional provides face-to-face care to a single patient.
   b. The service includes 4 required components.
   c. The service is provided to a patient who exhibits destructive behavior.
   d. The service environment is customized to the patient's behavior.

5. **Which of the following is not true for a physician reporting psychiatric collaborative care management (PCCM) services (99492–99494)?**
   a. Must have an arrangement for the services of a psychiatric consultant
   b. Must provide supervision of a behavioral health manager
   c. May include his/her time personally spent providing PCCM services in code selection
   d. Must be a psychiatrist

Part 3
Primarily for Hospital Settings

Part 3. Primarily for Hospital Settings

CHAPTER 15

Hospital Care of the Newborn

Contents

Perinatal Care

This chapter focuses on coding for care of the typical newborn and those with conditions not requiring intensive monitoring or critical care.

The American Academy of Pediatrics (AAP) Section on Neonatal-Perinatal Medicine, in conjunction with state chapters and councils of the AAP, has developed strategies that have been successful in addressing payment concerns for neonatal care. Contact your state chapter, its pediatric council, your section district AAP Executive Committee representative, a neonatal trainer, or the AAP Committee on Coding and Nomenclature for assistance in addressing any payment inequities for neonatal services in your state.

Definitions of the Perinatal and Neonatal Periods

For coding purposes, the *perinatal period* commences at 32 completed weeks of gestation through the 28th day following birth (the World Health Organization definition). Based on this definition, the *neonatal period* begins at birth and continues through *the completed 28th day after birth*, ending on the 29th calendar day after birth. The day of birth is considered day 0 (zero). Therefore, the day after birth is considered day 1. This definition is important for selecting the correct diagnosis code for conditions that originate in the perinatal period. (It is also important for selection of codes for neonatal critical care and initial intensive care.)

Attendance at Delivery and Newborn Resuscitation

99464   Attendance at delivery (when requested by the delivering physician or other qualified health care professional) and initial stabilization of newborn

99465   Delivery/birthing room resuscitation, provision of positive pressure ventilation and/or chest compressions in the presence of acute inadequate ventilation and/or cardiac output

Code **99464** is not reported when hospital-mandated attendance is the only underlying basis for providing the service. When physician on-call services are mandated by the hospital (eg, attending all repeat cesarean deliveries) and not physician requested, report code **99026** (hospital-mandated on-call service; in hospital, each hour) or **99027** (hospital-mandated on-call service; out of hospital, each hour). Refer to **Table 15-1** for coding examples.

> See chapters 16 and 18 for guidelines for codes **99026** and **99027**.
>
> Standby services requiring prolonged attendance, each 30 minutes (**99360**), are *not* reported in addition to attendance at delivery (**99464**) but *may be* reported with the newborn resuscitation services (**99465**) per *Current Procedural Terminology®* guidelines.

Attendance at delivery (**99464**)

- Service is only reported when requested by the delivering physician and indicated for a newborn who may require immediate intervention (ie, stabilization, resuscitation, or evaluation for potential problems).
- Medical record documentation must include the request for attendance at the delivery and substantiate the medical necessity of the services performed. If there is no documentation by the delivering physician for attendance at delivery, the verbal request and the reason for the request should be documented in the attendance note.
- Includes initial drying, stimulation, suctioning, blow-by oxygen, or continuous positive airway pressure or high-flow air/oxygen without positive-pressure ventilation (PPV); a cursory visual inspection of the neonate; assignment of Apgar scores; and discussion of the care of the newborn with the delivering physician and parents. A quick look into the delivery room or examination after stabilization is not sufficient to report **99464**.
- Any *medically necessary* procedures to complete the resuscitation that are provided in the delivery room may be reported separately (eg, direct laryngoscopy without intubation). Procedures performed solely due to hospital protocol (eg, protocol for arterial or venous catheterization prior to admission to the neonatal intensive care unit [NICU]) would not be separately reported.
- May be reported in addition to initial normal newborn (**99460**), initial sick newborn (**99221–99223**), initial intensive care of the neonate (**99477**), or critical care (**99468**; **99291, 99292**) codes.

> See Chapter 16 for guidelines for coding intensive or critical care services.

Table 15-1. Coding Examples for Attendance at Delivery	
Code(s)	**Example**
99464 and **99460**	A physician is called at the request of an obstetrician to stand by during a delivery and spends 30 minutes waiting for the delivery (**99464**) before the physician attends the delivery of a typical newborn and admits the newborn to her service (**99460**).
99464	A neonatologist is asked to be present at delivery by the delivering physician. The neonatologist documents a comprehensive examination of the neonate, in addition to the maternal and fetal history, and provides all the elements required for reporting of attendance at delivery. The neonate is typical and admitted to the newborn nursery under the orders of the general pediatrician.
	Although a history and examination were performed, this does not equate to initial hospital care of the newborn, which is reported by the attending physician who provides a comprehensive history and examination, orders screening tests and prophylactic interventions, and counsels the family on topics such as newborn feeding, sleep, and safety.

When qualifying resuscitative efforts including PPV are provided to a neonate with respiratory or cardiac instability, code **99465** (delivery/birthing room resuscitation) is reported instead of **99464**. Codes **99464** and **99465** *cannot be* reported on the same day of service. See **Chapter 18** for more information on attendance at delivery with neonatal resuscitation.

Coding Conundrum: What Service Can Be Reported When a Physician Arrives After Delivery?

There are no specific time requirements for reporting attendance at delivery. Remember, this service requires a request for attendance at delivery by the delivering physician and includes physician work to perform the initial drying, stimulation, suctioning, blow-by oxygen, or continuous positive airway pressure without positive-pressure ventilation; a cursory visual inspection of the neonate; assignment of Apgar scores; and discussion of the care of the newborn with the delivering physician and parents. When a physician arrives in the delivery room after the delivery and some or all this work has been performed, should attendance at delivery be reported? Physicians might want to consider

- When the newborn continues to require intervention or stabilization in the delivery room, code **99464** (attendance at delivery) may be reported if the physician work and medical necessity are related to the delivery and are not a component of a sick, intensive, or critical admission, and the nature of the intervention is documented in the medical record.
- When the work provided in the delivery room is related more to the initial hospital care (eg, neonate is examined and the physician sends the neonate to the well-baby nursery), only the initial normal newborn care code (**99460**) is reported.

    For example, attendance at delivery was requested by the delivering physician and the physician arrives after the delivery.

- The 1-minute Apgar score has been assigned and the neonate has been dried, stimulated, and suctioned by the nurses and is ready to be sent to the newborn nursery by the time the pediatrician appears in the delivery room. The delivering physician acknowledges that assistance is no longer needed. The attending pediatrician will report initial normal newborn care (**99460**) after completing the initial examination of the newborn. However, if the pediatrician is not the attending pediatrician, no service can be reported.
- In the previous example, the delivering physician wants continued assistance. The pediatrician assigns the 5-minute Apgar score, performs a cursory examination, and discusses the care of the newborn with the delivering physician and parents. Code **99464** can be reported because most of the basic elements of the attendance at delivery were performed and documented in the medical record.

    A stillborn neonate for whom unsuccessful resuscitation services are provided will be billed to the mother's insurer.

    A stillborn neonate examined after birth at the request of the obstetrician should be reported on the mother's insurance as a consultation, with a report sent to the obstetrician.

Normal Newborn Care

99460	Initial hospital or birthing center care, per day, for evaluation and management of normal newborn infant
99461	Initial care, per day, for evaluation and management of normal newborn infant seen in other than hospital or birthing center
99462	Subsequent hospital care, per day, for evaluation and management of normal newborn
99463	Initial hospital or birthing center care, per day, for evaluation and management of normal newborn infant admitted and discharged on the same date
99238	Hospital discharge day management; 30 minutes or less
99239	more than 30 minutes

A *normal newborn* may be defined as a newborn who

- Transitions to life in the usual manner
- May require delivery room intervention but is normal after transition
- May require some testing or monitoring (eg, bilirubin, complete blood cell count [CBC], culture)
- Does not require significant intervention
- May be observed for illness but is not sick
- May be late preterm but requires no special care
- May be in house with sick mother/twin

Codes **99460**, **99462**, **99463**, **99238**, and **99239** are used to report evaluation and management (E/M) services provided to the healthy newborn in a health care facility such as a hospital (including birthing room deliveries) or birthing center. They are reported when the neonate is cared for in the mother's room (rooming-in), a labor and delivery room, a postpartum floor, or a traditional newborn nursery and when a normal neonate is cared for after the mother is discharged (eg, awaiting adoption).

> Normal newborn codes can be reported for care provided to neonates who are acting normally but recovering from fetal stress or a low Apgar score or who are being observed for a potential problem but are asymptomatic.

Guidelines for reporting include

- The neonate is considered admitted at the time of leaving the delivery room. There is no code for observation of a newborn.
- Code **99463** (history and examination of the normal newborn, including discharge) should be reported when an initial history and physical examination and the discharge management are performed *on the same calendar date* for a normal newborn.

  Do not report **99463** when discharge occurs on the next calendar date even if less than 24 hours have passed since the initial newborn care.
- Code **99460** (history and examination of the normal newborn, initial service) is reported only once on the first day that the physician provides a face-to-face service in the facility. This date may not necessarily correlate with the date the patient is born or the hospital admission date.
- Code **99462** (subsequent hospital care, normal newborn) is reported once per calendar date on the date(s) subsequent to the initial normal newborn care service but *not* on the discharge date.
- Discharge management services performed on a day subsequent to initial newborn care are reported with code **99238** (hospital discharge day management; 30 minutes or less) or **99239** (hospital discharge day management; more than 30 minutes) when discharging a normal newborn.

  Include time spent in final examination of the patient, discussion of the hospital stay, instructions for continuing care, and preparation of discharge records, prescriptions, and referral forms. Time must be documented when reporting **99239**.

> Discharge day management codes 99238 and 99239 are valued (2.06 and 3.02 total facility relative value units [RVUs]) to include the physician's time and work such as counseling parents about care of the neonate that is not captured by 99462, subsequent newborn hospital care (1.19 total facility RVUs).

- Any additional procedures (eg, circumcision) should be reported in addition to normal newborn care codes. Modifier **25** (significant, separately identifiable E/M service) should be appended to the E/M code when a procedure is performed on the same day of service.

  When reporting an E/M service based on time (eg, discharge day management), do not include the time spent in relation to a separately reported service (eg, circumcision) in the time of the E/M service.

ICD-10-CM Codes for Newborn Services

International Classification of Diseases, 10th Revision, Clinical Modification (ICD-10-CM) codes from category **Z38** are used to report live-born neonates according to type of birth and are the first-listed codes for care by the attending or admitting physician during the entire birth admission. Other physicians providing care during the birth admission do not report **Z38** codes but instead report codes for the conditions managed at each encounter. Category **Z38** codes for a single live-born infant are shown in **Table 15-2**.

See the *ICD-10-CM* manual for **Z38** codes for multiple-birth neonates.

●=New code   ▲=Revised code   #=Re-sequenced code   +=Add-on code

Chapter 15. Hospital Care of the Newborn

Report *ICD-10-CM* code **Z76.2** (encounter for health supervision and care of other healthy infant and child) when a healthy newborn continues to receive daily visits pending discharge of the mother, adoption, or for other reasons. Code **Z76.2** is useful for indicating the reason for an extended stay of a healthy newborn.

Table 15-2. *International Classification of Diseases, 10th Revision, Clinical Modification Codes for Single Live-born Neonates*	
Z38.00	Single liveborn infant, delivered vaginally
Z38.01	Single liveborn infant, delivered by cesarean
Z38.1	Single liveborn infant, born outside hospital
Z38.2	Single liveborn infant, unspecified as to place of birth

Examples

➤ **The physician is not present at a repeat cesarean delivery of a healthy term boy.** The nursery calls the office and relates that the newborn has been admitted and seems fine. The physician's standing admission orders are followed, and the physician examines the newborn the following morning. The physician reviews the record, examines the neonate, and speaks with the mother. The newborn and mother remain in the hospital 2 additional days, when both are then discharged home. Discharge management takes 25 minutes.

ICD-10-CM	Diagnosis code for all days **Z38.01** (single liveborn by cesarean section)
Current Procedural Terminology (CPT)	**Day 1:** No charge (no face-to-face services provided) **Day 2: 99460** (initial normal newborn care) **Day 3: 99462** (subsequent normal newborn care) **Day 4: 99238** (hospital discharge day management; 30 minutes or less)

➤ **A baby is born vaginally in the hospital on March 3 at 9:00 am.** The pediatrician first sees the baby on March 4 at 7:00 am and, later the same date, determines that the newborn is ready for discharge. A history and examination of the newborn, discussion of the hospital stay with the parents, instructions for continuing care, family counseling, and preparation of the final discharge records are performed.

ICD-10-CM	**Z38.00** (single liveborn, delivered vaginally)
CPT	**99463** (initial normal newborn care and discharge on the same date)

➤ **A baby is born vaginally in the hospital on March 3 at 9:00 am.** The pediatrician provides initial newborn care on that date. On March 4 at 7:00 am, the pediatrician determines that the newborn is ready for discharge and spends 25 minutes in discharge day management. Each service is appropriately documented.

ICD-10-CM	Diagnosis code for each day **Z38.00** (single liveborn, delivered vaginally)
CPT	**Day 1: 99460** (initial normal newborn care and discharge on the same date) **Day 2: 99238** (discharge day management)

Teaching Point: Because the services were provided on different calendar dates, initial hospital care and discharge day management services are separately reported.

➤ **A subsequent hospital visit is performed in the well-baby nursery on a 2-day-old who is being observed due to risk of jaundice; however, no interventions are noted, and baby is doing well.**
Code **99462** (subsequent normal newborn care) is reported.

➤ **A neonate fails a routine hearing examination.** During a subsequent newborn care visit, the attending physician spends 15 minutes discussing the results with the parents and refers to an audiologist for testing to confirm or rule out hearing abnormality.

ICD-10-CM	**Z38.00** (single liveborn, delivered vaginally) **R94.120** (abnormal auditory function study)
CPT	**99462** (subsequent normal newborn care)

    Teaching Point: Only code **Z38.00** would be reported when the result of an auditory screening is normal. An audiologist performing auditory screening would report code **Z13.5**, encounter for screening for eye and ear disorders, and then **Z01.110** (encounter for hearing examination following failed hearing screening) in conjunction with the confirmatory testing.

Hospital Care of the Ill Neonate

Diagnosis Codes for Perinatal Conditions,

There are some important guidelines for reporting conditions that originate in the perinatal period. In *ICD-10-CM*, these conditions are classified to Chapter 16 and codes **P00–P96**. Codes in this chapter are used only on the neonate's record and not that of the mother.

The ordering of codes for neonates at the birth hospital are as follows:

1. **Birth outcome (Z38-, reported only by the attending/admitting physician)**
2. **Codes from the perinatal chapter (P00–P96)**
3. **Codes from the congenital anomalies chapter (Q00–Q99)**
4. **All other chapters**

    Other important guidelines include

- Perinatal condition codes are assigned for any condition that is clinically significant.
- In addition to clinical indications for reporting codes from other chapters, perinatal conditions are considered clinically significant if the condition has implications for future health care needs. Other clinical indications that apply to all conditions are those requiring
  — Clinical evaluation
  — Therapeutic treatment
  — Diagnostic procedures
  — Extended hospital stay
  — Increased nursing care and/or monitoring
- Should a condition originate in the perinatal period and continue past the 28th day after birth, the perinatal code should continue to be used regardless of the patient's age.
    Typical scenarios that may require exclusive use of perinatal or neonatal codes beyond the perinatal period are those related to care of a critically ill or recovering neonate, such as necrotizing enterocolitis in newborn (**P77.-**), chronic respiratory disease arising in the perinatal period (**P27.-**), and preterm birth (**P07.-**).
- Note that these codes are not reported for conditions with *onset after the patient is 28 days old*. For example, necrotizing enterocolitis with onset after the neonatal period is reported with codes **K55.30–K55.33**.
- If a newborn has a condition that could be due to the birth process or community acquired and documentation does not indicate which it is, the condition is reported as due to the birth process. Community-acquired conditions are reported with codes other than those in *ICD-10-CM* Chapter 16.
- Codes in categories **P00–P04**, newborn affected by maternal factors and by complications of pregnancy, labor, and delivery, may be reported when the conditions are suspected but have not yet been ruled out.

If a neonate is suspected of having an abnormal condition that, after examination and observation, is ruled out, assign codes for signs and symptoms or, in the absence of signs or symptoms, a code from category **Z05** (encounter for observation and evaluation of newborn for suspected diseases and conditions ruled out).

Examples

➤ **A neonate was born to a mother who tested positive for group B β-hemolytic streptococcal infection and received 4 doses of prophylactic intravenous administration of penicillin prior to delivery.** The newborn appeared typical in the delivery room and was admitted to the newborn nursery. A comprehensive maternal history and physical examination with review of intrapartum laboratory values were performed. The newborn was monitored for 48 hours with no indication of illness. On day 2, the patient was found to be a normal newborn.

ICD-10-CM	**Day 1: Z38.00** (single liveborn, delivered vaginally), **P00.89** (newborn affected by other maternal conditions) **Day 2: Z38.00** (single liveborn, delivered vaginally), **Z05.1** (observation and evaluation of newborn for suspected infectious condition ruled out)
CPT	**Day 1: 99460** **Day 2: 99462**

Teaching Point: On day 1, the patient was suspected of being affected by a localized maternal infection (**P00.89**), but by day 2, the condition was ruled out (**Z05.1**). Normal newborn care codes are reported rather than hospital care because the neonate, while at risk for infection in this case, was not treated but observed and did not develop infection.

Hospital Evaluation and Management Services to the Newborn

Levels of hospital E/M services are based on all hospital care services on the same date by the same physician or physicians of the same group practice (billing under the same tax identification number) and same exact specialty.

When multiple physicians of the same specialty and same group practice provide separate initial or subsequent hospital care to a newborn on the same date, report with a single code representing the combined work (eg, comprehensive history and examination with high-complexity medical decision-making [MDM]).

Normal Newborn Care or Hospital Care?

The choice between coding for normal newborn care and coding for hospital care is based on a physician's judgment. Services to newborns that require an increased level of physician care, nursing observation, or physiologic monitoring (but not intensive care as described by codes **99477–99480**) are typically reported with codes for initial or subsequent hospital care. **Table 15-3** shows the differences in relative value units and potential monetary values for normal and sick newborn care services.

Table 15-3. Comparison Values of Newborn and Hospital Care		
Code	**Total Facility RVUs[a]**	**Monetary Value Example (Based on $40 per RVU)**
99460	2.70	$108.00
99221 99222 99223	2.88 3.89 5.71	$115.20 $155.60 $228.40
99462	1.19	$47.60
99231 99232 99233	1.11 2.04 2.94	$44.40 $81.60 $117.60

Abbreviation: RVU, relative value unit.

[a] Not geographically adjusted.

- A sick visit will have a presenting problem that supports the need for diagnostic investigation or therapy. Therapeutic intervention is typically necessary for the sick newborn.
- The nature of the presenting problem and extent of work required to diagnose and manage the problem should be considered when determining the appropriate procedure code to describe the service.

Initial Hospital Care

Codes **99221–99223** are used to report the initial hospital care of a sick neonate who does not require intensive observation and monitoring or critical care services.

> Refer to Chapter 16 and Table 16-2 for the specific coding and documentation requirements for reporting initial hospital care.

Examples

➤ **The pediatrician sees a newborn boy admitted to the well-baby nursery.** The baby is A+ DAT+. He was born to a mother with blood type O+ who has a history of 2 previous newborns with jaundice secondary to ABO incompatibility. At 8 hours of age, the neonate appears jaundiced. A bilirubin and CBC with a reticulocyte count are ordered, results are evaluated, the newborn's risks for kernicterus are discussed with the family, and phototherapy is started. The pediatrician performs a comprehensive history (maternal history of pregnancy and delivery, significant family history) and physical examination. Medical decision-making is of moderate complexity for this new problem with moderate risk.

ICD-10-CM	**Z38.00** (single liveborn, delivered vaginally) **P55.1** (hemolytic disease due to ABO isoimmunization)
CPT	**99222** *MDM:* Moderate *History:* Comprehensive *Physical examination:* Comprehensive

Teaching Point: When reporting initial hospital care, all 3 key components (ie, history, physical examination, MDM), or average total floor/unit time if more than 50% of time spent is in counseling and/or coordination of care, must be met. The level of service is based on all hospital care services on the same date by the same physician or physicians of the same group practice and same specialty. If the minimum key components are not sufficiently met (eg, an expanded history is performed), the initial care must be reported using subsequent hospital care codes (**99231–99233**).

While code **P55.1** does not specifically mention "jaundice," the *ICD-10-CM* Index entry for jaundice due to ABO incompatibility directs only to code **P55.1**.

➤ **The pediatrician admits a term neonate, born vaginally, with ABO incompatibility (mom AB– and baby B+/ Coombs test result negative).** The otherwise normal neonate is monitored for elevated bilirubin.

ICD-10-CM	**Z38.00** (single liveborn, delivered vaginally) **P55.1** (ABO incompatibility)
CPT	**99460** (initial newborn care)

Teaching Point: The neonate is being observed but not treated, supporting **99460**.

Subsequent Hospital Care

Subsequent hospital care codes (**99231–99233**) are reported for each day of service subsequent to initial care for the newborn who continues to be sick (ie, not a typical neonate but not in critical condition and not requiring intensive observation and interventions).

> Refer to Chapter 16 and Table 16-3 for detailed coding and documentation requirements for codes 99231–99233.

- When a neonate is not treated but only observed for the potential development of illness, normal newborn codes would be reported.
- Report the appropriate code for the highest acuity on each date of service. On subsequent dates when a previously sick neonate is improved and requires no more care than a normal newborn, the subsequent normal newborn care code (**99462**) should be reported.

●=New code ▲=Revised code #=Re-sequenced code +=Add-on code

It is useful to consider the typical patient when reporting subsequent hospital care. These are
- **99231**: Usually, the patient is stable, recovering, or improving.
- **99232**: Usually, the patient is responding inadequately to therapy or has developed a minor complication.
- **99233**: Usually, the patient is unstable or has developed a significant complication or a significant new problem.

Example

➤ **On day 2 of the birth admission, the attending pediatrician provides subsequent hospital care to a term neonate, born vaginally, with ABO incompatibility (mom O+/AB− and baby B+/Coombs test result negative).** The total serum bilirubin is elevated and the pediatrician orders phototherapy. An expanded problem-focused interval history and examination are documented.

ICD-10-CM	**Z38.00** (single liveborn, delivered vaginally) **P55.1** (ABO incompatibility)
CPT	**99232** (subsequent hospital care)

Teaching Point: On day 2, the neonate requires MDM of moderate complexity (new diagnosis with prescription of phototherapy). This, along with the expanded problem-focused history or examination, supports code **99232**.

Discharge Day Management

Either code **99238** or **99239** (hospital day discharge management) is reported on the day the newborn is discharged (when on a separate day from the initial hospital care).
- A newborn who dies on the date of birth is not discharged from the hospital. The attending physician should report a code for the level of hospital care provided (ie, initial hospital care, intensive care, or critical care) as appropriate. Codes for discharge services are not reported.
- When a neonate is transferred to another facility, the physician providing care prior to transfer reports the appropriate code for the type of care provided on that date (eg, **99291**, **99292**; hourly critical care) prior to the transfer, not discharge day management.
- Time must be documented to support code **99239** (ie, time of >30 minutes).

> Chapter 16 includes more information on discharge day management codes **99238** and **99239**.

Example

➤ **The physician performs a follow-up visit for a neonate who will be discharged with a home apnea monitor.** The parents are counseled on their neonate's condition and given instructions for home care and follow-up. Forty-five minutes was spent on the floor reviewing the hospital course and expected follow-up and in counseling the parents.

CPT	**99239** (more than 30 minutes) Time (45 minutes unit/floor time dedicated to the patient) is the key controlling factor.

Teaching Point: If time spent in discharge day management is not documented, code **99238** must be reported.

Prolonged Services

+99356	Prolonged service in the inpatient or observation setting, requiring unit/floor time beyond the usual service; first hour (30–74 min)
+99357	each additional 30 minutes
99358	Prolonged evaluation and management service before and/or after direct patient care; first hour
+99359	each additional 30 minutes

- If direct (face-to-face) prolonged services in the inpatient setting (**99356**, **99357**) are required on the same day as a consultation (**99241–99245**, **99251–99255**), an initial hospital service (**99221–99223**), or a subsequent hospital service (**99231–99233**), they may be reported in addition to the basic E/M service (an add-on code).

- Direct prolonged services are not reported with normal newborn codes, intensive care codes, or neonatal/pediatric critical care codes because these services do not include an assigned typical time by *CPT*.
- *Time must be documented.*

   Prolonged clinical staff services (**99415** and **99416**) are not reported for inpatient care.

> The specific coding guidelines for reporting face-to-face (99354–99357) and non–face-to-face (99358, 99359) prolonged service codes are detailed in Chapter 16.

Examples

➤ **The physician performs an expanded problem-focused history and physical examination on a term neonate born via cesarean delivery who is experiencing mild tachypnea on a subsequent day.** The physician obtains and reviews a chest radiograph and CBC and requests that an oxygen saturation (SpO_2) monitor be placed on the neonate for 5 minutes. The chest radiograph and CBC are normal and the SpO_2 is persistently greater than 95%. The physician spends 65 minutes of total time on the floor with the patient, speaking with the mother and reviewing the chart.

CPT	**99232** (average time is 25 minutes)
	MDM: Low complexity
	History: Expanded problem focused
	Physical examination: Expanded problem focused
	99356 (direct prolonged services, first 30–74 minutes)

   Teaching Point: In addition to code **99232**, code **99356** will be reported based on total documented time spent on the floor or unit dedicated to the 1 patient. Time is not the controlling factor in selection of the subsequent hospital care code because there is no documentation of time spent counseling and coordinating care.

➤ **An infant is transferred from a Level III NICU, following a 30-day hospital stay, to a community Level II unit to complete recovery before home discharge.** A large volume of records accompanies the infant. A comprehensive history and physical examination are performed on admission; MDM is moderately complex. The physician spends another 1 hour and 20 minutes reviewing the extensive transfer records while off the unit.

CPT	**99222**
	MDM: Moderate complexity
	History: Comprehensive
	Physical examination: Comprehensive
	99358 (prolonged non–face-to-face services, first hour)
	99359 (each additional 30 minutes)

   Teaching Point: This service included 80 minutes of prolonged services. Code **99358** represents the first 60 minutes. Code **99359** is reported for the final 20 minutes of prolonged service. If fewer than 75 minutes of prolonged services were provided, code **99359** would not be reported because this code is reported for time that goes at least 15 minutes beyond the first hour or final 30 minutes.

Consultations

A consultation is reported when a physician or other appropriate source requests an opinion and/or advice from another physician or appropriate source. This request must be in writing or given verbally by the requestor and documented in the consultation record. The consulting physician renders advice, records it, and returns a report to the requesting physician or appropriate source.

> Chapter 16 details the specific reporting, documentation, and coding requirements for inpatient consultations. See Table 16-4 for inpatient consultation codes.

Example

➤ **At the request of a primary care physician, a neonatologist evaluates a 35-weeks' gestation neonate with recurrent hypoglycemia.** A detailed history is obtained from the mother noting she has no history of diabetes. Family history is negative for previous neonates with hypoglycemia or other metabolic diseases. Review of labor and delivery records is unremarkable. After birth, the newborn had 3 documented preprandial blood glucose concentrations less than 40 mg/dL and responded well to oral feeding. A detailed physical examination was performed. Physical examination and growth parameters are consistent with 35 weeks' gestation. The neonatologist recommends more frequent feeding and rechecking blood glucose before feeds until 4 consecutive preprandial glucose concentrations are greater than 60 mg/dL. The neonatologist spends 10 minutes explaining the findings and reassuring the baby's parents. The neonatologist writes a detailed chart note and discusses her recommendations with the pediatrician by phone.

ICD-10-CM	**P70.4** (hypoglycemia, newborn) **P07.38** (preterm newborn, gestational age 35 completed weeks)
CPT	**99253** MDM: Moderate complexity History: Detailed Physical examination: Detailed Or, if payer does not recognize consultations, **99221** (initial hospital care)

Coding for Transitions to Different Levels of Neonatal Care

During a hospital stay, a newborn or readmitted neonate may require multiple levels of care. A normal newborn may end up becoming sick, intensively ill, or critical during the same hospital stay. Neonates who were initially sick may also improve to require lower levels of care (eg, normal neonatal care).

It is important to remember

- When a patient qualifies for normal newborn care and, at a subsequent encounter on the same day, becomes ill and requires an additional encounter at a higher service level, normal newborn care (**99460** or **99462**) may be reported in addition to the following on the same day:
  — Hospital care (**99221–99223**)
  — Initial intensive care (**99477**)
  — Initial critical care (**99468**)
  — Time-based critical care (**99291, 99292**)
- *CPT* instructs to report the appropriate E/M code with modifier **25** for these services in addition to the normal newborn code.

Examples

➤ **A neonate who was initially normal becomes ill 5 hours after birth.** A pediatrician, who provided initial newborn care earlier the same day, provides a second E/M service to evaluate the neonate's condition and determines that a transfer to a NICU is necessary. Following transfer, a neonatologist provides initial intensive care to the newborn.

The pediatrician reports **99460** and **99223 25**	The neonatologist reports **99477**

Teaching Point: The second E/M service on the same date as the initial newborn care is reported with modifier **25** appended.

➤ **A neonate who was initially normal becomes ill several hours after Physician A provided normal newborn care.** Physician B of another specialty assumes management of the newborn's care and provides an initial hospital care service with a comprehensive history and examination and moderate MDM.

| Physician A reports
99460 | Physician B reports
99222 |

> **Teaching Point:** No modifier is required because the physicians are not of the same specialty.

- Once an initial-day care code for a higher service level has been reported, an *initial* code for a lower service level within the same hospital stay will not be reported.
  - If a patient has required intensive care (**99477**) but no longer qualifies for intensive care and is transferred to the care of a primary care pediatrician, the receiving physician will report subsequent hospital care (**99231–99233**) based on the level of service provided.
  - The receiving physician *will not report* initial hospital care (**99221–99223**) for the first encounter after the transfer.

Example

➤ **A neonate (2,600 g) is transferred from neonatal intensive care by an intensivist to a pediatric hospitalist to complete recovery before home discharge.** On the day of transfer, the intensivist provides intensive care from midnight to noon and determines the neonate no longer requires intensive care. The hospitalist provides a face-to-face visit to the neonate, documenting a detailed interval history, comprehensive examination, moderate-complexity MDM, and 75 minutes of time on the unit reviewing the patient's record and consulting with the family.

| The intensivist reports
99480 (subsequent intensive care, per day, for the E/M of the recovering infant [present body weight of 2501-5000 grams]) | The hospitalist reports
99233 (subsequent hospital care, typical time 35 minutes)
99356 (direct prolonged services, first 30–74 minutes) |

> **Teaching Point:** The hospitalist may not report initial hospital care for services to the patient who has received prior initial hospital services (eg, initial neonatal intensive care). The typical time of code **99233** was exceeded by more than 30 minutes, supporting code **99356**.

Payers that use the Medicare or Medicaid National Correct Coding Initiative (NCCI) will not allow separate payment of

- **Normal newborn hospital care (99460, 99462, 99463) by the same physician or a physician of the same specialty and same group practice on the same date as initial hospital care (99221–99223)**
- **Initial hospital care (99221–99223) by the same physician or a physician of the same specialty and same group practice on the same date as initial inpatient neonatal critical care (99468)**
- **Subsequent hospital care (99231–99233) by the same physician or a physician of the same specialty and same group practice on the same date as subsequent normal newborn care (99462)**

When reporting to these payers, report only the most extensive level of care provided; the code in column 1 of the NCCI edit table is considered the more comprehensive code. See Chapter 2 for more information on NCCI edits and where to find them.

Other Newborn Hospital Care

Circumcision

54150   Circumcision, using clamp or other device with regional dorsal penile or ring block

- If the circumcision using a clamp or other device is performed without dorsal penile or ring block, append modifier **52** (reduced services) to **54150**.
- Medicare has a global period of 0 (zero) assigned to code **54150**.
- When performing a circumcision and a separately identifiable E/M service on the same day (eg, **99462**, subsequent normal newborn care; **99238**, discharge services <30 minutes), append modifier **25** to the E/M code. Link the appropriate *ICD-10-CM* code (eg, **Z38.00**) to the E/M service and to the circumcision code.

- The American Hospital Association *Coding Clinic* instructs that code **Z41.2** (encounter for routine and ritual male circumcision) *is not assigned* during the birth admission, as circumcision is a routine part of the newborn's hospital care.

54160   Circumcision, surgical excision other than clamp, device, or dorsal slit; neonate (28 days of age or less)

54161   older than 28 days

Unlike code **54150**, Medicare has a global period of 10 days assigned to codes **54160** and **54161**. A physician who performs a procedure with a 10-day global period must append modifier **24** (unrelated E/M service by the same physician or other qualified health care professional during a postoperative period) to the E/M code for subsequent newborn or hospital care or discharge management (eg, **99238 24**) provided in the 10-day period following the procedure for general care of the newborn unrelated to the procedure.

> See Chapter 10 for information on coding for circumcisions performed in the office.

Frenotomy

40806   Incision of labial frenum (frenotomy)

Often, a newborn will experience issues with latching or feeding due to a tight frenulum. If the issues are severe enough to warrant intervention by means of incising the frenulum, report code **40806**. This may be completed in the hospital before discharge.

- If the physician performing the incision is also performing newborn care on the same date, be sure to append modifier **25** to the hospital care service also being reported.
- Do not report *CPT* code **41115** (excision of lingual frenum [frenectomy]) when the frenulum is only incised or clipped.

Car Safety Seat Testing

Codes **94780** and **94781** (car seat testing) are reported for monitoring to determine if *an infant through 12 months of age* may be safely transported in a car seat or must be transported in a car bed. These services are most commonly provided to infants who required critical care during their initial hospital stay.

- Car seat testing codes may be reported in addition to the subsequent hospital or discharge day management codes when performed and documented. *Note:* These codes cannot be reported in addition to critical or intensive care services.
- Time spent in car seat testing is not counted as time spent in discharge day management.
- Car seat testing may also be provided to an infant in an outpatient setting to determine if the infant can safely move from car bed to car seat transportation.

> See Chapter 18 for more information on car seat testing.

Resources

Discharge Day Management

"Hospital Discharge Day Management: Are You Coding Correctly?" February 2019 *AAP Pediatric Coding Newsletter*™ (https://coding.solutions.aap.org/article.aspx?articleid=2720944; subscription required)

Hospital Care of the Newborn

"You Code It! Assigning Appropriate Codes for Hospital Care of Newborns" January 2020 *AAP Pediatric Coding Newsletter* (https://coding.solutions.aap.org/article.aspx?articleid=2758028, subscription required)

Newborn Coding Decision Tool

American Academy of Pediatrics *Newborn Coding Decision Tool* (available for purchase online at https://shop.aap.org/newborn-coding-decision-tool-2021)

Test Your Knowledge!

1. **A neonate is born on September 1. How old is the neonate on September 30?**
   a. 30 days old
   b. 29 days old
   c. 28 days old
   d. 31 days old

2. **What code or codes does an attending pediatrician use to report initial face-to-face care of a normal newborn (born late on February 15, 2021) on February 16, 2021, and discharge management within 24 hours on February 17, 2021?**
   a. **99460**, **99462**, and **99238** or **99239**
   b. **99460** and **99238** or **99239**
   c. **99462** and **99238** or **99239**
   d. **99463**

3. **What code is reported by a pediatrician providing subsequent care to a neonate who is being observed for jaundice but is asymptomatic?**
   a. **99231**
   b. **99462**
   c. **99221**
   d. **99460**

4. **What is the basis for selecting discharge day management code 99239?**
   a. Documentation of more than 30 minutes spent face-to-face with the patient/caregivers
   b. The continuous time devoted to the care of the patient on the date of discharge
   c. The status of the neonate (normal or sick)
   d. Physician time of more than 30 minutes on unit/floor devoted to care of the individual patient

5. **What codes does a pediatrician report for assuming management of a neonate who no longer requires critical or intensive care but is not a normal newborn?**
   a. **99231–99233** (subsequent hospital care)
   b. **99251–99255** (inpatient consultation)
   c. **99221–99223** (initial hospital care)
   d. Any of the above if supported by documentation

Chapter 15. Hospital Care of the Newborn

Noncritical Hospital Evaluation and Management Services

Contents

●=New code   ▲=Revised code   #=Re-sequenced code   +=Add-on code

Coding for Noncritical Hospital Evaluation and Management Services

This chapter includes tables with descriptions of the required key components (ie, history, physical examination, medical decision-making [MDM], and time) for all evaluation and management (E/M) services that are described in the observation and inpatient hospital setting.

As a reminder, the 2021 changes to codes and guidelines for office evaluation and management services *only* affect codes 99202–99215.

Codes and selection requirements for observation and inpatient hospital care are unchanged from 2020.

See Chapter 6 for specific documentation requirements. See also the American Academy of Pediatrics Pediatric Evaluation and Management: Coding Quick Reference Card 2021 (available for purchase at https://shop.aap.org).

The following are basic guidelines for reporting noncritical/non-intensive observation and inpatient hospital E/M services. There are no distinctions between new and established patients.
- Codes are reported based on the cumulative services (performance of the required key components and/or time when appropriate) provided by an individual physician or any combination of physicians or other qualified health care professionals (QHPs)
  — Of the same specialty within a group
  — With the same tax identification number
  — During a single calendar day
- Services may be performed and reported by any physician of any specialty (eg, hospitalist, primary care physician, specialist) or other QHPs.
- Any procedure or other service with a *Current Procedural Terminology* (*CPT®*) code may be reported separately when performed by the reporting provider or group and documented.

Table 16-1 provides specific detail of required elements within each level of history and physical examination (eg, problem focused, detailed) and MDM (eg, straightforward, moderate) of an E/M code. Services may be reported using either the 1995 or 1997 documentation guidelines. The nature of the presenting problem (ie, reason for the encounter) is included as a contributory factor for levels of MDM but is not 1 of the 3 required elements.

Time-Based Code Selection
- Time in the observation and inpatient setting is defined as *floor or unit time* (dedicated to the 1 patient) and includes time spent
  — At the patient's bedside
  — Counseling family or patient (or those who may have assumed responsibility for the care of the patient [eg, foster parents, legal guardians, persons acting in loco parentis])
  — On the floor, performing and documenting the history and examination, and reviewing diagnostic tests
  — Coordinating care with care team members
- Time is the basis for code selection in lieu of key components only when more than 50% of the unit/floor time is spent in counseling and/or coordination of care.
- When time is used as the controlling factor in the selection of the code, the cumulative time spent and the notation that *more than half* the time was spent in counseling and/or coordination of care *must be documented* in the medical record.
- When time is spent off the unit/floor (eg, reviewing and/or discussing medical imaging studies in radiology), do not include that time in the unit/floor time.

See also the Prolonged Evaluation and Management Services Provided in the Inpatient Setting section later in this chapter for discussion of prolonged services.

Observation Care
- Hospital observation services are provided to patients who require monitoring and treatment to determine if inpatient admission will be required. For example, a patient with dehydration who requires rehydration, is not quite sick enough for immediate inpatient care, and may be able to later be discharged home would be admitted to observation.

Chapter 16. Noncritical Hospital Evaluation and Management Services

Table 16-1. Evaluation and Management Key Components[a]

History (must meet or exceed HPI, ROS, and PFSH)	Problem focused HPI: 1–3 elements ROS: 0 PFSH: 0	Expanded HPI: 1–3 elements ROS: 1 PFSH: 0	Detailed HPI: 4+ elements or status of 3 chronic or inactive conditions ROS: 2–9 PFSH: 1	Comprehensive HPI: 4+ elements or status of 3 chronic or inactive conditions ROS: 10+ PFSH: 3
Physical Examination (only required to choose from either the 1995 or 1997 guidelines)	**Problem focused** 1995: 1 body area/organ system 1997: Performance and documentation of 1–5 elements identified by a bullet (●) in ≥1 areas or systems	**Expanded** 1995: Limited examination—affected body area/organ system and other related areas/systems (total 2–7) 1997: Performance and documentation of at least 6 elements identified by a bullet (●) in ≥1 areas or systems	**Detailed** 1995: Extended examination—affected body area(s) and other symptomatic or related organ system(s) (total 2–7) 1997: Performance and documentation of at least 2 elements identified by a bullet (●) in at least 6 areas or systems or at least 12 elements identified by a bullet (●) in at least 2 areas or systems	**Comprehensive** 1995: 8+ organ systems or complete examination of a single organ system 1997: <u>Multisystem examination</u>—9 systems or areas with performance of all elements identified by a bullet (●) in each area/system examined and documentation of at least 2 elements identified by a bullet (●) of each area(s) or system(s) <u>Single organ system</u> <u>examination</u>—Performance of all elements identified by a bullet (●) and documentation of every element in box with shaded border and at least 1 element in box with unshaded border
MDM (must meet 2 of 3—diagnoses/options, data, and risk)	**Straightforward** # Diagnoses/options: Minimal Data: Minimal Risk: Minimal PP: Usually self-limited or minor severity	**Low complexity** # Diagnoses/options: Limited Data: Limited Risk: Low PP: Usually moderate severity	**Moderate complexity** # Diagnoses/options: Multiple Data: Moderate Risk: Moderate PP: Usually moderate to high severity	**High complexity** # Diagnoses/options: Extensive Data: Extensive Risk: High PP: Usually moderate to high severity

Abbreviations: HPI, history of present illness; MDM, medical decision-making; PFSH, past, family, and social history; PP, presenting problem; ROS, review of systems.

[a] See **Chapter 6** for a detailed description of the guidelines and components of evaluation and management services with documentation requirements and tips.

- Hospitals do not need to designate a separate area for these patients; rather, designation of observation versus inpatient status is dependent on the physician's order and the likelihood that the patient's treatment may avoid inpatient admission.
- Initial observation care is reported by the admitting physician or QHP using codes **99218–99220**. Subsequent-day observation care is reported with codes **99224–99226** and observation care discharge management with code **99217**.
- Consulting physicians of specialties (ie, other than the attending physician) who provide care in the observation setting report outpatient consultation (**99241–99245**) or subsequent observation care codes (**99224–99226**). (See the "Coding Conundrum: 2 Physicians Providing Initial Observation or Inpatient Hospital Day Services" box later in this chapter for Medicare and *CPT* guidance.)
- Admission (ie, initial care) and discharge services (observation or inpatient status) provided on the same day are reported with codes **99234–99236**.

- When the patient's status changes from observation to inpatient status or vice versa (eg, utilization review staff request that the physician change status from inpatient to observation), the physician should write an order to reflect the change and report only the code that reflects care consistent with the patient's final status on that date.
- Typical time has not been established for code **99217**, so time spent in discharge management is not a factor in the selection of this code.

Coding Conundrum: 2 Physicians Providing Initial Observation or Inpatient Hospital Day Services

When Payers Follow Medicare Rules

Initial observation services: The admitting physician will report the initial observation care codes (**99218–99220**). Other physicians (ie, physicians belonging to a different group practice and/or of a different specialty) providing initial services to a patient in observation will report a new or established office or outpatient evaluation and management (E/M) code (**99202–99215**) based on the performance and documentation of the required key components.

Initial inpatient hospital services: Initial inpatient hospital care codes (**99221–99223**) may be reported by every physician who performs initial hospital care. The admitting physician will append modifier **AI** (principal physician of record) to codes **99221–99223**.

When Payers Do Not Follow Medicare Rules

Initial observation services: The admitting physician will report the initial observation care codes (**99218–99220**). The office or outpatient consultation codes (**99241–99245**) may be reported by other physicians if the service was requested by a physician or other appropriate source, opinion and/or advice was rendered by the consulting physician, and a written report was generated from the consulting physician to the referring physician. When the criteria for reporting a consultation are not met, the subsequent observation E/M codes (**99224–99226**) would be reported based on the level of care provided and documented.

Initial inpatient hospital services: The admitting physician will report the initial hospital care codes (**99221–99223**). Inpatient consultation codes (**99251–99255**) may be reported by other physicians if the requirements for reporting the services are met (ie, requested, opinion/advice rendered, written report to requesting source). Otherwise, subsequent hospital care E/M codes (**99231–99233**) are reported.

Initial Observation Care

99218–99220 Initial observation care, per day, for the evaluation and management of a patient

See the full code requirements in **Table 16-2**. The examples included here and throughout the chapter are coded based on the 1995 E/M documentation guidelines.

When reporting based on key components

- The history and physical examination to support code **99218** may be detailed or comprehensive. The MDM is of straightforward to low complexity.
- Comprehensive history and physical examination in conjunction with moderate-complexity MDM support code **99219**. Code **99220** requires comprehensive history and examination with high-complexity MDM.

Initial observation care codes are reported

- On the first day that the admitting physician provides face-to-face services to the patient in the observation setting.
- Using the code that reflects the overall care provided by the admitting physician to the patient on that calendar date. When "observation status" is initiated in the course of an encounter in another site of service (eg, emergency department [ED], physician's office), all E/M services performed by the same physician (or physicians of the same specialty in the same group practice) are considered part of the initial observation care when performed on the same calendar date.

See the "Unique Considerations for Hospital Services" box later in this chapter for more details about coding for initial observation care initiated elsewhere (eg, office, emergency department).

Important guidelines to remember include

- If the patient is admitted for observation and subsequently is formally admitted to the hospital on the same day, only the initial inpatient hospital code (**99221–99223**) is reported.
- Physicians from other groups providing services on the same date will report other appropriate outpatient E/M services based on the services provided and payer requirements.
- Observation services are reported with place of service code **22** (on campus—outpatient hospital).

Chapter 8 addresses the guidelines for selection of codes 99241–99245 and Chapter 7 for 99202–99215; see Chapter 4 for more information on place of service codes.

- Code selection is dependent on the performance and documentation of all 3 key components. Time may be used as the key or controlling factor in the selection of the code if more than 50% of the total face-to-face encounter and/or floor/unit time is spent in counseling and/or coordination of care.
- Observation care codes are not reported for initial transitional care of hospital-born neonates.

Table 16-2. Observation Care

Key Components (For a description of key components, see Table 16-1.)

Initial Day: 3 of 3 key components must be performed to at least the degree specified for the codes in each row. A chief complaint is required for each level of history.

CPT Code/Time[a]	Medical Decision-making[b]	History	1995 Examination[c]
99218 30 min	Straightforward to low complexity PP: Usually low severity	HPI: ≥4 or 3 CC; ROS: 2–9; PFSH: 1/3	2–7 detailed
99219 50 min	Moderate complexity PP: Usually responding inadequately to therapy or minor complication	HPI: ≥4 or 3 CC; ROS: ≥10; PFSH: 3/3	≥8 body areas/ systems
99220 70 min	High complexity PP: Usually patient is unstable or develops significant complication or new problem.	HPI: ≥4 or 3 CC; ROS: ≥10; PFSH: 3/3	≥8 body areas/ systems

Subsequent Day: 2 of 3 key components must be performed to at least the degree specified for the codes in each row. A chief complaint is required for each level of service.

99224 15 min	Straightforward to low complexity PP: Usually stable, recovering, or improving	HPI: 1–3; ROS: 0; PFSH: 0	1 body area/system
99225 25 min	Moderate complexity PP: Usually responding inadequately to therapy or minor complication	HPI: 1–3; ROS: 1; PFSH: 0	2–7 limited
99226 35 min	High complexity PP: Usually patient is unstable or develops significant complication or new problem.	HPI: ≥4 or 3 CC; ROS: 2–9; PFSH: 0	2–7 detailed

Abbreviations: CC, chronic condition; CPT, Current Procedural Terminology; HPI, history of present illness; PFSH, past, family, and social history; PP, presenting problem; ROS, review of systems.

[a] Typical time is an average and represents a range of times that may be higher or lower depending on clinical circumstances.

[b] The presenting problem is considered to be a contributory factor and does not need to be present to the degree specified.

[c] Number of body areas or organ systems examined; see **Table 16-1** for details.

Use **Table 16-2** to help you in the selection of the appropriate codes in the following clinical examples:

Examples

➤ **A 5-month-old boy is admitted to observation due to suspected viral bronchiolitis.**

History: Patient presented to the ED with respiratory distress, cough, and wheezing. History of present illness: duration, several days; quality, coughing and now wheezing today; severity, trouble breathing with retractions; timing, especially while feeding; associated signs and symptoms, runny nose and fever; irritability; and feeding intolerance. Review of systems: all systems reviewed and notable for temperature as high as 38.8°C (101.8°F) today, alternately sleepy and fussy, a productive and deep-sounding cough, clear runny nose, taking longer to feed because of cough and nasal drainage but able to finish some bottles, and no vomiting or diarrhea; urinary, fewer wet diapers but still urinating every 4 to 6 hours. Past history: immunizations are up to date, normal obstetric and perinatal course, milestones met, no known allergies. Family history: asthma in mother and sister and seasonal allergies in father; no genetic or immunologic disease. Social history: no tobacco exposure; goes to child care 3 days a week; lives with mother and father.

Physical examination: Comprehensive examination of constitutional (temperature, 38.6°C [101.5°F]; pink with mild cyanosis with coughing spasm; respiratory rate, 60 breaths per minute; oxygen saturation, 88%), eyes, ears, mouth, nose, throat, cardiovascular, respiratory, gastrointestinal, genitourinary, musculoskeletal, skin, neurologic, and lymphatic systems performed. Tachypnea with retractions, heart rate at the high end of reference range, and mild dehydration are noted.

Laboratory tests: Respiratory viral panel, basic metabolic panel, complete blood cell count (CBC), and chest radiograph are ordered.

Assessment/plan: Assessment is respiratory distress, probable viral bronchiolitis without pneumonia. The plan is to give albuterol every 3 hours, admit to observation status, and continue to suction secretions and supply supplemental oxygen and intravenous (IV) fluids.

International Classification of Diseases, 10th Revision, Clinical Modification (ICD-10-CM)	*CPT*
R06.03 (respiratory distress) **R09.02** (hypoxemia) **E86.0** (dehydration)	**99219** (requires comprehensive history and examination and moderate MDM) *MDM:* Moderate complexity (new problem with additional workup and acute illness with systemic symptoms) *History:* Comprehensive *Physical examination:* Comprehensive

Teaching Point: Remember, all 3 key components must be met for the level of initial observation care reported. The level of history and examination are comprehensive. Medical decision-making is moderate. This supports code **99219**. If MDM were of high complexity, code **99220** would be reported.

➤ **An established patient presents to her physician's office on Monday.** During the evaluation of the patient, the physician decides to admit to observation care for further treatment and monitoring for fever, acute pyelonephritis, and dehydration. The physician does not see the patient in the observation setting until the next morning (Tuesday) but phones in orders and coordinates care with the nursing staff on Monday. On Tuesday, the physician performs a face-to-face initial observation care service (detailed history and examination, moderate-complexity MDM) on the patient and determines the patient is not improving enough to be discharged.

ICD-10-CM	*CPT*
N10 (acute pyelonephritis) **E86.0** (dehydration)	Monday's visit **99212–99215** (office E/M, established patient)
	Tuesday's visit **99218** (initial observation care) or, if admitted as an inpatient on Tuesday, **99221** (initial hospital care)

Teaching Point: Initial observation care and initial inpatient care (**99218–99220**, **99221–99223**) require a face-to-face service with the patient by the reporting physician in the facility. Entry of the history, physical examination, and orders directly into a facility electronic health record (EHR) by online connection without a face-to-face visit in the facility does not support reporting (and could be interpreted as fraudulent). Also, an outpatient office building connected physically to the hospital does not count as the patient being seen in the hospital.

➤ **Same patient; however, the physician sees the patient in the office and in the hospital on the same day.** The combined E/M service in the office and hospital results in a comprehensive history and physical examination with moderately complex MDM.

Teaching Point: Only the initial observation care (**99219**) is reported because that code represents all of the physician's E/M services to the patient on the date of admission.

●=New code   ▲=Revised code   #=Re-sequenced code   +=Add-on code

Subsequent Observation Care

99224–99226 Subsequent observation care, per day, for the evaluation and management of a patient

- Codes include all E/M services by a physician, QHP, or physicians in the same group and same specialty provided on a given day.
- Level of service reported will be dependent on the total services provided and documented.
- Codes require that 2 of the 3 key components be performed and documented.

> **Some payers may require medical decision-making as 1 of the 2 key components performed and documented.**

- Time may be used as the key or controlling factor in code selection if more than 50% of the total encounter (ie, floor/unit time) is spent in counseling and/or coordination of care.
- An interval history is required for subsequent observation visits (ie, additional or updated history obtained since the last physician assessment, including history of present illness and problem-pertinent system review). A past, family, and social history is not required.
- Individual documentation for each encounter should contain all information necessary to determine the level of service provided. It is important to document the chief complaint and other factors of the patient presentation that affect management at each encounter.

> **Be careful to avoid the temptation to simply cut and paste your previous day's note.**

The complexity of the presenting problems is often an indicator of the medically necessary level of subsequent observation services required. *CPT* indicates the patient presentation for each level of subsequent observation care. See the MDM row of **Table 16-1** for presenting problems for each code.

Use **Table 16-2** to help you select the appropriate codes in the following clinical example:

Example

➤ **7:00 am: A 13-year-old girl is seen by her hospitalist for subsequent observation care following an observation admission the previous evening for a concussion with loss of consciousness (LOC) of less than 5 minutes after being hit by a softball.** She was admitted to observation due to recurrent vomiting and confusion. She is now also experiencing a severe headache with nausea. The hospitalist discusses the case with a neurologist and orders computed tomography (CT) in addition to obtaining an expanded problem-focused history and examination.

ICD-10-CM	*CPT*
S06.0X1A (concussion with LOC of 30 minutes or less, initial encounter)	**99225**
G44.309 (posttraumatic headache, unspecified, not intractable)	*MDM:* Moderate complexity
R11.10 (vomiting)	*History:* Expanded problem focused
	Physical examination: Expanded problem focused

Teaching Point: The condition of the patient in this example is worsening. Medical decision-making is moderate based on discussion of the case with another physician and an order for a CT scan in conjunction with the risk of an acute complicated injury. Additional diagnosis codes for the external cause of injury (**W21.07XA**, struck by softball, initial encounter; **Y93.64**, activity, baseball [includes softball]) may be required by state or facility policy. Seventh character **A** is appropriate for active management of the injury.

Observation Care Discharge Day Management

99217   Observation care discharge day management

Code **99217** is to be used to report all services provided to a patient on discharge from observation status (ie, final examination of the patient, discussion of the hospital stay, counseling, instructions for continuing care, and preparation of discharge records) if the discharge *is on a day other than the initial date of observation status.*

Chapter 16. Noncritical Hospital Evaluation and Management Services

- Performance of the key components is not required.
- Observation care discharge services are not assigned a typical time.
- A face-to-face encounter is required on the date that code **99217** is reported. Even if some of the discharge work was performed on the day prior to discharge, code **99217** would be reported on the discharge date if a face-to-face encounter occurred on that date.

Example

➤ **A 13-year-old girl is seen by her hospitalist for subsequent observation care (third day of admission) for a concussion with LOC of less than 5 minutes after being hit by a softball.** She experienced no vomiting overnight and headache has resolved. The CT scan result was negative, and neurology found no evidence of complications from her injury. The patient ate a light breakfast without nausea or vomiting. She is discharged with home care instructions and precautions. Code **99217** (observation care discharge day management) is reported and linked to diagnosis code **S06.0X1A**. Additional codes (**W21.07XA**, struck by softball, initial encounter; **Y93.64**, activity, baseball [includes softball]) may be reported to indicate the cause of the condition.

Observation or Inpatient Hospital Care Services (Including Admission and Discharge Services)

When a patient is admitted and discharged from observation or inpatient services on the *same date of service,* report codes **99234–99236**. (See code **99463** for initial E/M of a normal newborn admitted and discharged on the same date.)
- Code selection is based on the performance and documentation of all 3 key components.
  - Include the combined services provided by the same physician or physicians of the same specialty within a group during a calendar day.
  - At times, an attending physician may see the patient only once (eg, when admitted by phone and not seen face-to-face until the discharge on the next date). However, the documentation should support that initial observation care and discharge day management services were both provided (eg, describe physician's involvement over course of the stay).
- Time may be used as the key or controlling factor in the selection of the code if more than 50% of the total face-to-face encounter (eg, floor/unit time) is spent in counseling and/or coordination of care.
- Except where payer guidance specifies otherwise, reporting of initial observation or inpatient care is based on the date of the face-to-face assessment and not the date of admission or designation of a status by a facility on physician order.

Reporting to Payers Using Medicare Policy

Medicaid and private payers may adopt a Medicare policy that limits reporting of codes **99234–99236** to services provided to a patient who was admitted to observation or inpatient status for *at least 8 hours and not more than 24 hours.* Under this policy, when a patient is admitted to observation or inpatient care for fewer than 8 hours on the same calendar date, only the initial observation (**99218–99220**) or inpatient care (**99221–99223**) shall be reported by the physician. A separate code for discharge services is not reported.

Medicare also requires that there must be a medical observation record for the patient that contains dated and timed physician's orders for the observation services the patient is to receive, nursing notes, and progress notes prepared by the physician indicating physical presence and personal performance of services. This record must be in addition to (and not a copy and paste of) any record prepared as a result of an ED or outpatient clinic encounter.

Use **Table 16-3** to review the required components used to select level of service in the following examples:

Table 16-3. Observation or Inpatient Care Admission and Discharge on the Same Day (99234–99236)

Key Components (For a description of key components, see Table 16-1.)

3 of 3 key components must be performed to at least the degree specified for the codes in each row. A chief complaint is required for each level of history.

CPT Code/Time[a]	Medical Decision-making[b]	History	1995 Examination[c]
99234 (A&D) 40 min	Straightforward to low complexity PP: Usually low severity	HPI: ≥4 or 3 CC; ROS: 2–9; PFSH: 1/3	2–7 detailed
99235 (A&D) 50 min	Moderate complexity PP: Usually responding inadequately to therapy or minor complication	HPI: ≥4 or 3 CC; ROS: ≥10; PFSH: 3/3	≥8 body areas/systems
99236 (A&D) 55 min	High complexity PP: Usually patient is unstable or develops significant complication or new problem.	HPI: ≥4 or 3 CC; ROS: ≥10; PFSH: 3/3	≥8 body areas/systems

Abbreviations: A&D, admission and discharge on same day; CC, chronic conditions; *CPT, Current Procedural Terminology*; HPI, history of present illness; PFSH, past, family, and social history; PP, presenting problem; ROS; review of systems.

[a] Typical time is an average and represents a range of times that may be higher or lower depending on clinical circumstances.

[b] The presenting problem is considered to be a contributory factor and does not need to be present to the degree specified.

[c] Number of body areas or organ systems examined; see **Table 16-1** for details.

Examples

➤ **6:00 am: An 8-year-old girl is admitted to observation for continuous nebulizer treatment due to an exacerbation of asthma.** Encounter includes comprehensive history and examination and MDM of moderate complexity. The physician monitors the patient periodically until symptoms are resolved. Decision for discharge to home is made at 11:00 am. Diagnosis is moderate persistent asthma with exacerbation.

ICD-10-CM	CPT
J45.41 (moderate persistent asthma with [acute] exacerbation)	**99235** *MDM:* Moderate complexity *History:* Comprehensive *Physical examination:* Comprehensive

Teaching Point: Face-to-face services performed include initial care and discharge management. A code from the **99234–99236** series would be reported because observation admission and discharge services were provided on the same date. Alternatively, if the payer requires an observation stay of 8 hours to report **99234–99236**, code **99222** (initial observation care) would be reported for this 5-hour stay.

➤ **An established patient is seen in the physician's office with acute viral laryngotracheitis (croup) and admitted for observation at 6:00 pm on Tuesday.** The attending physician telephones the observation admission orders and does not see the child again until the next morning (Wednesday). On Wednesday, the physician completes a history and physical examination and, later that afternoon, discharges the child.

ICD-10-CM	CPT
J05.0 (croup) (same for both dates of service)	Tuesday's visit **99212–99215** (office E/M, established patient) Wednesday's visit **99234–99236** (observation care, same-day admission and discharge)

Teaching Point: Because the physician first saw the patient in observation on Wednesday, the office visit on Tuesday and the admission and discharge on Wednesday are separately reported.

➤ **A 4-year-old patient with croup is admitted from the ED at 6:00 am on Monday.** An attending physician, from a different group than the ED physician, sees the child that morning and performs the initial history and physical examination. Another physician from the attending physician's same specialty and group practice returns to the hospital at 5:00 pm and, after evaluation of the child, discharges the patient home. The combined service is a comprehensive history and physical examination with moderate-level MDM.

ICD-10-CM	CPT
J05.0 (croup)	**99235** (observation care, same-day admission and discharge) *MDM:* Moderate complexity *History:* Comprehensive *Physical examination:* Comprehensive

Teaching Point: Because the 2 physicians who provided care in the observation setting are of the same specialty and same group practice, the code representing the combined work of the 2 visits is reported. If more than 50% of the total unit/floor time of the 2 physicians who provided observation care were spent in counseling and/or coordination of care, the level of service would be selected based on time (eg, 50 minutes for **99235**).

➤ **A 10-year-old patient is seen in the ED at 5:00 am on Monday after experiencing a seizure while sleeping.** Workup in the ED indicated a first-time generalized tonic-clonic seizure in an otherwise healthy patient. A pediatric neurologist is consulted in the ED and admits the patient to observation. The neurologist's combined services include a comprehensive history and examination and moderate-complexity MDM. Assessment is benign childhood epilepsy with centrotemporal electroencephalographic spikes. The child is discharged to home that afternoon.

ICD-10-CM	CPT
G40.009 (localization-related [focal] [partial] idiopathic epilepsy and epileptic syndromes with seizures of localized onset, not intractable, without status epilepticus) **G84.83** (Todd's paralysis [postepileptic])	**99235** (observation care, same-day admission and discharge) *MDM:* Moderate complexity *History:* Comprehensive *Physical examination:* Comprehensive

Teaching Point: The neurologist reports only the observation admission and discharge because the consultation in the ED is included in the work of the observation services. An Excludes2 note at **G40.009** indicates that Todd paralysis (**G84.83**) may be separately reported.

Inpatient Hospital Care

Initial Inpatient Hospital Care

99221–99223 Initial hospital care, per day, for the evaluation and management of a patient
- Initial inpatient hospital service codes are used to report initial face-to-face services provided to a hospital inpatient.
- Initial inpatient encounters by more than 1 physician must be reported based on payer guidelines. (See the "Coding Conundrum: 2 Physicians Providing Initial Observation or Inpatient Hospital Day Services" box earlier in this chapter.)
- Selection of the code is based on performance and documentation of the 3 required key components or on time if more than 50% of the encounter is spent in counseling and/or coordination of care (**Table 16-4**).
- The lowest level of initial hospital care (**99221**) requires at least a detailed history and detailed physical examination. If the level of history and/or physical examination performed and documented is expanded or problem focused, initial inpatient hospital care must be reported using subsequent hospital visit codes (**99231–99233**) because the required key components for code **99221** have not been met.
- The code is reported on the first day that a face-to-face (physician–patient) service is provided.
- The date of initial hospital care that the physician reports does not need to correlate with the facility's date of admission.
- Report only an initial hospital care code when a patient is admitted to inpatient status from observation status.

Use **Table 16-4** to review the required components used to select level of service in the following examples:

Chapter 16. Noncritical Hospital Evaluation and Management Services

Table 16-4. Inpatient Hospital Care

Initial Day: 3 of 3 key components (see **Table 16-1**) must be performed to at least the degree specified for the codes in each row. A chief complaint is required for each level of history.

CPT Code/Time[a]	Medical Decision-making[b]	History	1995 Examination[c]
99221 30 min	Straightforward to low complexity PP: Usually low severity	HPI: ≥4 or 3 CC; ROS: 2–9; PFSH: 1/3	2–7 detailed
99222 50 min	Moderate complexity PP: Usually responding inadequately to therapy or minor complication	HPI: ≥4 or 3 CC; ROS: ≥10; PFSH: 3/3	≥8 body areas/systems
99223 70 min	High complexity PP: Usually patient is unstable or develops significant complication or new problem.	HPI: ≥4 or 3 CC; ROS: ≥10; PFSH: 3/3	≥8 body areas/systems

Subsequent Day: 2 of 3 key components (see **Table 16-1**) must be performed to at least the degree specified for the codes in each row.

CPT Code/Time[a]	Medical Decision-making[b]	History	1995 Examination[c]
99231 15 min	Straightforward to low complexity PP: Usually stable, recovering, or improving	HPI: 1–3; ROS: 0; PFSH[d]: 0	1 body area/system
99232 25 min	Moderate complexity PP: Usually responding inadequately to therapy or minor complication	HPI: 1–3; ROS: 1; PFSH[d]: 0	2–7 limited
99233 35 min	High complexity PP: Usually patient is unstable or develops significant complication or new problem.	HPI: ≥4 or 3 CC; ROS: 2–9; PFSH[d]: 0	2–7 detailed

Abbreviations: CC, chronic conditions; *CPT, Current Procedural Terminology;* HPI, history of present illness; PFSH, past, family, and social history; PP, presenting problem; ROS; review of systems.

[a] Typical time is an average and represents a range of times that may be higher or lower depending on clinical circumstances.
[b] The presenting problem is considered to be a contributory factor and does not need to be present to the degree specified.
[c] Number of body areas or organ systems examined; see **Table 16-1** for details.
[d] Past, family, and social history is not required for interval history.

Examples

➤ **An 8-week-old is seen in the ED and admitted by Physician A.** Over the past 2 days, the mother reported that the infant seemed warm to the touch, fed much less than normal, and was harder to arouse. The mother had noticed only 2 wet diapers and 1 stool in the past 24 hours.

Review of systems: Fever; no history of heart murmur; no apnea or cyanosis; no wheeze or respiratory distress.

Past, family, and social history: Full-term male; no reported problems with pregnancy or delivery; delivered by repeat cesarean. No maternal complications with delivery; rupture of membranes at the time of cesarean delivery, no fever prior to cesarean delivery. Discharged on day 4 with mother feeding well. No prior ED visits or hospitalizations since birth hospitalization, no sick contacts at home, and lives with parents and 2 older female siblings. Two-month well-child vaccinations were received last week.

Physical examination: Comprehensive examination includes vital signs with rectal temperature 38.0°C (100.4°F) and general appearance with examination of head, mucous membranes, clavicles, heart, lungs, abdomen, hips, genitalia, skin, and general neurologic assessment.

Assessment: Laboratory evaluation: CBC with white blood cells 12,000, no left shift on differential; urinalysis normal or negative with pH 7.0, specific gravity 1.020; fever. Concern for sepsis or serious bacterial infection; doubt pyelonephritis given normal urinalysis; less likely meningitis given normal examination and not ill appearing; doubt bronchiolitis given lack of viral symptoms. Urine and blood culture results pending.

Plan: 8-week-old with fever, dehydration, and lethargy. Admit for IV antibiotics and IV fluids, pending culture results. Continue breastfeeding ad lib. Discussed current diagnostic and treatment plans with parents and advised that Dr B will visit later today to discuss further.

Unit/floor time is 35 minutes with 15 minutes spent in counseling and/or coordination of care. Moderate-complexity MDM, detailed history, and comprehensive examination support the reporting of code **99221**.

●=New code   ▲=Revised code   #=Re-sequenced code   +=Add-on code

➤ **Later that same calendar day, Physician B from the same group practice sees the infant.** She adds to the history (particularly under review of systems), examines the infant, and spends 25 minutes of a 40-minute visit talking with the parents.

ICD-10-CM	CPT
R50.9 (fever, unspecified) **E86.0** (dehydration) **R53.83** (lethargy)	**99222** *MDM:* Moderate complexity *History:* Comprehensive *Physical examination:* Comprehensive *Combined unit/floor time:* 75 minutes with 40 minutes spent in counseling and/or coordination of care

Teaching Point: The total E/M services provided on this date now include key components supporting code **99222**. However, Physician A and Physician B provided hospital care on the admission date with a combined time of 75 minutes with documentation that more than 50% of the unit/floor time was spent in counseling and/or coordination of care. This supports code **99223**. Physician A submits no bill, and Physician B submits the bill for the calendar day's service.

> See Chapter 1 for more information on code selection based on time.

Subsequent Hospital Care

99231–99233 Subsequent hospital care, per day, for the evaluation and management of a patient
- Codes include all E/M services by a physician or QHP of the same specialty and same group practice provided on a subsequent day. The level of service reported will be dependent on the total services provided and documented.
- Selection of the code is based on performance and documentation of *2 of 3 key components* or time if more than 50% of the encounter is spent in counseling and/or coordination of care (see **Table 16-4**).
- An interval history is required for subsequent hospital visits (ie, additional or updated information obtained since the last physician assessment, including chief complaint, history of present illness, and problem-pertinent system review).

> Past, family, and social history is not required as part of an interval history.

Use **Table 16-4** to help you in the selection of the appropriate codes in the following examples:

Examples

➤ **Same patient as previous example (ie, 8-week-old with fever, dehydration, and lethargy).** No reported problems overnight; breastfeeding well; continues to have low-grade fever (38.2°C [100.8°F] maximum temperature) overnight; no reported apnea or cyanosis; no respiratory distress. Drinking better, more wet diapers, more alert.

Physical examination: Expanded problem-focused examination, including vital signs and general appearance, heart, lungs, genitourinary, and skin.

Laboratory: No growth in blood or urine cultures at less than 24 hours.

Assessment/plan: Continued fever. Concern for sepsis; suspect viral etiology given negative workup so far for common serious bacterial infections, such as pyelonephritis and bacteremia. Continue IV antibiotics until culture results are negative for 48 hours; continue breastfeeding ad lib. Spoke with mother and reviewed overnight events, morning laboratory results, current plan, and possible discharge home tomorrow.

ICD-10-CM	CPT
R50.9 (fever)	**99232** *MDM:* Straightforward *History:* Expanded interval history *Physical examination:* Limited (2–7 systems or body areas)

Teaching Point: In this example, the MDM is straightforward based on 2 of 3 MDM elements being limited: a limited number and complexity of problems and management options (stable established problem); limited amount and complexity of data reviewed (laboratory results); and moderate risk of an undiagnosed problem requiring IV antibiotics. A payer may require MDM as 1 of 2 key components supporting subsequent hospital care. This example would be limited to code **99231** if MDM were a required component.

Time cannot be used as the controlling factor in selection of the code because the documentation does not indicate the total floor/unit time or time spent in counseling and/or coordination of care.

➤ **Same progress note as in previous vignette but with the following additional documentation: Spoke with mother for 30 minutes and reviewed overnight events, morning laboratory results, and current plan; anticipate discharge home tomorrow.** Total visit time: 40 minutes.

Time would be used as the controlling factor in selection of the code because a total of 40 minutes was spent on the unit/floor with the patient and more than 50% of the time was spent in counseling. The appropriate code would be **99233**.

Hospital Discharge Day Management

99238	Hospital discharge day management; 30 minutes or less
99239	more than 30 minutes

Codes **99238** (≤30 minutes) and **99239** (>30 minutes) are reported by the attending physician providing discharge services on a day subsequent to the date of the admission service. Discharge codes are not reported when a patient is transferred to another physician or another unit in the same facility.

> **If the total time spent in performing discharge management is not documented in the medical record, code 99239 cannot be supported.**

- Subsequent hospital care is reported in lieu of discharge day management (and initial hospital care) when a patient is transferred to another hospital and receives care from the same physician or a physician of the same group and specialty.
- When a patient is transferred to another facility and into the services of a physician who is not in the same group practice and same specialty as the transferring physician, each physician reports the appropriate E/M code for the service provided.
- A face-to-face physician-patient encounter in the hospital is required, although time is unit/floor time.
- Reporting is based on the total time (does not have to be continuous) spent performing all final discharge services, including, as appropriate, examination of the patient, discussion of the hospital stay, patient and/or family counseling, instructions for continuing care to all relevant caregivers, and preparation of referral forms, prescriptions, and records.

> **Only unit or floor time spent on the date of the discharge management is reported with codes 99238 and 99239. Do not include time spent documenting discharge on a date after the service was rendered.**

- May be used to report discharge services provided to patients who die during their hospital stay.
- Services are reported on the day the physician sees the patient and performs discharge services, even if the patient leaves the hospital on a different day.
- Only the attending physician or physician providing services on behalf of the attending physician (eg, covering physician, physician of same group and same specialty) may report discharge management services. If another physician is providing concurrent care, his or her services would be reported using subsequent hospital visit codes (**99231–99233**).
- Time spent in discharge services must be documented in the medical record to report code **99239**. If the total time spent performing the discharge management is not documented in the medical record, report code **99238** instead of **99239**. Only time spent on the day of discharge may be counted.
- Time spent on the day of discharge performing separately reported services (eg, car safety seat testing) is not included in the discharge day management time.

Examples

➤ **Same patient as previous example (ie, 8-week-old with fever, dehydration, and lethargy). Patient is continued on IV antibiotics until this morning, is breastfeeding well, and has no more fever.** Examination performed includes vital signs, general appearance, heart, lungs, abdomen, and skin. Blood and urine culture results remain negative after 48 hours. Intravenous antibiotics are discontinued. Patient is discharged home with instructions for home care and follow-up. The physician spends 35 minutes on the floor reviewing the hospital course, expected follow-up, and signs and symptoms of possible sepsis or infection with the mother.

This visit would be reported with code **99239** because 35 minutes were spent in the provision of discharge management services and the time was documented in the medical record.

➤ **An attending physician is notified by phone of the death of a patient who was an inpatient.** The physician comes into the facility the next morning and completes documentation. Discharge day management services (**99238–99239**) are not reported when no face-to-face encounter (eg, pronouncement of death or hospital discussion with family) is provided by the attending physician.

Discharge Versus Subsequent Hospital Services

Codes **99238** and **99239** are underused and often reported incorrectly. Subsequent hospital visit codes should not be reported on the day of discharge alone or in addition to the discharge code. Code **99239** is one of the most underreported *CPT* codes, even though it often more accurately reflects the service performed than codes for subsequent hospital care. Physicians often spend longer than 30 minutes in discharge management, especially when the patient is seen several times that day. Time spent in charting *on the day of discharge* is counted in the total unit/floor time. *Note:* The 2021 relative value units (RVUs) were not available at time of publication.

CPT Code	2019 Medicare RVUs
99231	1.11
99232	2.04
99233	2.94
99238	2.06
99239	3.02

Teaching Point: The RVUs for discharge service codes reflect the additional services provided on the day of discharge.

Unique Considerations for Hospital Services

Unusual circumstances can be created by a patient being admitted to the hospital following an office visit and then being seen on hospital rounds by another physician. Proper coding in these situations will be contingent on whether the attending physician and colleagues provide coverage and whether billing is under the same group practice. A group practice is typically distinguished by tax identification (ID) number, but it is important to note any payer contract that defines group practice differently (eg, by group National Provider Identifier).

Coordinating billing is important. The office billing manager should have all hospital charges for each patient by the end of the next business day to coordinate billing and avoid delays in claims submissions.

Office Visit and Initial Hospital Care on Same Day of Service

The primary care physician examines the patient in the office and a colleague admits the patient to the hospital later the same day for the same problem. If using independent tax ID numbers, each physician would submit a separate bill (ie, the primary care physician would bill for the office visit; the colleague would bill for the observation or inpatient hospital admission). If using the same tax ID number, services should be combined into 1 initial hospital care code encompassing the combined work of the 2 encounters. If the 2 encounters are not related and have different diagnoses, there is a legitimate reason to submit a claim for 2 distinct evaluation and management (E/M) services on the same day, even by the same provider, but be prepared to justify payment. If 2 distinct E/M services are reported on the same day of service by the same provider, append modifier **25** to the second service. Alternatively, bundle the 2 encounters, including all appropriate *International Classification of Diseases, 10th Revision, Clinical Modification* codes.

Two Hospital Visits on Same Day of Service

The primary care physician admits the patient to the hospital in the morning and a colleague (same group practice and specialty) is called to see the patient in the evening. The services are combined and billed as a single service. If the physicians are from different group practices or different specialties, the services are separately reportable.

When office or outpatient E/M and hospital admissions occur on the same calendar day, coding will depend on whether the admitting physician and/or physician of the same group and specialty provides face-to-face care in the hospital setting.

Consultations

CPT defines *consultations* as services provided by a physician at the request of another physician or "other appropriate source" to provide advice or opinion about the management or evaluation of a specific problem. Medicare does not recognize consultation codes but pays for the services using codes for other E/M services. Detailed information on the *CPT* and Centers for Medicare & Medicaid Services Medicare guidelines for reporting consultations for office and outpatient consultations appears in **Chapter 7**. Please review those guidelines carefully as general guidelines that apply for all consultations.

Consultation codes should not be reported by the physician who has agreed to accept transfer of care before an initial evaluation. Consultation codes are appropriate to report if the decision to accept transfer of care cannot be made until after the initial consultation evaluation, regardless of site of service.

Guidelines Used by Payers That Follow Medicare Consultation Guidelines

Medicare guidelines require that consultations provided to patients in observation status will be reported with office or outpatient E/M codes **99202–99215**. If the patient is new to the physician (ie, has not received any face-to-face professional services from the physician or another physician of the same specialty who belongs to the same group practice *within the past 3 years*), codes **99202–99205** are reported based on the performance and documentation of the required key components. If the patient does not meet the requirements of a new patient, an established patient office or outpatient E/M code is reported.

Consultations provided to inpatient hospital patients are reported using initial inpatient hospital care codes (**99221–99223**). The admitting physician must report the initial hospital care services with modifier **AI** (principal physician of record) appended to the appropriate code to distinguish the services from the consulting physician. Subsequent face-to-face services, including new consultations within the same admission, are reported with subsequent hospital care codes **99231–99233**.

Check with your commercial payers to learn if they follow Medicare consultation guidelines or have otherwise adopted consultation guidelines that differ from *CPT*. See **Table 16-5**.

Table 16-5. Consultation Codes Using *Current Procedural Terminology* and Medicare Guidelines			
Codes Used by Payers That Follow *CPT* Consultation Guidelines		**Codes Used by Payers That Follow Medicare Consultation Guidelines**	
Observation	**Inpatient**	**Observation**	**Inpatient**
99241–99245	99251–99255	99202–99205, 99212–99215	99221–99223, 99231–99233
Abbreviation: *CPT, Current Procedural Terminology.*			

Guidelines Used by Payers That Follow *Current Procedural Terminology* Consultation Guidelines

Consultations for Patients in Observation

99241–99245 Office consultation for a new or established patient (Includes consultations in other outpatient settings. See key components and time in **Table 16-6**.)

●=New code   ▲=Revised code   #=Re-sequenced code   +=Add-on code

Table 16-6. Observation Consultation Codes

Key Components (For a description of key components, see Table 16-1.)
3 of 3 key components must be performed to at least the degree specified under the code.

CPT Code/Time[a]	Medical Decision-making	History[b]	1995 Examination[c]
99241 15 min	Straightforward	HPI: 1–3; ROS: 0; PFSH: 0	1 body area/system
99242 30 min	Straightforward	HPI: 1–3; ROS: 1; PFSH: 0	2–7 limited
99243 40 min	Low complexity	HPI: ≥4 or 3 CC; ROS: 2–9; PFSH: 1/3	2–7 detailed
99244 60 min	Moderate complexity	HPI: ≥4 or 3 CC; ROS: ≥10; PFSH: 3/3	≥8 body areas/systems
99245 80 min	High complexity	HPI: ≥4 or 3 CC; ROS: ≥10; PFSH: 3/3	≥8 body areas/systems

Abbreviations: CC, chronic conditions; *CPT, Current Procedural Terminology;* HPI, history of present illness; PFSH, past, family, and social history; ROS; review of systems.

[a] Typical time is an average and represents a range of times that may be higher or lower depending on clinical circumstances.

[b] A chief complaint is required for all levels of history.

[c] Number of body areas or organ systems examined; see **Table 16-1** for details.

- Level of care is determined by performing and documenting the required 3 key components (ie, history, physical examination, and MDM) or time as described for other E/M services that are assigned a typical time. Follow-up visits that are initiated by the physician consultant are reported using codes for subsequent observation care services (**99224–99226**).
- If an additional request for an opinion or advice on the same or a new problem is received from the attending physician and documented in the medical record, office or outpatient consultation codes, unlike inpatient consultation codes, may be used again.
- In the observation care setting, report prolonged service in the outpatient setting with a direct patient contact code (**99354, 99355**) in addition to the appropriate outpatient consultation code (**99241–99245**) when the typical time of the consultation is exceeded by 30 minutes or more.

When reporting codes 99202–99205 or 99212–99215 in lieu of consultation codes, see 99417 (prolonged service with or without direct patient contact on the date of an office or other outpatient service). See Chapter 7 for more information on reporting code 99417.

Use **Table 16-6** to help you in the selection of the appropriate codes in the following example:

Example

➤ **A 14-year-old is admitted to observation after an episode of syncope while playing basketball.** The patient's mother notes that her paternal uncle died suddenly at age 19 due to an undetected heart problem and she is quite concerned. The attending physician consults a pediatric cardiologist for her opinion and advice after finding no abnormalities. The cardiologist performs a comprehensive history and physical examination, reviews electrocardiogram tracings, and orders an echocardiogram. Documentation of the written report is included in the shared medical record. Assessment is syncope of unknown origin and family history of sudden cardiac death. The cardiologist reports the service with

ICD-10-CM	CPT
R55 (syncope and collapse) **Z82.41** (family history of sudden cardiac death)	**99244** *MDM:* Moderate *History:* Comprehensive *Physical examination:* Comprehensive Or, if payer does not recognize consultations, office or other outpatient E/M service with moderate-complexity MDM **99204** (new patient) **99214** (established patient)

Teaching Point: If the payer does not allow payment for consultation codes, the appropriate office or other outpatient E/M code is reported. Level 4 (**99204, 99214**) codes are supported based on the moderate complexity of MDM (supported by evaluation of an undiagnosed new problem with uncertain prognosis and a moderate amount and complexity of data to review and analyze). See **Chapter 7** for more information on office and other outpatient E/M code selection.

Inpatient Consultations

99251–99255 Inpatient consultation for a new or established patient

- Codes **99251–99255** are to be used only once by the reporting physician for an individual hospital patient for a particular admission. There are no specific guidelines for the length of stay.
- Follow-up visits provided in the hospital by the same physician must be reported using subsequent care codes (**99231–99233**). Examples of a follow-up visit might be to complete the initial consultation when test results become available or in response to a change in the patient's status.
- If a second consultation by a physician or physicians of the same specialty and same group practice is requested by the attending physician to address a completely different problem during the same hospital stay, subsequent hospital care codes (**99231–99233**) must be reported. The subsequent role of a consultant in the ongoing care of the patient must be clearly stated in the medical record by the attending physician. If the attending physician turns over the care of the patient to the consultant, the consultant, now the new attending physician, should use subsequent hospital care codes (**99231–99233**) to indicate the level of service provided.
- The attending physician and consultant may continue to provide care to the patient. Each would code for subsequent hospital care as long as the problems they manage are different. (The attending and consulting physicians should use different *diagnosis* codes to indicate they are managing different problems.) When 2 physicians provide care for the same diagnosis on 1 date, the medical necessity for each service must be clearly documented.
- If a patient is readmitted for the same or a different problem (ie, a new hospital stay), an initial inpatient consultation code may be reported if it meets the definition and requirements for reporting a consultation.
- When an inpatient consultation is performed on a date a patient is admitted to the hospital, all E/M services provided by the consultant (including any outpatient encounters) related to the admission are reported with the inpatient consultation service code. If a patient is admitted after an outpatient consultation (eg, office, ED) and the patient is not seen on the unit on the date of admission, only the outpatient consultation code is reported.

Use **Table 16-7** to help you in the selection of the appropriate codes in the following examples:

Examples

➤ **A 3-month-old patient is seen by the pediatrician in the ED and is subsequently admitted for bilious vomiting, dehydration, and possible bowel obstruction.** A pediatric surgeon is consulted and, following workup, diagnoses volvulus due to malrotation of the intestine. He documents his written report in the medical record, speaks to the parents, and arranges for immediate surgery. The surgeon reports his consultation service with

ICD-10-CM	CPT
K56.2 (volvulus) Or, if diagnosed as congenital volvulus, **Q43.3** (congenital malformations of intestinal fixation)	**99255 57** Or, if payer does not recognize consultations, **99223 57** (initial hospital visit) *MDM:* High complexity *History:* Comprehensive *Physical examination:* Comprehensive

Table 16-7. Inpatient (99251–99255) Consultation Codes

Key Components (For a description of key components, see Table 16-1.)
3 of 3 key components must be performed to at least the degree specified under the code.

CPT Code/Time[a]	Medical Decision-making[b]	History[c]	1995 Examination[d]
99251 20 min	Straightforward	HPI: 1–3; ROS: 0; PFSH: 0	1 body area/system
99252 40 min	Straightforward	HPI: 1–3; ROS: 1; PFSH: 0	2–7 limited
99253 55 min	Low complexity	HPI: ≥4 or 3 CC; ROS: 2–9; PFSH: 1/3	2–7 detailed
99254 80 min	Moderate complexity	HPI: ≥4 or 3 CC; ROS: ≥10; PFSH: 3/3	≥8 body areas/systems
99255 110 min	High complexity	HPI: ≥4 or 3 CC; ROS: ≥10; PFSH: 3/3	≥8 body areas/systems

Abbreviations: CC, chronic conditions; *CPT, Current Procedural Terminology;* HPI, history of present illness; PFSH, past, family, and social history; ROS, review of systems.

[a] Typical time is an average and represents a range of times that may be higher or lower depending on clinical circumstances.
[b] The presenting problem is considered to be a contributory factor and does not need to be present to the degree specified.
[c] A chief complaint is required for all levels of history.
[d] Number of body areas or organ systems examined; see **Table 16-1** for details.

Teaching Point: Follow-up visits by the gastroenterologist are reported using the appropriate-level subsequent inpatient hospital codes (**99231–99233**). Modifier **57** indicates a decision for surgery at the encounter and may prevent bundling of the consultation with the preservice work of the procedure.

➤ **A neonatologist is asked by an obstetrician to consult with a mother in preterm labor with triplets at 23 weeks' gestation.** She is being treated with steroids and magnesium sulfate. The neonatologist reviews the maternal prenatal and hospital record, interviews the mother, and meets with both parents to discuss fetal and neonatal risks and likely hospital course and complications if delivered in the next few days. The neonatologist spends a total of 65 minutes of floor/unit time devoted to this patient's consultation, which is dominated by discussing morbidity and mortality risks as well as resuscitation and possible treatment.

ICD-10-CM	CPT
O60.02 (preterm labor without delivery, second trimester) **O30.102** (triplet pregnancy, unspecified number of placenta and unspecified number of amniotic sacs, second trimester)	**99253** (typical time 55 minutes) Inpatient floor/unit time (65 minutes) is the key or controlling factor. Or, if payer does not recognize consultations, **99223** (average 70 minutes)

Teaching Point: Pediatric hospital care may, at times, begin prior to birth with services provided to the mother during the peripartum period. Although it is atypical for pediatric claims to be submitted for services to adult patients, these services rendered to the mother are an exception. Services provided prior to delivery are reported as services to the mother (ie, to the mother's health insurance plan).

Code **99223** (typical time 70 minutes) is selected based on *CPT* instruction that the higher-level code is selected when the time of service passes the midpoint between consecutively timed services. Code **99222** (typical time 50 minutes) would be reported to a payer that requires meeting or exceeding the typical time assigned to an E/M code.

Concurrent Care

Concurrent care is defined by *CPT* as the provision of similar services to the same patient by more than 1 physician on the same day. Concurrent care may be provided by physicians from different practices or physicians from the same practice but different specialties. When concurrent care is provided, the diagnosis code(s) reported by each physician should reflect the medical necessity for the provision of services by more than 1 physician on the same *date* of service. Although it is easier to justify concurrent care when each treating physician reports different diagnoses, if the *diagnosis* code is reported for the same condition, it does not prevent billing for the services.

Example

➤ **The attending physician wants the consultant to provide ongoing management of 1 problem (eg, heart failure) while the attending physician provides ongoing management for other active problems (eg, pneumonia, inadequate weight gain).**

Both physicians would report subsequent hospital care codes and link the *CPT* codes to the appropriate *diagnosis* codes.

> See the claim form example in Chapter 1 for an example of linking diagnoses to procedure codes on a claim.

Interprofessional Telephone/Internet/Electronic Health Record Consultation

A consultation request by a patient's attending or primary physician or other QHP soliciting opinion and/or treatment advice by telephone, internet, or EHR from a physician with specialty expertise (consultant) is reported by the consultant with interprofessional consultation codes **99446–99451**. This consultation does not require face-to-face contact between the patient and consultant. The patient may be in the inpatient or outpatient setting.

> For information on reporting interprofessional consultation or on services provided via an interactive audiovisual telemedicine system, see Chapter 20.

Teaching Points: Progression of Care

Selecting the appropriate level of service from the appropriate family of codes will be dependent on the documentation of the child's condition, type of service (observation vs inpatient), and intensity of the service provided on a particular day of service. The following scenarios indicate the category of codes that should be reported based on the progression of care provided (**Figure 16-1**). Remember that the level of service reported is based on all the face-to-face care provided during the calendar day.

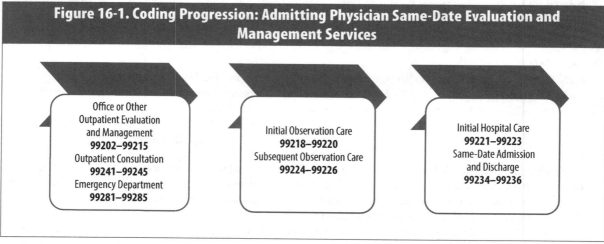

Figure 16-1. Coding Progression: Admitting Physician Same-Date Evaluation and Management Services

Office or Other Outpatient Evaluation and Management
99202–99215
Outpatient Consultation
99241–99245
Emergency Department
99281–99285

Initial Observation Care
99218–99220
Subsequent Observation Care
99224–99226

Initial Hospital Care
99221–99223
Same-Date Admission and Discharge
99234–99236

Report only the applicable service that is farthest to the right (applies to encounters for the same or related problem by the same individual or physicians and/or other QHPs of the same group practice and specialty).

One Physician or Physicians of the Same Specialty and Group

Examples

➤ **A patient receives E/M services in the office and is sent to the hospital on the same day.**

If the patient is examined in the office or outpatient setting, admitted to the hospital for observation or as an inpatient, and not seen in the hospital on the same day, report the appropriate office or outpatient code (**99202–99215**) or consultation code (**99241–99245**) as applicable.

If the patient is examined in the office or outpatient setting, admitted to the hospital for observation or as an inpatient, and seen in the hospital on the same day, report the appropriate initial observation or inpatient hospital code (**99218–99220** or **99221–99223**) based on all the E/M services provided on that calendar day.

If the patient is admitted by Physician A and discharged on the same day by Physician B (from the same practice and of the same specialty), a code for same-day admission and discharge observation or inpatient services (**99234–99236**) is reported based on the combined services.

➤ **A patient receives an initial face-to-face E/M service in the observation setting.**

If the patient is admitted to observation and not discharged or admitted to inpatient status on the same date, the appropriate initial observation code (**99218–99220**) is reported by the attending physician.

If the patient is admitted and discharged on the same day, a code for admission and discharge observation or inpatient services (**99234–99236**) is reported.

If the patient is admitted for observation and subsequently formally admitted to the hospital on the same day, only the initial inpatient hospital code (**99221–99223**) is reported.

If the patient was admitted to observation care status and is seen the following day and not discharged, codes **99224–99226** are reported for the subsequent-day encounter.

If the patient is placed in observation status and then admitted as an inpatient the next day, initial observation (**99218–99220**) and initial hospital care (**99221–99223**) codes are reported with the appropriate dates of service. If the level of service performed during the initial hospital care does not meet the requirements for the initial hospital care (all 3 key components or time requirements), report the appropriate subsequent hospital care code (**99231–99233**).

If the patient is discharged from observation status on a day subsequent to the admission, observation care discharge management (**99217**) is reported.

➤ **A patient receives face-to-face E/M services in the inpatient hospital setting by the attending physician or physicians of the same group and same specialty.**

If the patient is evaluated in the hospital and not discharged on the same date, the appropriate initial hospital care code (**99221–99223**) is reported for the first face-to-face E/M service.

If the patient is admitted and discharged on the same day, a code for admission and discharge observation or inpatient services (**99234–99236**) is reported.

If the patient is followed on subsequent days, codes **99231–99233** are reported for each subsequent day of service.

If the patient is discharged on a day subsequent to the initial service, discharge code **99238** or **99239** is reported.

If the patient's condition deteriorates and he or she requires *critical care services,* coding will be dependent on the age of the child. If the child is 6 years or older, hourly critical care services will be reported (**99291** and **99292**) in addition to codes **99231–99233**. See Chapter 18 for guidelines used to report critical care, including transfers of care and concurrent critical care.

For infants weighing 5,000 g or less, if the patient's condition declines and he or she requires intensive care services, see Chapter 18 for specific details about coding intensive care services.

See examples of transfers from one physician to another physician of a different specialty and/or group practice in **Table 16-8.**

Table 16-8. Transfer of Service in the Observation or Inpatient Status

Example	Physician A reports	Physician B reports as appropriate
The patient is examined by physician A in the office and sent to the hospital to be admitted by physician B, a hospitalist or other physician from a group with a different tax identification number than physician A.	All E/M and other services provided in the office (eg, **99202–99215**)	Initial hospital observation or inpatient service (**99218–99220, 99221–99223**), or same-day admission and discharge if discharged on the same date (**99234–99236**)
Physician A admits the patient during a face-to-face visit and then transfers care (not a consultation) to a physician of a different specialty.	Initial hospital observation or inpatient service (**99218–99220** or **99221–99223**) and, if care is provided on subsequent days prior to transfer, subsequent observation care (**99224–99226**) or subsequent inpatient care (**99231–99233**)	Subsequent observation care (**99224–99226**) or subsequent inpatient care (**99231–99233**) until the day of discharge (observation [**99217**] or hospital [**99238, 99239**])
Physician A admits the patient (face-to-face visit) and requests an opinion or advice from physician B, who may be from the same or different group or specialty, and the requirements for a consultation are performed.	Initial hospital care (**99221–99223**) and, if care is provided on subsequent days prior to discharge, subsequent inpatient care (**99231–99233**) until the day of discharge (**99238** or **99239**)	In observation setting, outpatient consultation or outpatient E/M (**99241–99245** or **99202–99215**); in inpatient setting, inpatient consultation or initial hospital care (**99251–99255** or **99221–99223**) and subsequent care if provided (**99231–99233**); if care is transferred, discharge day management services (**99238** or **99239**)
Physician A admits the patient by phone and then transfers care (not a consultation) to a physician of a different group in the hospital.	There is nothing to report for an admission by phone unless the time spent could be reported by a non–face-to-face code such as non-direct prolonged services (**99358, 99359**) if >30 min is spent.	The appropriate initial hospital observation or inpatient service (**99218–99220, 99221–99223**), or same-day admission and discharge if discharged on the same date (**99234–99236**)

Abbreviation: E/M, evaluation and management.

Prolonged Evaluation and Management Services Provided in the Inpatient Setting

Prolonged service codes are reported when a physician provides services that *are 30 minutes or more beyond the usual service duration* described in an E/M code or other codes with a published maximum time. The code categories for prolonged service are subdivided into service with direct (ie, face-to-face) patient contact and service without direct patient contact.

Direct Prolonged Service

+99356   Prolonged service in the inpatient or observation setting, requiring unit/floor time beyond the usual service; first hour (30–74 min) (List separately in addition to the code for inpatient or observation evaluation and management service.) (Use code **99356** in conjunction with codes **90837, 99218–99220, 99221–99223, 99224–99226, 99231–99233, 99234–99236, 99251–99255, 99304–99310**.)

+99357   each additional 30 minutes (List separately in addition to the code for prolonged physician service.) (Use code **99357** in conjunction with code **99356**.)

According to *CPT*, the prolonged services inpatient add-on codes **99356** and **99357** may be reported in addition to observation codes (**99218–99220, 99224–99226, 99234–99236**) because, although observation care services are performed in an outpatient setting, the intraservice times for the codes are defined as unit or floor time.

● Direct inpatient/observation setting prolonged services (**99356** and **99357**) may only be reported in conjunction with the following codes:

●=New code   ▲=Revised code   #=Re-sequenced code   +=Add-on code

- **99221–99223** (initial hospital care)
  - **99218–99220** (initial observation care)
  - **99234–99236** (admission/discharge same day)
  - **99224–99226** (subsequent observation care)
  - **99231–99233** (subsequent hospital care)
  - **99251–99255** (inpatient consultations)
  - **99304–99310** (nursing facility services)
  - **90837** (psychotherapy without E/M, 60 minutes)
  - **90847** (family psychotherapy [conjoint psychotherapy] [with patient present], 50 minutes)
  - If a code does not have a typical time listed (eg, hospital discharge [**99238**, **99239**]), direct prolonged services may not be reported in conjunction with it.
- Time in the inpatient facility is defined as unit/floor time dedicated to the patient. (*Note:* It is Medicare's policy that time spent reviewing charts or discussion of a patient with house medical staff and not with direct face-to-face contact with the patient cannot be billed as prolonged service. It is important to be aware of Medicaid and private payers that adopt Medicare policy [ie, allow only face-to-face time].)
- When an E/M service is reported using time as the key or controlling factor, prolonged services can be reported only when the prolonged service exceeds 30 minutes beyond the highest level of E/M service (eg, **99220**, **99223**).
- The medical record must reflect the total time of the service and medical need for the service. **Table 16-9** shows the time requirements for codes **99356** and **99357**.

Table 16-9. Coding Direct Prolonged Services for Inpatient and Observation Care

Total Duration of Prolonged Services, min	Code(s)
<30	Not reported separately
30–74	**99356** × 1
75–104	**99356** × 1 and **99357** × 1
≥105 (≥1 h 45 min)	**99356** × 1 and **99357** × 2 (or more for each additional 30 min)

Example

➤ **A 10-year-old patient is admitted to the care of a neurologist following a first-time seizure that occurred shortly after waking in the morning.** The neurologist completes a comprehensive history and physical examination. Results of an electroencephalogram are reviewed. The diagnosis is juvenile myoclonic epilepsy. Later that same day, the neurologist visits the patient and spends 60 minutes discussing the patient's test results and the anticipated plan of care with the parents and documents the total unit/floor time of 120 minutes in the medical record.

The neurologist reports her services with codes **99223** and **99356**.

Teaching Point: The neurologist reports initial inpatient hospital code **99223** based on the key components of comprehensive history and examination and high-complexity MDM. The typical time assigned to code **99223** is 70 minutes. This leaves an additional 50 minutes of unit/floor time that may be appropriately reported with prolonged services code **99356**.

Prolonged Service Before or After Direct Patient Care

99358   Prolonged evaluation and management service before and/or after direct patient care; first hour
99359   each additional 30 minutes (Use code **99359** in conjunction with code **99358**.)

- Non-direct (non–face-to-face) prolonged physician services (**99358** and **99359**) may be reported on a different date than the related primary service. The related primary service may be an E/M service (with or without an assigned typical time), a procedure, or other service.
- Non-direct prolonged E/M services must relate to a face-to-face service that has occurred or will occur and must be relevant to ongoing care.

Example

➤ **The pediatrician spends 40 minutes reviewing extensive medical records that are received the day after a patient is admitted.**

Code **99358** would be reported. Prolonged service of less than 30 minutes' total duration would not be separately reported.

> Refer to Chapter 7 for details of the specific requirements for reporting physician prolonged services in conjunction with office or outpatient evaluation and management services (99202–99205, 99212–99215).

Split/Shared Billing

A split/shared E/M service is one in which a physician and a QHP, such as a nurse practitioner or physician assistant, from the *same group practice* each personally perform a medically necessary and substantive portion of 1 or more face-to-face E/M encounters on the same date.

The following requirements apply to all split/shared services:

- A portion of the key components of the service must be provided face-to-face by the physician to report under the physician's National Provider Identifier.
- Split/shared services were defined and implemented for services to Medicare beneficiaries. Private payers may adopt the same or a similar policy.
- The physician and QHP must each document and sign their portion of the service.
- A physician cannot merely sign off on the documentation of the work by the QHP.
- If the E/M service is reported based on counseling and/or coordination of care, the physician and the QHP must each document their time supporting the level of service reported.
- Documentation must support the total time, the portion of time (ie, >50%) spent in counseling and/or coordination of care, and a summary of the issues discussed and/or coordination of care provided.
- Shared services are not permitted if the QHP is a hospital employee.
- Services may be reported by the QHP or physician (if QHP may bill).
- Shared services are allowed when sick hospital care services are reported (combined physician and QHP time) and with discharge services.
- *Critical care is never a split/shared service* because critical care services reflect the work of only 1 individual.

> Split/shared billing differs from incident-to billing, which is only allowed in a non-facility setting. See Chapter 13 for more information on incident-to rules.

Example

➤ **A pediatrician and QHP from the same group practice see a patient on the same date.** The QHP provides and documents initial hospital care, including a comprehensive history, detailed examination, and MDM of moderate complexity. Later that day, the pediatrician is called to see the patient, who is exhibiting new symptoms, and to review new laboratory test results. Taking into account both services, which have been individually documented and signed, the examination and history are comprehensive and MDM is of high complexity.

Teaching Point: Because both providers are from the same group practice and have signed off on their individually provided services, the services may be shared and billed under the physician as code **99223**. The combined times spent by the physician and QHP may also be used in code selection when more than 50% of that time was spent in counseling and/or coordination of care.

Medical Team Conferences

| 99366 | Medical team conference with interdisciplinary team of health care professionals, face-to-face with patient and/or family, 30 minutes or more, participation by nonphysician qualified health care professional |
| 99367 | Medical team conference with interdisciplinary team of health care professionals, patient and/or family not present, 30 minutes or more; participation by physician |

●=New code ▲=Revised code #=Re-sequenced code +=Add-on code

99368   Medical team conference with interdisciplinary team of health care professionals, patient and/or family not present, 30 minutes or more; participation by nonphysician qualified health care professional

Codes **99366–99368** are used to report participation by physicians or other health care professionals in conferences to coordinate or manage care and services for established patients with chronic or multiple health conditions (eg, cerebral palsy) or with congenital anomalies (eg, craniofacial abnormalities).

> See Chapter 12 for a complete summary of the reporting requirements for medical team conferences.

Code **99367** is the only code that may be reported by a physician, and it can only be reported *when the patient and/or family is not present* at the team conference. When the physician or QHP who may report E/M services (eg, advanced practice nurse) participates in a medical team conference with the patient and/or family present, the appropriate-level E/M code (eg, **99231–99233**) will be reported based on the place of service and total face-to-face time spent in counseling and/or coordination of care.

Advance Care Planning

99497   Advance care planning, including the explanation and discussion of advance directives such as standard forms (with completion of such forms, when performed), by the physician or other qualified health care professional; first 30 minutes, face-to-face with the patient, family member(s) and/or surrogate

+99498   each additional 30 minutes (List separately in addition to code for primary procedure)

Codes **99497** and **99498** include

- Face-to-face service by a physician or QHP to a patient, family member, or surrogate spent in counseling and discussion of advance directives
- Completion of forms, when applicable (eg, Health Care Proxy, Durable Power of Attorney for Health Care, Living Will, Medical Orders for Life-Sustaining Treatment)

Face-to-face time spent by the physician or QHP is required and the total time must be documented.

Active management of problems is not included in advance care planning. Other E/M services provided on the same date as advance care planning may be separately reported, with the exceptions of hourly critical care services (**99291** and **99292**), inpatient neonatal and pediatric critical care (**99468** and **99469**; **99471–99476**), and initial and continuing intensive care services (**99477–99480**).

Do not report codes **99497** and **99498** in conjunction with codes **99291** and **99292**, **99468** and **99469**, **99471–99476**, or **99477–99480**.

Example

➤ **An adolescent with metastatic cancer wishes to discuss and be involved in planning her care.** Her oncologist spends 50 minutes face-to-face with the patient and her parent assessing their understanding of the diagnosis and prognosis, the continued hope that treatment is successful, and the patient's wishes to be included in decisions about her care. A plan of care is developed and documented and an appointment with the supportive care team at the hospital is scheduled to provide additional counseling and support services to the patient and family.

The oncologist may report codes **99497** and **99498** for the 50 minutes of face-to-face time spent providing the advance care planning. Because the *CPT* prefatory language and code descriptors for advance care planning do not include other instruction on the time required for reporting, these services may be reported based on general *CPT* instruction to report when the midpoint is passed (eg, 1 unit of **99498** may be reported for 46–75 minutes). Exceptions may apply for payers with policy requiring that the time be met or exceeded.

Continuing Care After Hospitalization

A key goal of many quality improvement programs is avoidance of readmittance and/or ED visits following hospitalization. In recent years, *CPT* and payers have recognized a need for codes to capture services related to care coordination and management of chronic and episodic conditions that may lead to emergency and inpatient care. For physicians continuing patient care after hospital discharge, services such as transitional care management and chronic care management offer opportunities to provide and be compensated for care aimed at reducing the risk of decline, exacerbation, and/or functional decline.

See Chapter 12 for more information on transitional and chronic care management services.

Hospital-Mandated On-Call Services

99026	Hospital mandated on-call service; in-hospital, each hour
99027	out of hospital, each hour

- Codes **99026** and **99027** describe services provided by a physician who is on call per hospital mandate as a condition of medical staff privileges.
- Used to report on-call time spent by the physician when he or she is not providing other services.
- Time spent performing separately reportable services should not be included in time reported as mandated on-call services.
- Most payers do not cover these services because they consider this a contract issue between the hospital and physician. However, these codes may be used for tracking purposes.

Resources

Hospital Discharge Day Management

"Hospital Discharge Day Management: Are You Coding Correctly?" February 2019 *AAP Pediatric Coding Newsletter* (https://coding.solutions.aap.org/article.aspx?articleid=2720944; subscription required)

Observation Services

"Observation Services: Reporting Care by Multiple Physicians" May 2019 *AAP Pediatric Coding Newsletter* (https://coding.solutions.aap.org/article.aspx?articleid=2731589; subscription required)

Test Your Knowledge!

1. **Which is true of code selection for initial hospital evaluation and management services when based on time?**
   a. Codes are always selected based on time.
   b. Physicians should include only time spent face-to-face with the patient.
   c. Physicians select codes based on the total unit/floor time dedicated to 1 patient.
   d. Unit/floor time includes time spent off the unit/floor (eg, in radiology).

2. **Which key component distinguishes code 99219 from 99220?**
   a. History
   b. Examination
   c. Medical decision-making
   d. None; only the typical time distinguishes the codes.

3. **Which of the following codes is correct when a patient is admitted to inpatient care at 4:00 am and discharged at 3:00 pm on the same date?**
   a. 99238
   b. 99239
   c. 99234–99236
   d. 99217

4. **Which codes would a physician report when a consultation to a patient in observation results in a transfer of care to the consulting physician and admission to inpatient status later on the same date?**
   a. Inpatient consultation (**99251–99255**) and subsequent hospital care (**99231–99233**)
   b. Initial observation care (**99218–99220**)
   c. Subsequent hospital care (**99231–99233**)
   d. Initial hospital care (**99221–99223**)

5. **What additional codes would a pediatrician report for 90 minutes' total unit/floor time when reporting code 99232 (25-minute typical time) based on key components?**
   a. None; there is no face-to-face time noted.
   b. **99356** × 1
   c. **99356** × 1, **99357** × 1
   d. **99358** × 1

●=New code ▲=Revised code #=Re-sequenced code +=Add-on code

Emergency Department Services

Contents

Reporting the Diagnosis Code for Emergency Department (ED) Visits

Emergency department (ED) physicians play critical roles in care and documentation. While multiple symptoms may be listed as the chief complaint during the ED triage process, the physician must designate only 1 sign, symptom, disease, or injury as the chief complaint. Hospitals depend on the physician's designation of the chief complaint because only 1 diagnosis code may be reported for this category on the hospital claim form. This diagnosis is used to help support the urgency of the ED visit under prudent layperson guidelines. This may be different from conditions that are "present on admission" that must now be tracked by hospitals.

The diagnoses on the physician's claim for professional services are equally important. Some health plans now compare diagnosis codes submitted on physician claims that include codes **99284** and **99285** to a predetermined list of diagnosis codes indicating conditions that typically require these levels of service. When a claim for **99284** or **99285** is submitted with diagnosis codes not included on the list, the claim may be down-coded (eg, **99283**) and paid at the rate of the lesser code.

Some Medicaid plans also significantly limit the amount paid for any condition not included on a diagnosis list, regardless of the level of service reported. To receive the payment most appropriate under the health plan contract

- List first the diagnosis that is most responsible for the level of service provided and report the code for that diagnosis first on your claim. Some plans consider only the first 2 diagnoses listed on the claim.
- Document and report codes for all current conditions that require or affect patient care treatment or management. Some plans take into account all diagnoses on the claim, including
- Complicating factors (eg, **F84.0**, autism spectrum disorder)
- Social determinants of health (eg, **Z59.0**, homelessness)
- External cause of injury (eg, **W13.0XXA**, fall [on] [from] balcony)

Physicians should document all diagnoses including factors that increased the complexity of medical decision-making (MDM) of an encounter. To appeal the down-coded claim, medical records supporting the higher level of service must be submitted to the health plan.

Reporting External Cause of Injury

States may require EDs to report codes describing the circumstances of an injury. These codes are referred to as *external cause* codes in *International Classification of Diseases, 10th Revision, Clinical Modification* (*ICD-10-CM*). These codes capture the cause, intent, place of occurrence, activity of the patient at the time of the event, and patient status (eg, employee, military, volunteer, student).

> External cause of injury codes are found in the *International Classification of Diseases, 10th Revision, Clinical Modification* External Cause of Injuries Index. For example, under the term *struck,* sub-terms allow reporting of common causes such as a struck by baseball (W21.03) or even uncommon accidents such as struck by hailstones (X39.8) or lightning (T75.0-). Combination codes allow for reporting multiple details, such as striking against an object with subsequent fall (W18.0-).

External cause codes provide information that is valuable for research on the cause and occurrence of injuries as well as evaluation of injury prevention strategies (eg, reduced reporting of injuries due to automobile crashes following prohibition of cell phone use while driving). This is particularly important in pediatrics, as injuries remain the leading cause for death and disability. While the physician may not be required to add the specific external cause code with the discharge diagnosis, there should be sufficient documentation in the record to allow a coder to extract the proper diagnosis code.

Key points for reporting external cause codes include

- External cause codes may be reported in conjunction with any health condition that is related to an external cause (eg, adverse effect of medical treatment).
- External cause codes are never the principal or first-listed diagnosis code.
- In *ICD-10-CM*, only external cause codes for the cause and intent of an injury or illness are reported for the duration of treatment, with the seventh character of the code indicating whether an encounter is for initial care, subsequent care, or care for sequela (late effect) of the injury or illness.

> Seventh character **A** is often reported for management of injuries other than fracture in the emergency department. It may be helpful to remember that seventh character **A** (initial encounter) is reported for active treatment and not for care during the healing phase of an injury. For example, **S61.411A** (laceration without foreign body of right hand, initial encounter) is reported for active management of the wound versus care during the healing phase or to address a late effect.

●=New code   ▲=Revised code   #=Re-sequenced code   +=Add-on code

Chapter 17. Emergency Department Services

- External cause codes indicating place of occurrence, activity, and patient status are reported only at the initial encounter for treatment.
- If the intent (eg, accident, self-harm, assault) of the cause of an injury or other condition is unknown or unspecified, code the intent as *accidental.*
- No external cause code should be assigned when the cause and intent of an illness or injury are included in another reported code (eg, **T58.11XA**, initial encounter for toxic effect of carbon monoxide from utility gas, accidental).
- No external cause code should be assigned when an injury is ruled out after examination and observation (eg, **Z04.1**, encounter for examination and observation following transport accident).

Reporting Suspected or Confirmed Abuse

Suspected (**T76.-**) or confirmed abuse (**T74.-**) is reported as the first-listed diagnosis when this is the reason for the encounter. Codes for associated mental health or injury are reported secondary to the code for suspected or confirmed abuse. See **Table 17-1** for *ICD-10-CM* codes for abuse that may be reported by ED physicians caring for children.

Table 17-1. Abuse or Neglect: *ICD-10-CM* Codes for Suspected, Confirmed, or Ruled Out

The appropriate seventh character is to be added to each code from categories **T74** and **T76**. **A**, initial encounter; **D**, subsequent encounter; **S**, sequela

Suspected Abuse/Neglect	Confirmed	Ruled Out
T76.02X- Child neglect or abandonment, suspected	**T74.02X-** Child neglect or abandonment, confirmed	Encounter for examination and observation
T76.12X- Child sexual abuse, suspected	**T74.12X-** Child physical abuse, confirmed	**Z04.42** following alleged child rape (ruled out)
T76.32X- Child psychological abuse, suspected	**T74.22X-** Child sexual abuse, confirmed	**Z04.72** following alleged child physical abuse (ruled out)
T76.52X- Child sexual exploitation, suspected	**T74.32X-** Child psychological abuse, confirmed	**Z04.81** of victim following forced sexual exploitation
T76.62X- Child forced labor exploitation, suspected	**T74.4XX-** Shaken infant syndrome	**Z04.82** of victim following forced labor exploitation
	T74.52X- Child sexual exploitation, confirmed	
	T74.62X- Child forced labor exploitation, confirmed	

- Codes are selected based on documentation. The record should clearly state whether abuse is suspected, ruled out, or confirmed.
- If a suspected case of child abuse, neglect, or mistreatment is ruled out during an encounter, code **Z04.72** (encounter for examination and observation following alleged child physical abuse, ruled out) should be used, not a code from **T76**.
- If a suspected case of forced sexual exploitation or forced labor exploitation is ruled out during an encounter, code **Z04.81** (encounter for examination and observation of victim following forced sexual exploitation) or **Z04.82** (encounter for examination and observation of victim following forced labor exploitation) should be used, not a code from **T76**.
- When reporting confirmed abuse, report also codes for assault (**X92–Y04**; **Y08**, **Y09**) and perpetrator (**Y07.-**).

ED Evaluation and Management Codes

- Evaluation and management (E/M) codes **99281–99285** are only reported when care is provided in an ED. An ED is defined as an organized hospital-based facility for the provision of unscheduled episodic services to patients who present for immediate medical attention. The facility must be available 24 hours a day, 7 days a week.
  - Some states allow for freestanding EDs that are not hospital affiliated. Payers may or may not allow the use of ED codes in these circumstances.
  - Physician services provided in a freestanding hospital-affiliated ED may be subject to specific billing rules. Check payer contracts for payment and billing policies.
- Services performed in an urgent care center, a nonhospital facility, or a facility that is not open 24 hours a day should be reported with the appropriate *Current Procedural Terminology* (CPT®) office or outpatient visit codes (**99202–99215**) and with the appropriate place of service code (eg, **20** for urgent care facility). These facilities are not considered freestanding EDs.

- Selection of the appropriate E/M code is primarily driven by the risk involved in the presenting problem, evaluation measures, and/or treatment options.
- Performance and documentation of all 3 key components (ie, history, physical examination, and MDM) are used to select the level of an ED E/M code.

Emergency Department Caveat: Code 99285

The emergency department evaluation and management code 99285 allows an exception to the "3 key components" rule (Level 5 caveat) for patients whose clinical condition, mental status, or lack of available history may not permit obtaining a comprehensive history and/or physical examination. Therefore, code 99285 may be reported for patients presenting with a high-severity condition that requires a high level of medical decision-making when circumstances prevent the physician from obtaining a comprehensive history and/or completing a comprehensive physical examination. When such urgency exists, the physician must document the condition or reason why a comprehensive history and/or comprehensive physical examination could not be obtained.

- Time spent in counseling and/or coordination of care *cannot* be used as a key or controlling factor in the selection of the E/M code; nor can prolonged services be reported with ED codes. Because of the unpredictability and inconsistency in the intensity of these services, there are presently no time values assigned to this family of codes.
- There is no differentiation between new or established patients for ED encounters. All problems for encounters in the ED are considered new to the attending physician for purposes of determining MDM.
- The ED codes are not reported if the treating ED physician admits the patient to his or her service for observation or inpatient status on the same date of service as the ED encounter. Only the appropriate initial observation (**99218–99220**), initial hospital care (**99221–99223**), or initial observation or inpatient hospital admission and discharge, same day (**99234–99236**), codes are reported instead of ED codes. All the E/M work performed in the ED should be combined with any additional work performed for admission (and, when appropriate, discharge) when selecting the correct code and level of care.

Table 17-2 summarizes the key components required for each ED E/M code based on the 1995 and 1997 Centers for Medicare & Medicaid Services *Documentation Guidelines for Evaluation and Management Services*. Also refer to **Chapter 6**, Evaluation and Management Documentation Guidelines, for more details on E/M coding guidelines. Medical necessity is an overarching criterion for selecting the level of E/M service. Physicians should always consider whether the nature of the presenting problem supports the medical necessity of services rendered when selecting the level of E/M service.

Use **Table 17-2** to help you in the selection of the appropriate level of ED E/M service in the examples for each level of service that follow.

For more information on coding evaluation and management services in the emergency department, see "Evaluation and Management Coding in the Emergency Department" in the May 2018 *AAP Pediatric Coding Newsletter* ™ (https://coding.solutions.aap.org/article. aspx?articleid=2679117; subscription required).

Examples

➤ **A 9-month-old presents with a rash.** History of present illness (HPI): Rash noted by mother this evening after arriving home from a trip to visit relatives. All systems are reviewed and results are normal other than rash. Immunizations are up to date. Current temperature is 36.4°C (97.5°F). The infant appears well with vesicles characteristic of heat rash on neck, back, and inner thighs. Examination of head, eyes, ears, nose, oropharynx, cardiovascular, and respiratory systems are normal. The diagnosis of miliaria rubra is discussed with parents, who are instructed to follow up with the primary care pediatrician if they have any concerns.

Chapter 17. Emergency Department Services

Table 17-2. Emergency Department Services

Key Components

3 of 3 key components must be performed to at least the degree specified for each code. All patients in the emergency department are considered new patients.

Code	MDM	History	Physical Examination
99281	**Straightforward** # Diagnoses/options: Minimal Data: Minimal Risk: Minimal	**Problem focused** HPI: 1–3 elements ROS: 0 PFSH: 0	**Problem focused** **1995:** One body area/organ system **1997:** 1–5 elements identified by a bullet (●) in ≥1 areas or systems
99282	**Low complexity** # Diagnoses/options: Limited Data: Limited Risk: Low	**Expanded problem focused** HPI: 1–3 elements ROS: 1 PFSH: 0	**Expanded problem focused** **1995:** Limited examination—affected body area/organ system and 1–6 other related areas/systems **1997:** ≥6 elements identified by a bullet (●) in ≥1 areas or systems
99283	**Moderate complexity** # Diagnoses/options: Multiple Data: Moderate Risk: Moderate	**Expanded problem focused** HPI: 1–3 elements ROS: 1 PFSH: 0	**Expanded problem focused** **1995:** Limited examination—affected body area/organ system and 1–6 other related areas/systems **1997:** ≥6 elements identified by a bullet (●) in ≥1 areas or systems
99284	**Moderate complexity** # Diagnoses/options: Multiple Data: Moderate Risk: Moderate	**Detailed** HPI: 4+ elements or status of 3 chronic or inactive conditions ROS: 2–9 PFSH: 1	**Detailed** **1995:** Extended examination—affected body area(s) and 1–6 other symptomatic or related organ system(s) **1997:** ≥2 elements identified by a bullet (●) in ≥6 areas or systems or ≥12 elements identified by a bullet (●) in ≥2 areas or systems
99285	**High complexity** # Diagnoses/options: Extensive Data: Extensive Risk: High	**Comprehensive** HPI: 4+ elements or status of 3 chronic or inactive conditions ROS: 10+ PFSH: 2 Or clinical condition or mental status did not permit performance of history (must document reason that comprehensive history could not be performed).	**Comprehensive** **1995:** 8+ organ systems or complete examination of a single organ system **1997:** <u>Multisystem examination</u>—≥9 organ systems or body areas with performance of all elements identified by a bullet (●) in each area/system examined Documentation is expected for ≥2 elements identified by a bullet (●) of each area(s) or system(s). <u>Single organ system examination</u>—Performance of all elements identified by a bullet (●) and documentation of every element in each box with a shaded border and at least 1 element in a box with an unshaded border Or clinical condition or mental status did not permit performance of examination.

Abbreviations: HPI, history of present illness; MDM, medical decision-making; PFSH, past, family, and social history; ROS, review of systems.

> **ICD-10-CM**
> **L74.0** (miliaria rubra)
>
> **CPT**
> **99281**
> *Documentation must support all 3 elements (ie, MDM, history, and examination).*
> MDM: Straightforward (no. of diagnoses/options: minimal [self-limiting condition]; data: limited; risk: minimal)
> History: Detailed (HPI: 1–3 elements [duration of rash, associated fever]; review of systems [ROS]: 14 systems; past, family, and social history [PFSH]: past history [immunization history])
> Examination: Expanded problem focused (1995) (limited examination of affected body area/organ system plus 1–6 other related areas/systems)

Teaching Point: The straightforward MDM supports code **99281**. Low-complexity MDM is required to support **99282**.

➤ **An 11-month-old presents with fever and cough.** The parents note that the infant has had nasal congestion for several days and now has fever and cough. The ROS is notable for irritability, rhinorrhea, and cough. Temperature at home was 38.0°C (100.4°F) and is now 37.2°C (99.0°F). No medications were given at home. The infant has no known drug allergies, and all immunizations are up to date. A detailed examination is performed. The diagnosis is upper respiratory infection. Parents are instructed to manage with humidifier and use of saline and nasal bulb and to monitor for dehydration.

> **ICD-10-CM**
> **J06.9** (acute upper respiratory infection, unspecified)
>
> **CPT**
> **99282**
> *Documentation must support all 3 elements (ie, MDM, history, and examination).*
> MDM: Low complexity (no. of diagnoses/options: multiple [new problems without additional workup planned]; data: limited [history obtained from others]; risk: low)
> History: Detailed (HPI: 4 elements; ROS: 3; PFSH: past history [no known drug allergies, immunizations])
> Examination: Detailed (1995) (extended examination of affected body area/organ system plus 1–6 other related body areas/organ systems)

Teaching Point: The low-complexity MDM supports code **99282**.

➤ **An 8-month-old presents with poor feeding and crankiness.** HPI: Mother suspects ear infection; the infant has not eaten well for the past 2 days and cried several times during the night. ROS: The infant is pulling at her left ear. There has been a normal number of wet diapers today. The pediatrician diagnosed bilateral otitis media 1 month ago, which was treated with amoxicillin. The patient is fully immunized and has no known drug allergies. A detailed examination is performed with findings supporting acute recurrent suppurative otitis media of the left ear. The plan of amoxicillin/clavulanate, 600 mg/5 mL twice daily for 10 days, with follow-up with primary care in 14 days, is discussed with the parents, who are provided a patient education handout on otitis media.

ICD-10-CM
H66.005 (acute suppurative otitis media without spontaneous rupture of ear drum, recurrent, left ear)

CPT
99283
Documentation must support all 3 elements (ie, MDM, history, and examination).

MDM: Moderate complexity (no. of diagnoses/options: multiple [new problem without additional workup planned]; data: limited [history from someone other than the patient]; risk: moderate [prescription drug management])

History: Expanded problem focused (HPI: 1–3 elements; ROS: 2–9; PFSH: past history [otitis media, no known drug allergies, immunization history])

Examination: Detailed (1995) (extended examination of affected body area[s] and other symptomatic or related organ systems)

Teaching Point: The expanded problem-focused history supports code **99283**.

➤ **A 6-month-old presents with fever and crankiness.** HPI: The infant has a temperature of 38.9°C (102.0°F). Ibuprofen was given at home about 2 hours ago. The infant is pulling at his left ear, is not eating well, and has been cranky since last evening. ROS: The infant has mild nasal congestion. There has been a normal number of wet diapers today. There has been no vomiting or diarrhea. All other systems are reviewed and results are negative. The ED physician uses an electronic exchange to review primary pediatric records for the infant, who was diagnosed with bilateral otitis media 1 month ago, which was treated with amoxicillin. The patient is fully immunized and has no known drug allergies. A detailed examination is performed, noting an ill-appearing infant. The diagnosis is acute suppurative otitis media of the right ear and fever with no indications of other potential cause. The plan of amoxicillin/clavulanate, 600 mg/5 mL twice daily for 10 days, with follow-up with primary care in 14 days or sooner if symptoms persist, is discussed with the parents, who are provided a patient education handout on otitis media.

ICD-10-CM
H66.001 (acute suppurative otitis media without spontaneous rupture of ear drum, right ear)
R50.9 (fever)

CPT
99284
Documentation must support all 3 elements (ie, MDM, history, and examination).

MDM: Moderate complexity (no. of diagnoses/options: multiple [new problems without additional workup planned]; data: moderate; risk: moderate)

History: Detailed (HPI: 4+ elements or status of 3 chronic or inactive conditions; ROS: complete; PFSH: 1 [past medical])

Examination: Detailed (1997) (≥2 elements identified by a bullet [●] in ≥6 areas or systems or ≥12 elements identified by a bullet [●] in ≥2 areas or systems)

Teaching Point: The patient's presentation required evaluation for the cause of the fever, which may have been due to a process other than the otitis media. If the physician documented the otitis media as recurrent, the *ICD-10-CM* code would be **H66.004**.

➤ **The ED physician evaluates a 10-month-old for fever, vomiting, and lethargy.** A comprehensive history and physical examination are performed and there is high-complexity MDM for this new problem requiring additional workup and hospitalization. Because of a concern for meningitis, the on-call pediatrician is consulted and is asked to perform a lumbar puncture and to determine the child's disposition. The pediatrician does the procedure, confirms the course of treatment by the ED physician, and admits the infant as an inpatient to her service.

> **ICD-10-CM**
> **R50.9** (fever)
> **R11.10** (vomiting)
> **R53.83** (lethargy)
>
> **CPT**
> **99285** (ED visit code)
> *Documentation must support all 3 elements (ie, MDM, history, and examination).*
> MDM: High complexity (no. of diagnoses/options: extensive; data: moderate; risk: high)
> History: Comprehensive (HPI: 4+ elements or status of 3 chronic or inactive conditions; ROS: 10+; PFSH: 2)
> Examination: Comprehensive (1995) (8+ organ systems or complete examination of a single organ system)

Teaching Point: The ED physician reports **99285**. The admitting pediatrician reports codes **99221–99223 25** (initial inpatient hospital care) and **62270** (lumbar puncture) in conjunction with the same diagnosis codes reported by the ED physician. See the Comanagement of ED Patients section later in this chapter. A code for meningitis is not reported until the encounter at which the condition is confirmed.

➤ **The ED physician is treating a 6-year-old who was struck by a car while riding a bicycle on a neighborhood street.** The patient is brought in by emergency medical services (EMS) from the scene with concern for closed head trauma (no known loss of consciousness [LOC] is reported) with vomiting and multiple friction burns and bruises. The child is not accompanied by a parent. The child was wearing a helmet. Despite initial concern that the child might be in imminent risk of a life-threatening condition, after further assessment and comprehensive examination, imaging studies, and consultation with a trauma surgeon, the ED physician determines there is no risk of deterioration and the child is clinically stable. No history, other than that obtained from EMS, is available prior to the *trauma service* evaluation. There was high-complexity MDM. No separately billable procedures were performed. The child is admitted for observation by a hospitalist for a concussion.

> **ICD-10-CM**
> **S06.0X0A** (concussion with no LOC, initial encounter)
> **T22.151A** (friction burn, first degree, right shoulder, initial encounter)
> **S50.811A** (abrasion, right forearm, initial encounter)
> **S50.311A** (abrasion, right elbow, initial encounter)
> **S70.02XA**, **S70.12XA** (contusions, left hip and thigh, initial encounter)
> **V13.4XXA** (bicycle driver collision with car, traffic accident, initial encounter)
> **Y92.414** (local residential or business street as the place of occurrence)
>
> **CPT**
> **99285** (ED visit code)

Teaching Point: The Level 5 caveat regarding unobtainable history would apply because this patient's condition was initially felt to be unstable and no other history, other than that from EMS, was available. Evaluation and management services by the trauma surgeon would be reported with office or other outpatient consultation codes (likely **99244** or **99245**). The admitting hospitalist will report initial observation care (**99218–99220**). All diagnoses are reported by each physician.

Comanagement of ED Patients

Only 1 physician should report an ED E/M service for a patient who receives care in the ED. In general, this will be the emergency physician or pediatric emergency medicine specialist who is staffing the ED. At times, other physicians (eg, generalists, specialists) may provide care for a patient in the ED.

The type of service reported will depend on whether the other physician is providing consultative services, a specific intervention (eg, diagnostic or therapeutic procedure), or primary management of the patient. The ED physician will typically report the ED E/M code or time-based critical care (when provided) and the other physician will report services as follows:

●=New code ▲=Revised code #=Re-sequenced code +=Add-on code

Chapter 17. Emergency Department Services

- *Consultation:* An outpatient consultation (**99241–99245**) may be reported with place of service **23** (ED) when the ED physician requests the opinion of and/or advice from the other physician. See **Chapter 8** for full requirements for codes **99241–99245**.
- If a payer follows Medicare guidelines and does not cover consultations or the second physician is called in to assume management of the patient's care, services should be reported using the office or outpatient E/M codes (**99202–99215**) with place of service **23**. See **Chapter 7**, Office and Other Outpatient Evaluation and Management Services, for detailed requirements for reporting consultations.
- *Observation or inpatient admission:* See **Chapter 16** for discussion of codes reported when a consulting physician admits the child to the hospital for observation or inpatient services after stabilization and/or provision of care in the ED. For inpatient intensive or critical care services, see codes discussed in **Chapter 18**.
- *Critical care:* If the patient is critically ill or injured, the physicians providing critical care services may report the services using time-based critical care codes **99291** and **99292** (see **Table 18-2**).

Directing Emergency Medical Technicians

99288   Physician or other qualified health care professional direction of emergency medical systems (EMS) emergency care, advanced life support

- Report code **99288** (physician direction of EMS) when
  - The physician directing the services is in the hospital and in 2-way communication with EMS personnel who are in the prehospital setting providing advanced life support that requires direct or online medical control.
  - The documentation includes the times of all contacts, any orders provided, and/or directions provided to the EMS team.
- Code **99288** may be reported on the same day as ED E/M or hourly critical care services. Modifier **25** would be appended to code **99288** to alert payers that this was a significant and separately identifiable service from ED E/M (**99281–99285**) or the critical care (**99291, 99292**) service provided.
- The supervising physician cannot report the actual procedures and interventions performed by the EMS team because he or she is not physically present during the transport.
- Code **99288** is designated as a bundled procedure (included in the work value of other services) by Medicare. There are no relative values assigned under the Medicare Resource-Based Relative Value Scale. Check with your major payers and negotiate for coverage of this service.
- See codes **99485** and **99486** in **Chapter 18**, Critical and Intensive Care, for information on supervision of inter-facility transport of a critically ill or injured patient, 24 months or younger, via direct 2-way communication with a transport team.
- When a qualified health care professional (QHP) (eg, nurse practitioner) provides critical care services during transport, and those services will be reported under the QHP's National Provider Identifier or by the employing hospital, the ED physician does not report **99288**.

Critical Care in the ED

99291   Critical care, E/M of the critically ill or critically injured patient; first 30 to 74 minutes
+99292   each additional 30 minutes (Use in conjunction with **99291**.)

To report **99291** and **99292**, the patient's condition must meet the specific *CPT* definition of a critically ill or injured patient. A *critical illness* or *injury* is defined in *CPT* as one that acutely impairs 1 or more vital organs such that there is a high probability of imminent or life-threatening deterioration of the patient's condition. Guidelines for reporting critical care codes **99291** (critical care, E/M of the critically ill or injured patient; first 30–74 minutes) and **99292** (each additional 30 minutes) are described in detail in **Chapter 18**, Critical and Intensive Care.

- Time-based critical care codes (**99291, 99292**) should be used to report the provision of critical care when performed in the ED. The global codes for pediatric or neonatal critical care should not be reported by a physician providing critical care in the ED unless that physician (eg, an intensivist) will continue to provide critical care services in the inpatient setting.
- Time spent providing critical care does not need to be continuous and includes time at the bedside as well as time in the ED reviewing data specific to the patient, discussing the patient with other physicians, and discussing the patient's management or condition with the patient's family.

> Time of any learner (eg, student, resident) involved in the patient's care may not be reported by the attending physician. Only the time specifically spent by the attending physician may be reported.

- Time reported for critical care must be devoted to the critically ill or injured patient. Therefore, the "critical care clock" stops when attention is turned to the care of another patient or the physician is not readily available in the ED.
- See **Table 18-1** for a list of services and procedures that are included in hourly critical care codes.
- Those procedures not bundled with codes **99291** and **99292** and personally performed by the reporting provider may be reported separately (eg, starting an intravenous line on a child younger than 3 years, placing an intraosseous or central venous line, endotracheal intubation, cardiopulmonary resuscitation [CPR], cardioversion). Time spent performing these separately reported services must be subtracted from the critical care time calculated and reported.

Example

➤ **A 13-month-old with apparent sepsis and hypotension is brought to the ED.** The child requires placement of an intraosseous needle to achieve vascular access and subsequently receives parenteral fluids, antibiotics, and vasopressors. The child experiences cardiopulmonary arrest, prompting the ED physician to intubate the child. Cardiopulmonary resuscitation is performed for 20 minutes. The child is in the ED for a total of 45 minutes before transfer to the intensive care unit.

ICD-10-CM
I46.9 (cardiac arrest)
This code would be reported if the physician included sepsis in the diagnosis; for example, **A41.9** (sepsis, unspecified organism), **R65.21** (severe sepsis with septic shock), **I46.8** (cardiac arrest due to other underlying condition).

CPT
99285 25
92950 (CPR)
36680 (placement of intraosseous needle)
31500 (endotracheal intubation, emergency)

    Teaching Point: Critical care time does not accrue during the performance of non-bundled, separately billable procedures. Because CPR is a separately billable, non-bundled procedure, the ED physician did not spend a minimum of 30 minutes providing critical care. Because the E/M service is reported rather than critical care, coding is based on documented key components of history, examination, and MDM. However, the caveat for code **99285** allows reporting based on the extent of history and examination possible within the constraints imposed by the urgency of the patient's clinical condition and mental status.

- Critical care may be reported on the same day as an ED E/M code when provided by the same physician as long as 2 independent services are provided. Modifier **25** should be appended to the ED E/M code when this occurs.

Examples

➤ **The ED physician performs a comprehensive history and physical examination on a 13-month-old patient with severe stridor and respiratory distress believed to be secondary to croup.** Medical decision-making is highly complex. The patient's condition does not improve with nebulized epinephrine and then worsens, evidenced by progressive lethargy. The patient goes into respiratory failure and 75 minutes of critical care is provided. Ten minutes of the critical care time is spent performing endotracheal intubation.

ICD-10-CM
J96.00 (acute respiratory failure)
J05.0 (croup)

CPT
99285 25 (ED visit code)
99291 25 (critical care, first 30–74 minutes)
31500 (endotracheal intubation, emergency)

●=New code ▲=Revised code #=Re-sequenced code +=Add-on code

Teaching Point: Endotracheal intubation is not bundled with critical care; therefore, time spent in the provision of the service (10 minutes for this patient) is not considered in the total critical care time, so only the base code, **99291**, can be used. Modifier **25** is appended to codes **99285** and **99291** to indicate they were significant and separately identifiable services.

➤ **The ED physician saw a 10-year-old for moderate asthma exacerbation in the morning.** The child responded well to an aerosolized bronchodilator treatment and was discharged home. The child returns to the ED a few hours later with a more severe exacerbation and is seen by the same physician. The child now has respiratory failure with hypoxia. The child receives oxygen, a continuous bronchodilator nebulizer treatment, and, subsequently, a parenteral broncho-dilation drug. The child improves enough to be admitted to a monitored medical ward bed with diagnosis of respiratory failure due to status asthmaticus. The ED physician spends a total of 60 minutes in patient-directed critical care.

ICD-10-CM **J96.01** (acute respiratory failure with hypoxia) **J45.42** (moderate persistent asthma with status asthmaticus)
CPT **99284 25** **99291**

Teaching Point: The patient received oxygen, continuous inhalation treatment, and parenteral bronchodilator in the ED. However, these services include no professional component. The facility will report the services because the cost of supplies and clinical staff time are an expense to the facility.

International Classification of Diseases, 10th Revision, Clinical Modification codes for severe sepsis (R65.20) and septic shock (R65.21) are reported secondary to the underlying infection (eg, A41.9, sepsis, unspecified organism) and followed by codes for related organ failure (eg, J96.01, acute respiratory failure with hypoxia).

Reporting Procedures in the ED

Many procedures performed in the ED have an associated global period assigned by Medicare and other payers and/or are subject to the *CPT* surgical package. The global period affects reporting of pre- and post-procedural care. The *CPT* surgical package defines the work included in each surgical procedure. (See **Chapter 19**, Common Surgical Procedures and Sedation in Facility Settings, for the definition of the *CPT* surgical package and Medicare global period and examples of reporting procedures when follow-up care is provided by another physician.)

To report an E/M service in addition to a procedure, there must be documentation of performance of a significant and separately identifiable E/M service beyond the pre- and post-procedural work typical for the procedure (eg, evaluation for a concussion and repair of wounds at 1 encounter). Post-procedural prescriptions for pain control or prophylactic antibiotics may be included in the procedure performed.

Table 17-3 contains a list of procedures (with assigned Medicare global periods) commonly performed in the ED.

Any separately identifiable procedure that is personally performed by the physician may be reported, with the exception of

- Procedures that are bundled in time-based critical care codes (See **Table 18-1** for a list of services and procedures that are included in hourly critical care codes.)
- Services performed by hospital personnel because they are billed by the hospital facility (If a nurse or other clinical staff assist in part of a procedure, the ED physician may bill for the professional services if the ED physician provides the primary or key component of the procedure.)
- Hydration, infusion, and/or injection procedures (**96360–96379**) because the physician work associated with the procedures involves only confirmation of the treatment plan and not direct supervision of staff
- Procedures involving use of hospital-owned equipment (eg, pulse oximetry), unless the procedure includes a technical and professional component (If performed and documented, the professional component may be reported with modifier **26** [professional component] appended to the procedure code.)
- Modifier **54** is appropriately appended to procedure codes with 10- or 90-day global periods when the patient will not return to the ED for follow-up care (eg, removal of sutures or fracture care follow-up visits).

Table 17-3. Common Emergency Department Procedures

Procedures Not Assigned a Global Period

These procedures have an X or M status in the Medicare Physician Fee Schedule.

Arterial puncture **36600**

Venipuncture, >3 y requiring physician skill **36410**

Venipuncture, <3 y requiring physician skill, femoral/jugular **36400**

Procedures With 0-Day Global Period

Bladder aspiration **51100**

Burn care, <5% TBSA **16020**, 5%–10% TBSA **16025**, >10% TBSA **16030**

Cardiopulmonary resuscitation **92950**

Cardioversion **92960**

Chest tube insertion **32551**

Endotracheal intubation, emergency **31500**

Foreign body removal, conjunctiva **65205**, ear **69200**

Gastric intubation and aspiration(s), therapeutic, including lavage (if performed) **43753**

Intraosseous needle placement **36680**

Laceration repair, simple ≤2.5 cm, face/ears/lips **12011**

    Repair, simple, scalp/trunk/extremities ≤2.5 cm, **12001**, 2.6–7.5 cm **12002**

    Repair, simple 2.6–5.0 cm, face/ears/lips **12013**

Lumbar puncture **62270**, with fluoroscopic or CT guidance **62328**

Pleural drainage, percutaneous, with insertion of indwelling catheter; without imaging guidance **32556**, with imaging guidance **32557**

Splint, finger **29130**, short arm **29125**, short leg **29515**, ankle **29540**

Strap, knee **29530**, shoulder **29240**

Subungual hematoma evacuation **11740**

Thoracentesis, needle or catheter, without imaging **32554**, with imaging **32555**

Procedures With 10-Day Global Period

Foreign body removal, nose **30300**

Foreign body removal with incision, subcutaneous, simple **10120**

Incision and drainage, abscess, simple **10060**

Incision and drainage, finger, complicated (eg, felon) **26011**

Incision and drainage, perianal abscess **46050**

Laceration repair, intermediate, face/ears/lips ≤2.5 cm **12051**, 2.6–5.0 cm **12052**

    Repair, intermediate, hands/feet/neck ≤2.5 cm **12041**, 2.6–7.5 cm **12042**

    Repair, intermediate, scalp/trunk/arms/legs ≤2.5 cm **12031**, 2.6–7.5 cm **12032**

Nursemaid elbow reduction **24640**

Puncture aspiration of abscess, hematoma, bulla, or cyst **10160**

Repair, nail bed **11760**

Procedures With 90-Day Global Period

Fracture, clavicle **23500**

Fracture, finger distal, each **26750**

Fracture, finger shaft, each **26720**

Dislocation, shoulder, reduction **23650**

Abbreviations: *CPT, Current Procedural Terminology;* CT, computed tomography; TBSA, total body surface area.

Point-of-Care Ultrasound

Point-of-care ultrasound services performed by the ED physician (**Table 17-4**) are separately reportable in addition to the ED E/M service when *all 3 of the following conditions apply:*

- Thorough evaluation of organ(s) or anatomical region is performed.
- There is permanent image documentation (with measurements, when clinically indicated).
- A written report equivalent to that typically produced by a radiologist is documented.

●=New code ▲=Revised code #=Re-sequenced code +=Add-on code

Use of handheld or portable ultrasound that does not include all 3 of the listed elements is not separately reported.

Without all these elements, the examination is not separately reported and would be considered part of any E/M service provided. (*Exception:* Permanent image documentation is not required for ophthalmic ultrasound for biometric measurement.)

Table 17-4. Codes for Common Point-of-Care Ultrasound Procedures
76536 Soft tissues of head and neck (eg, thyroid, parathyroid, parotid)
76604 Chest (includes mediastinum when performed)
76700 Abdominal; complete
76705 Abdominal; limited (eg, single organ, quadrant, follow-up)
76770 Retroperitoneal (eg, renal, aorta, nodes), complete
76775 Retroperitoneal (eg, renal, aorta, nodes), limited
76857 Pelvis (nonobstetric); limited or follow-up
76870 Scrotum and contents[a]
76881 Complete joint (eg, joint space and periarticular soft tissue structures)[b]
76882 Joint or other nonvascular extremity structure(s), limited[b]
76885 Infant hips; dynamic (requiring physician or other QHP manipulation)
76886 Infant hips; limited, static (not requiring physician or other QHP manipulation)
+76937 Ultrasound guidance for vascular access requiring ultrasound evaluation of potential access sites, documentation of selected vessel patency, concurrent real-time ultrasound visualization of vascular needle entry, with permanent recording and reporting (List separately in addition to code for primary procedure.)
93976 Duplex scan of arterial inflow and venous outflow of abdominal, pelvic, scrotal contents and/or retroperitoneal organs; limited study[a]

Abbreviation: QHP, qualified health care professional.

[a] Evaluation of vascular structures using color and spectral Doppler is separately reportable. However, color Doppler alone, when performed for anatomical structure identification in conjunction with a real-time ultrasound examination, is not reported separately.

[b] Code **76881** requires ultrasound examination of all the following joint elements: joint space (eg, effusion), periarticular soft-tissue structures that surround the joint (eg, muscles, tendons, other soft tissue structures), and any identifiable abnormality. When fewer than all the required elements for a "complete" examination (**76881**) are performed, report the "limited" code (**76882**).

Point-of-care ultrasound services in the ED are reported by the physician with the professional service only modifier (**26**). (See **Table 17-5** and the Modifiers Used With ED Codes section later in this chapter for more information.) The technical component (eg, equipment cost, facility overhead costs) is typically reported by the facility. (Payers may limit physicians to reporting the professional component only for all facility-based services even if the physician performs the ultrasound and/or owns the equipment used for the service. The technical component includes all associated overhead costs. Check individual payer policies for reporting.)

One use of point-of-care ultrasound in the ED is the focused assessment with sonography for trauma (FAST) examination. This may consist of 2 distinct components: limited transthoracic echocardiogram and limited abdominal ultrasound. When 2 distinct procedures are performed, 2 codes are reported.

76705   Ultrasound, abdominal, real-time with image documentation; limited

93308   Echocardiography, transthoracic, real-time with image documentation (2D), includes M-mode recording, when performed, follow-up or limited study

When a limited ultrasound examination of the chest is included (eg, for pneumothorax), report code **76604** (ultrasound, chest [includes mediastinum when performed], real-time with image documentation). Limited studies are defined in *CPT* as those that include examination of less than the required elements for a "complete" examination (eg, limited number of organs, limited portion of region evaluated). See your *CPT* reference for required components of complete examinations.

Please see the discussion of central venous access in **Chapter 19** for appropriate reporting of ultrasound guidance for vascular access (**76937**). This code is reported separately in addition to a code for primary vascular access procedure (eg, **36555**).

When ultrasound guidance is used for needle placement for procedures such as aspiration of an abscess, code **76942** is reported. Do not report code **76942** in conjunction with a service for which the code descriptor includes ultrasound guidance (eg, joint aspiration). Code **76937** (ultrasound guidance for vascular access) is not reported in conjunction with code **76942**.

Example

➤ **A child is seen in the ED for injuries sustained in a traffic accident.** The physician performs a trauma assessment, including a FAST examination. This examination may consist of 2 distinct components: limited transthoracic echocardiogram and limited abdominal ultrasound. When 2 distinct procedures are performed, 2 codes are reported.

In addition to the appropriate E/M service code, the physician reports **76705 26** (ultrasound, abdominal, real-time with image documentation; limited) and **93308 26** (echocardiography, transthoracic, real-time with image documentation [2D], includes M-mode recording, when performed, follow-up or limited study). Modifier **26** signifies the physician is reporting the professional component of each service. The facility will report the same codes with modifier **TC** to indicate reporting of the technical component of each service. When applicable and all requirements for reporting are met, an ultrasound performed with physician-owned equipment is reported without a modifier (ie, modifier **26** is not applicable).

Modifiers Used With ED Codes

Physicians need to understand when it is appropriate to report modifiers in addition to E/M or procedural service codes. Modifiers **25** (significant, separately identifiable E/M service) and **57** (decision for surgery) may be appended to ED E/M codes to indicate E/M beyond the preservice work of a procedure. Procedures performed in the ED may require reporting of modifiers such as **26** (professional component), **54** (surgical care only), or **59** (distinct procedural service) or, when accepted by the payer in lieu of modifier **59**, modifier **XE** (separate encounter), **XP** (separate practitioner), **XS** (separate structure), or **XU** (unusual nonoverlapping service). **Table 17-5** lists modifiers commonly used in the ED. (See **Chapter 2**, Modifiers and Coding Edits, for more detail on the use of modifiers.)

Examples

➤ **A child is seen in the ED for left shoulder pain that occurred following a fall while playing soccer at a community sports field.** The child is examined for additional injuries (expanded problem-focused history, detailed examination). A radiograph interpreted by a radiologist reveals a displaced mid-shaft clavicle fracture. The physician places the patient in a sling and refers the patient to another physician for follow-up care.

ICD-10-CM
S42.022A (displaced fracture of left clavicle, initial encounter)
W18.30XA (unspecified fall on same level, initial encounter)
Y93.66 (activity, soccer)
Y92.322 (soccer field as place of occurrence)

CPT
99283 25
23500 54 (closed treatment of clavicular fracture, without manipulation)

Teaching Point: The use of modifier **54** (surgical care only) alerts payers that another physician will report postsurgical care. Alternatively, the ED physician may report the ED E/M code based on the level of service performed and documented and allow another physician to report the global fracture care. Medical decision-making for the ED visit is moderate based on a new problem without additional workup (the diagnosis is known at the end of the encounter, although treatment will follow) and moderate risk related to the decision for closed treatment of a fracture without manipulation.

●=New code   ▲=Revised code   #=Re-sequenced code   +=Add-on code

Modifier	When to Use
Table 17-5. Common Modifiers Used in the Emergency Department	
24	An unrelated E/M service is provided during the global period of a previously performed procedure by the same physician or group.
25	A significant, separately identifiable E/M service is performed by the same physician on the same day of the procedure or other service.
26	Reporting professional component only of a service for which payment includes equipment (or technical services) cost (eg, radiograph)
32	A service is mandated by third-party payer, regulation, or governmental entity.
51	Multiple procedures are performed on the same day other than E/M, physical medicine and rehabilitation services, or provision of supplies (eg, vaccines).
54	Only the surgical care component of a procedure was provided. Another physician will provide postoperative care.
57	Decision for surgery was made. Some payers may require this modifier be appended to the E/M code only with procedures with 90-day global periods.
59	Distinct procedural service (non-E/M) was performed on the same day as another procedural service and was at a different encounter or a different surgery or procedure or was performed on a different body site or organ system.
63	Procedures (**20000–69999**) and certain procedures in the Medicine section of *CPT*) performed on an infant weighing <4 kg if the code descriptor does not include a descriptor of "young infant or neonate"
76	The same physician repeats a procedure or service on the same date of service.
77	Another physician repeats a procedure or service already performed by another physician on the same day of service.
79	An unrelated procedure is performed during the global period of a previously provided procedure by the same physician or group.
XE	The service was provided at a separate encounter on the same date.
XP	The non-E/M service or procedure was performed by a separate practitioner of the same group on the same date.
XS	The procedure or service was performed on a separate structure.
XU	Unusual nonoverlapping service

Abbreviations: *CPT, Current Procedural Terminology*; E/M, evaluation and management.

➤ **The ED physician is caring for a 9-year-old who has a 4-cm–long, deep laceration of the right calf and a separate 1-cm–long laceration of the right ankle from broken glass in his backyard.** The physician performs a detailed history and physical examination. A radiograph of the extremity shows no retained radiopaque foreign bodies. The child's immunizations are current, with the last tetanus booster less than 5 years ago. The physician irrigates, carefully explores both wounds, and performs a 2-layer repair on the calf. The ankle laceration requires only single-layer closure. The child is discharged with appropriate follow-up plans.

ICD-10-CM
S81.811A (laceration without foreign body, right lower leg, initial encounter)
S91.011A (laceration without foreign body, right ankle, initial encounter)
W25.XXXA (contact with sharp glass, initial encounter)
Y92.007 (garden or yard of noninstitutional residence)

CPT
99283 25
12032 (intermediate repair of the extremities, 2.6–7.5 cm)
12001 59 or **XS** (simple repair of the extremity, ≤2.5 cm)

●=New code ▲=Revised code #=Re-sequenced code +=Add-on code

Teaching Point: Modifier **25** is used to indicate the ED E/M service was significant and separately identifiable from the preservice work of the laceration repairs. Append modifier **25** only when providing an E/M and other service with an E/M component (pre- and post-service work) on the same date.

A modifier is required to indicate the simple repair was performed on a separate site from the intermediate or layered closure. Verify payer policy on reporting of modifier **59** (distinct procedural service) versus **XS** (separate structure). (See **Chapter 2**, Modifiers and Coding Edits, for more information on these modifiers.)

See **Chapter 10**, Surgery, Infusion, and Sedation in the Outpatient Setting, for more examples of coding for laceration repairs. See also "You Code It! Integumentary Repair," in the April 2020 *AAP Pediatric Coding Newsletter* (https://coding.solutions.aap.org/article.aspx?articleid=2763375; subscription required).

Sedation

Moderate Sedation

Moderate sedation (**99151–99157**) (**Table 17-6**) is a drug-induced depression of consciousness during which patients may respond purposefully to verbal commands, either alone or accompanied by light tactile stimulation. Moderate sedation may be necessary for the performance of certain procedures in the ED.

Table 17-6. Moderate Sedation		
Moderate Sedation	**First 10–22 min Intraservice Time**	**Each Additional 15 min Intraservice Time**
Moderate sedation services provided by the same physician or other qualified health care professional performing the diagnostic or therapeutic service that the sedation supports, requiring the presence of an independent trained observer to assist in the monitoring of the patient's level of consciousness and physiological status; initial 15 minutes of intra-service time, patient younger than 5 years of age	99151	+99153
5 years or older	99152	+99153
Moderate sedation services (other than those services described by codes **00100–01999**) provided by a physician other than the health care professional performing the diagnostic or therapeutic service that the sedation supports; younger than 5 years	99155	+99157
5 years or older	99156	+99157

- Codes are selected based on intraservice time. Intraservice time
  - Begins with the administration of the sedating agent(s)
  - Ends when the procedure is completed, the patient is stable for recovery status, and the physician or other QHP providing the sedation ends personal continuous face-to-face time with the patient
  - Includes ordering and/or administering the initial and subsequent doses of sedating agents
  - Requires continuous face-to-face attendance of the physician or other QHP
  - Requires monitoring patient response to the sedating agents, including
    - Periodic assessment of the patient
    - Further administration of agent(s) as needed to maintain sedation
    - Monitoring of oxygen saturation, heart rate, and blood pressure
- Moderate sedation services of less than 10 minutes' intraservice time are not separately reported.

Coding and documentation requirements for reporting this service are detailed in **Chapter 19**, Common Surgical Procedures and Sedation in Facility Settings.

Example

➤ **A 10-year-old presents to the ED with left forearm pain after falling from her bicycle.** She fell onto a concrete patio at her house but did not hit her head. The injury occurred 1 hour ago and was iced by the mother, but pain and swelling continued. Evaluation and management service includes a detailed history, expanded problem-focused examination, and moderate-complexity MDM. Imaging shows a Salter-Harris type II physeal fracture of the left distal radius (interpreted by the radiologist). An orthopedic surgeon is consulted and requests that the ED physician provide moderate sedation for closed reduction in the ED. The ED physician documents 25 minutes of moderate sedation, beginning with administration of the sedating agent and ending when the patient is sufficiently recovered so that the physician's continuous face-to-face monitoring is no longer necessary. The ED physician reports

ICD-10-CM **S59.222A** (Salter-Harris type II physeal fracture, lower left radius) **V18.000A** (pedal cycle rider injured noncollision transport accident, nontraffic accident) **Y92.018** (other place of single-family house)
CPT **99283 25** **99156** (moderate sedation by other than physician performing procedure, first 15 minutes) **99157** (moderate sedation, each additional 15 minutes)

Teaching Point: The orthopedic surgeon will separately report the fracture reduction procedure (eg, **25605**, closed treatment with manipulation) and, if applicable, any medically necessary E/M service beyond the preservice work of the procedure (modifier **57** may be required to indicate that the physician determined the need for the procedure at this encounter).

Deep Sedation

Deep sedation or analgesia is a drug-induced depression of consciousness during which patients cannot be easily aroused but respond purposefully after repeated verbal or painful stimulation (eg, purposefully pushing away the noxious stimuli). The ability to independently maintain ventilatory function may be impaired. Patients may require assistance in maintaining a patent airway, and spontaneous ventilation may be inadequate. Cardiovascular function is usually maintained. A state of deep sedation may be accompanied by partial or complete loss of protective airway reflexes.

Although ED physicians may provide deep sedation, payment for these services is limited.

Deep sedation provided by a physician also performing the services for which the sedation is being provided is reported by appending modifier **47** (anesthesia by surgeon) to the procedure code for the service for which sedation is required. Many health plans do not pay separately for anesthesia by the physician or surgeon performing the procedure.

National Correct Coding Initiative (NCCI) edits do not allow payment of an ED visit (**99281–99285**) and deep sedation when provided by the same ED physician or 2 ED physicians of the same group practice. No modifier will override the NCCI edits. Payers that have adopted Medicare or Medicaid NCCI edits will deny the ED visit when reported on the same date as deep sedation.

Please see **Chapter 19**, Common Surgical Procedures and Sedation in Facility Settings, for more information on deep sedation.

Special Service Codes

99053	Service(s) provided between 10:00 pm and 8:00 am at 24-hour facility, in addition to basic service
99056	Service(s) typically provided in office, provided out of office at request of patient, in addition to basic service
99060	Service(s) provided on an emergency basis, out of office, which disrupts other scheduled office services, in addition to basic service

Special service codes may be used to report services that are an adjunct to the basic service provided. *CPT* guidelines do not restrict the reporting of adjunct special service codes in the ED. However, third-party payers will have specific policies for coverage and payment. Communicate with individual payers to understand their definition or interpretation of the service and coverage and payment policies.

These codes are intended to describe services that are provided outside the normal time frame and location.

Code **99053** would be reported when services are provided between the designated time limits in an ED.

CPT does not restrict reporting of any procedure or service to any specific specialty. However, it would be inappropriate for an ED physician to report code **99056** or **99060** for services provided in the ED.

If appropriate, a non-ED physician could report *CPT* code **99056** or **99060** when he or she provides services in the ED in addition to an outpatient office or clinic visit, ED visit, or consultation E/M code.

Continuum Models for Asthma, Head Injury, and Laceration

The continuum model is a teaching tool that gives examples of how common conditions in the ED might be reported based on the severity and/or complexity of the presenting problem(s).

Following are 3 common conditions—asthma, head injury, and laceration—described across the continuum of codes **99281–99285** plus critical care. Although the actual assignment of a code for an individual patient may vary from the examples, members of the American Academy of Pediatrics Committee on Coding and Nomenclature generally agree that these examples provide an accurate representation of how 1 condition typically flows across the family of codes.

It is important to remember that all 3 key components (ie, history, examination, and MDM) must be met to support the code selected. Past, family, and social history elements are required only for codes **99284** (1 of 3) and **99285** (2 of 3).

Continuum Model for Asthma			
***CPT* Code Vignette**	**History**	**Physical Examination (systems)**	**Medical Decision-making (1. diagnoses; 2. data; 3. risk)**
99281 Stable asthma, out of medication	***Problem focused*** CC: asthma medication concern HPI: duration of medication use, no side effects ROS: constitutional, respiratory	***Problem focused*** Constitutional (vitals, general appearance) and respiratory systems (effort and auscultation)	***Straightforward*** 1. Established problem, stable 2. Asthma control test reviewed 3. Anticipatory guidance with routine follow-up
99282 Stable asthma, out of medication and noncustodial parent concerned about continuous use of control medication	***Expanded problem focused*** CC: out of asthma medication HPI: stable but out of medication, no use of rescue inhaler ROS: normal ENMT, infrequent nighttime cough, all others reviewed and normal PFSH: current medications reviewed, no hospitalizations	***Expanded problem focused*** Constitutional (height, weight, temperature), respiratory system (effort and auscultation), eyes, and ENMT (nasal and oral mucosa)	***Low complexity*** 1. Established problem, stable 2. Review and evaluation of asthma control test 3. Alteration in medication regimen and/or refills
99283 Known asthma with URI symptoms	***Expanded problem focused*** CC: asthma with stuffy nose and sinus pressure HPI: stuffy nose for 2 days, sinus pressure today, dry cough this afternoon relieved by inhalation treatment ROS: no fever; denies postnasal drip, shortness of breath, and wheezing; no body aches PFSH: current medications and allergies updated, asthma diagnosed in 2016, to ED twice last year for asthma symptoms	***Expanded problem focused*** Constitutional (temperature, weight, height, pulse oxygen), eyes, ENMT, respiratory (effort and auscultation), and other pertinent organ systems	***Moderate complexity*** 1. Self-limited problem and 1 established problem with mild exacerbation or new problem with no additional workup 2. Asthma control test, pulse oxygen 3. ≥1 chronic illnesses with mild exacerbation, progression *or* side effects of treatment and/or prescription drug management

●=New code   ▲=Revised code   #=Re-sequenced code   +=Add-on code

Chapter 17. Emergency Department Services

Continuum Model for Asthma (*continued*)

CPT Code Vignette	History	Physical Examination (systems)	Medical Decision-making (1. diagnoses; 2. data; 3. risk)
99284 Known asthma with moderate exacerbation	**Detailed** CC: shortness of breath, wheezing HPI: timing of symptom onset, context (exposure to flowers), modifying factors (used rescue inhaler and inhalation treatment at home), severity (worse than prior episodes) ROS: feels tired and scared, no fever, denies dizziness or fainting, no ear or throat pain, chest feels tight, no GI or GU complaints PFSH: medications and allergies updated	**Detailed** Constitutional (temperature, blood pressure, pulse oxygen, general appearance), ENMT, neck, respiratory, cardiovascular, and skin	**Moderate complexity** 1. New problem to examiner with or without additional workup planned 2. Pulmonary function testing, chest radiograph 3. Continuous or back-to-back inhalation treatments until improved
99285 Known asthma with moderate to severe exacerbation and hypoxia	**Comprehensive** CC: unable to catch breath HPI: duration and severity of symptoms, medications used, other signs and symptoms ROS: constitutional, eyes, ENMT, respiratory, cardiovascular, and at least 5 more (all others reviewed and negative) PFSH: medications and allergies updated, no tobacco use or exposure	**Comprehensive** Constitutional, eyes, ENMT, respiratory, cardiovascular, GI, neurologic, skin	**High complexity** 1. New problem, additional workup planned (Transfer to hospitalist for observation care.) 2. Blood gases, pulse oxygen, pulmonary function testing, chest radiograph 3. Severe exacerbation of chronic condition
99291, 99292 **Critical Care** Known asthma unstable with marked distress and (impending) respiratory failure			**High complexity** 1. Severe exacerbation with high probability of imminent or life-threatening deterioration requires >30 min of directed patient care. 2. Assess, manipulate, and support vital system function(s) to treat respiratory failure and/or to prevent further life-threatening deterioration of the patient's condition. (Usually requires use of additional therapies such as ketamine, magnesium sulfate, parenteral adrenergic agents, and/or heliox; ET intubation; or BiPAP.)

Abbreviations: BiPAP, bi-level positive airway pressure; CC, chief complaint; *CPT, Current Procedural Terminology;* ED, emergency department; ENMT, ear, nose, mouth, throat; ET, endotracheal; GI, gastrointestinal; GU, genitourinary; HPI, history of present illness; PFSH, past, family, and social history; ROS, review of systems; URI, upper respiratory infection.

Continuum Model for Head Injury

CPT Code Vignette	History	Physical Examination (systems)	Medical Decision-making (1. diagnoses; 2. data; 3. risk)
99281 Repaired scalp laceration, well healed, presents for suture removal	**Problem focused** CC: suture removal HPI: wound repair 10 days ago, no complaints	**Problem focused** Limited skin	**Straightforward** 1. Established problem, improved 2. No tests ordered/reviewed 3. Suture removal
99282 Minor head trauma without local bruising, swelling, or laceration, no neurologic changes	**Expanded problem focused** CC: bumped head HPI: context (injury mechanism), timing	**Expanded problem focused** Examination of skin and neurologic system	**Low complexity** 1. New problem, no additional workup 2. No tests ordered/reviewed 3. Acute uncomplicated injury
99283 Minor head trauma with local bruising, swelling, or laceration, no neurologic changes; GCS 15	**Expanded problem focused** CC: hit in head HPI: injury mechanism, timing, associated signs and symptoms ROS: neurologic, musculoskeletal	**Expanded problem focused** Eyes, ENMT, skin, and neurologic system	**Moderate complexity** 1. New problem, no additional workup 2. No tests ordered/reviewed 3. Acute complicated injury
99284 Head trauma with signs of concussion	**Detailed** CC: head injury with LOC HPI: mechanism of injury, associated signs and symptoms (pain, loss of recall), duration of LOC (<5 min), severity (no focal neurologic changes; GCS ≥13) PFSH: medications, allergies, past illnesses/injuries	**Detailed** Eyes, ENMT, neck, respiratory, cardiovascular, skin, neurologic, and other pertinent systems	**Moderate complexity** 1. New problem, no additional workup planned. 2. Radiology and laboratory tests may be obtained. Neurology or neurosurgical consultation may be obtained. 3. Acute complicated injury.
99285 Head trauma with signs of concussion including LOC (<5 min), brief seizure, and/ or persistent emesis; closed skull fracture and/or focal neurologic changes may be present; GCS 9–12	**Comprehensive** CC: head trauma with LOC HPI: mechanism of injury, associated signs and symptoms (pain, emesis), duration of LOC (<5 min), severity (GCS 9–12) ROS: ≥10 systems PFSH: medications, allergies, past illnesses/injuries, family or social history (eg, bleeding disorders, use of drugs or alcohol)	**Comprehensive** Constitutional, eyes, ENMT, respiratory, cardiovascular, gastrointestinal, neurologic, skin	**High complexity** 1. New problem, no additional workup planned. 2. History obtained from someone other than patient. Radiology and laboratory tests may be obtained/reviewed. Neurology or neurosurgical consultation may be obtained. 3. Acute injuries that may pose a threat to life or bodily function.
99291, 99292 Critical Care Head trauma with persistent LOC and/or seizures; open or closed skull fracture and/ or focal neurologic changes may be present; GCS ≤8			**High complexity** 1. Critically ill, unstable patient; requires >30 min of directed patient care. 2. Physician assesses, manipulates, and supports vital system function(s) to treat single or multiple vital organ system failure and/or to prevent further life-threatening deterioration of the patient's condition.

Abbreviations: CC, chief complaint; *CPT, Current Procedural Terminology;* ENMT, ear, nose, mouth, throat; GCS, Glasgow Coma Scale; HPI, history of present illness; LOC, loss of consciousness; PFSH, past, family, and social history; ROS, review of systems.

Chapter 17. Emergency Department Services

●=New code   ▲=Revised code   #=Re-sequenced code   +=Add-on code

Continuum Model for Laceration

These codes reflect E/M services only and not any procedure the same physician may provide. The physician needs to be aware that the pre-procedural and intra-procedural global periods may include some of the medical decision-making indicated with each code, thus reducing the level of E/M service provided, and that any E/M service reported with a procedure must meet the requirement for a significant, separately identifiable service.

CPT Code Vignette	History	Physical Examination (systems)	Medical Decision-making (1. diagnoses; 2. data; 3. risk)
99281 Repaired scalp laceration, well healed, presents for suture removal	***Problem focused*** CC: suture removal HPI: wound repair 10 days ago, no complaints	***Problem focused*** Limited skin	***Straightforward*** 1. Established problem, stable 2. No tests ordered/reviewed 3. Minimal risk—suture removal
99282 Uncomplicated laceration of single body area or organ system	***Expanded problem focused*** CC: laceration HPI: location, context (mechanism of injury), timing ROS: skin or musculoskeletal	***Expanded problem focused*** Skin and/or musculoskeletal, neurologic systems	***Low complexity*** 1. New problem, laceration 2. No tests ordered/reviewed 3. Acute uncomplicated injury
99283 Uncomplicated laceration of single body area or organ system with minor associated injury (eg, minor head injury) *or* Uncomplicated lacerations of >1 body area or organ system *or* Minimally complicated laceration (eg, small foreign body, delay in seeking care) of single body area or organ system	***Expanded problem focused*** CC: laceration(s) HPI: location, context (mechanism of injury), timing ROS: skin or musculoskeletal	***Expanded problem focused*** Constitutional, skin and/or musculoskeletal, neurologic systems	***Moderate complexity*** 1. New problem(s). 2. Radiograph of affected area may be ordered/viewed. 3. Acute complicated injury.
99284 Uncomplicated laceration of single body area or organ system with other associated injury (eg, mild concussion) *or* Minimally complicated lacerations (eg, small foreign body) of >1 body area or organ system *or* Complicated laceration (eg, infection, GSW, deep knife wound) of single body area or organ system without immediate threat to life or limb	***Detailed*** CC: injuries HPI: location, context (mechanism of injury), timing, associated signs and symptoms ROS: constitutional, skin, musculoskeletal, neurologic PFSH: medications and allergies	***Detailed*** Eyes, neck, respiratory, cardiovascular, skin, musculoskeletal, neurologic	***Moderate complexity*** 1. New problem. 2. Radiograph of affected area may be ordered/viewed. 3. Acute complicated injury.
99285 Uncomplicated laceration of ≥1 body area or organ system with significant associated injury (eg, multiple trauma) *or* Complicated laceration (eg, GSW, deep knife wound) of >1 body area or organ system without immediate threat to life or limb	***Comprehensive*** CC: injuries HPI: location, context (mechanism of injury), timing, associated signs and symptoms ROS: ≥10 systems PFSH: medications, allergies, and pertinent family history of tobacco, alcohol, or substance use	***Comprehensive*** Constitutional, eyes, ENMT, respiratory, cardiovascular, musculoskeletal, neurologic, skin	***High complexity*** 1. New problem 2. Tests ordered/reviewed (radiology and/or laboratory) 3. Acute injury that may pose a threat to life or bodily function or emergency major surgery

Continuum Model for Laceration (*continued*)

CPT Code Vignette	History	Physical Examination (systems)	Medical Decision-making (1. diagnoses; 2. data; 3. risk)
99291, 99292 **Critical Care** Uncomplicated or complicated laceration of ≥1 body area or organ system with significant associated injury (eg, multiple trauma) with immediate threat to life or limb			**High complexity** 1. Critically ill, unstable patient; requires >30 min of directed patient care. 2. Physician assesses, manipulates, and supports vital system function(s) to treat single or multiple vital organ system failure and/or to prevent further life-threatening deterioration of the patient's condition.

Abbreviations: CC, chief complaint; *CPT, Current Procedural Terminology;* E/M, evaluation and management; ENMT, ear, nose, mouth, throat; GSW, gunshot wound; HPI, history of present illness; PFSH, past, family, and social history; ROS, review of systems.

Resources

Evaluation and Management

"Evaluation and Management Coding in the Emergency Department," May 2018 *AAP Pediatric Coding Newsletter* (https://coding.solutions.aap.org/article.aspx?articleid=2679117; subscription required)

Repair of Integumentary Lacerations

"You Code It! Integumentary Repair," April 2020 *AAP Pediatric Coding Newsletter* (https://coding.solutions.aap.org/article.aspx?articleid=2763375; subscription required)

●=New code   ▲=Revised code   #=Re-sequenced code   +=Add-on code

Test Your Knowledge!

1. **In the emergency department (ED), what must the physician designate as the chief complaint?**
   a. The diagnosis, after workup, determined to be chiefly responsible for services provided
   b. All presenting signs, symptoms, or injuries
   c. Only 1 sign, symptom, disease, or injury
   d. A suspected condition based on presenting signs, symptoms, or injury

2. **Which of the following is true for ED services (99281–99285)?**
   a. No history is required for Level 5 encounters.
   b. All 3 key components must support code selection except when the ED caveat applies.
   c. The ED physician must select a level of service based on time.
   d. The level of service may be selected based on the complexity of medical decision-making alone.

3. **Which of the following is true of critical care in the ED?**
   a. Procedures performed during the time of critical care are never separately reported.
   b. Critical care time includes time spent performing separately reported procedures.
   c. Time spent discussing the patient's management or condition with the patient's family is not included in critical care time.
   d. Certain procedures, as specified in *CPT*, are included in critical care services.

4. **Which of the following must be included to support billing for ultrasound in the ED?**
   a. There is permanent image documentation (with measurements, when clinically indicated).
   b. Thorough evaluation of organ(s) or anatomical region is performed.
   c. A written report equivalent to that typically produced by a radiologist is documented.
   d. All of the above

5. **Which modifier may be required when an ED physician performs the professional component of a diagnostic service (eg, interprets and creates a report for an ultrasound)?**
   a. **XE** (separate encounter)
   b. **59** (distinct procedural service)
   c. **26** (professional component)
   d. **TC** (technical component)

CHAPTER 18

Critical and Intensive Care

Contents

●=New code   ▲=Revised code   #=Re-sequenced code   +=Add-on code

This chapter focuses on correctly coding critical and intensive care, including attendance at delivery; neonatal resuscitation; hourly critical care; critical care of the neonate, infant, and child younger than 6 years; and intensive care of the recovering or low birth weight neonate and infant. Services commonly reported before and after intensive or critical care services, such as consultations and care during emergency transport, are included.

Evaluation and management (E/M) of the child who no longer requires intensive or critical care is discussed in **Chapter 16**, Noncritical Hospital Evaluation and Management Services.

Critical Care Services

Critical Illness or Injury

- A *critical illness or injury* is defined by *Current Procedural Terminology* (*CPT*®) as one that acutely impairs 1 or more vital organs such that there is a high probability of imminent or life-threatening deterioration of the patient's condition.
- Services qualify as critical care *only if both* the injury or illness *and* the treatment being delivered meet the following criteria:
  — The illness or injury acutely impairs 1 or more vital organs as defined previously.
  — The treatment delivered involves high-complexity medical decision-making (MDM) to prevent life-threatening deterioration of the patient's condition.
- Critical care involves high-complexity MDM to assess, manipulate, and support vital organ system function(s); treat single or multiple organ system failure; and/or prevent further life-threatening deterioration of the patient's condition.
- Immaturity alone, or any of the specific procedures, equipment, or therapies associated with care of the immature neonate, does not define critical care.
- Coding critical care is not determined by the location in which the care is delivered but by the nature of the care being delivered and the condition of the patient requiring care.
- Critical care is not limited to an inpatient setting or a critical care area, and a physician of any specialty can provide these services. Services must be provided directly by the physician or other qualified health care professional (QHP).
- Many typically performed procedures are included (bundled) in the work valuation of each critical care code and cannot be reported separately (**Table 18-1**). (See also the Procedures *Not* Bundled With Critical/Intensive Care Services section later in this chapter for commonly provided services not bundled with hourly and/or neonatal and pediatric critical care service.)

Table 18-1. Critical Care Bundled Services			
CPT **Code and Procedure**	**Hourly Critical Care** 99291, 99292	**Pediatric Transport** 99466, 99467	**Neonatal/Pediatric Critical and Intensive Care** 99468–99476, 99477–99480
Interpretation and Monitoring			
71045 X-ray, chest; single view **71046** X-ray, chest; 2 views	X	X	X
93561 Cardiac output measurement **93562** subsequent measurement of cardiac output	X X	 X	X X
94760 Pulse oximetry; single determination **94761** multiple determinations (eg, during exercise) **94762** by continuous overnight monitoring	X	X	X
Vascular Access Procedures			
36000 Introduction of needle or intracatheter, vein	X	X	X
36140 Catheterization extremity artery			X
36400 Venipuncture, <3 years, requiring physician or QHP skill; femoral or jugular vein **36405** scalp vein **36406** other vein		X	X

●=New code   ▲=Revised code   #=Re-sequenced code   +=Add-on code

Table 18-1 (*continued*)

CPT Code and Procedure	Hourly Critical Care 99291, 99292	Pediatric Transport 99466, 99467	Neonatal/Pediatric Critical and Intensive Care 99468–99476, 99477–99480
Vascular Access Procedures (*continued*)			
36410 Venipuncture, ≥3 years, requiring physician or QHP skill	X		X
36415 Collection of venous blood by venipuncture	X	X	X
36420 Venipuncture, cutdown; younger than age 1 year			X
36430 Transfusion, blood or blood components **36440** Push transfusion, blood, 2 years or younger			X
36510 Catheterization of umbilical vein, newborn			X
36555 Insertion of non-tunneled CICC; <5 years of age			X
36591 Collection blood from venous access device	X	X	X
36600 Arterial puncture, withdrawal of blood for diagnosis	X	X	X
36620 Arterial catheterization, percutaneous **36660** Catheterization, umbilical artery, newborn			X
Other Procedures			
31500 Endotracheal intubation, emergency			X
43752 Nasogastric/orogastric intubation, fluoroscopic guidance	X	X	X
43753 Gastric intubation including lavage if performed	X	X	X
51100 Aspiration of bladder; by needle			X
51701 Insertion of non-indwelling bladder catheter **51702** Temporary indwelling bladder catheter; simple			X
62270 Spinal puncture, lumbar, diagnostic			X
92953 Temporary transcutaneous pacing	X	X	X
94002 Ventilation initiation; inpatient/observation, initial day **94003** each subsequent day	X	X	X
94004 Ventilation initiation; nursing facility, per day	X		X
94375 Respiratory flow volume loop			X
94610 Intrapulmonary surfactant administration			X
94660 CPAP initiation and management **94662** CNP, initiation and management	X	X	X
94780 Car seat/bed testing, infants through 12 months; 60 minutes **94781** each additional full 30 minutes			X

Abbreviations: CICC, centrally inserted central venous catheter; CNP, continuous negative pressure ventilation; CPAP, continuous positive airway pressure; *CPT, Current Procedural Terminology*; QHP, qualified health care professional.

Hourly Critical Care

99291   Critical care, E/M of the critically ill or critically injured patient; first 30 to 74 minutes

+99292   each additional 30 minutes (Use in conjunction with **99291**.)

   Guidelines for reporting codes **99291** and **99292**

- Reported when critical care is provided for 30 minutes or more
  - In the outpatient setting (eg, emergency department [ED], office, clinic) *regardless of age*
  - To an inpatient 6 years or older (Daily critical care of a child younger than 6 years is discussed later in this chapter.)
  - Concurrently by a second physician from a different specialty to a critically ill or injured patient, regardless of age
  - To an inpatient aged 5 years or younger when the patient is being transferred to another facility where a receiving physician of the same specialty but different medical group will be reporting the daily inpatient critical care service codes (**99468** and **99469**; **99471** and **99472**; **99475** and **99476**)
  - By the physician physically transporting a critically ill child older than 2 years or when payer policy does not recognize codes **99466** and **99467** (face-to-face transport care of the critically ill or injured patient 24 months or younger, discussed later in this chapter)
- Many procedures typically performed are included (*bundled*) in the work valuation of the code and cannot be reported separately (see **Table 18-1**). (See also the Procedures *Not* Bundled With Critical/Intensive Care Services section later in this chapter for commonly provided services not bundled with hourly and/or neonatal and pediatric critical care services.)
- Procedures not included as bundled may be reported separately (eg, lumbar puncture, endotracheal intubation, thoracentesis).

> **The reported time of critical care *cannot* include any time spent performing procedures or services that are reported separately.**

- Critical care is not permitted to be reported as a split/shared service (ie, the times of a physician and QHP cannot be combined and reported as a single service). When the physician and neonatal nurse practitioner (NNP) provide critical care services to a patient, only one may report the code.
- Codes **99291** and **99292** may be reported by an individual of a *different specialty* from either the same or a different group on the same day that neonatal or pediatric critical care services are reported by another individual (**99468–99476**).
- A teaching physician may report time-based critical care services only when he or she was present for the entire period for which the claim is submitted and that time is supported in documentation of the service.
- When inpatient and outpatient critical care services are provided to a neonate, infant, or child younger than 6 years on the same date by the same physician (or physician of the same group and specialty), only the *inpatient* critical care codes are reported (**99468–99476**). See exceptions included in the Neonatal and Pediatric Daily Critical Care Codes and Emergency Medical Services Supervision and Patient Transport sections later in this chapter.
- Other significant, separately identifiable E/M services (eg, **99212–99215**, **99281–99285**) can be reported in addition to time-based critical care services as appropriate. Do not count time spent in separately reported E/M services in critical care time.
  National Correct Coding Initiative (NCCI) edits bundle ED E/M codes **99281–99285** with codes **99291** and **99292**. Appending a modifier will not override the edits. Payers who use these edits will not pay for both services on the same date by the same physician or physicians of the same group practice and same specialty.

Time Units of Hourly Critical Care

- Reporting is time based. **Table 18-2** lists times and billing units. The total floor or unit time devoted to the patient in the provision of critical care is used in code selection. Critical care time includes physician–patient face-to-face time or time spent on the patient's *unit or floor* directly related to the patient's care (eg, hands-on care at the bedside, reviewing test results, discussing care with other medical staff or family, documenting services in the medical record).
- Time spent in the provision of critical care does not need to be continuous. The cumulative time of critical care provided on a single date of service is used to calculate the units of service provided.

> **When a *continuous period* of critical care occurs before and after midnight, report the total time on the date that the period of care was initiated. Do not report a second initial hour of critical care for the period beginning at midnight.**

- The physician must be immediately available to the patient during time reported as critical care. No time spent in activities that take place out of the unit, off the patient's floor, or consulting with other caregivers from home is included in critical care time.
- The time required to report code **99291** must be met by a single physician. If multiple physicians and other QHPs from the same group practice and same specialty care for a patient after a single physician has provided the initial 30 minutes of critical care, combine the total time and report with code **99292** as appropriate. Do not report **99291** more than once per day. All services must be reported under the name and National Provider Identifier of a single physician.
- Code **99291** is reported once on a given date of service when 30 to 74 minutes of critical care is performed. If less than 30 minutes of critical care is provided, an appropriate E/M service (eg, **99202–99215** for office services, **99221–99233** for inpatient hospital care) is reported.
- Code **99292** is reported with 1 unit for each additional period up to 30 minutes beyond the previous period. *Time spent providing critical care services must be documented in the medical record.*

Table 18-2. Reporting Hourly Critical Care Services					
Do not report services of <30 minutes as critical care; report the appropriate E/M service for the site where service is provided.					
Duration of Face-to-face Critical Care	30–74 min	75–104 min	105–134 min	135–164 min	165–194 min
CPT **Codes and Units of Service**	99291	99291 × 1, 99292 × 1	99291 × 1, 99292 × 2	99291 × 1, 99292 × 3	99291 × 1, 99292 × 4
Abbreviations: *CPT, Current Procedural Terminology;* E/M, evaluation and management.					

Examples

➤ **A 13-year-old with cystic fibrosis is seen in the ED for respiratory distress.** The ED physician provides an hour of critical care before the child is admitted to the intensive care unit by an intensivist.

Code **99291** with 1 unit of service (30–74 minutes) is reported by the ED physician. The intensivist will report the appropriate level of daily hospital and/or hourly critical care.

➤ **A 4-month-old is admitted with fever, lethargy, and poor feeding. Laboratory tests, cultures, and intravenous (IV) fluids are started.** Later that afternoon, the infant decompensates, developing desaturation, apnea, and falling blood pressures. The pediatrician returns to the bedside; 3 hours are spent at the hospital stabilizing the infant, directing nursing staff, discussing management options with the tertiary care facility, speaking with the parents, and monitoring the infant while awaiting the transport team to take the infant to a hospital where the pediatrician does not practice.

The transferring physician reports initial hospital care code (**99221–99223**) along with **99291** and **99292** with 4 units of service for the 180 minutes of critical care services.

Procedures *Not* Bundled With Critical/Intensive Care Services

When reporting hourly critical or neonatal and pediatric critical and intensive care services, many services commonly performed in the provision of critical care are not bundled into the intensive or critical care services. However, claim edits may require appending a modifier to indicate the services were distinct. Examples of procedures that are not bundled with critical care services include (not all-inclusive)

- Thoracentesis (**32554, 32555**) (via needle or pigtail catheter)
- Percutaneous pleural drainage with insertion of indwelling catheter (**32556, 32557**)
- Complete (double volume) exchange transfusion (**36450**, newborn; **36455**, other)
- Partial exchange transfusion (**36456**)
- Abdominal paracentesis (**49082, 49083**)
- Bone marrow aspiration (**38220**)
- Circumcision (**54150**)
- Cardioversion (**92960**)
- Cardiopulmonary resuscitation (**92950**)
- Extracorporeal membrane oxygenation (ECMO) (**33946–33949**)

Chapter 18. Critical and Intensive Care

- Peripherally inserted central catheter (**36568–36573**)
- Insertion of non-tunneled centrally inserted central venous catheter, older than 5 years (**36556**)
- Replacement (rewire) of non-tunneled centrally inserted central venous catheter (**36580**)
- Therapeutic apheresis (**36511–36514**)
- Insertion of cannula for hemodialysis, other purpose (separate procedure); vein to vein (**36800**)
- Placement of needle for intraosseous infusion (**36680**)
- Initiation of selective head or total body hypothermia in the critically ill neonate (**99184**) (Report only once at initiation of service.)

Payer edits may vary, and certain services are bundled unless performed for diagnostic purposes rather than monitoring. The following instructions from the Medicaid NCCI manual demonstrate reporting of diagnostic services:

Lumbar puncture (**62270**, **62328**) and suprapubic bladder aspiration (**51100**) are *separately reportable* with hourly critical care (**99291**, **99292**) but are *not separately reportable* with the pediatric and neonatal critical care service codes (**99468–99472**, **99475**, **99476**) and the intensive care services codes (**99477–99480**).

> Emergency cardiac defibrillation is included in cardiopulmonary resuscitation (**92950**). Per the Medicaid National Correct Coding Initiative manual, if emergency cardiac defibrillation without cardiopulmonary resuscitation is performed in the emergency department or critical/intensive care unit, the cardiac defibrillation service is not separately reportable. Report code **92960** only for elective cardioversion.

Example

➤ **During an encounter with a child who was found unconscious in a swimming pool, a physician spends 10 minutes performing cardiopulmonary resuscitation (CPR) and then another 45 minutes providing critical care before the patient is transferred to another facility.** Critical care service (**99291**) time is documented and distinctly identifiable in the patient record from the time spent performing the separately reportable CPR (**92950**), for which start and stop times were documented.

Diagnostic rhythm electrocardiogram (ECG) codes **93040–93042** are reported only when there is a sudden change in a patient status associated with a change in cardiac rhythm that requires a diagnostic rhythm ECG and return to the critical care unit. When separately reporting a diagnostic ECG, do not include the time for this service in the time spent providing critical care. Modifier **59** is appended to the ECG code when indicated by patient status and performed on the same date as critical care services.

Transesophageal echocardiography (TEE) monitoring (**93318**) *without probe placement* is not separately reportable by a physician performing critical care E/M services. However, if a physician places a transesophageal probe to be used for TEE monitoring on the same date of service that the physician performs critical care E/M services, code **93318** may be reported with modifier **59**. The time necessary for probe placement *shall not be included* in the critical care time reported with *CPT* codes **99291** and **99292**. This is true for all separately reportable procedures performed on a patient receiving critical care E/M services. Diagnostic TEE services may be separately reportable by a physician performing critical care E/M services.

> American Academy of Pediatrics Tip: Payers may require modifier **25** to be appended to the codes for critical care services rather than appending modifier **59** to the procedure code. Modifier **59** is intended to distinguish 2 distinct non–evaluation and management services.

Many practice management and billing systems include claim scrubbers that provide an alert that claim edits apply and a modifier may be appropriate based on clinical circumstances. Payers may also offer online tools for determining when code pair edits apply.

Definition of Neonatal/Perinatal Periods

For coding purposes, the *neonatal period* begins at birth and continues through the completed 28th day after birth, ending on the 29th calendar day after birth. The day of birth is considered day 0 (zero). Therefore, the day after birth is considered day 1.

This definition is important in selecting the initial- and subsequent-day neonatal critical care codes **99468** and **99469** as well as code **99477** for the initial hospital care of the neonate, 28 days or younger, who requires intensive observation, frequent interventions, and other intensive care services.

Chapter 18. Critical and Intensive Care

ICD-10-CM Guidelines and Neonatal Critical Care

It is important to correctly assign *International Classification of Diseases, 10th Revision, Clinical Modification* (ICD-10-CM) codes that reflect the diagnoses for which critical care services were required. Assign codes for neonatal conditions that require treatment or further investigation, prolong the length of stay, or require resource utilization as well as codes for conditions that have implications for future health care needs.

> When care is provided by the attending physician during the birth admission, report first a code from category **Z38** (liveborn infants according to place of birth and type of delivery). Codes for abnormal conditions are reported secondary to the code for live birth. When a neonate is transferred to another facility after birth, the admission to the receiving facility is not a birth admission and **Z38** codes are not reported.

- *ICD-10-CM* contains codes (**P00–P96**) for conditions originating in the perinatal period described as having their origin in the fetal or perinatal period (before birth through the first 28 days after birth) even if morbidity occurs later. Again, this period includes the completed 28th day after birth with the day of birth being counted as day 0 (zero).
  - These codes are only to be reported when the condition originates in this time, but they can be reported beyond the perinatal period if the condition(s) causes morbidity or is the primary reason for or contributing to the reason the patient is receiving health care.
  - The perinatal code should continue to be used regardless of the patient's age if a condition originates in the perinatal period and continues throughout the patient's life.

Example

➤ **A 24-month-old who was a 26-weeks' gestation preterm neonate is referred to audiology for an annual hearing evaluation due to the history of preterm birth.** The *ICD-10-CM* code that is linked to the audiology referral is **P07.25** (extreme immaturity of newborn, gestational age 26 completed weeks).

- Any condition *originating* after the perinatal period (29th calendar day after birth and beyond) is not reported with codes for perinatal conditions.
- A diagnosis of prematurity must be documented to support reporting of a code for prematurity. Coders cannot assign codes for prematurity based solely on documented gestational age.
- Codes in category **P05** are reported for the newborn affected by fetal growth restriction or slow intrauterine growth.
  - Codes in subcategory **P05.0** are used to report that the neonate is light for dates but not small. These neonates have often been said to exhibit *asymmetrical growth restriction*. (See definitions in the "*ICD-10-CM* Codes for Small and/or Light for Gestational Age" box later in this chapter.)
  - Codes in subcategory **P05.1** are used to report the neonate is small or small and light for dates. These newborns have often been said to exhibit *symmetrical growth restriction*.
- Code **P05.2** is provided for reporting fetal (intrauterine) malnutrition affecting a newborn who is not light or small for gestational age.

ICD-10-CM Codes for Small and/or Light for Gestational Age

International Classification of Diseases, 10th Revision, Clinical Modification (ICD-10-CM) codes for small and/or light for gestational age are aligned to the World Health Organization definitions of these conditions. In the United States, many clinicians use the term *small for gestational age* for all newborns below the 10th (or 5th) percentile for gestational age and then subcategorize as *symmetrical* when weight, length, and head circumference are all below the 10th percentile and *asymmetrical* when only the weight is below the 10th percentile. Asymmetrical fetal growth would fall in the light for gestational age group, whereas symmetrical fetal growth would fall in the small for gestational age group. Note that head circumference percentile is not a factor in choosing the correct code.

The World Health Organization provides definitions to support diagnostic selection for these conditions.
- *Light for gestational age:* usually referred to as weight below but length above the 10th percentile for gestational age
- *Small for gestational age:* usually referred to as weight and length below the 10th percentile for gestational age

ICD-10-CM includes codes **P05.09** (newborn light for gestational age, ≥2,500 g) and **P05.19** (newborn small for gestational age, other) to allow for identification of all neonates with fetal growth and malnutrition, fetal growth retardation, and preterm birth.

●=New code   ▲=Revised code   #=Re-sequenced code   +=Add-on code

Chapter 18. Critical and Intensive Care

- Codes from category **P07** (disorders of newborn related to short gestation and low birth weight) are reported based on the recorded birth weight and estimated gestational age to indicate these conditions are the cause of morbidity or reason for additional care of the newborn.
  - When both are documented, weight is sequenced before age.
  - These codes may be reported for a child as well as for an adult who was preterm or had a low birth weight as a newborn and this is affecting the patient's current health status.

Codes in subcategory **P07.3-** (preterm newborn) should be reported for neonates born at 36 weeks' gestation who stay in the newborn nursery or who are cared for in the neonatal intensive care unit (NICU).

> Codes in subcategory **P07.0-** (extremely low birth weight newborn) and **P07.1-** (other low birth weight newborn) are not reported in conjunction with codes in category **P05** (disorders of the newborn due to slow fetal growth and fetal malnutrition). However, subcategory **P07.2-** (extreme immaturity of newborn) and **P07.3-** (preterm newborn) may be reported in addition to category **P05**.

Attendance at Delivery and Newborn Resuscitation

Attendance at Delivery

99464   Attendance at delivery (when requested by the delivering physician or other qualified health care professional) and initial stabilization of newborn

Attendance at delivery (**99464**) is only reported when the physical presence of the provider is requested by the delivering physician and indicated for a newborn who may require immediate intervention (ie, stabilization, resuscitation, or evaluation for potential problems).

- Includes initial drying, stimulation, suctioning, blow-by oxygen, or continuous positive airway pressure (CPAP) without positive-pressure ventilation (PPV); a cursory visual inspection of the neonate; assignment of Apgar scores; and discussion of the care of the newborn with the delivering physician and parents. A quick look in the delivery room or examination after stabilization is not sufficient to support reporting of **99464**.
  - When qualifying resuscitative efforts are provided, code **99465** (delivery/birthing room resuscitation) is reported instead. Codes **99464** and **99465** cannot be reported on the same day of service.

See **Chapter 15**, Hospital Care of the Newborn, for further discussion and coding examples.

Neonatal Resuscitation

99465   Delivery/birthing room resuscitation, provision of positive pressure ventilation and/or chest compressions in the presence of acute inadequate ventilation and/or cardiac output

Attendance at delivery with neonatal resuscitation (**99465**)

- Requires PPV delivered by any means (resuscitation bag or T-piece resuscitator) and/or cardiac compressions.
- Do *not* report when T-piece resuscitator is used to provide CPAP only (see the "Coding Conundrum: T-Piece Positive-Pressure Ventilation" box later in this chapter).
- May be reported in addition to any initial care service, including initial critical care (**99468**), hourly critical care (**99291**, **99292**), initial neonatal intensive care (**99477**), or normal newborn care (**99460**) if the resuscitation results in a stable term neonate.

> Payers may require modifier **25** (significant, separately identifiable evaluation and management [E/M] service) appended to the code for E/M services reported in addition to code **99464** or **99465**. However, National Correct Coding Initiative edits do not bundle these services.

- Medically necessary procedures (eg, **31500**, intubation, endotracheal, emergency procedure; **31515**, laryngoscopy, direct, for aspiration; **36510**, catheterization of umbilical vein for diagnosis or therapy, newborn; **94610**, surfactant administration) essential to successful resuscitation that are performed in the delivery room prior to admission may also be reported in addition to codes **99465** and **99468** or **99477** (initial neonatal critical or intensive care).
  - Do not separately report services performed as a convenience before admission to the NICU.
  - Medical record documentation must clearly support that the services are provided as a required measure for emergency resuscitation and not as part of an admission protocol.

Coding Conundrum: T-Piece Positive-Pressure Ventilation
A frequently asked question is whether code **99465** can be reported if the T-piece resuscitator is used to provide continuous positive airway pressure (CPAP) only. Clearly, from the definitions given previously, the answer is no. If the neonate responds to provision of CPAP with an adequate respiratory effort, code **99464** should be reported.

On the other hand, if the neonate is apneic or, in the judgment of the provider, exhibiting inadequate respiratory effort, positive-pressure breaths administered by the T-piece resuscitator in lieu of a manual bag-mask resuscitator would justify reporting code **99465**. It is important for the documentation to explicitly state that the neonate demonstrated respiratory and/or cardiac instability requiring intervention, including apnea or inadequate respiratory effort to support gas exchange; that the provider instituted positive-pressure ventilation (PPV); and the neonate's response to the PPV.

Example

➤ **A neonatologist attends an emergency cesarean delivery of a term neonate with non-reassuring fetal heart tracing at the request of an obstetrician.** The neonate has no spontaneous activity. The resuscitation includes PPV, intubation, and placement of an umbilical vein catheter. The newborn is stabilized and admitted to the NICU, where the neonatologist administers surfactant and performs an umbilical artery catheterization.

The intubation and umbilical vein catheterization are separately reported procedures provided as part of the resuscitation and not as a convenience to the physician prior to admission.	**CPT** **99465** (delivery/birthing room resuscitation) **31500** (endotracheal intubation, emergency) **36510** (catheterization of umbilical vein for diagnosis or therapy, newborn) **99468 25** (initial neonatal critical care)

Teaching Point: Modifier **25** is appended to code **99468** to signify a significant, separately identifiable E/M service provided in addition to codes **31500** and **36510** because these services are bundled by NCCI edits. (For more on edits, see **Chapter 2**, Modifiers and Coding Edits.) Codes **99465** and **99468** are not bundled by NCCI edits, but individual payers may require modifier **25** to designate separately identifiable critical care services on the same date. The surfactant administration and umbilical artery catheterization are not separately reported when performed in conjunction with neonatal critical care.

Neonatal and Pediatric Daily Critical Care Codes

Codes are
- Reported for critical care of children younger than 6 years in the inpatient setting.
- Global—they encompass all E/M services by a single provider (or provider of the exact same specialty in the same group) on 1 calendar date. Other physicians and QHPs providing critical care must report hourly critical care code **99291** or **99292**. (See exceptions under the Guidelines for Reporting Neonatal or Pediatric Inpatient Critical Care section later in this chapter.)
- Bundled—they have commonly performed procedures included in the E/M codes. See **Table 18-1** for services and procedures that are included with neonatal critical care codes.
- Not time based. Prolonged services *may not* be reported in conjunction with neonatal or pediatric critical care services.
- Not based on typical E/M rules and the performance and documentation of key components (ie, history, physical examination, MDM, and/or time).
- Reported based on postnatal age (see the Definition of Neonatal/Perinatal Periods section earlier in this chapter) and initial or subsequent care (**Table 18-3**).

Table 18-3. Neonatal and Pediatric Global Critical Care			
Inpatient Neonatal Critical Care	**28 Days or Younger**	**29 Days Through 24 Months of Age**	**2 Through 5 Years of Age**
Initial inpatient neonatal critical care	99468	99471	99475
Subsequent inpatient neonatal critical care	99469	99472	99476

Neonatal Critical and Intensive Care Supervision Requirements

The American Medical Association/Specialty Society Relative Value Scale Update Committee (RUC) makes valuation recommendations based on surveys in which physicians who perform services are presented with a vignette describing the typical patient and the face-to-face physician work associated with that service. The neonatal and pediatric critical and intensive care code vignettes describe hands-on care by the attending physician (intraservice work) as well as the preservice and post-service work associated with this service. Neither the vignette nor the intent of the codes was to imply that 24-hour in-house attendance was a requirement of this code set. However, the codes' values were established assuming the physician is physically present and participating directly in the patient's care for a significant portion of the reported service. Documentation in the patient's chart should reflect this active participation, including documentation of hands-on care, such as a personal physical examination. *Supervision of all the care from a distance without face-to-face care is not reported as critical or intensive care.* (Refer to **Appendix IV,** Global Per Diem Critical Care Codes: Direct Supervision and Reporting Guidelines.)

The vignettes also include the phrase "repeated examinations over a 24-hour period," which was included to indicate that these neonates or infants do not receive "continuous" care but rather are typically evaluated during numerous intervals over a 24-hour period, depending on the clinical needs of the patient. In some cases, the neonate's or infant's level of illness requires in-house attending presence for extended periods, while only daytime presence is required in other situations. While the critical care team is present with the neonate or infant for the full 24 hours, overnight in-house care by the reporting physician is determined by the complexity of the total population of neonates cared for in a nursery or the changes in a specific neonate's or infant's condition that cannot be adequately assessed or managed over the telephone.

Under the heading Inpatient Neonatal and Pediatric Critical Care Service, *CPT* states that codes **99468, 99469,** and **99471–99476** are used to report services provided by a physician "directing the inpatient care" of a critically ill neonate, infant, or child through 5 years of age. The medical record documentation must support the physician's presence and supervision of the team as well as the critical nature of the child's disease. As noted previously, the directing physician is not required to be present or in the facility for the total 24 hours of daily care. Rather, because neonatal and pediatric critical and intensive care may require numerous encounters to reevaluate and manage the patient each day, neonatal and pediatric critical and intensive care codes encompass all the sick care provided within a calendar day.

Coding Conundrum: Selecting the Appropriate Code

Many diagnoses or conditions, such as respiratory distress, infection, seizures, mild to moderate hypoxic-ischemic encephalopathy, and metabolic disorders, can be reported with codes **99468, 99477,** or **99221–99223.** The patient's clinical status, required level of monitoring and observation, and present body weight will determine which of these code sets is chosen. Selection of the service must be justified by medical record documentation.

Guidelines for Reporting Neonatal or Pediatric Inpatient Critical Care

- The physician or NNP (subject to state regulations, scope of practice, and hospital privilege credentials) primarily responsible for the patient on the date of service should report the neonatal or pediatric critical care codes. When both the physician and NNP provide critical care services to a patient, only one may report the code.
- If critical care is provided in both the outpatient and inpatient settings by the same physician or a physician of the same specialty and group, only the inpatient code is reported.
- Codes are reported only once per day, per patient.
- When the same physician or physicians of the same specialty and group practice provide pediatric critical care during transport of a child 24 months or younger (**99466, 99467, 99485, 99486**) and critical care after admission to the receiving facility, both services are reported and modifier **25** is appended to the transport code.
- Initial critical care codes (**99468, 99471, 99475**) are only reported once per calendar day and once per hospital stay for a given patient. If the patient is readmitted to critical care during the same hospital stay, report a subsequent critical care code (**99469, 99472, 99476**).
- Subsequent critical care may be reported on multiple days even if there is no change in the patient's condition if the patient continues to meet the critical care definition and documentation supports this level of service.
- Care may be provided on any unit of a hospital facility.
- Care must be provided by the reporting physician, but it also includes the services provided by the health care team functioning under the direct supervision of the physician or an advanced nurse practitioner who is employed by the physician or physician group and when allowed under state licensure requirements. See the Neonatal Critical and Intensive Care Supervision Requirements section earlier in this chapter and **Appendix IV**, Global Per Diem Critical Care Codes: Direct Supervision and Reporting Guidelines.
- Medical record documentation must support the need for and meet the definition of critical care (eg, complex MDM, high probability of imminent or life-threatening deterioration, organ system failure).

Subsequent-day neonatal and pediatric intensive care codes (**99478–99480**) are reported when critical care is no longer required and the neonate who weighs 5,000 g or less on the day of service requires more intensive care than what is typically provided under routine subsequent hospital care (**99231–99233**). Once the neonate weighs at least 5,001 g and critical care services are no longer required, report subsequent-day inpatient hospital visit codes (**99231–99233**).

Neonatal Critical Care

99468   Initial inpatient neonatal critical care, per day, for the evaluation and management of a critically ill neonate, 28 days of age or younger

99469   Subsequent inpatient neonatal critical care, per day, for the evaluation and management of a critically ill neonate, 28 days of age or younger

Selection of the appropriate code will depend on the newborn's or infant's condition and the intensity of the service provided and documented on a particular day of service.

- Codes may be reported in addition to normal newborn care (**99460** or **99462**) or neonatal consultation (**99251–99255**) when the patient receives normal newborn care or consultation and then, at a subsequent separate encounter on the same day, requires critical care. However, the neonatologist would report only critical or intensive care services if a transfer of care occurs at the initial consultation. Each service should be reported with the appropriate diagnosis code to support the service (eg, diagnosis codes for well newborn and the defined illness).

> National Correct Coding Initiative edits bundle normal newborn care to neonatal critical care, but you may use modifier 25 (significant, separately identifiable evaluation and management service) to override the edit under appropriate circumstances (eg, separate encounters).

- Only a single code representing the highest level of service performed and documented is reported if all the care was provided by a single physician or physicians of the same specialty and group practice. However, if the intensity of care progresses over the day and services are provided by physicians from different groups or specialties, or the patient is transferred to another facility, each physician reports a different level of service.

Coding Conundrum: Applying the Critical Care Definition

While immaturity commonly leads to many levels of organ dysfunction that will increase the risk of a critical illness in a newborn, neither immaturity alone nor any of the specific procedures or therapies associated with care of the immature neonate or infant qualifies alone for reporting critical care. The physician must use his or her experience and judgment in assigning the *Current Procedural Terminology* definition of *critical care*. In summary, these are patients presently at clear risk of death or serious morbidity, requiring close observation and frequent interventions and assessments, and high-complexity medical decision-making (MDM) is apparent in the medical record documentation. No single criterion places or excludes a patient from this category, and the patient is not required to demonstrate all the characteristics listed in this chapter. The most convincing way to demonstrate the appropriate application of a critical care code is to clearly document the neonate's condition in the medical record, noting the risks to the patient, frequency of needed assessments and interventions, degree and type of organ failure(s) the patient is presently experiencing, and complexity of the MDM.

Examples

➤ **A term 3,500-g neonate is born cyanotic following a vaginal delivery.** He has minimal respiratory distress and appears otherwise vigorous. He is brought to the NICU, where a chest radiograph shows dramatic cardiomegaly and a marked increase in pulmonary markings. An umbilical artery catheter and umbilical vein catheter are inserted to determine blood gases. An ECG is performed, and a pediatric cardiologist is consulted to obtain an emergency echocardiogram.

It is important to remember that respiratory support (ie, mechanical ventilation) is not required to report critical care services. In this case, serious cyanosis and clear evidence of cardiac decompensation qualify as critical care. Code **99468** would be reported for initial date of neonatal critical care services. The umbilical vessel catheterizations are bundled with **99468**. Depending on the findings on the echocardiogram and a need for cardiac intensive care, the cardiologist may report hourly critical care for any additional time beyond the echocardiogram. If critical care is not provided, the cardiologist would report consultative services (**99251–99255**) or subsequent hospital care (if requirements for reporting a consultation are not met). (See **Chapter 16**, Noncritical Hospital Evaluation and Management Services, for more information on reporting consultations and reporting to payers who do not recognize consultation codes.) If the neonate were transferred to a cardiac center by the neonatologist, the neonatologist would report time-based critical care codes (**99291, 99292**) for the care provided prior to the transfer rather than **99468**.

➤ **A 6-day-old born at 31 weeks' gestation with unstable apnea is weaned off the ventilator to CPAP.** She is continued on caffeine, partial parenteral nutrition by central vein, and IV antibiotics.

Code **99469** is reported because the medical record continues to document the neonate's instability and the continued need for critical care services.

Coding Conundrum: Apnea in Neonates

Apnea in neonates may be an expected component of preterm birth and may be effectively managed by manual stimulation, pharmacological stimulation, high-flow nasal oxygen, or continuous positive airway pressure. At other times, this symptom is associated with a serious underlying problem(s) and reflects the instability of a critically ill neonate. When this is the case, one or more of the same interventions will be required. The physician must employ his or her best clinical judgment and clearly document the factors that make the patient's present condition critical (or require intensive care). The same requirements for organ failure, risk of imminent deterioration, and complex medical decision-making apply. With apnea and many other conditions, the following drive correct code selection: the total picture of the neonate with the diagnosis, clinical presentation, and immediate threat to life; amount of hands-on and supervisory care provided by the physician; and the level of intervention needed to manage that neonate's conditions on a given day. When critical care codes are reported, the documentation must support the physician's judgment that the patient is critically ill and services provided are commensurate with the condition on that day of service on which critical care codes are reported.

Pediatric Critical Care

99471 Initial inpatient pediatric critical care, per day, for the evaluation and management of a critically ill infant or young child, 29 days through 24 months of age

99472 Subsequent inpatient pediatric critical care, per day, for the evaluation and management of a critically ill infant or young child, 29 days through 24 months of age

99475 Initial inpatient pediatric critical care, per day, for the evaluation and management of a critically ill infant or young child, 2 through 5 years of age

99476 Subsequent inpatient pediatric critical care, per day, for the evaluation and management of a critically ill infant or young child, 2 through 5 years of age

Codes **99471–99476** are used to report direction of the inpatient care of a critically ill infant or young child outside of the neonatal period. Services are provided to patients who are at least 29 days of age (postnatal age with day of birth being 0 [zero]) until the child reaches 6 years of age. Initial pediatric critical care for children of these ages is reported with code **99471** (29 days through 24 months of age—up to, but not including, the second birthday) or **99475** (2 through 5 years of age—up to, but not including, the sixth birthday).

Initial pediatric critical care codes (**99471, 99475**) are only reported once per calendar day, per hospital stay for a given patient. If the patient is sent to another inpatient unit for continued care and then requires readmission to critical care during the same hospital stay, report a subsequent critical care code (**99472, 99476**) on the readmission date and each subsequent date the child remains critical. These subsequent-day codes may be reported only by a single individual and only once per day, per patient, in a given setting.

Examples

➤ **A 22-month-old girl with status epilepticus is initially treated by the ED physician (1 hour of critical care).** Although seizures were initially controlled, pharmacologic management led to irregular respiratory activity, lethargy, and hypotension. The patient was admitted to the pediatric intensive care unit at 11:00 pm that evening by the critical care attending physician, who intubated her, placed her on a ventilator, began fluid expansion, used dobutamine to control her blood pressure, and made arrangements for a bedside electroencephalogram (EEG).

The ED physician would report 1 hour of critical care (**99291**). The pediatrician or intensivist would report his or her services with the initial inpatient pediatric critical care code (**99471**) for that calendar day, even though only 1 hour of care was provided. One hour later, after midnight, a new date of service would begin. The intubation is bundled with **99471** and cannot be separately billed.

➤ **A hospitalist admits a 5-year-old to observation for exacerbation of asthma that initially improved with treatment.** Later the same day, the patient is found to be in respiratory failure and the hospitalist provides 35 minutes of critical care services before transferring the patient's care to a pediatric intensivist. The pediatric intensivist assumes management of the critically ill patient at 10:00 pm.

The hospitalist reports initial observation care (**99218–99220**) based the level of service provided and appends modifier **25** to indicate that this service is significant and separately identifiable from critical care services reported with code **99291**. The intensivist reports code **99475** (initial inpatient pediatric critical care, per day, for the E/M of a critically ill infant or young child, 2 through 5 years of age).

Patients Critically Ill After Surgery

Postoperative care of a surgical patient is included in the surgeon's global surgical package. For some neonatal surgical care, critical care days are included in the work values assigned to surgical procedures (eg, **39503** [repair of diaphragmatic hernia], **43314** [esophagoplasty, thoracic approach; with repair of tracheoesophageal fistula], **49605** [repair of large ompha-locele or gastroschisis; with or without prosthesis]).

However

- If a second physician provides care for the routine postoperative patient, the surgeon must append modifier **54** (surgical care only) to the surgical code. (A formal transfer of care should be documented.)
- If the surgeon provides and reports the complete surgical care package, a request for consultation from another specialist may be made.
- If the patient's course is not typical and an unexpected complication occurs that requires concurrent care from another specialist, both may report their service.

Example

➤ **If a surgeon first requests a consultation, an initial consultation code (or other appropriate E/M code based on the payer's payment policy for consultations) would be reported by the consultant.** If the surgeon requests concurrent care for a specific medical problem, time-based critical care (**99291**, **99292**) or subsequent hospital care (**99231–99233**) codes would be reported dependent on the child's condition and care provided. The diagnosis code representing the condition or symptom being treated should be reported with the concurrent *CPT* code. The rationale for the need for concurrent care must be documented in the surgeon's notes.

Remote Critical Care Services

G0508   Telehealth consultation, critical care, physicians typically spend 60 minutes communicating with the patient via telehealth (initial)

G0509   Telehealth consultation, critical care, physicians typically spend 50 minutes communicating with the patient via telehealth (subsequent)

Remote critical care is the direct delivery of medical care by a physician(s) for a critically ill or critically injured patient from an off-site location (ie, when a critically ill or injured patient requires additional critical care resources that are not available on-site). *CPT* instructs to report code **99499** (unlisted E/M service) appended with modifier **95** (synchronous telemedicine service rendered via a real-time interactive audio and video telecommunications system) for neonatal and pediatric critical care via telemedicine. Other payers may allow reporting with codes **G0508** or **G0509** with place of service **02**. It is recommended that practices verify health plan policies for provision of critical care services via telemedicine before initiating these services.

See **Chapter 20**, Digital Medicine Services: Technology-Enhanced Care Delivery, for more information on reporting telemedicine services, including remote critical care.

Initial and Continuing Intensive Care

99477   Initial hospital care, per day, for the evaluation and management of the neonate, 28 days of age or younger, who requires intensive observation, frequent interventions, and other intensive care services

99478   Subsequent intensive care, per day, for the evaluation and management of the recovering very low birth weight infant (present body weight less than 1500 grams)

99479   Subsequent intensive care, per day, for the evaluation and management of the recovering low birth weight infant (present body weight of 1500–2500 grams)

99480   Subsequent intensive care, per day, for the evaluation and management of the recovering infant (present body weight of 2501–5000 grams)

Continuing intensive care services provided to an infant weighing more than 5,000 g (approximately 11.02 lb) are reported with subsequent hospital care codes (99231–99233). Documentation of these services must support 2 of 3 key components or the total unit or floor time and time spent counseling and/or coordinating care.

Neonatal and pediatric intensive care codes (**99477–99480**) may be used to report care for neonates or infants who are not critically ill but have a need for intensive monitoring, observation, and frequent assessments by the health care team and supervision by the physician. This includes

- Neonates who require intensive but not critical care services from birth
- Neonates who are no longer critically ill but require intensive physician and health care team observation and interventions
- Recovering low birth weight infants who require a higher level of care than that defined by other hospital care services

These neonates often have a continued need for oxygen, parenteral or gavage enteral nutrition, treatment for apnea of prematurity, and thermoregulation from an Isolette or radiant warmer, and may be recovering from cardiac or surgical care. The intensive services described by these codes include intensive cardiac and respiratory monitoring, continuous and/or frequent vital sign monitoring, heat maintenance, enteral and/or parenteral nutritional adjustments, and laboratory and oxygen saturation monitoring when provided.

- These are bundled services and include the same procedures that are bundled with neonatal and pediatric critical care services (**99468–99476**). See **Table 18-1** for a list of all the services and procedures that are included.
- Code **99477** is used to report the more intensive services that an ill but not critically ill neonate (28 days or younger) requires on the day of admission to inpatient care. Code **99477** includes all E/M services on that date, excluding
  — Attendance at delivery (**99464**) or newborn resuscitation (**99465**), which may be reported in addition to code **99477**, when performed.
  — Normal newborn care (**99460–99462**), when performed.
  — Append modifier **25** to code **99477** when reporting on the same date as **99460–99462**, **99464**, or **99465**.

Payers that have adopted the Medicare National Correct Coding Initiative (NCCI) edits will not allow payment of codes 99460–99462 and 99477 for services by the same physician or physicians of the same specialty and group practice on the same date. Only code 99477 is reported under these circumstances. See more about NCCI edits in Chapter 2, Modifiers and Coding Edits.

- Code **99477** should also be used to report readmission to a facility (after initial discharge) of an ill neonate (aged 28 days or younger) if the neonate requires intensive (not critical) care services.
- If the infant is older than 28 days at admission but weighs less than 5,000 g, codes **99221–99223** should be used for intensive care on the date of hospital admission (typically **99223**, assuming documentation of comprehensive history and physical examination and high-level MDM). Codes **99478–99480** are typically used for subsequent days, as long as the infant continues to require intensive care.
- Services are typically (but not required to be) provided in a NICU or special care unit and require a higher intensity of care than would be reported with codes **99221–99223** (initial hospital care of sick patient).
- Patients are under constant observation by the health care team under direct physician supervision.
- Codes **99478–99480** include all the E/M services (and bundled procedures) provided to the neonate on the date of service.
- **Table 18-4** illustrates codes for subsequent-day neonatal and pediatric intensive care services (**99478–99480**) by present body weight.

Table 18-4. Neonatal and Pediatric Subsequent-Day Intensive Care				
Description	**Present Weight <1,500 g**	**Present Weight 1,500–2,500 g**	**Present Weight 2,501–5,000 g**	**Present Weight ≥5,001 g**
Subsequent intensive care	99478	99479	99480	99231–99233

- Codes **99478–99480** are reported once per calendar day of subsequent intensive (but not critical) care for the E/M of the recovering infant weighing 5,000 g or less. Selection of the code will be dependent on the *present* body weight of the infant, not the infant's age, on the date of service. Therefore, code selection may change from one day to the next depending on the infant's present body weight and condition.

Chapter 18. Critical and Intensive Care

- Once the baby's weight exceeds 5,000 g, subsequent hospital care codes (**99231–99233**) are reported until the date of discharge (**99238**, **99239**).

Examples

➤ **A 1,500-g neonate has mild respiratory distress.** She is on 30% oxygen by nasal cannula, a cardiorespiratory monitor, and continuous pulse oximetry. Laboratory tests and radiographs are ordered, and IV fluids and antibiotics are started. Frequent monitoring and observation are required and ordered.

   Code **99477** (initial hospital care for the ill neonate, 28 days of age or less, who requires intensive observation and monitoring) would be reported by the admitting physician.

➤ **A 1,150-g neonate, now 5 days old, is receiving 30% oxygen and also continues to receive IV fluids, small trophic feeds, and caffeine for apnea.**

   Code **99478** would be reported.

➤ **A 15-day-old, 1,600-g neonate remains in an Isolette for thermoregulation and is on methylxanthines for intermittent apnea and bradycardia, for which the neonate requires continuous cardiorespiratory and pulse oximetry monitoring.** The physician adjusts the neonate's continuous gavage feeds based on tolerance and weight.

   Code **99479** would be reported.

➤ **A baby requires intensive care and weighs 2,500 g on Monday.** The following day, she continues to require intensive care and her weight is 2,504 g.

   Code **99479** would be reported for the care provided on Monday. Code **99480** would be reported for the continuing intensive care provided the following day.

In these examples, the neonate is not critically ill but continues to require intensive monitoring and constant observation by the health care team under direct physician supervision.

Coding for Transitions to Different Levels of Neonatal Care

During a hospital stay, a newborn or readmitted neonate may require different levels of care. A normal newborn may end up becoming sick, intensively ill, or critical during the same hospital stay. Neonates who were initially sick may also improve to require lower levels of care (eg, normal neonatal care).

An initial-day critical or intensive care code (eg, **99468**, **99477**) is reported only once per hospital stay. If the patient recovers and is later stepped up again to that higher level of care, only the subsequent-level codes (**99469**, **99478–99480**) are reported.

Figure 18-1 provides an illustration of coding for a newborn who transitions from critical care to intensive care and hospital care before discharge. Note that all services take place during the same admission and the physicians are of 2 different specialties (eg, general pediatrics and neonatology). Each physician individually reports the services provided, and each may only report 1 initial hospital or intensive or critical care service. You can also refer to the American Academy of Pediatrics (AAP) *Newborn Coding Decision Tool* (available for purchase at https://shop.aap.org) for numerous scenarios of coding for newborn care throughout admissions and transfers of care.

Example

➤ **A neonate (2,600 g) becomes critically ill after being transferred from neonatal critical care by a neonatologist to a hospitalist pediatrician (same facility) to complete her recovery before home discharge.** Care is again transferred to the same neonatologist or neonatologist of the same group practice for critical care services.

The neonatologist reports	The hospitalist reports
99469 (subsequent inpatient neonatal critical care, per day, for the E/M of a critically ill neonate, 28 days of age or younger)	**99233** (subsequent hospital care) or, if ≥30 minutes of critical care services were rendered, **99291**, **99292** (hourly critical care services)

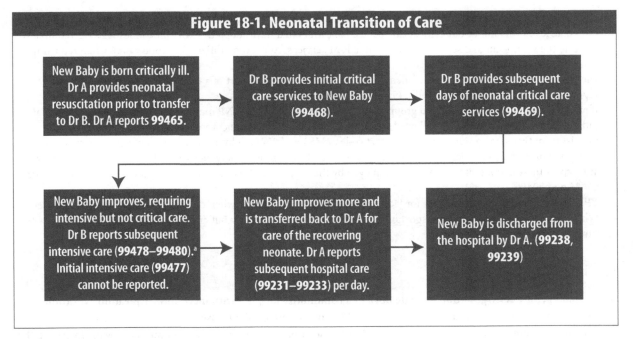

Figure 18-1. Neonatal Transition of Care

New Baby is born critically ill. Dr A provides neonatal resuscitation prior to transfer to Dr B. Dr A reports **99465**.

→ Dr B provides initial critical care services to New Baby (**99468**).

→ Dr B provides subsequent days of neonatal critical care services (**99469**).

New Baby improves, requiring intensive but not critical care. Dr B reports subsequent intensive care (**99478–99480**).[a] Initial intensive care (**99477**) cannot be reported.

→ New Baby improves more and is transferred back to Dr A for care of the recovering neonate. Dr A reports subsequent hospital care (**99231–99233**) per day.

→ New Baby is discharged from the hospital by Dr A. (**99238**, **99239**)

[a] Assumes patient's current weight supports code assignment.

Teaching Point: The neonatologist may not report initial neonatal critical care for services to the patient who has received prior initial hospital services (eg, initial neonatal intensive care). If the patient initially met the requirements for subsequent intensive care rather than subsequent hospital care, code **99480** would be reported in lieu of code **99233**.

Emergency Medical Services Supervision and Patient Transport

Pediatric Critical Care Patient Transport

Face-to-face Critical Care Patient Transport

99466   Critical care face-to-face services, during an interfacility transport of critically ill or critically injured pediatric patient, 24 months of age or younger; first 30–74 minutes of hands-on care during transport

99467   each additional 30 minutes (List separately in addition to code **99466**)

Codes **99466** and **99467** are used to report the physical attendance and direct face-to-face care provided by a physician or QHP during the inter-facility transport of a critically ill or injured patient aged 24 months or younger.

● The patient's condition must meet the *CPT* definition for critical care.
● Face-to-face time begins when the physician or practitioner assumes primary responsibility for the patient at the referring hospital or facility and ends when the receiving hospital or facility accepts responsibility for the patient's care. Only the time the physician spends in direct face-to-face contact with the patient during transport should be reported.
  — Less than 30 minutes of face-to-face time cannot be reported.
  — Time must be documented.
  — Code **99467** is used to report each additional 30 minutes of physician face-to-face time of critical care provided on the same day of service beyond the first 74 minutes.
● Codes include the bundled services listed in **Table 18-1**. Codes **99466** and **99467** may be reported separately from any other procedures or services that are not bundled and performed on the date of transfer. The time involved in performing any procedures that are not bundled and are reported separately should not be included in the face-to-face transport time.
● Procedures or services that are performed by other members of the transport team with the physical presence, participation, and supervision of the accompanying physician may be reported by the physician. Documentation must support the physician's participation.
● Medical record documentation must include the total face-to-face time spent with the patient, the critical nature of the patient's condition, and any performed procedures that are not bundled.

- The pediatric critical care transport codes are preadmission codes and may be reported in addition to neonatal (**99468**) or pediatric (**99471**) initial-day critical care codes. For payers that have adopted NCCI edits, modifier **25** is required to indicate the significant and separately identifiable E/M services. Append modifier **25** to code **99466** when reporting in conjunction with daily critical care codes.

- Face-to-face critical care services provided during an inter-facility transport of a child older than 24 months are reported with hourly critical care codes (**99291** and **99292**).

- If an NNP employed by the neonatal group is on the transport team, the NNP may report codes **99466** and **99467** if independent billing by an NNP is allowed by the state and the activities are covered in the scope of practice. The neonatologist from that same group would not report codes **99485** and **99486** (physician direction of pediatric critical care transport) or **99288** (physician direction of emergency medical systems emergency care). The facility (hospital) could also report these services if the NNPs are employed by the hospital. In this case, the neonatologist would report codes **99485** and **99486**.

- *CPT* does not include specific codes for face-to-face transport of a patient when criteria for critical care are not met. When face-to-face care during transport of a patient is medically necessary but critical care is not, report code **99499** (unlisted E/M service).

Example

➤ **A 3,000-g, 38-weeks' gestation neonate born at a community hospital with meconium aspiration syndrome requires ventilator care and transport to a Level III unit where ECMO is also available.** The receiving neonatologist accompanies the transport nurse and therapist. Ground transport takes 40 minutes one way. On arrival, the neonatologist spends 60 minutes face-to-face evaluating and stabilizing the newborn. The newborn is intubated, surfactant is administered, umbilical venous and arterial catheters are inserted, and parents are counseled. The neonatologist spends 5 minutes intubating and administering the surfactant and 20 minutes placing the umbilical venous and arterial catheters. The newborn is then transferred to the neonatal transport van and back to the receiving nursery. Total time from bedside back to the receiving nursery is 60 minutes. Frequent assessments and alterations in drugs, fluids, and ventilator settings are performed on the transport back. The neonatologist spent a total of 120 minutes of face-to-face critical care time with the neonate; 25 minutes is subtracted for the performance of non-bundled procedures. The neonatologist continues care of the newborn in the NICU.

99466 25	(first 74 minutes)
99467 25 × 1 unit	(final 21 minutes)
31500	(endotracheal intubation, emergency)
94610	(surfactant administration)
36510	(catheterization of umbilical vein)
36660	(catheterization of umbilical artery)
99468 25	(initial neonatal critical care)

Modifier **25** is appended to each of the services to designate a significant and separately identifiable E/M service provided by the same physician on the same date of service. Endotracheal intubation is bundled with daily neonatal critical care but is separately reported when provided during transport of the critically ill or injured neonate.

Non–face-to-face Pediatric Critical Care Patient Transport

#99485   Supervision by a control physician of interfacility transport care of the critically ill or critically injured pediatric patient, 24 months of age or younger, includes two-way communication with transport team before transport, at the referring facility and during the transport, including data interpretation and report; first 30 minutes

#99486   each additional 30 minutes (List separately in addition to code **99485**)

Code **99485** is used to report the first 16 to 45 minutes of a control physician's documented non–face-to-face supervision of inter-facility critical care transport of a patient 24 months or younger, which includes all 2-way communication between the control physician and the specialized transport team prior to transport, at the referring facility, and during transport to the receiving facility.

Each additional 30-minute period of communication is reported with add-on code **99486**.

- The patient's condition must meet the *CPT* definition of critical care.
- Only report for patients 24 months or younger who are critically ill or injured.
- The control physician does not report any services provided by the specialized transport team.

- The control physician only reports cumulative time spent communicating with the specialty transport team members during an inter-facility transport. Communication between the control physician and the referring facility before or following patient transport *is not* counted.
- Reportable time begins with the initial discussions with the transport team, including discussions of the best mode of transport and strategies for therapy on arrival. Time ends when the patient's care is handed over to the receiving facility team.
- Do not report **99485** or **99486** for services of 15 minutes or less or for any time spent in supervision of a QHP from the same group who is reporting **99466** or **99467**.
- Time spent with the individual patient's transport team and reviewing data submissions should be recorded. Time spent discussing the patient with the referring physician or facility is not counted.
- Codes **99485** and **99486** represent preadmission services and may be reported by the same or different individual(s) of the same specialty and same group when neonatal or pediatric critical care services (**99468–99476**) are reported for the same patient on the same day.

Example

➤ **A community pediatrician asks to refer a newborn with cyanosis, tachycardia, and possible congenital cardiac disease.** The neonatologist dispatches the transport team, consisting of a hospital-employed transport nurse and a respiratory therapist. On the trip to the referring hospital, the neonatologist converses by telephone for 10 minutes with the team, explaining the newborn's condition and formulating an initial treatment plan. After arrival, the nurse evaluates the neonate and telephones the neonatologist to discuss the findings. The decision is made to provide prostaglandin to maintain ductal patency and avoid oxygen therapy. Because of the critical nature of the newborn, the neonatologist elects to remain on the telephone until therapy is completed (15 minutes). The team then leaves the referring hospital. On the return trip, telephone contact lasting 10 minutes is again made to update the physician on the neonate's condition, vital signs, and overall physical status. The team then completes the transport without further incident.

The neonatologist spent a total of 35 minutes in direct 2-way telephone communication with the team in 3 discrete episodes. The neonatologist carefully documents the time spent in the medical record, including what decisions were made during each contact. Code **99485** is used to report this service.

Direction of Emergency Medical Services

99288   Physician or other qualified health care professional direction of emergency medical systems (EMS) emergency care, advanced life support

See the Non–face-to-face Pediatric Critical Care Patient Transport section earlier in this chapter for discussion of physician non–face-to-face supervision of inter-facility transport of a critically ill or injured pediatric patient 24 months or younger (**99485, 99486**).

Code **99288**

- May be reported by any physician of any specialty or QHP when advanced life support services are provided via 2-way voice communications (eg, cardiac and/or pulmonary resuscitation; administration of IV fluids, antibiotics, or surfactant).
- This code reflects all the services provided by the directing physician and is not based on any time requirements. Code **99288** may be reported when less than 16 minutes is spent in physician non–face-to-face supervision of inter-facility transport of a critically ill or injured pediatric patient (ie, requirements for reporting **99485** are not met).
- The directing physician should maintain documentation of the times of all contacts, orders, and/or directions for treatment or management of the patient.
- Services or procedures performed by emergency medical services (EMS) personnel are not reported by the physician because he or she was not physically present.
- When an advance practice professional provides and reports face-to-face services during transport, the physician would not report **99288**.
- The appropriate diagnoses are linked to the service.
  - If, after directing EMS personnel, the physician performs the initial critical care, the appropriate critical care code (eg, **99468**, initial inpatient neonatal critical care) would also be reported with modifier **25** appended to indicate that 2 separate and distinct E/M services were provided by the same physician on the same day of service.

Chapter 18. Critical and Intensive Care

There is no assigned Medicare relative value unit to this service, so it is carrier priced and payments will vary by payer. Medicare considers code **99288** a bundled service and does not pay separately for the service. Check with your state Medicaid program and other payers to determine their coverage policy.

Total Body Systemic and Selective Head Hypothermia

99184   Initiation of selective head or total body hypothermia in the critically ill neonate, includes appropriate patient selection by review of clinical, imaging and laboratory data, confirmation of esophageal temperature probe location, evaluation of amplitude EEG, supervision of controlled hypothermia, and assessment of patient tolerance of cooling

(Do not report **99184** more than once per hospital stay)

Examples

➤ **A term neonate born with evidence of hypoxic-ischemic encephalopathy is admitted to the NICU and receives critical care services.** Laboratory, EEG, blood gas, and imaging studies confirm the neonate meets objective criteria for *total body cooling*. Continuous total body cooling is undertaken.

   Code **99184** is reported for total body systemic hypothermia in addition to **99468**, initial day of neonatal critical care.

➤ **A term neonate born with evidence of hypoxic-ischemic encephalopathy is admitted to the NICU and receives critical care services.** Laboratory, EEG, blood gas, and imaging studies confirm the neonate meets objective criteria for *selective head cooling*. Continuous selective head cooling is undertaken.

   Code **99184** is reported for selective head hypothermia in addition to **99468**, initial day of neonatal critical care.

When total body systemic or selective head hypothermia is used in treatment of a critically ill neonate, code **99184** represents the work of initiating the service.

Documentation for use of total body systemic hypothermia and selective head hypothermia should include the neonatal criteria that support initiating this service.
- During either cooling approach, monitoring includes
  — Radiographic confirmation of core temperature probe
  — Continuous core temperature assessment and adjustment
  — Repeated assessment of skin integrity
  — Recurrent objective evaluation of evolving neurologic changes (eg, Sarnat stage), which may also include assessment of continuous amplitude EEG monitoring
- In addition, cooling-related laboratory evaluations are required to monitor for cooling-specific complications, including metabolic and coagulation alterations.

Extracorporeal Membrane Oxygenation (ECMO) or Extracorporeal Life Support (ECLS) Services

Prolonged ECMO and extracorporeal life support (ECLS) services provide cardiac and/or respiratory support, allowing the heart and/or lungs to rest and recover when sick or injured. These services commonly involve multiple physicians and supporting health care personnel to manage each patient. ECMO and ECLS codes differentiate components of initiation and daily management of ECMO and ECLS from daily management of a patient's overall medical condition.

These services include cannula insertion (**33951–33956**), ECMO or ECLS initiation (**33946** or **33947**), daily ECMO or ECLS management (**33948** or **33949**), repositioning of the ECMO or ECLS cannula(e) (**33957–33964**), and cannula removal (**33965–33986**). Each physician providing part of the ECMO/ECLS services may report the services they provide except when prohibited by *CPT* instruction (eg, cannula repositioning is not reported by the same or another physician on the same date as initiation of ECMO/ECLS).

Example

➤ **Venoarterial ECMO is initiated for a patient with cardiac and respiratory failure.** Physician A inserts the cannulae. Physician B manages the initial transition to ECMO, including working with physician A, ECMO specialists, and others to initiate an ongoing assessment of anticoagulation, venous return, cannula positioning, and optimal flow. Physician B also provides daily management of the patient's overall care. When ECMO is discontinued, physician A returns and removes the cannulae.

Physician A will report codes for insertion and removal of the ECMO cannulae (eg, **33952** and **33966**). Physician B will report initiation of venoarterial ECMO (**33947**), the appropriate hospital and/or critical care codes for overall management of the patient for each day provided (eg, **99291**, **99292**, or **99231–99233**), and daily management of ECMO (**33949**) for each day provided.

ECMO/ECLS Cannula Insertion, Repositioning, and Removal

Codes for insertion, repositioning, and removal of ECMO and ECLS are reported based on the patient's age, with separate codes for procedures performed on newborns through 5 years of age and on patients 6 years and older. Codes for these services are shown in **Table 18-5**. While typically only performed by surgeons, other pediatric providers may perform them as well.

> Each physician providing a part of extracorporeal membrane oxygenation/extracorporeal life support services may report the part they provided except as prohibited by *Current Procedural Terminology* instruction.

Table 18-5. Extracorporeal Membrane Oxygenation or Extracorporeal Life Support Cannula(e) Procedures

Approach	Birth Through 5 Years of Age	6 Years and Older	Do Not Report With
Insertion			
Percutaneous peripheral (arterial/venous) cannula(e)[a]	33951	33952	33957–33964
Open peripheral (arterial/venous) cannula(e)	33953	33954	33957–33964, 34812, 34820, 34834
Central cannula(e) by sternotomy or thoracotomy	33955	33956	33957–33964, 32100, 39010
Reposition[b]			
Percutaneous, reposition peripheral (arterial and/or venous) cannula(e)[a]	33957	33958	33946, 33947, 34812, 34820, 34834
Open, reposition peripheral (arterial and/or venous) cannula(e)[a]	33959	33962	33946, 33947, 34812, 34820, 34834
Central cannula(e) reposition by sternotomy or thoracotomy[a]	33963	33964	33946, 33947, 32100, 39010
Removal[c]			
Removal of peripheral (arterial and/or venous) cannula(e), percutaneous	33965	33966	Not applicable
Removal of peripheral (arterial and/or venous) cannula(e), open	33969	33984	34812, 34820, 34834, 35201, 35206, 35211, 35216, 35226
Removal of central cannula(e) by sternotomy or thoracotomy	33985	33986	35201, 35206, 35211, 35216, 35226

[a] Includes fluoroscopic guidance when performed.
[b] Repositioning of cannula(e) at the same session, as insertion is not separately reported.
[c] Report only the insertion when cannula(e) is replaced in the same vessel.

●=New code   ▲=Revised code   #=Re-sequenced code   +=Add-on code

Chapter 18. Critical and Intensive Care

- Do not separately report repositioning of the ECMO or ECLS cannula(e) (**33957–33964**) at the same session as insertion (**33951–33956**).
- Report replacement of ECMO or ECLS cannula(e) in the same vessel using the insertion code (**33951–33956**) only.
- If a cannula(e) is removed from one vessel and a new cannula(e) is placed in a different vessel, report the appropriate cannula(e) removal (**33965–33986**) and insertion (**33951–33956**) codes.
- Fluoroscopic guidance used for cannula(e) repositioning (**33957–33964**) is included in the procedure when performed and should not be separately reported.
- Extensive repair or replacement of an artery may be additionally reported (eg, **35226**, **35286**, **35371**, **35665**).
- Direct anastomosis of a prosthetic graft to the artery sidewall to facilitate arterial perfusion for ECMO or ECLS is separately reported with code **33987** in addition to codes **33953–33956**.

+33987   Arterial exposure with creation of graft conduit (eg, chimney graft) to facilitate arterial perfusion for ECMO/ ECLS (List separately in addition to code for primary procedure)

   Do not report **33987** in conjunction with **34833** (open iliac artery exposure with creation of conduit for delivery of aortic or iliac endovascular prosthesis, by abdominal or retroperitoneal incision, unilateral).

ECMO/ECLS Initiation and Daily Management

33946   Extracorporeal membrane oxygenation (ECMO)/extracorporeal life support (ECLS) provided by physician; initiation, venovenous

33947   initiation, venoarterial

33948   daily management, each day, venovenous

33949   daily management, each day, venoarterial

Initiation of the ECMO or ECLS circuit and setting parameters (**33946**, **33947**) involves determining the necessary ECMO or ECLS device components, blood flow, gas exchange, and other necessary parameters to manage the circuit.

Daily care for a patient on ECMO or ECLS includes managing the ECMO or ECLS circuit and related patient issues. These services may be performed by one physician while another physician manages the overall patient medical condition and underlying disorders, but a single physician may provide both services. Regardless of the patient's condition, the basic management of ECMO and ECLS is similar. Documentation for each service should be distinct in the medical record.

- Do not report modifier **63** (procedure performed on infants <4 kg) when reporting codes **33946–33949**.
- The physician reporting daily ECMO or ECLS oversees the interaction of the circuit with the patient, management of blood flow, oxygenation, carbon dioxide clearance by the membrane lung, systemic response, anticoagulation and treatment of bleeding, cannula positioning, alarms and safety, and weaning the patient from the ECMO or ECLS circuit when heart and/or lung function has sufficiently recovered.
- Daily management of the patient may be separately reported using the relevant hospital observation services, hospital inpatient services, or critical care E/M codes (**99218–99220**, **99221–99223**, **99231–99233**, **99234–99236**, **99291**, **99292**, **99468–99480**).
- Daily management (**33948** or **33949**) or cannula repositioning (**33957–33959**, **33962–33964**) may not be reported on the same date as initiation (**33946** or **33947**) by the same or different physician.

Sedation

Refer to **Chapter 19**, Common Surgical Procedures and Sedation in Facility Settings, for specific guidelines for reporting sedation services, including moderate (conscious) sedation (**99151–99157**) and deep sedation.

Car Seat/Bed Testing

94780   Car seat/bed testing for airway integrity, for infants through 12 months of age, with continual clinical staff observation and continuous recording of pulse oximetry, heart rate and respiratory rate, with interpretation and report; 60 minutes

+94781   each additional full 30 minutes (List separately in addition to **94780**.)

Neonates who required critical care during their initial hospital stay are most often those patients who require monitoring to determine if they may be safely transported in a car seat or must be transported in a car bed. While these codes are bundled under neonatal and pediatric critical and intensive care codes (**99468–99472**, **99477–99480**), the services most often take place when a neonate is about to go home and, therefore, can be reported if hospital care services (**99231–99233**) or hospital discharge services (**99238**, **99239**) are being reported instead.

●=New code   ▲=Revised code   #=Re-sequenced code   +=Add-on code

Report codes **94780** and **94781** when the following conditions are met:

- The patient must be an infant (ie, 12 months or younger). Assessment after the patient is 29 days or older may be necessary.
- Continual clinical staff observation with continuous recording of pulse oximetry, heart rate, and respiratory rate is required.
- Inpatient or office-based services are reported.
- Vital signs and observations must be reviewed and interpreted and a written report generated by the physician.
- Codes are reported based on the total observation time spent and documented.
- If less than 60 minutes is spent in the procedure, code **94780** may not be reported.
- Each additional full 30 minutes (ie, not less than 90 minutes) is reported with code **94781**.
- Do not include the time of car seat/bed testing in time attributed to discharge day management services (**99238**, **99239**).
- These codes may be reported with discharge day management (**99238**, **99239**), normal newborn care services (**99460**, **99462**, **99463**), or subsequent hospital care codes (**99231–99233**).

Examples

➤ **A neonate born at 26 weeks' gestation requires a car seat test on the date of discharge from the hospital.**
Code **94780** is reported in addition to hospital discharge management code **99238** or **99239**.

➤ **A neonate born at 26 weeks' gestation requires a car seat test prior to discharge from the hospital.** The newborn has received 60 minutes of testing reported with **94780** and now receives an additional 30 minutes.
Codes **94780** and **94781** are reported.

Values and Payment

The typical times for E/M services most commonly provided to newborns can be used as an excellent and quick internal audit mechanism to judge coding adequacy. The times are based on RUC survey results.

Although not exact or applicable for every patient, they are the average times (in minutes) spent by neonatologists for the typical or average patient. RUC Survey Times for Hospital Care and Critical Care Services are available online at www.aap.org/cfp (access code AAPCFP26).

Payment Advocacy

The AAP encourages chapter development of pediatric councils as forums to discuss pediatric issues with payers. Pediatric councils have the potential to facilitate better working relationships between pediatricians and health insurance plans and to improve quality of care for children. Learn more about AAP pediatric councils at www.aap.org/en-us/professional-resources/practice-transformation/getting-paid/Pages/aap-pediatric-councils.aspx.

The AAP Section on Neonatal-Perinatal Medicine, in conjunction with state chapters and councils of the AAP, has developed strategies that have been successful in addressing payment concerns for neonatal care. Contact your state chapter, its pediatric council, your section district AAP Executive Committee representative, a neonatal trainer, or the AAP Committee on Coding and Nomenclature for assistance in addressing any payment inequities for neonatal services in your state.

Resources

Coding Education

AAP Section on Neonatal-Perinatal Medicine coding trainers are available to provide coding education through local educational seminars and continuing education events. Contact section manager Jim Couto (jcouto@aap.org) for additional information about these valuable services.

Critical Care Supervision

Global Per Diem Critical Care Codes: Direct Supervision and Reporting Guideline (**Appendix IV**)

Newborn Coding Decision Tool

AAP *Newborn Coding Decision Tool* (available for purchase at https://shop.aap.org)

Payment Advocacy

AAP pediatric councils (www.aap.org/en-us/professional-resources/practice-transformation/getting-paid/Pages/aap-pediatric-councils.aspx)

Test Your Knowledge!

1. **Which of the following is true for critical care services (99291, 99292)?**
   a. The time required to report code **99291** must be met by a single physician.
   b. Code **99291** can be reported based on the combined times spent by a physician and other qualified health care professional.
   c. A teaching physician may not report time-based critical care services.
   d. All procedures performed are separately reported in addition to critical care services.

2. **Which of the following supports reporting delivery/birthing room resuscitation (99465)?**
   a. Continuous positive airway pressure without positive-pressure ventilation
   b. Use of blow-by oxygen
   c. Provision of positive-pressure ventilation in response to respiratory instability
   d. A neonate responds to provision of continuous positive airway pressure with an adequate respiratory effort

3. **Which of the following supports reporting code 99291?**
   a. The services provided must meet the definition of critical care.
   b. At least 30 minutes must be spent by 1 person providing critical care services.
   c. The time of the critical care services cannot include time spent providing separately reported services.
   d. All of the above

4. **What code is reported when a neonate, weighing 2,550 g, requires intensive care services after prior step-down to hospital services during the same hospital stay?**
   a. **99233** (level 3 subsequent hospital care)
   b. **99479** (subsequent intensive care)
   c. **99480** (subsequent intensive care)
   d. **99477** (initial intensive care services)

5. **Which may be reported in conjunction with initiation of extracorporeal membrane oxygenation (ECMO) (33946, 33947)?**
   a. **33948** (ECMO/extracorporeal life support daily management, each day, venovenous)
   b. **99468** (initial neonatal critical care) by the same physician
   c. Modifier **63** (procedure performed on infants <4 kg)
   d. Repositioning of cannula at same session as insertion

Common Surgical Procedures and Sedation in Facility Settings

Contents

●=New code   ▲=Revised code   #=Re-sequenced code   +=Add-on code

Chapter 19. Common Surgical Procedures and Sedation in Facility Settings

Surgical Package Rules

Current Procedural Terminology (*CPT*®) surgical codes (**10004–69990**) are packaged or global codes including all the necessary services normally furnished by a surgeon before, during, and after a procedure. *CPT* defines only a surgical package, whereas the Centers for Medicare & Medicaid Services (CMS) defines the surgical package in terms of global periods based on the pre-, intra-, and postoperative work values assigned to each procedure.

● Most state Medicaid programs follow the CMS definition.

● Each commercial insurance company will have its own policy for billing and payment of global surgical care, and most will designate a specific number of follow-up days for surgical procedures.

Both *CPT* and the CMS agree that

● Surgical codes include local infiltration, metacarpal/metatarsal/digital block, or topical anesthesia by the physician performing the procedure.

● Preoperative care

— Includes evaluation and management (E/M) service(s) *subsequent to the decision for surgery* (eg, assessing the site and condition, explanation of procedure, obtaining informed consent) on the day before and/or on the date of the procedure (including history and physical).

— When the initial decision to perform surgery is made on the day prior to or on the day of surgery, the appropriate-level E/M visit may be reported separately with modifier **57** (decision for surgery) appended. This modifier shows the payer that the E/M service was necessary to make the decision for surgery (ie, not the routine preoperative evaluation).

— When an E/M service performed on the day of the procedure is unrelated to the decision to perform surgery and is significant and distinct from the usual preoperative care associated with the procedure, it may be reported with modifier **25** (significant, separately identifiable E/M service by the same physician on the same day of the procedure or other service) appended.

— Medical record documentation must support that the service was significant, separately identifiable, and medically necessary. An E/M service performed prior to the decision to perform the procedure is separately reportable.

— Different diagnoses are not required when reporting an E/M visit and procedure.

> **Centers for Medicare & Medicaid Services Addresses Preoperative Care Differently for Minor and Major Procedures**
>
> For "minor" procedures (ie, procedures assigned a 0- or 10-day global period or endoscopies), the evaluation and management (E/M) visit on the date of the procedure is considered a routine part of the procedure regardless of whether it is prior or subsequent to the decision for surgery. In these cases, modifier **57** is not recognized.
>
> An E/M code may be reported on the same day as a minor surgical procedure only when a significant, separately identifiable E/M service is performed; modifier **25** is appended to the E/M code.
>
> When the initial decision to perform a major surgical procedure (ie, procedures assigned a 90-day global period) is made on the day prior to or on the day of a procedure, the E/M service may be reported appended with modifier **57**. Medical record documentation should support that the decision for surgery was made during the encounter and that additional time was spent in performing counseling of the risks, benefits, and outcomes.

● Postoperative care

— Includes all associated typical postoperative care (eg, dictation of progress notes; counseling with the patient, family, and/or other physicians; writing orders; evaluating the patient in the postanesthesia recovery area).

— Care for therapeutic surgical procedures includes only the care that is usually part of the surgical service.

— Care for diagnostic procedures (eg, endoscopies, arthroscopies, injection procedures for radiography) includes only the care that is related to the recovery from the diagnostic procedure.

— Care resulting from complications of surgery.

— Any complications, exacerbations, recurrence, treatment of unrelated diseases or injuries, or the presence of other diseases or injuries that require additional services may be reported separately.

> **Centers for Medicare & Medicaid Services Criteria for Reporting Postoperative Medical or Surgical Services**
>
> • All additional medical or surgical services required of the surgeon during the postoperative period of the surgery because of complications *that do not require additional trips to the operating room* are included in the global package (not separately reported).
>
> • Does not include treatment for the underlying condition or an added course of treatment that is not part of normal recovery from surgery. (See modifiers **24**, **58**, and **79** discussed in the Global Periods and Modifiers for Reporting Postoperative Care section.)

Chapter 19. Common Surgical Procedures and Sedation in Facility Settings

●=New code ▲=Revised code #=Re-sequenced code +=Add-on code

Global Periods and Modifiers for Reporting Postoperative Care

The CMS-designated global periods for each *CPT* procedure code can be found on the Resource-Based Relative Value Scale of the Medicare Physician Fee Schedule (MPFS) at www.cms.gov/medicare/medicare-fee-for-service-payment/physicianfeesched.

- It designates specific postoperative periods for certain procedure codes (ie, 0, 10, or 90 days). When determining the postoperative period, the day after surgery is day 1 of a 10- or 90-day period.
- In addition to the *CPT* code, physicians use modifier **78** for return to the operating room for a related procedure during a postoperative period. This includes return to the operating room for treatment of complications of the first procedure.
- For return to the operating room for staged or more extensive procedures and therapeutic procedures following a diagnostic procedure, append modifier **58**.
- Report procedures during the postoperative period that are unrelated and not due to complications of the original procedure with modifier **79** and unrelated E/M services with modifier **24** (documentation is typically required prior to payment).
- Other codes are designated YYY, which means the postoperative period is set by the carrier. There are no associated postoperative days included in the payment for codes assigned with status codes XXX (the global concept does not apply) or ZZZ (assigned to an add-on code for a service that is always related to another service to which the global period is assigned).

Reporting Postoperative Care

- Report *CPT* code **99024** (postoperative follow-up visit) for follow-up care provided by the physician who performed a procedure (or the covering physician) during the global surgery period.
  - Reporting of inpatient or observation follow-up visits is typically not required.
  - Reporting code **99024** allows a practice to track the number of visits performed by individuals during the postoperative period of specific procedures, calculate office overhead expenses (eg, supplies, staff, physician time) associated with the procedure, and potentially use the data to negotiate higher payment rates.

> Payers track the postoperative care provided. If a physician is not providing or reporting the postoperative care (99024) typically performed for a procedure, payers may reduce payment for the surgical service because payment includes postoperative care as part of the procedure.

- Append modifier **24** (unrelated E/M service by the same physician during a postoperative period) to the code for an E/M service provided by the physician who performed a procedure during the postoperative period.
- When physicians from different practices perform part of a surgical package, the procedure should be reported with one of the following modifiers:
  - **54** (surgical care only)
  - **55** (postoperative management only)
  - **56** (preoperative management only)

> See Chapter 2 for a more detailed description of modifiers. For critical care following surgery, see the Patients Critically Ill After Surgery section in Chapter 18.

These situations require communication among the surgeon, the physician providing preoperative or postoperative care, and each physician's respective billing personnel to ensure accurate reporting and payment.

- No modifier is required when a physician (different specialty or group practice) other than the surgeon provides unrelated services to a patient during the postoperative period.

Despite the use of different National Provider Identifiers and diagnosis codes, some payers with assigned follow-up surgical periods will deny the service. The claim should be appealed for payment with a letter advising the payer that the service was unrelated to any surgery.

Multiple Procedures on the Same Date

Often, multiple, separately reportable services are provided in one session or on one date of service. However, it is important to recognize which surgical services are considered a component of another procedure and which are separately reported.

- It is not appropriate to report multiple Healthcare Common Procedure Coding System (HCPCS)/*CPT* codes when a single, comprehensive HCPCS/*CPT* code describes the procedures performed.

Example

> ➤ **Code 42820 describes tonsillectomy and adenoidectomy in a patient younger than 12 years.** It would not be appropriate to separately report **42825** (tonsillectomy) and **42830** (adenoidectomy).

- Surgical access (eg, laparotomy) is integral to more comprehensive procedures (eg, appendectomy) and not separately reported.
- When the surgical approach fails, report only the code for the approach that resulted in the completed procedure. For example, if laparoscopy fails and an open approach is used to complete the procedure, report only the open procedure.
- It is advisable to adopt a process for checking the National Correct Coding Initiative (NCCI) edits prior to submitting multiple procedure codes for services on the same date, as the NCCI edits are used by many payers.

> See Chapter 2, Modifiers and Coding Edits, for more information on the National Correct Coding Initiative.

- For Medicaid, the NCCI manual is also informative regarding correct reporting and use of modifiers to override NCCI edits.
- When more than 1 procedure/service is performed on the same date, during the same session, or during a postoperative period, several *CPT* modifiers may apply. Documentation must support the reason for applying a modifier (eg, indicate a separate incision).
  - Modifier **59** is often appended to surgical procedure codes to override payer edits that otherwise would not allow payment for services that may be components of other services.

> See also modifiers **XE** (separate encounter), **XP** (separate provider), **XS** (separate structure), and **XU** (unusual nonoverlapping service) in Chapter 2.

  - It is important to carefully consider whether other modifiers are more appropriate (eg, **50**, bilateral service; an anatomical modifier such as **E4**, lower right eyelid) to indicate a distinct service.

Separate Procedure Designation

One designation in *CPT* helps identify procedures that are commonly performed as an integral component of another procedure. The parenthetical comment "(separate procedure)" follows the code descriptor for these services.

- Services designated as a separate procedure should not be reported in addition to the code for the total procedure or service of which they are considered an integral component.
- A procedure or service that is designated as a separate procedure may be
  - Carried out independently and be the only code reported
  - Considered to be unrelated or distinct from other procedures/services provided at that time and reported in addition to other procedures/services by appending modifier **59** (distinct procedural service)

Increased or Decreased Procedural Services

Increased Procedural Service

Modifier **22** (increased procedural service) may be appended to the code for a surgical procedure when the work required to provide the service was *significantly greater* than typically required for that procedure. To substantiate modifier **22**, documentation must support that the procedure was more difficult due to 1 or more of the following conditions:

- Increased intensity or time
- Technical difficulty
- The severity of the patient's condition
- Significantly increased physical and mental effort

Example

➤ **A child undergoes surgery for acute appendicitis with rupture.** The procedure takes 45 minutes longer than typical due to subhepatic location and rupture of the appendix. The surgeon documents the increased work and time of the procedure and reports

> **44970 22**   Laparoscopy, surgical, appendectomy
>
> **Teaching Point:** Because the work of the procedure was significantly increased by the location and rupture of the appendix, modifier **22** is appropriately appended.

> See Chapter 2 for discussion of other surgical modifiers (eg, **62**, 2 surgeons; **66**, surgical team) and general information on modifiers.

Reporting Terminated or Partial Procedures

- When a procedure is started but cannot be completed due to extenuating circumstances, physicians should consider the individual situation, including the reason for termination of the procedure and the amount of work that was performed, when determining how to report the service rendered.
- When a procedure was performed but not entirely successful (eg, portion of foreign body removed), it may be appropriate to report the procedure code that represents the work performed without modification.
- Only report reduced services (modifier **52**) or discontinued procedure (modifier **53**) when the service was significantly reduced from the typical service and as instructed in *CPT.*

Examples

➤ *CPT* instructs to append modifier **52** (reduced service) to the code for circumcision, using clamp or other device with regional dorsal penile or ring block (**54150**), when performed without dorsal penile or ring block.

- If the work performed prior to discontinuation was insignificant, it may be appropriate to not report the procedure.
- When not reporting the procedure, consider whether the level of a related E/M service was increased due to the complexity of medical decision-making associated with the attempted procedure, any complicating factors, and the revised management or treatment plan.

> For more information on reporting discontinued or incomplete procedures, see "Reporting Terminated Procedural Services" in the November 2014 *AAP Pediatric Coding Newsletter*™ (https://coding.solutions.aap.org/article.aspx?articleid=1921435; subscription required).

Reporting by Assistant Surgeon

An assistant surgeon is a physician or other qualified health care professional (QHP) who provides active assistance in the performance of a procedure when clinically indicated (eg, technically complex procedure).

- See the Assistant Surgeon in a Teaching Facility section later in this chapter for guidance on reporting assistant surgeon services by a physician in a teaching facility.
- Global rules do not apply to services performed by an assistant surgeon. Payment is based on a percentage of the fee schedule amount allowed for the procedure performed (eg, Medicare allows 16%).
- Modifiers are appended to the code(s) for the procedure on the assistant's claim. See **Table 19-1** for modifiers for reporting services by an assistant surgeon.

Table 19-1. Modifiers for Reporting Assistant Surgeon Services	
80	Assistant surgeon (use for MD or DO)
81	Minimum assistant surgeon
82	Assistant surgeon (when qualified resident surgeon not available)
AS	Physician assistant, nurse practitioner, or clinical nurse specialist services for assistant at surgery

- Reductions for multiple procedures on the same date may apply.
- See individual payer policies for assistant at surgery, as many limit payment to only specific procedures and/or may require documentation substantiating the need for assistance.

Procedures Performed on Infants Less Than 4 kg

Modifier **63** is used to identify procedures performed on neonates and infants with present body weight of up to 4 kg.

- This modifier signals significantly increased complexity and physician or other QHP work commonly associated with these patients.
- Append modifier **63** to codes for procedures performed on these infants only when there is no instruction prohibiting reporting.
- Services that cannot be reported with modifier **63** are those that have been valued based on the intensity of the service in patients weighing less than 4 kg. See "Summary of *CPT* Codes Exempt from Modifier **63**" in your *CPT* reference for a list of codes exempt from modifier **63**.
- Unless otherwise designated, this modifier may only be appended to procedures or services listed in the **20100–69999** code series and codes **92920, 92928, 92953, 92960, 92986, 92987, 92990, 92997, 92998, 93312–93318, 93452, 93463, 93505, 93530–93533, 93561–93564, 93568, 93580, 93582, 93590–93592, 93615,** and **93616**. Modifier **63** is not appended to codes from the E/M, anesthesia, radiology, or pathology/laboratory section of *CPT*.
- Use of modifier **63** may require submission of an operative note with the claim. The operative note should include the patient's weight. It is also beneficial to report the patient's weight on the claim.
- Payer acceptance of modifier **63** may be limited to specific procedures and increased payment allowance (above the payment for the same procedure in a patient weighing more than 4 kg) varies. Verify policies of individual health plans for reporting this modifier.

Examples

➤ **A 13-day-old weighing 2.4 kg requires peripheral cannulae insertion for extracorporeal membrane oxygenation (ECMO).** The physician reports

    33951 63   Extracorporeal membrane oxygenation (ECMO)/extracorporeal life support (ECLS) provided by physician; insertion of peripheral (arterial and/or venous) cannula(e), percutaneous, birth through 5 years of age (includes fluoroscopic guidance, when performed)

    Teaching Point: The patient weighed less than 4 kg, and the procedure is not listed as modifier **63** exempt. Therefore, modifier **63** is appropriately appended to indicate the increased intensity and/or work of performing the procedure on the neonate. Note that modifier **63** cannot be appended to codes for initiation or daily management of ECMO/ECLS (**33646–33949**).

➤ **An infant weighing 3 kg undergoes transventricular valvotomy of the pulmonary valve.** The physician reports

    33470   Valvotomy, pulmonary valve, closed heart; transventricular

    Teaching Point: The parenthetical instruction below code **33470** ("Do not report modifier **63** in conjunction with **33470**") prohibits reporting modifier **63**, including when this procedure is performed on an infant weighing less than 4 kg.

Chapter 19. Common Surgical Procedures and Sedation in Facility Settings

    ●=New code ▲=Revised code #=Re-sequenced code +=Add-on code

Physicians at Teaching Hospitals Guidelines for Billing Procedures

The CMS established and maintains guidelines for documentation and billing by teaching physicians. Physicians at Teaching Hospitals guidelines for billing procedures are less complex than those for billing E/M services. Guidelines specify that

- When a procedure is performed by a resident, teaching physician attendance and participation are required and must be documented. See examples of appropriate documentation in **Table 19-2**.
- The level of participation required by the teaching physician depends on the type of procedure being performed.
- A resident, nurse, or teaching physician may document the teaching physician's attendance.

The rules for supervising physicians in teaching settings can be obtained on the CMS website at http://cms.hhs.gov/manuals/downloads/clm104c12.pdf, section 100.

> Modifier **GC** (services have been performed by a resident under the direction of a teaching physician) must be appended to procedure codes for services performed by a resident under the direction of a teaching physician.

Minor Procedures

- The CMS defines a minor procedure as one taking *5 minutes or less* to complete with relatively little decision-making once the need for the procedure is determined.
- Minor procedures are usually assigned a 0- to 10-day global period.
- Teaching physicians may bill for a minor procedure when they personally perform the service or when a resident performs the service and they are present for the entire procedure.
- The resident may document the procedure but must attest to the teaching physician's presence.

Interpretation of Diagnostic Radiology and Other Diagnostic Tests

- The teaching physician may bill for interpretation of the diagnostic service if he or she interprets tests or reviews findings with the resident.

Table 19-2. Examples of Appropriate Documentation of Teaching Physician Presence	
Minor procedures	*"Dr Teaching Physician was present during the entire procedure."* —Nurse *"Dr Teaching Physician observed me performing this procedure."* —Dr Resident
Interpretation of diagnostic radiology and other diagnostic tests	*"I personally reviewed the MRI with Dr Resident and agree with his findings."* —Dr Teaching Physician *"I personally reviewed the CAT scan with Dr Resident. Findings are indicative of (insert)."* —Dr Teaching Physician
Endoscopy	*"I was present during the entire viewing of this endoscopy."* —Dr Teaching Physician
Surgery other than minor procedures	*"Dr Teaching Physician was present during entire surgery."* —Dr Resident *"I was present and observed Dr Resident perform the key portion of this procedure."* —Dr Teaching Physician
Complex or high-risk surgeries and procedures	*"I was physically present during this entire procedure with the exception of the [opening and/or closing], as that overlapped with the key portion of another case."* —Dr Teaching Physician *"Dr Y was immediately available during the overlapping portions of this case, which included [cite specifics]."* —Dr Teaching Physician
Abbreviations: CAT, computerized axial tomography; MRI, magnetic resonance imaging.	

- Documentation must support a personal interpretation or a review of the resident's notes with indication of agreement with the resident's interpretation.
- Changes to the resident's interpretation must be documented.

Endoscopy

- The teaching physician must be present for the entire viewing starting at the time of insertion and ending at the time of removal of the endoscope.
- Viewing the procedure through a monitor located in another room does not meet the requirements for billing.
- The presence of the teaching physician must be documented in the medical record. The teaching physician's presence must be stated.

Complex or High-risk Surgeries and Procedures

- A complex procedure or surgery (eg, cardiac catheterization), requires the direct or personal supervision of a physician as specified in Medicare or local policy or in the *CPT* description.
- A teaching physician must be present with a resident for the entire procedure when billing for a service identified by the CMS or local policy as complex and requiring personal supervision by a physician.
- Documentation must support that the teaching physician was present.

Surgery Other Than Minor, Complex, or High-risk Procedures

- The teaching physician must assume the responsibility of preoperative, operative, and postoperative care of the patient. He or she must be present during all critical and key portions (as determined by the teaching physician) of the procedure. For example, if opening or closing is not considered to be key or critical, the teaching physician does not need to be present.
- The teaching physician must be immediately available to furnish services during the entire procedure.
- If circumstances prevent the physician from being immediately available, arrangements must be made with another qualified surgeon to be immediately available to assist with the procedure.
- The physician's presence for single surgical procedures may be demonstrated in notes made by the teaching physician, resident, or nurse.
- When the teaching physician is present for the entire procedure, only the written attestation of his or her presence is required.
- If the teaching physician is present during only the key or critical portions of the surgery, documentation must indicate his or her presence at those portions of the procedure (the resident may still document the operative report).
- When billing for 2 overlapping (concurrent) surgeries, the teaching physician must be present for the key or critical portions of both procedures and must personally document his or her presence. The surgeon cannot be involved in a second case until all key or critical portions in the first case have been completed.
- Arrangements may be made with another qualified surgeon to be present at one of the surgeries. The name of the other surgeon who was immediately available during overlapping surgeries must be documented.

Postoperative Care

- The teaching physician determines which postoperative visits are considered key or critical and require his or her presence.
- If the teaching physician is not providing postoperative care included in the global surgery package, he or she will report the procedure(s) with modifiers **54** (surgical care only) and **56** (preoperative management only).
- Postoperative care is reported by another physician with the same surgical procedure code with modifier **55** (postoperative management only).
- The surgeon and physician providing postoperative care must keep a copy of a written transfer agreement in the patient's medical record.

Assistant Surgeon in a Teaching Facility

Medicare will not pay for the services of assistants at surgery furnished in a teaching hospital that has a training program related to the medical specialty required for the surgical procedure and has a qualified resident available to perform the service. This policy may be applied by Medicaid and other payers.

- When the MPFS allows payment for an assistant surgeon and a physician assists a teaching physician because no qualified resident was available, modifier **82** (assistant surgeon [when qualified resident surgeon not available]) is appended to the code for the procedure performed on the assistant surgeon's claim.
- The unavailability of a qualified resident surgeon is a prerequisite for use of modifier **82**. Documentation must specify that no qualified resident was available or that there was no residency program related to the medical specialty required for the surgical procedure.
- This modifier is only used in teaching hospitals and only if there is no approved training program related to the medical specialty required for the surgical procedure or no qualified resident was available.

Burn Care

CPT code **16000** (initial treatment, first-degree burn, where no more than local treatment is required) is reported when initial treatment is performed for the symptomatic relief of a first-degree burn that is characterized by erythema and tenderness.

16020	Dressings and/or debridement of partial-thickness burns, initial or subsequent; small or less than 5% total body (eg, finger)
16025	medium or 5%–10% total body surface area (eg, whole face or whole extremity)
16030	large or greater than 10% total body surface area (eg, more than 1 extremity)
16035	Escharotomy; initial incision
+16036	each additional incision

Codes **16020–16030**

- Are used to report treatment of burns with dressings and/or debridement of small to large partial-thickness burns (second degree), whether initial or subsequent.
- Are reported based on the percentage of total body surface area (TBSA) affected.
- The percentage of TBSA involved must be calculated and documented when reporting care of second- or third-degree burns.

    Pediatric physicians often use the Lund-Browder classification method for estimating the TBSA based on patient age. (The Lund-Browder diagram and classification method table are in *CPT 2021 Professional Edition*.)
- An E/M visit (critical care, emergency department [ED] services, inpatient or outpatient E/M) may be provided for evaluation of the patient's injuries and management of complications such as dehydration, shock, infection, multiple organ dysfunction syndrome, electrolyte imbalance, cardiac arrhythmias, and respiratory distress.

    Report the E/M code appropriate to the setting and care provided with modifier **25** appended to indicate the significant, separately identifiable E/M service is medically indicated, performed, and documented in addition to the burn care.
- Other services (eg, pulmonary testing/therapy, physical/occupational therapy) and procedures (eg, mechanical ventilation, central line placement and hyperalimentation, grafting, hyperbaric oxygenation, dialysis, tracheotomy, pacemaker insertion) should be additionally reported beyond that of local treatment of the burned surface reported by codes **16000–16036**.
- Codes **16020–16030** include dressing application (whether initial or subsequent) and any associated debridement or curettement.
- It is advisable to use *International Classification of Diseases, 10th Revision, Clinical Modification* (ICD-10-CM) category **T31**, burns classified according to extent of body surface involved, as an additional code for reporting purposes when there is mention of a third-degree burn involving 20% or more of the body surface.

Codes **16035** and **16036**

- Are reported per incision of eschar (dead tissue cast off from the surface of the skin in full-thickness burns).
- Are not reported based on anatomical site; report with 1 unit of code **16035** for the first incision only and 1 unit of code **16036** for each additional incision regardless of body area.

Surgical Preparation and Skin Grafting

15002	Surgical preparation or creation of recipient site by excision of open wounds, burn eschar, or scar (including subcutaneous tissues), or incisional release of scar contracture, trunk, arms, legs; first 100 sq cm or 1% of body area of infants and children
+15003	each additional 100 sq cm, or part thereof, or each additional 1% of body area of infants and children

15004   Surgical preparation or creation of recipient site by excision of open wounds, burn eschar, or scar (including subcutaneous tissues), or incisional release of scar contracture, face, scalp, eyelids, mouth, neck, ears, orbits, genitalia, hands, feet and/or multiple digits; first 100 sq cm or 1% of body area of infants and children

+15005   each additional 100 sq cm, or part thereof, or each additional 1% of body area of infants and children

- Surgical preparation codes **15002–15005** for skin replacement surgery describe removal of nonviable tissue to treat a burn, traumatic wound, or necrotizing infection.
  — Report codes **15002–15005** for preparation of a clean and viable wound surface for placement of an autograft, flap, or skin substitute graft or for negative pressure wound therapy (NPWT).

> An incisional release of scar contracture may also be used to create a clean wound bed.

  — Code selection for surgical preparation codes is based on the location and size of the defect.
  — Measurements apply to the recipient area. See measurements based on patient age in **Table 19-3**.

Table 19-3. Application of Skin Replacement Codes by Size of the Recipient Area

Adults and Children ≥10 y	Infants and Children <10 y
100 cm²	Each percentage of body surface area

  — Codes **15002–15005** are always preparation for healing by primary intention. Do not report codes **15002–15005** for chronic wounds left to heal by secondary intention.
  — Report the appropriate codes when closure is achieved by adjacent tissue transfer (codes **14000–14061**) or a complex repair (codes **13100–13153**) rather than skin grafts or substitutes.

Example

➤ **An 8-year-old patient undergoes surgical preparation for skin grafting of face, front of right arm, and right hand.** The body areas are measured as face, 4% of body area; right arm, 4%; and right hand, 1%.

ICD-10-CM	CPT
Appropriate codes for burns by depth and body area	**15004** (first 1% of body areas of face and hand) **15005** × 4 (each additional 1%) **15002 59** (first 1% body area of arm) **15003** × 3 (each additional 1%)

  Teaching Point: Because the face and hand are both included in the descriptor for codes **15004** and **15005**, the percentages of body areas are combined. Because the preparation of an area on the arm is described by codes **15002** and **15003**, the body area of the arm is not added to that of the face and hand. Modifier **59** indicates that the procedure reported with code **15002** was performed on distinct body areas not described by code **15004**.

- Codes **16020–16030** include the application of materials (eg, dressings) not described in codes **15100–15278** (skin grafts and substitutes). See skin graft code descriptors online at www.aap.org/cfp (access code AAPCFP26).
  — When burn wounds are treated and subsequently require skin grafting at the same session, report the burn code along with the appropriate skin graft code.
  — A skin graft procedure may be a staged procedure (delayed) with the preparation of the recipient site and the graft procedure being performed on different dates.
        In these cases, modifier **58** (staged procedure) is appended to the grafting procedure code performed during the global period.
  — The appropriate code for harvesting cultured skin autograft is **15040** (harvest of skin for tissue cultured skin autograft, 100 sq cm or less).
  — Debridement is considered a separate procedure only when
    ▪ Gross contamination requires prolonged cleansing.
    ▪ Appreciable amounts of devitalized or contaminated tissue are removed.
    ▪ Debridement is carried out separately without immediate primary closure.

— Measurements apply to the recipient area.
- For patient aged 10 years and older report 1 unit per 100 sq cm.
- Report 1 unit per 1% of body area of children 9 years and younger.
— Procedures involving the wrist and/or ankle are reported with codes that include "arm" or "leg" in the descriptor.
— The physician should select the skin substitute graft application code based on the actual size of the wound, after wound preparation has been performed, and not the amount of the skin graft substitute used.
— The party supplying skin substitute graft products reports HCPCS codes for the products.

Musculoskeletal Procedures

Fracture and Dislocation Care Codes

Codes for fracture/dislocation care
- Are listed by anatomical location.
- Are provided (in most cases) for closed or open treatment, with or without manipulation, and with or without internal fixation.
- Most include a 90-day period of follow-up care under the Medicare global package. Append modifier **57** (decision for surgery) to an E/M code when the decision for the procedure is made during a visit on the day before or day of the procedure.
- Include the initial casting, splinting, or strapping.
- Do not include radiographs.
- Routine follow-up visits during the global period are reported with no charge with code **99024** (post-op follow-up visit related to the original procedure).
- Append modifier **76** to the usual procedure number to indicate repeat procedure or service by the same physician or other QHP for re-reduction of a fracture and/or dislocation.

Example

➤ **A child is evaluated in the ED for an injury to the left elbow following a fall caused by overturning her bicycle on the sidewalk of her apartment complex.** An orthopedic surgeon is consulted to determine if the injury requires percutaneous fixation. The orthopedic surgeon evaluates the child and diagnoses a displaced supracondylar humerus fracture. A decision is made to proceed with closed reduction and pinning. The procedure takes place on the same date. The child is admitted to the hospital for postoperative monitoring and discharged to home the next day. The orthopedic surgeon provided consultation, procedure, and discharge-day E/M services.

ICD-10-CM	CPT
S42.412A (displaced simple supracondylar fracture without intercondylar fracture of left humerus, initial encounter for closed fracture) **V18.0XXA** (pedal cycle driver injured in noncollision transport accident in nontraffic accident, initial encounter) **Y92.480** (sidewalk as the place of occurrence of the external cause)	**99251–99255 57** (inpatient consultation) or, if the payer does not pay consultation codes, **99221–99223 57** (initial hospital care)
Same as previous	**24538** (percutaneous skeletal fixation of supracondylar or transcondylar humeral fracture, with or without intercondylar extension)

Teaching Point: Because code **24538** is assigned a 90-day global period in the MPFS, many payers may require modifier **57** (decision for surgery) appended to the E/M code reported for the same date of service. Individual payers may have different policies. The postoperative care in the hospital is not separately reported. Follow-up visits in the office should be reported with code **99024** (postoperative follow-up visit).

Osteotomy Humerus With Intramedullary Lengthening Device

A Category III (emerging technology) code became effective July 1, 2020, for osteotomy with insertion of an externally controlled lengthening device used in treatment of a limb length discrepancy. Note that these codes are not reported for insertion of an intramedullary rod in treatment of a fracture.

●**0594T**   Osteotomy, humerus, with insertion of an externally controlled intramedullary lengthening device, including intraoperative imaging, initial and subsequent alignment assessments, computations of adjustment schedules, and management of the intramedullary lengthening device

● Category III codes may not be covered by all health plans or may be covered under limited circumstances. Verify health plan coverage prior to providing these procedures.

● Do not report **0594T** in conjunction with application of multiplane, unilateral, external fixation with stereotactic computer-assisted adjustment (**20696**), osteotomy (**24400, 24410**), osteoplasty (**24420**), or treatment of humeral shaft fracture with insertion of intramedullary implant (**24516**).

● Revision of externally controlled intramedullary lengthening device is reported with unlisted procedure code **24999**.

Removal of Musculoskeletal Hardware

20665   Removal of tongs or halo applied by another individual

20670   Removal of implant; superficial (eg, buried wire, pin or rod) (separate procedure)

20680   deep (eg, buried wire, pin, screw, metal band, nail, rod or plate)

Removal of a halo or tongs is included in the placement procedure. However, removal of a halo or tongs by another physician is separately reported with code **20665**. (*Note:* Physicians of the same specialty and same group practice are typically considered as the same physician for billing purposes.)

Codes **20670** and **20680** may be reported for removal of orthopedic hardware. If it is necessary to remove an implant within the global period (eg, due to breakage), report the appropriate removal code with modifier **78** (unplanned return to the operating/procedure room by the same physician or other QHP following initial procedure for a related procedure during the postoperative period.)

Respiratory

Intubation and Airway Management

31500   Intubation, endotracheal, emergency

● Moderate sedation (**99151–99157**) may be reported in addition to the intubation if used to sedate the patient prior to and during the intubation procedure (eg, in rapid sequence intubation) and reporting criteria are met.

● See the Sedation section later in this chapter for more on moderate sedation.

31502   Tracheostomy tube change prior to establishment of fistula tract

Report code **31502** when an indwelling tracheostomy tube is replaced.

> Routine changing of a tracheostomy tube after a fistula tract has been established is included in a related evaluation and management service.

31505–31520 Indirect laryngoscopy

Report code **31505** for indirect diagnostic laryngoscopy. If, while performing this procedure, a foreign body is removed, report code **31511** (laryngoscopy with removal of foreign body).

31515   Direct laryngoscopy with or without tracheoscopy

Code **31515** is reported when laryngoscopy is performed for aspiration.

When diagnostic direct laryngoscopy, with or without tracheoscopy, is performed on a newborn, report code **31520**. Do not report modifier **63** (procedure performed on infant <4 kg) in conjunction with code **31520**.

31525   Laryngoscopy, direct, with or without tracheoscopy; diagnostic except newborn

Thoracostomy, Thoracentesis, and Pleural Drainage

32551	Tube thoracostomy, includes connection to drainage system (eg, water seal), when performed, open (separate procedure)
32554	Thoracentesis, needle or catheter, aspiration of the pleural space; without imaging guidance
32555	with imaging guidance
32556	Pleural drainage, percutaneous, with insertion of indwelling catheter; without imaging guidance
32557	with imaging guidance

- Thoracostomy (**32551**) represents an open procedure involving incision into a rib interspace with dissection extending through the chest wall muscles and pleura. Thoracentesis and percutaneous pleural drainage may be more commonly performed in pediatrics with the exception of neonatal and pediatric critical care.
- Percutaneous image guidance cannot be reported in conjunction with code **32551**, which represents an open procedure.
    Diagnostic ultrasound performed prior to thoracostomy to localize a collection in the pleural space is separately reportable only when the complete ultrasound study of the chest (**76604**) is performed with permanent recording of images.
- Thoracentesis codes **32554** and **32555** represent a procedure in which the surgical technique is puncture of the pleural space to remove fluid or air. Although a catheter (eg, pigtail catheter) may be used, it is not left in place at the end of the procedure.
- Percutaneous pleural drainage codes **32556** and **32557** represent procedures in which an indwelling catheter is inserted into the pleural space and remains at the end of the procedure. The catheter is secured in place and connected to a suction drainage system.
- Removal of chest tubes and non-tunneled indwelling pleural catheters is included in a related E/M service and not a separately reportable procedure.
- For insertion of a tunneled pleural catheter with cuff, see code **32550**. For removal of a tunneled pleural catheter with cuff, see **32552**.

Cardiovascular Procedures

Cardiac Catheterization

Cardiac catheterization includes introduction, positioning, and repositioning, when necessary, of catheter(s) within the vascular system; recording of intracardiac and/or intravascular pressure(s); and final evaluation and report of procedure.

Several procedures include heart catheterization when performed. Verify that multiple procedures are separately reportable per the prefatory and parenthetical instruction for these codes in your *CPT* coding reference. Explicit guidance regarding separately reportable diagnostic cardiac catheterization is provided for many procedures (eg, atrial septostomy).

Diagnostic heart catheterization in a patient without congenital anomaly is reported with the following codes:

93451	Right heart catheterization including measurement(s) of oxygen saturation and cardiac output, when performed
93452	Left heart catheterization including intraprocedural injection(s) for left ventriculography, imaging supervision and interpretation, when performed
93453	Combined right and left heart catheterization including intraprocedural injection(s) for left ventriculography, imaging supervision and interpretation, when performed

Catheterization for Congenital Anomalies

93530	Right heart catheterization, for congenital cardiac anomalies
93531	Combined right heart catheterization and retrograde left heart catheterization, for congenital cardiac anomalies
93532	Combined right heart catheterization and transseptal left heart catheterization through intact septum with or without retrograde left heart catheterization, for congenital cardiac anomalies
93533	Combined right heart catheterization and transseptal left heart catheterization through existing septal opening, with or without retrograde left heart catheterization, for congenital cardiac anomalies

It is important to note that codes **93530–93533** are reported *only when cardiac catheterization is performed for evaluation of congenital cardiac anomalies.*

- There is no age limit mentioned in the narrative description of codes **93530–93533**. As long as there is a congenital cardiac anomaly, it is appropriate to report these codes. These codes take into account

— The added technical difficulty presented when structures may be in abnormal positions and locations.
— Additional preservice time in reviewing noninvasive data, previous cardiac catheterizations, and previous surgeries.
— Procedures may be more time consuming due to small vessels, multiple measurements that must be made, instability of patients, frequency of multiple sites of arterial-venous admixture, and performance of other required interventions.
— Procedures such as percutaneous transcatheter closure of patent ductus arteriosus (**93582**) include right and left heart catheterization for congenital cardiac anomalies. Be sure to read the *CPT* instructions for procedures performed in conjunction with congenital cardiac catheterization to determine if the catheterization is separately reportable.

Pericardiocentesis and Pericardial Drainage

33016   Pericardiocentesis, including imaging guidance, when performed
33017   Pericardial drainage with insertion of indwelling catheter, percutaneous, including fluoroscopy and/or ultrasound guidance, when performed; 6 years and older without congenital cardiac anomaly
33018   birth through 5 years of age or any age with congenital cardiac anomaly
33019   Pericardial drainage with insertion of indwelling catheter, percutaneous, including CT guidance

● Codes **33016–33019** include imaging guidance when performed. Do not separately report imaging guidance (eg, **75989**, **76942**, **77002**, **77012**, **77021**) with codes **33016–33019**.
— For thoracoscopic (video assisted) pericardial procedures, see code **32601**, **32604**, **32658**, **32659**, or **32661**.
— For purposes of reporting percutaneous pericardial drainage with insertion of indwelling catheter, congenital cardiac anomaly is defined as
▪ Abnormal situs (heterotaxy, dextrocardia, mesocardia)
▪ Single ventricle anomaly/physiology
▪ Any patient in the first 90-day postoperative period after repair of a congenital cardiac anomaly defect
● Report **33017–33019** only when the catheter remains in place when the procedure is completed and not when a catheter is placed to aspirate fluid and then removed at the conclusion of the procedure.
● Do not separately report transthoracic, transesophageal, or Doppler echocardiography in addition to codes **33016–33018** when echocardiography is performed solely for the purpose of pericardiocentesis guidance.

Atrial Septostomy

●**33741**   Transcatheter atrial septostomy (TAS) for congenital cardiac anomalies to create effective atrial flow, including all imaging guidance by the proceduralist, when performed, any method (eg, Rashkind, Sang-Park, balloon, cutting balloon, blade)
●**33745**   Transcatheter intracardiac shunt (TIS) creation by stent placement for congenital cardiac anomalies to establish effective intracardiac flow, all imaging guidance by the proceduralist when performed, left and right heart diagnostic cardiac catherization for congenital cardiac anomalies, and target zone angioplasty, when performed (eg, atrial septum, Fontan fenestration, right ventricular outflow tract, Mustard/Senning/Warden baffles); initial intracardiac shunt
+●**33746**   each additional intracardiac shunt location (List separately in addition to code for primary procedure)

New codes **33741–33746** are used to report creation of effective intracardiac blood flow in the setting of congenital heart defects. Codes **92992** (atrial septectomy or septostomy; transvenous method, balloon) and **92993** (atrial septectomy/septostomy, blade method) have been deleted.

Code **33741**
● Involves the percutaneous creation of improved atrial blood flow (eg, balloon/blade method), typically in infants weighing 4 kg or less with congenital heart disease.
    Do not append modifier **63** (procedures performed on infants <4 kg) with **33741**.
● Includes percutaneous access, placing the access sheath(s), advancement of the transcatheter delivery system, and creation of effective intracardiac atrial blood flow.
    Ultrasound guidance for vascular access and fluoroscopic guidance for the intervention is included, when performed.
● Diagnostic cardiac catheterization is separately reported when performed at the same session as **33741**, but it is not typically performed at the same session. See instructions in *CPT* addressing when it is appropriate to separately report cardiac catheterization.
    Do not separately report cardiac catheterization that is fluoroscopic guidance for the intervention or limited hemodynamic and angiographic data used solely for purposes of accomplishing the intervention.

●=New code   ▲=Revised code   #=Re-sequenced code   +=Add-on code

Chapter 19. Common Surgical Procedures and Sedation in Facility Settings

- Use **93462** to report transseptal puncture performed in conjunction with **33741**.

  Codes **33745** and **33746**
- Include intracardiac stent placement, target zone angioplasty preceding or after stent implantation, and *complete diagnostic right and left heart catheterization* (not separately reported), when performed.
  - Ultrasound guidance for vascular access and fluoroscopic guidance for the intervention is included, when performed.
  - Includes any and all balloon angioplasties performed in the target lesion, including any pre-dilation or post-dilation following stent placement, or use of larger/smaller balloon to achieve therapeutic result.
  - Angioplasty in a separate and distinct intracardiac lesion may be reported separately with modifier **59** (distinct procedural service) appended to the angioplasty code.
- Cardiovascular injection procedures for diagnostic angiography (**93563**, **93565–93568**) are typically performed during **33745** and, *when performed for an evaluation separate and distinct from the shunt creation,* may be reported separately.

  Append modifier **59** to codes for diagnostic angiography performed at the same session for angiographic evaluation separate and distinct from the shunt creation.
- When additional, different intracardiac locations are treated in the same session, code **33746** may be reported for each additional intracardiac shunt creation by stent placement at a separate location.

> Multiple stents placed in a single location may only be reported with a single code and not a first or additional unit of 33746.

Aortic Valve Replacement

#33440   Replacement, aortic valve; by translocation of autologous pulmonary valve and transventricular aortic annulus enlargement of the left ventricular outflow tract with valved conduit replacement of pulmonary valve (Ross-Konno procedure)

33411   with aortic annulus enlargement, noncoronary sinus

33412   with transventricular aortic annulus enlargement (Konno procedure)

33413   by translocation of autologous pulmonary valve with allograft replacement of pulmonary valve (Ross procedure)

Code **33440** allows for reporting aortic valve replacement by translocation of the autologous pulmonary valve and transventricular aortic annulus enlargement of the left ventricular outflow tract with valved conduit replacement of pulmonary valve (combined Ross-Konno procedure).

- Do not report separate codes for the Konno procedure (**33412**) and Ross procedure (**33413**) performed at the same session in lieu of code **33440**.
- See the parenthetical instruction following code **33440** in your *CPT* coding reference for other procedures not separately reported in conjunction with code **33440**.

Example

➤ **A 4-year-old established patient undergoes autologous pulmonary valve replacement of the aortic valve and a Konno aortoventriculoplasty to correct a mixed aortic valvular stenosis with regurgitation and multilevel ventricular outflow obstruction.**

ICD-10-CM	CPT
Q23.0 (congenital stenosis of aortic valve)	**#33440**

Teaching Point: A single code, **33440**, is reported for the combined Ross-Konno procedure. It would be inappropriate to separately report these procedures or other aortic valve, aortic root, pulmonary valve, or ventricular reconstruction procedures.

Valvuloplasty

33390   Valvuloplasty, aortic valve, open, with cardiopulmonary bypass; simple (ie, valvotomy, debridement, debulking, and/or simple commissural resuspension)

33391   complex (eg, leaflet extension, leaflet resection, leaflet reconstruction, or annuloplasty)

Do not report code **33391** in conjunction with code **33390**.

●=New code   ▲=Revised code   #=Re-sequenced code   +=Add-on code

Codes for open valvuloplasty of the aortic valve

- Are descriptive of currently performed valvuloplasty procedures
  — Code **33390** is specifically for reporting valvotomy, debridement, debulking, and/or simple commissural resuspension.
  — Code **33391** represents more complex procedures not limited to the examples in the code descriptor.
- May be reported in conjunction with the code for transmyocardial revascularization (**33141**), operative tissue ablation and reconstruction of atria (**33255–33259**), and reoperation, valve procedure, more than 1 month after original operation (**33530**), when appropriate

Open procedures for aortic valve replacement are reported with codes **33405**, **33406**, and **33410** based on the type of replacement valve (ie, prosthetic, homograft, or stentless).

Transcatheter Pulmonary Valve Implantation

33477   Transcatheter pulmonary valve implantation, percutaneous approach, including pre-stenting of the valve delivery site, when performed

The key instructions for reporting code **33477** are

- Should only be reported once per session
- Includes, when performed
  — Percutaneous access, placing the access sheath, advancing the repair device delivery system into position, repositioning the device as needed and deploying the device(s), angiography, all cardiac catheterization(s) for hemodynamic measurements, intraprocedural contrast injections, radiologic supervision, and interpretation performed to guide transcatheter pulmonary valve implantation
  — Percutaneous balloon angioplasty of the conduit or treatment zone, valvuloplasty of the pulmonary valve conduit, and stent deployment within the pulmonary conduit or an existing bioprosthetic pulmonary valve
- **Does not include** (Report separately, when performed.)
  — Codes **92997** and **92998** when pulmonary artery angioplasty is performed at a site separate from the prosthetic valve delivery site
  — Codes **37236** and **37237** when pulmonary artery stenting is performed at a site separate from the prosthetic valve delivery site
  — Same-session/same-day *diagnostic* cardiac catheterization services (See your *CPT* reference for further instruction and append catheterization code with modifier **59**.)
  — Diagnostic coronary angiography performed at a separate session from an interventional procedure
  — Percutaneous coronary interventional procedures
  — Percutaneous pulmonary artery branch interventions
  — Percutaneous ventricular assist device procedure codes (**33990–33993**), ECMO/ECLS procedure codes (**33946–33989**), or balloon pump insertion codes (**33967**, **33970**, **33973**)
  — Percutaneous peripheral bypass (**33367**), open peripheral bypass (**33368**), or central bypass (**33369**)

Percutaneous Transcatheter Closure of Patent Ductus Arteriosus

93582   Percutaneous transcatheter closure of patent ductus arteriosus

- Includes, when performed
  — Introduction of catheter, right heart or main pulmonary artery (**36013**)
  — Selective catheter placement, left or right pulmonary artery (**36014**)
  — Introduction of catheter, aorta (**36200**)
  — Aortography, thoracic, without serialography, radiological supervision and interpretation (**75600**)
  — Aortography, thoracic, by serialography, radiological supervision and interpretation (**75605**)
  — Heart catheterization or catheter placement for coronary angiography (**93451–94361**)
  — Heart catheterization for congenital cardiac anomalies (**93530–93533**)
  — Injection procedure during cardiac catheterization including imaging supervision, interpretation, and report; for supravalvular aortography (**93567**)
- Separately report
  — Left heart catheterization by transseptal puncture through intact septum or by transapical puncture (**93462**)
  — Add-on codes for injection procedures during cardiac catheterization, including imaging supervision, interpretation, and report, for
    ▪ Selective coronary angiography during congenital heart catheterization (**93563**)

●=New code   ▲=Revised code   #=Re-sequenced code   +=Add-on code

- Selective opacification of aortocoronary venous or arterial bypass graft(s) to one or more coronary arteries and in situ arterial conduits, whether native or used for bypass to one or more coronary arteries during congenital heart catheterization, when performed (**93564**)
- Selective left ventricular or left atrial angiography (**93565**)
- Selective right ventricular or right atrial angiography (**93566**)
- Pulmonary angiography (**93568**)

Vascular Access

Many vascular access procedures are included in the services reported with critical or intensive care codes. Please see **Chapter 18** for a list of procedures that are not separately reported by a physician or QHP who is reporting critical care services on the same date.

Central Venous Access

There is no distinction between venous access achieved percutaneously or via cutdown. Report the venous access code (**tables 19-4** and **19-5**) appropriate to the

- Type of insertion (ie, centrally inserted or peripherally inserted).
- Type of catheter (eg, non-tunneled vs tunneled).
- Device (eg, with or without port).
- Age of child.
- In non-facility settings, code **96522** may be reported for refilling and maintenance of an implantable pump or reservoir for systemic (intravenous, intra-arterial) drug delivery.
- Irrigation of an implanted venous access device for drug delivery (**96523**) is only reported in non-facility settings and when no other service is reported by the same individual on the same date.
- Codes for refilling and maintenance and/or irrigation are not reported by physicians in facility settings.

> If an existing central venous access device is removed and a new one *placed via a separate venous access site,* appropriate codes for both procedures (removal of old, if code exists, and insertion of new device) should be reported. See replacement codes for removal with replacement *via the same venous access site.*

Insertion or Replacement of Centrally Inserted Central Venous Access Device

- To qualify as a centrally inserted central venous access device, both of the following must be true:
  - The entry site must be the *jugular, subclavian, or femoral vein or the inferior vena cava.*
  - The tip of the catheter must terminate in the *subclavian, brachiocephalic (innominate), or iliac veins; the superior or inferior vena cava; or the right atrium.*
- Moderate sedation services are separately reportable with codes **99151–99157.** For more information on reporting moderate sedation, see the Sedation section later in this chapter.
- Report imaging guidance for gaining access to venous entry site or manipulating the catheter into final central position (in addition to codes **36555–36558**) with either of the following codes:
  - **76937** (ultrasound guidance for vascular access requiring ultrasound evaluation of potential access sites, documentation of selected vessel patency, concurrent real-time ultrasound visualization of vascular needle entry, with permanent recording and reporting)
  - **77001** (fluoroscopic guidance for central venous access device placement, replacement [catheter only or complete], or removal [includes fluoroscopic guidance for vascular access and catheter manipulation, any necessary contrast injections through access site or catheter with related venography radiologic supervision and interpretation, and radiographic documentation of final catheter position])
- Documentation of ultrasound guidance for peripherally inserted central catheter (PICC) placement should include evaluation of the potential puncture sites, patency of the entry vein, and real-time ultrasound visualization of needle entry into the vein.
- *Do not separately report ultrasound for vessel identification only.*

Insertion of Peripherally Inserted Central Venous Access Device

Midline catheters terminate in the peripheral venous system. Midline catheter insertion is not reported as a peripherally inserted central venous catheter insertion. See codes **36400**, **36406**, and **36410** for midline catheter insertion.

Table 19-4. Insertion and Replacement of Central Venous Catheter

Insertion	Child <5 y	Child ≥5 y
Insertion non-tunneled centrally inserted central venous catheter	36555	36556
Insertion tunneled centrally inserted central venous catheter, without subcutaneous port or pump	36557	36558
Insertion tunneled centrally inserted central venous access device, with subcutaneous port	36560	36561
Insertion	**Any Age**	
Insertion tunneled centrally inserted central venous access device with subcutaneous pump	36563	
Insertion of tunneled centrally inserted central venous access device, requiring 2 catheters via 2 separate venous access sites; without subcutaneous port or pump (eg, Tesio-type catheter)	36565	
Insertion of tunneled centrally inserted central venous access device, requiring 2 catheters via 2 separate venous access sites; with subcutaneous port(s)	36566	
Replacement		
Replacement, *catheter only,* of central venous access device, with subcutaneous port or pump, central or peripheral insertion site	36578	
Replacement, *complete,* of a non-tunneled centrally inserted central venous catheter, without subcutaneous port or pump, through same venous access	36580	
Replacement, *complete,* of a tunneled centrally inserted central venous catheter, without subcutaneous port or pump, through same venous access	36581	
Replacement, *complete,* of a tunneled centrally inserted central venous access device, with subcutaneous port, through same venous access	36582	
Replacement, *complete,* of a tunneled centrally inserted central venous access device, with subcutaneous pump, through same venous access	36583	

Table 19-5. Insertion or Replacement of Peripherally Inserted Central Venous Catheter

Insertion Procedure	Child <5 y	Child ≥5 y
Insertion of peripherally inserted central venous catheter, without subcutaneous port or pump, *without imaging guidance*	36568	36569
Insertion of peripherally inserted central venous access device, with subcutaneous port	36570	36571
Insertion of peripherally inserted central venous catheter, without subcutaneous port or pump, including all imaging guidance, image documentation, and all associated radiological supervision and interpretation required to perform the insertion	#36572	#36573
Replacement Procedure	**Any Age**	
Replacement, catheter only, of central venous access device, with subcutaneous port or pump, central or peripheral insertion site	36578	
Replacement, complete, of a peripherally inserted central venous catheter, without subcutaneous port or pump, through same venous access, including all imaging guidance, image documentation, and all associated radiological supervision and interpretation required to perform the replacement	36584	
Replacement, complete, of a peripherally inserted central venous access device, with subcutaneous port, through same venous access	36585	

CPT copyright 2020 American Medical Association. All rights reserved.   ●=New code   ▲=Revised code   #=Re-sequenced code   +=Add-on code

- To qualify as a PICC, both of the following must be true:
  — The entry site must be a peripheral vein (eg, axillary, basilic, or cephalic).
  — The tip of the catheter must terminate in the subclavian, brachiocephalic (innominate), or iliac veins; the superior or inferior vena cava; or the right atrium.
- Codes **36568** and **36569** are reported for PICC insertion without a subcutaneous port *and without imaging guidance* based on the patient's age.
    Do not report imaging guidance (**76937**, **77001**) in conjunction with codes **36568** and **36569**.
- If imaging guidance is used in PICC insertion, see codes **36572**, **36573**, and **36584**. Imaging guidance is included in the placement (**36572**, **36573**) or complete replacement (**36584**) of a PICC without subcutaneous port or pump.
- Using magnetic guidance or any other guidance modality that does not include imaging or image documentation for insertion of a PICC is reported with codes **36568** and **36569**.
- Chest radiographs (**71045–71048**) should not be reported for the purpose of documenting the final catheter position by the same physician on the same day of service as the PICC insertion (**36572**, **36573**, or **36584**).
    If PICC insertion is performed without confirmation of the catheter tip location, append modifier **52** (reduced service) to the code for catheter insertion (**36572**, **36573**, or **36584**).
- Documentation of services includes
  — Images from all modalities used (eg, ultrasound, fluoroscopy) stored to the patient record
  — Associated supervision and interpretation
  — Venography performed through the same venous puncture
  — The final central position of the catheter with imaging
- Report PICC insertion *with a subcutaneous port* with codes **36570** and **36571**.
  — Ultrasound (**76937**) or fluoroscopic guidance (**77001**) may be separately reported when performed and documented.
  — Documentation of ultrasound guidance for PICC placement should include evaluation of the potential puncture sites, patency of the entry vein, and real-time ultrasound visualization of needle entry into the vein.

Repair of Central Venous Catheters

36575   Repair of tunneled or non-tunneled central venous access catheter, without subcutaneous port or pump, central or peripheral insertion site

36576   Repair of central venous access device, with subcutaneous port or pump, central or peripheral insertion site

36593   Declotting by thrombolytic agent of implanted vascular access device or catheter

36595   Mechanical removal of pericatheter obstructive material (eg, fibrin sheath) from central venous device via separate venous access

> For radiologic supervision and interpretation of mechanical removal of pericatheter obstructive material from a central venous device via separate venous access, report **75901**.

36596   Mechanical removal of intraluminal (intracatheter) obstructive material from central venous device through device lumen

36598   Contrast injection(s) for radiologic evaluation of existing central venous access device, including fluoroscopy, image documentation and report

  Repair of a central venous catheter includes fixing the device without replacement of the catheter or port/pump.
- For the repair of a multi-catheter device, with or without subcutaneous ports or pumps, use the appropriate code describing the service with 2 units of service.
- Repair of any central venous access catheter *without a port or pump* is reported with code **36575**.
- Repair of any central venous catheter *with a port or pump* is reported with code **36576**.
- Code **36593** is reported for declotting of an implanted vascular device or catheter *by thrombolysis.*
- Code **36593** *is not reported* for declotting of a pleural catheter. Use unlisted procedure code **32999** for declotting of a pleural catheter.
- Code **36595** and **36596** are reported for a procedure with *mechanical removal* of pericatheter or intraluminal obstructive material.
  — Radiologic supervision and interpretation is separately reported with code **75901**.
  — Do not report code **36595** or **36596** in conjunction with code **36593** or **36598**.

- When the patency of a central line is evaluated under fluoroscopy, code **36598** is reported for the contrast injection, image documentation, and report.
  — Fluoroscopy (**76000**) is not separately reported.
  — See codes **75820–75827** for complete venography studies.

Removal of Central Venous Catheters

36589   Removal of tunneled central venous catheter, without subcutaneous port or pump

36590   Removal of tunneled central venous access device, with subcutaneous port or pump, central or peripheral insertion

Removal codes are reported for removal of the entire device. See replacement codes for partial replacement (catheter only) or complete exchange *in the same venous access site* of central venous access devices.

- For removal of both catheters (placed from separate venous access sites) of a multi-catheter device, with or without subcutaneous ports/pumps, use the appropriate code describing the service with 2 units of service.
- When removal of an existing central venous access device is performed in conjunction with placement of new device *via a separate venous access site,* report both procedures.

Arterial Access

36600   Arterial puncture, withdrawal of blood for diagnosis

36620   Arterial catheterization or cannulation for sampling, monitoring or transfusion (separate procedure); percutaneous

36625   cutdown

- An arterial puncture for diagnosis is reported with code **36600**.
- Code **36620** is reported when a percutaneous peripheral arterial catheterization is performed. Code **36625** is reported when a cutdown is performed.

Transfusions

36430   Transfusion, blood or blood components

36440   Push transfusion; blood, 2 years or younger

36450   Exchange transfusion, blood, newborn

36455   other than newborn

36456   Partial exchange transfusion, blood, plasma, or crystalloid necessitating the skill of a physician or other qualified health care professional; newborn

> The placement of catheters to support exchange transfusions may be reported separately with the appropriate vascular access codes.

- Indirect transfusion of blood or blood products (**36430**) should be used only if the physician personally infuses the substance, and not if the blood is administered by nursing personnel and allowed to enter the vessel via gravity or meter flow.
  — Push transfusion (**36440**) is used only for patients younger than 2 years. This code should be used only if the physician personally performs the transfusion.
  — Codes **36430** and **36440** are not separately reported when the same physician or physicians of the same specialty and same group practice are reporting neonatal or pediatric critical care (**99468–99472**, **99475**, **99476**).
- Complete exchange transfusions (double volume) performed during the neonatal period are reported using code **36450**; exchange transfusions for all other age groups are reported using code **36455**.
  — The assumption is that the exchange for the neonate is performed via the umbilical vein, while an exchange for an older child or adult is performed via a peripheral vessel.
  — The actual placement of catheters to support the exchange transfusion may be reported separately with the appropriate vascular access codes.
- Partial exchange transfusions (eg, for hyperviscosity syndrome in the neonate) should be reported using code **36456**.
- Do not report other transfusion codes (**36430**, **36440**, or **36450**) with **36456**.
- Do not append modifier **63** (procedure performed on infants <4 kg) when reporting code **36450** or **36456**.

●=New code   ▲=Revised code   #=Re-sequenced code   +=Add-on code

Hydration, Intravenous Infusions

> See Chapter 10 for more information on coding for hydration and intravenous infusion services.

These codes *are not reported by a physician or other QHP when performed in a facility setting* because the physician work associated with these procedures involves only affirmation of the treatment plan and direct supervision of the staff performing the services. These codes may be reported by the facility.

Ear, Nose, and Throat Procedures

69421   Myringotomy including aspiration and/or eustachian tube inflation requiring general anesthesia

69436   Tympanostomy (requiring insertion of ventilating tube), general anesthesia

- For bilateral procedure, report code **69436** with modifier **50**.
- Insertion of ventilation tube(s) is not separately reported when performed in conjunction with another middle ear procedure (eg, tympanoplasty) without significant increase in work.
- Cleaning debris from the lateral drum, including a pars flaccida retraction pocket, is inclusive to the tube placement code.
- Use of an operating microscope is included in the procedure described by **69436**.

92511   Nasopharyngoscopy with endoscope (separate procedure)

   Code **92511** is designated as a "separate procedure" and should not be reported in addition to the code for the total procedure or service of which it is considered an integral component.
- When carried out independently, report code **92511**.
- When considered to be unrelated or distinct from other procedures or services provided at that time, report code **92511 59** in addition to other procedures or services.

Laryngoplasty

#31551   Laryngoplasty; for laryngeal stenosis, with graft, without indwelling stent placement, younger than 12 years of age

#31552   age 12 years or older

#31553   Laryngoplasty; for laryngeal stenosis, with graft, with indwelling stent placement, younger than 12 years of age

#31554   age 12 years or older

31580   Laryngoplasty; for laryngeal web, with indwelling keel or stent insertion

31584   Laryngoplasty; with open reduction and fixation of (eg, plating) fracture, includes tracheostomy, if performed

- Do not report graft separately if harvested through the laryngoplasty incision (eg, thyroid cartilage graft).
- Report only one of the following codes for a single operative session: **31551–31554** or **31580**.
- Codes for treatment of laryngeal stenosis by laryngoplasty with graft are selected based on whether or not the procedure includes indwelling stent placement and by the age of the patient (<12 years or ≥12 years) (**Table 19-6**).

Table 19-6. Laryngoplasty for Laryngeal Stenosis Codes by Patient Age		
Laryngoplasty; for laryngeal stenosis, with graft,	**Patient <12 y**	**Patient ≥12 y**
without indwelling stent placement	31551	31552
with indwelling stent placement	31553	31554

- Open treatment of a hyoid fracture is reported with code **31584** (repair procedure on the larynx).
- To report tracheostomy, see code **31600**, **31601**, **31603**, **31605**, or **31610**.
- Report laryngoplasty, not otherwise specified or for removal of a keel or stent, with code **31599**.

Adenoidectomy and Tonsillectomy

42820	Tonsillectomy and adenoidectomy; younger than age 12
42821	age 12 or over
42825	Tonsillectomy, primary or secondary; younger than age 12
42826	age 12 or over
42830	Adenoidectomy, primary; younger than age 12
42831	age 12 or over
42835	Adenoidectomy, secondary; younger than age 12
42836	age 12 or over

For partial ablation of tonsils with laser, report the appropriate code from **42820** or **42821**, or **42825** or **42826**, with modifier **52** (reduced service).

For control of hemorrhage following tonsillectomy or adenoidectomy, see codes **42960–42972**.

Digestive System Procedures

Gastric Intubation and Aspiration

43752	Naso- or orogastric tube placement, requiring physician's skill and fluoroscopic guidance (includes fluoroscopy, image documentation and report)
43753	Gastric intubation and aspiration(s), therapeutic (eg, for ingested poisons), including lavage if performed

Do not report code **43752** or **43753** in conjunction with

- Critical care codes (**99291, 99292**)
- Neonatal critical care codes (**99468, 99469**)
- Pediatric critical care codes (**99471–99476**)
- Pediatric intensive care service codes (**99477–99480**)

Note that code **43752** is reported when a physician's skill is required for placement of a nasogastric or orogastric tube using fluoroscopic guidance.

- This service is not separately reported when a physician's skill is not required or placement is performed without fluoroscopic guidance.
- Replacement of a nasogastric tube requiring physician's skill and fluoroscopic guidance may also be reported with code **43752**.

Examples

➤ **A 10-year-old is brought to the ED after having ingested drugs.** Gastric intubation and lavage are performed.
Code **43753** would be reported in addition to the appropriate E/M service (eg, ED services **99281–99285**). Code **43753** is not separately reported when performed in conjunction with critical care (eg, **99291, 99292; 99468–99476**) or by a physician during pediatric patient transport (**99466, 99467**).

➤ **A patient requires placement of a nasogastric tube.** Attempts by nursing staff are unsuccessful, so placement by the physician is required. The physician places the tube using fluoroscopic guidance.
Code **43752** would be reported in addition to the appropriate E/M service but is not reported when the service is performed by the physician out of convenience rather than necessity for a physician's skill. Use of fluoroscopic guidance is required and must be documented (ie, image documentation and report).

Gastrostomy Tube Replacement

43762	Replacement of gastrostomy tube, percutaneous, includes removal, when performed, without imaging or endoscopic guidance; not requiring revision of gastrostomy tract
43763	requiring revision of gastrostomy tract

- Codes **43762** and **43763** are used to report gastrostomy tube change without imaging or endoscopic guidance.

    Codes **43762** and **43763** include the gastrostomy tube kit.
- See code **49450** for replacement of gastrostomy tube with fluoroscopic guidance.

●=New code   ▲=Revised code   #=Re-sequenced code   +=Add-on code

- See code **43246** for placement with endoscopic guidance
- A significant, separately identifiable E/M service on the same date may be reported with modifier **25** appended to the E/M code (eg, **99213 25**). An E/M service should not be reported when the encounter is solely for replacement of the gastrostomy tube.

Enterostomy/Cecostomy With Colonic Lavage

44300   Placement, enterostomy or cecostomy, tube open (eg, for feeding or decompression) (separate procedure)

     (Do not report **44300** in conjunction with **44701** for cannulation of the colon for intraoperative colonic lavage)

     (For percutaneous placement of duodenostomy, jejunostomy, gastro-jejunostomy or cecostomy [or other colonic] tube including fluoroscopic imaging guidance, see **49441–49442**)

+44701   Intraoperative colonic lavage (List separately in addition to code for primary procedure)

     (Use **44701** in conjunction with **44140**, **44145**, **44150**, or **44604** as appropriate)

     (Do not report **44701** in conjunction with **44950–44960**)

Report code **44300** for enterostomy or cecostomy tube placement except when tube placement is for intraoperative colonic lavage.

Codes **44300** and **44701** may be separately reported except in instances when the tube placement is for intraoperative colonic lavage.

Appendectomy

44950   Appendectomy
+44955   when done for indicated purpose at time of other major procedure
44960   for ruptured appendix with abscess or generalized peritonitis
44970   Laparoscopy, surgical, appendectomy
44979   Unlisted laparoscopy procedure, appendix

Appendectomy is one of the most common procedures in pediatrics. As a sole procedure, appendectomy coding is fairly straightforward, with 3 code choices: **44950**, **44960**, and **44970**.

CPT instructs that incidental appendectomy (ie, not due to disease or symptom) during intra-abdominal surgery does not usually warrant reporting a code for the appendectomy procedure.

- If it is necessary to report an incidental appendectomy performed during another intra-abdominal procedure, append modifier **52** (reduced service).
- The Medicaid NCCI manual also instructs that incidental removal of a normal appendix during another abdominal surgery is not separately reportable. This instruction is likely followed by other payers.

Appendectomy performed for an indicated purpose (ie, problem with the appendix) in conjunction with another procedure is separately reported.

- Report add-on code **44955** in addition the code for the primary procedure when open appendectomy is performed (due to clinical indication) in conjunction with another procedure.
- Code **44979** must be reported for a laparoscopic appendectomy when done for an indicated purpose at the time of another major procedure.
- A separate diagnosis code (distinct from the diagnoses for which other intra-abdominal procedures were performed) should be linked to the appendectomy procedure code to indicate the medical necessity of the procedure.

Hernia Repair

49491   Repair, initial inguinal hernia, preterm infant (younger than 37 weeks gestation at birth), performed from birth up to 50 weeks postconception age, with or without hydrocelectomy; reducible
49492   incarcerated or strangulated
49495   Repair, initial inguinal hernia, full term infant younger than age 6 months, or preterm infant older than 50 weeks postconception age and younger than age 6 months at the time of surgery, with or without hydrocelectomy; reducible
49496   incarcerated or strangulated
49500   Repair initial inguinal hernia, age 6 months to younger than 5 years, with or without hydrocelectomy; reducible
49501   incarcerated or strangulated

Chapter 19. Common Surgical Procedures and Sedation in Facility Settings

49505	Repair initial inguinal hernia, age 5 years or older; reducible
49507	incarcerated or strangulated
49520	Repair recurrent inguinal hernia, any age; reducible
49521	incarcerated or strangulated

- For purposes of reporting inguinal hernia repair, postconception age equals gestational age at birth plus age of newborn/infant in weeks at the time of the hernia repair.
- Initial inguinal hernia repair performed on preterm newborns and infants who are older than 50 weeks' postconception age and younger than 6 months at the time of surgery should be reported using codes **49495** and **49496**.
- **Table 19-7** includes criteria for determining initial hernia repair codes by patient birth status, age, and hernia status.

Table 19-7. Code Selection Initial Hernia Repair in Infants

Patient Status	Hernia Reducible	Hernia Incarcerated or Strangulated
Preterm, <37 weeks gestation at birth, performed from birth up to 50 weeks postconception age	49491	49492
Term infant age <6 months, or preterm infant >50 weeks postconception age and <6 months at the time of surgery	49495	49496

- Modifier **63** (procedure performed on infants <4 kg) is not appended to code **49491**, **49492**, **49495**, or **49496**.
- Separately report inguinal hernia repair (**49495–49525**) performed in conjunction with inguinal orchiopexy (**54640**).

Genitourinary System Procedures

Anogenital Examination

| 99170 | Anogenital examination, magnified, in childhood for suspected trauma including image recording when performed |

Moderate sedation may be separately reported when performed by the same physician performing the anogenital examination. Moderate sedation service of less than 10 minutes of intraservice time is not separately reported.

Example

➤ **A 6-year-old girl is brought to the ED by her mother after the mother noted blood in the child's underpants and was concerned about sexual molestation.** The physician performs a comprehensive history and physical examination. Because of the findings on general examination, the physician elects to further examine the child's genitalia with magnification to document findings that may be consistent with abuse or trauma.

ICD-10-CM	CPT

Report confirmed abuse with all of the following:
T74.22XA (child sexual abuse, confirmed, initial encounter)
An appropriate injury code (eg, **S39.848A**, other specified injuries of external genitals, initial encounter)
A code from categories **X92–Y06** or **Y08** for assault
A code from category **Y07** to identify the perpetrator of assault
 	
    If abuse is suspected but not confirmed, report **T76.22XA** (child sexual abuse, suspected, initial encounter) and a code for injury.
 	
    If there are no findings, report **Z04.42** (encounter for examination and observation following alleged child rape or sexual abuse).
	99285 (comprehensive ED examination)
	99170 (anogenital examination)
	If the same physician performs moderate (conscious) sedation, also report code **99152**. See more on moderate sedation in the Sedation section later in this chapter.

●=New code   ▲=Revised code   #=Re-sequenced code   +=Add-on code

Chapter 19. Common Surgical Procedures and Sedation in Facility Settings

Lysis/Excision of Labial or Penile Adhesions

54162   Lysis or excision of penile post-circumcision adhesions

56441   Lysis of labial adhesions

Lysis of labial or penile adhesions performed by the application of manual pressure without the use of an instrument to cut the adhesions is considered part of the E/M visit and not reported separately.

Code **54162** is only reported when lysis is performed under general anesthesia or regional block, with an instrument, and under sterile conditions.

- This code has a 2020 total relative value of 5.79 when performed in a facility setting and a Medicare 10-day global surgery period, which payers may or may not use.
- If post-circumcision adhesions are manually broken during the postoperative period by the physician or physician of the same group and specialty who performed the procedure, it would be considered part of the global surgical package.

> **A code for repair (eg, 13131, repair, complex, forehead, cheeks, chin, mouth, neck, axillae, genitalia, hands and/or feet; 1.1 cm to 2.5 cm) is not reported in addition to code 54162 for the repair performed in conjunction with lysis or excision of penile post-circumcision adhesions.**

- Report the service with *ICD-10-CM* code **N47.0**, adherent prepuce in a newborn, or **N47.5**, adhesions of prepuce and glans penis (patients older than 28 days).
- For repair of incomplete circumcision with removal of excessive residual foreskin, see code **54163**.

Code **56441** is performed by using a blunt instrument or scissors under general or local anesthesia.

- The 2020 total relative value units for this procedure in a facility setting are 4.24.
- Code **56441** includes a Medicare 10-day global surgery period, which may or may not be used by payers.
- *ICD-10-CM* code **Q52.5** (fusion of labia) would be reported with *CPT* code **56441**.
- When provided without anesthesia, modifier **52** may be appended to indicate reduced services. Payer guidance may vary with regard to use of modifier **52**.

Repair of Penis

Correction of Chordee and Hypospadias

54300   Plastic operation of penis for straightening of chordee (eg, hypospadias), with or without mobilization of urethra

54304   Plastic operation on penis for correction of chordee or for first stage hypospadias repair with or without transplantation of prepuce and/or skin flaps

Code **54300** is appropriately reported for straightening of the chordee to correct congenital concealed penis (**Q55.64**). This procedure may also be performed to correct an entrapped penis after newborn circumcision (eg, release of concealed penis with coverage of deficient penile ventral skin using penile skin-raised Byars flaps and re-circumcision).

Codes **54304–54336** describe procedures performed to correct hypospadias in either single-stage or multiple-stage procedures.

- Do not separately report codes **54300**, **54304**, or **54360** (plastic operation on penis to correct angulation) when reporting single-stage repair of hypospadias.

Correction of penile chordee or penile curvature is included in all single-stage repairs of hypospadias.

- For more detailed information on reporting procedures to repair hypospadias, see the American Urological Association policy and advocacy brief, "Pediatric Hypospadias Repair: A New Consensus Document on Coding," at www.auanet.org/Documents/practices-resources/coding-tips/Pediatric-Hypospadias-Repair.pdf.

Negative Pressure Wound Therapy

97605   Negative pressure wound therapy (eg, vacuum assisted drainage collection), utilizing durable medical equipment (DME), including topical application(s), wound assessment, and instruction(s) for ongoing care, per session; total wound(s) surface area less than or equal to 50 square centimeters

97606   total wound(s) surface area greater than 50 square centimeters

97607   Negative pressure wound therapy (eg, vacuum assisted drainage collection), utilizing disposable, non-durable medical equipment including provision of exudate management collection system, topical application(s), wound assessment, and instructions for ongoing care, per session; total wound(s) surface area less than or equal to 50 square centimeters

97608   total wound(s) surface area greater than 50 square centimeters

●=New code   ▲=Revised code   #=Re-sequenced code   +=Add-on code

It has become common in recent years for physicians to include use of NPWT or vacuum-assisted closure in the management of traumatic and surgical wounds.

Negative pressure wound therapy
- Requires direct (one-on-one) physician or QHP contact with the patient.
- May be initiated in a hospital or surgical center setting and continued in the home setting after discharge.
- Includes application of dressings.
- Is separately reported when performed in conjunction with surgical debridement (**11042–11047**).
- Documentation should include current wound assessment, including
  — Quantitative measurements of wound characteristics (eg, site, surface area and depth)
  — Any previous treatment regimens
  — Debridement (when performed)
  — Prescribed length of treatment
  — Dressing types and frequency of changes
  — Other concerns that affect healing
- Encounters for ongoing NPWT may include documentation of progress of healing and changes in the wound, including measurement, amount of exudate, and presence of granulation or necrotic tissue.
- Codes **97605** and **97606** represent NPWT provided via a system that includes a *non-disposable* suction pump and drainage collection device.

Supplies, including dressings, are reportable with HCPCS codes (eg, **A6550**, wound care set, for NPWT electrical pump, includes all supplies and accessories).
- Codes **97607** and **97608**
  — Report NPWT that utilizes a *disposable* suction pump and collection system.
  — Are not reported in conjunction with codes **97605** and **97606**.
  — Payer policies may limit coverage to care of specific types of wounds that require NPWT to improve granulation tissue formation and to certain types of NPWT equipment.
  — Be sure to verify the coverage policy of the patient's health plan prior to provision of services.
  — Supplies for a disposable system are reported with code **A9272**, which also includes all dressings and accessories.

Sedation

Moderate Sedation

Moderate sedation codes **99151–99153** and **99155–99157** (**Table 19-8**) are used for reporting moderate sedation when intraservice time is 10 minutes or more.

Moderate sedation is a drug-induced depression of consciousness during which patients respond purposefully to verbal commands, either alone or accompanied by light tactile stimulation.
- Codes **99151–99157** are distinguished by service provider, patient age, and time spent.
- No interventions are required to maintain cardiovascular functions or a patent airway, and spontaneous ventilation is adequate.
- Moderate sedation codes are not used to report administration of medications for pain control, minimal sedation (anxiolysis), deep sedation, or monitored anesthesia care (**00100–01999**).
- Moderate sedation in the outpatient setting is typically performed by the same physician or QHP who is performing the diagnostic or therapeutic service and requires the presence of an independent trained observer.
- An *independent trained observer* is an individual qualified to monitor the patient during the procedure but who has no other duties (eg, assisting at surgery) during the procedure.

Codes **99151–99153** are reported when
- The administration of moderate sedation is provided by the physician who is simultaneously performing a procedure (eg, fracture reduction, vessel cutdown, central line placement, wound repair).
- An independent trained observer is present to assist the physician in the monitoring of the patient during the procedure or diagnostic service.

In the facility setting, a physician or QHP other than the person performing the diagnostic or therapeutic service may provide moderate sedation services.

Codes **99155–99157** are reported when a second physician or QHP other than the health care professional performing the diagnostic or therapeutic services provides moderate sedation.

Codes **99153** and **99157** are reported for each additional 15 minutes of intraservice time.

Chapter 19. Common Surgical Procedures and Sedation in Facility Settings

Table 19-8. Moderate Sedation		
Moderate Sedation *Moderate sedation of <10 minutes is included in the procedure performed. Report an additional unit when intraservice time extends at least 8 minutes beyond the first or last full 15 minutes of service.*	**First 10–22 min of Intraservice Time**	**Each Additional 15 min of Intraservice Time**
Moderate sedation services provided by the same physician or other qualified health care professional performing the diagnostic or therapeutic service that the sedation supports, requiring the presence of an independent trained observer to assist in the monitoring of the patient's level of consciousness and physiological status; initial 15 minutes of intraservice time, patient younger than 5 years of age	99151	+99153
5 years or older	99152	+99153
Moderate sedation services (other than those services described by codes **00100–01999**) provided by a physician other than the health care professional performing the diagnostic or therapeutic service that the sedation supports; younger than 5 years	99155	+99157
5 years or older	99156	+99157

The midpoint between the end of the previous 15-minute period must be passed to report an additional unit of intraservice time (ie, intraservice time must continue for at least 8 minutes beyond the last full 15 minutes of intraservice time).

Documentation Requirements for Moderate Sedation

Documentation must include

- A description of the procedure
- Name and dosage(s) of the sedation agent(s)
- Route of administration of the sedation agent(s)
- Who administered the agent (ie, physician or independent observer)
- Ongoing assessment of the child's level of consciousness and physiological status (eg, heart rate, oxygen saturation levels) during and after the procedure
- The presence, name, and title of the independent observer
- Total time from administration of the sedation agent(s) (start time) until the physician's face-to-face service is no longer required (end time)

Time of Moderate Sedation

- Codes are selected based on intraservice time. Intraservice time
  - Begins with the administration of the sedating agent(s)
  - Ends when the procedure is completed, the patient is stable for recovery status, and the physician or other QHP providing the sedation ends personal continuous face-to-face time with the patient
  - Includes ordering and/or administering the initial and subsequent doses of sedating agents
  - Requires continuous face-to-face attendance of the physician or other QHP
  - Requires monitoring patient response to the sedating agents, including
    - Periodic assessment of the patient
    - Further administration of agent(s) as needed to maintain sedation
    - Monitoring of oxygen saturation, heart rate, and blood pressure
- Moderate sedation service of less than 10 minutes' intraservice time is not separately reported.
- Preservice work of moderate sedation services is not separately reported or included in intraservice time. Preservice work includes
  - Assessment of the patient's past medical and surgical history with particular emphasis on cardiovascular, pulmonary, airway, or neurologic conditions
  - Review of the patient's previous experiences with anesthesia and/or sedation
  - Family history of sedation complications
  - Summary of the patient's present medication list
  - Drug allergy and intolerance history

— Focused physical examination of the patient, with emphasis on
- Mouth, jaw, oropharynx, neck, and airway for Mallampati score assessment
- Chest and lungs
- Heart and circulation
- Vital signs, including heart rate, respiratory rate, blood pressure, and oxygenation, with end-tidal carbon dioxide when indicated

— Review of any pre-sedation diagnostic tests
— Completion of a pre-sedation assessment form (with American Society of Anesthesiologists [ASA] physical status classification)
— Patient informed consent
— Immediate pre-sedation assessment prior to first sedating doses
— Initiation of intravenous access and fluids to maintain patency

● Do not separately report or include the time of post-service work in the intraservice time. Post-service work of moderate sedation includes
— Assessment of the patient's vital signs, level of consciousness, neurologic, cardiovascular, and pulmonary stability in the post-sedation recovery period
— Assessment of patient's readiness for discharge following the procedure
— Preparation of documentation for sedation service
— Communication with family or caregiver about sedation service

● Oxygen saturation (**94760–94762**) cannot be reported separately.

Example

➤ **A 5-year-old hospitalized child needs insertion of a tunneled central venous catheter (36558).** A second physician will provide the moderate sedation while the first physician performs the procedure. The sedating physician administers the agent(s) and assesses the patient continuously until a safe level of moderate sedation is achieved. He or she monitors the child closely and administers additional doses of sedating and/or analgesic agent(s) as needed. The service, from the time of administration of the agent until determination that the child is stable and face-to-face physician time is no longer required, takes a total of 35 minutes. The physician providing the moderate sedation will report

ICD-10-CM	CPT
Appropriate diagnosis code	**99156** (moderate [conscious] sedation services by second physician or QHP, patient 5 years or older, first 15 minutes) **+99157** (moderate [conscious] sedation, each additional 15 minutes of intraservice time)

Deep Sedation

Deep sedation/analgesia is a drug-induced depression of consciousness during which patients cannot be easily aroused but respond purposefully after repeated verbal or painful stimulation (eg, purposefully pushing away the noxious stimuli).
● The ability to independently maintain ventilatory function may be impaired.
● Patients may require assistance in maintaining a patent airway, and spontaneous ventilation may be inadequate.
● Cardiovascular function is usually maintained.
● A state of deep sedation may be accompanied by partial or complete loss of protective airway reflexes.

Anesthesia services include
● Preoperative evaluation of the patient
● Administration of anesthetic, other medications, blood, and fluids
● Monitoring of physiologic parameters
● Other supportive services
● Postoperative E/M related to the surgery (Ongoing critical care services by an anesthesiologist may be separately reportable.)

Pediatricians who provide deep sedation services for procedures performed outside the operating suite should follow the same anesthesia policies and coding instructions as other providers of anesthesia services.

> If surgery is canceled, subsequent to the preoperative evaluation, payment may be allowed to the anesthesiologist for an evaluation and management (E/M) service and the appropriate E/M code (eg, consultation) may be reported. See Chapter 16 for information on reporting these services.

CPT codes for reporting anesthesia services, including deep sedation, monitored anesthesia care, or general anesthesia, are **00100–01999**. These codes are not as specific as codes for other services and generally identify a body area or type of procedure.

00102	Anesthesia for procedures involving plastic repair of cleft lip
01820	Anesthesia for all closed procedures on radius, ulna, wrist, or hand bones

Add-on codes may be reported to identify special circumstances that increase the complexity of providing anesthesia care, including

99100	Patient under 1 year or older than 70 years (not reported in conjunction with codes **00326, 00561, 00834**, or **00836**)
99116	Anesthesia complicated by total body hypothermia
99135	Anesthesia complicated by controlled hypotension
99140	Emergency conditions

Emergency is defined by *CPT* as a situation in which delay in treatment of the patient would lead to a significant increase in the threat to life or body part.

Modifiers are reported in addition to anesthesia codes to indicate the physical status of the patient. The ASA classification of the patient's physical status is represented by the following HCPCS modifiers:

P1	Normal healthy patient
P2	Patient with mild systemic disease
P3	Patient with severe systemic disease
P4	Patient with severe systemic disease that is a constant threat to life
P5	Moribund patient who is not expected to survive without the operation
P6	Declared brain-dead patient whose organs are being removed for donor purposes

Other modifiers that may be required by payers for anesthesia services by pediatric physicians are those identifying the type of anesthesia or anesthesia provider.

AA	Anesthesia services performed personally by anesthesiologist

- Payers may require this modifier for services personally rendered by physicians other than anesthesiologists. This signifies that services were not rendered by a nonphysician provider, such as a certified registered nurse anesthetist.

GC	This service has been performed in part by a resident under the direction of a teaching physician
G8	Monitored anesthesia care for deep complex, complicated, or markedly invasive surgical procedure
G9	Monitored anesthesia care for patient who has history of severe cardiopulmonary condition
QS	Monitored anesthesia care service

- Medicare considers deep sedation equivalent to monitored anesthesia care. Private payers may vary.

Base units for anesthesia services are published in the ASA *Relative Value Guide* and by the CMS for each anesthesia procedure code. Payers typically do not require reporting of base units on the claim for services.

- Many private payers will allow additional base units for physical status modifiers **P3** (1 unit), **P4** (2 units), and **P5** (3 units).
- Anesthesia time is reported in minutes unless a payer directs to report units (1 unit per 15 minutes). Start and stop times must be documented, including multiple start and stop times when anesthesia services are discontinuous.

Postoperative Pain Management

Generally, the surgeon is responsible for postoperative pain management. However, a surgeon may request assistance with postoperative pain management (eg, epidural or peripheral nerve block).

- Payers may require a written request by the surgeon for postoperative pain management by the anesthesia provider.
- When a catheter is placed as the mode of anesthesia (eg, epidural catheter) and retained for use in postoperative pain management, this is not separately reported.
- When separately reporting postoperative pain management, append modifier **59** (distinct procedural service) to indicate the separate service and document this service distinctly (and preferably separately) from the anesthesia record.

- When an epidural catheter is used for postoperative pain management, code **01996** (daily management of epidural) may be reported on days subsequent to the day of surgery. Daily management of other postoperative pain management devices may be reported with subsequent hospital care codes (**99231–99233**).

Example

➤ **An orthopedic surgeon requests preanesthetic insertion of a catheter to provide a continuous infusion of the femoral nerve for postoperative pain relief for a patient undergoing an arthroscopy of the knee with lateral meniscectomy.** The anesthesiologist uses ultrasound guidance to insert a catheter for continuous infusion prior to inducing general anesthesia for the surgical procedure.

ICD-10-CM	CPT
Appropriate diagnosis code	**01400** (anesthesia for open or surgical arthroscopic procedures on knee joint; not otherwise specified) **64448 59** (injection, anesthetic agent[s] and/or steroid; femoral nerve, continuous infusion by catheter [including catheter placement])

Teaching Point: Because the anesthetist provided a distinct service separate from the anesthesia for the procedure, the catheter insertion is separately reported with modifier **59**. Had the procedure been performed under an epidural block and the epidural catheter left in place for postoperative pain management, no additional code would be reported.

Resources

Sedation

"Beyond Moderate Sedation: Coding for Anesthesia Services," April 2014 *AAP Pediatric Coding Newsletter* (https://coding.solutions.aap.org/article.aspx?articleid=1906504; subscription required)

"Documentation of Deep Sedation Services (Online Exclusive)," May 2014 *AAP Pediatric Coding Newsletter* (https://coding.solutions.aap.org/article.aspx?articleid=1906514; subscription required)

Surgery

CMS-designated global periods, Medicare Resource-Based Relative Value Scale Physician Fee Schedule (www.cms.gov/Medicare/Medicare-Fee-for-Service-Payment/PhysicianFeeSched/PFS-Relative-Value-Files.html; see column O)

"The Surgical Package and Related Services," May 2018 *AAP Pediatric Coding Newsletter* (https://coding.solutions.aap.org/article.aspx?articleid=2679119; subscription required)

"Coding Challenge: Modifiers and Procedural Services (Online Exclusive)," May 2018 *AAP Pediatric Coding Newsletter* (https://coding.solutions.aap.org/article.aspx?articleid=2679120; subscription required)

"Reporting Terminated Procedural Services," November 2014 *AAP Pediatric Coding Newsletter* (https://coding.solutions.aap.org/article.aspx?articleid=1921435; subscription required)

"Subspecialty Corner: Coding for Complications of Neonatal Circumcision," June 2017 *AAP Pediatric Coding Newsletter* (https://coding.solutions.aap.org/article.aspx?articleid=2629478; subscription required)

American Urological Association, "Pediatric Hypospadias Repair: A New Consensus Document on Coding" (www.auanet.org/Documents/practices-resources/coding-tips/Pediatric-Hypospadias-Repair.pdf)

Teaching Physician

Medicare Teaching Physician Services rules (http://cms.hhs.gov/manuals/downloads/clm104c12.pdf; see section 100)

●=New code   ▲=Revised code   #=Re-sequenced code   +=Add-on code

Test Your Knowledge!

1. **Which is not reported separately (outside the surgical package) when payers follow the Centers for Medicare & Medicaid Services global period rules?**
   a. Return to the operating room for treatment of complications of the first procedure
   b. Treatment for the underlying condition
   c. Management of complications that do not require return to the operating room
   d. An unrelated procedure performed during the postoperative period of a procedure

2. **Which modifier is required when the surgeon consults another physician who manages conditions unrelated to a surgery during the postoperative period?**
   a. No modifier is required.
   b. Modifier **54**
   c. Modifier **55**
   d. Modifier **56**

3. **For which surgical procedures may the teaching physician be immediately available rather than present during portions of the procedure?**
   a. A minor procedure
   b. A complex or high-risk procedure as identified by Medicare or *Current Procedural Terminology*
   c. All surgical procedures
   d. A surgery that is not a minor or a complex or high-risk procedure

4. **What code(s) is reported for peripherally inserted central venous catheter insertion without a subcutaneous port and without imaging guidance?**
   a. Code **36568** or **36569**
   b. Code **36400**
   c. Code **36572** or **36573** with modifier **52**
   d. Code **36570**

5. **Which of the following codes is reported when 24 minutes of intraservice time of moderate sedation is provided by a second physician (ie, not performing the procedure) to a 3-year-old patient?**
   a. **99151**
   b. **99151, 99153** x 1
   c. **99155, 99157** x 1
   d. **99155**

●=New code   ▲=Revised code   #=Re-sequenced code   +=Add-on code

Part 4
Digital Medicine Services

Part 4: Digital Medicine Services

Digital Medicine Services: Technology-Enhanced Care Delivery

Contents

    ●=New code   ▲=Revised code   #=Re-sequenced code   +=Add-on code

Digital Medicine Services

This chapter provides information on coding for services that reflect and support the use of technology in enhancing care delivery. This includes 3 distinct types of digital services.

- Services provided via digital communication technology involving separate written or recorded communications, such as secure email exchanges, as opposed to real-time audiovisual communication
- Remote physiologic monitoring and related treatment management services, including utilization of patient data acquired remotely in the diagnosis and/or management of health conditions
- Virtual face-to-face care facilitated by digital technology providing simultaneous audiovisual communication between a patient and a physician or other qualified health care professional (QHP) at remote locations

Due to the coronavirus disease 2019 (COVID-19) public health emergency, some of the information provided in this chapter may vary based on payers. During the public health emergency, allowances were made to use and report certain codes outside of *Current Procedural Terminology* (*CPT*®) instruction and/or typical payment policy. However, these allowances were limited to the duration of the emergency. Check with your payers before reporting any of the following services outside of their intention.

> *Current Procedural Terminology (CPT)* describes virtual face-to-face care as a synchronous telemedicine service. Telemedicine is defined by *CPT* as a *real-time* interaction between a physician or other qualified health care professional (QHP) and a patient who is located at a distant site from the physician or QHP.

Each of the services involving digital technology has distinct service elements and periods of service.

Before providing any digital medicine service, understand local and state laws, ensure that communications will be Health Insurance Portability and Accountability Act of 1996 (HIPAA) compliant, establish written guidelines and procedures, educate payers and negotiate for payment, and educate patients.

Review the payment policies of health plans and payers such as Medicaid prior to initiating digital medicine services, as coverage and payment may vary.

Online Digital Evaluation and Management Services

Digital communication technology (eg, secure patient portals, electronic health record [EHR]/health exchange communications) that do not meet the *CPT* definition of telemedicine are increasingly used to provide health care services. This category of services includes evaluation and management (E/M) services provided via digital communication such as secure email and interprofessional consultation via telephone, internet, and/or EHR.

Verify individual health plan policies for payment for digital medical services.

Online Digital Medical Services

#99421	Online digital evaluation and management service, for an established patient, for up to 7 days, cumulative time during the 7 days; 5–10 minutes
#99422	11–20 minutes
#99423	21 or more minutes
98970	Qualified nonphysician health care professional online digital assessment and management service, for an established patient, for up to seven days, cumulative time during the 7 days; 5-10 minutes
98971	11–20 minutes
98972	21 or more minutes

Codes **99421–99423** are reported by physicians and other QHPs whose scope of practice includes E/M services as described by codes **99202–99499**. Codes **98970–98972** are reported by health care professionals (eg, speech or physical therapist) whose scope of practice does not include E/M services as described by codes **99202–99499**.

Online digital E/M services are different from telemedicine services. The required delivery mechanism for telemedicine (ie, synchronous audiovisual communication) is not required for online digital E/M services. Online digital E/M services may be provided using asynchronous communication such as messaging in a patient portal or via secure email.

Online digital E/M services must be patient or caregiver initiated. Online digital E/M includes

- Cumulative physician or other QHP time devoted to the patient's care over a period of 7 days whether the time is spent addressing single or multiple different problems within the 7-day period

- Cumulative service time includes
  - Review of the initial inquiry by the physician or QHP
  - Review of patient records or data pertinent to assessment of the patient's problem
  - Physician's or QHP's personal interaction with clinical staff focused on the patient's problem
  - Development of management plans including physician or QHP generation of prescriptions or ordering of tests
  - Subsequent communication with the patient through online, telephone, email, or other digitally supported communication that does not otherwise represent a separately reported E/M service
- Permanent documentation storage (electronic or hard copy) of the encounter
     Do not report online digital services
- Of less than 5 minutes' total time.
- Based on time spent by clinical staff.
- During the postoperative period of a procedure.
- If another E/M service (in person or telemedicine) for the same or related problem occurred within 7 days prior to the online digital service.

> **If a patient generates the initial online digital inquiry for a new problem within 7 days of a previous evaluation and management (E/M) visit that addressed a different problem, the online digital E/M service may be reported separately.**

- If a separately reported E/M visit occurs within 7 days following the initiation of the online service. Instead, combine all work of the online digital E/M service into selection of the code for the other E/M service.

Examples

➤ **On January 1, a pediatrician provides an online E/M service to a patient with a rash, which includes obtaining history, reviewing digital photographs of the rash, and advising the caregiver on home treatment.** The time of service is 10 minutes and is reportable with code **99421**. The service is reported when the 7-day service period is complete and no other E/M service has been rendered.

➤ **For the same patient as in the previous example, the caregiver sends a new photograph with concern that the rash is not responding to treatment on January 3.** The pediatrician sees the patient in the office later that day. Code **99421** is not reported for the prior online digital E/M services, but the level of service reported for the office encounter (eg, **99213**) includes the medical decision-making (MDM) or time of the online encounters.

➤ **A patient is seen in the office by a pediatrician for complaint of a foreign body in the ear on January 9.** On January 14, the same patient receives an online digital E/M service for advice on treating a mild sunburn on the child's shoulders and face. Because the problem addressed by the online service is not related to the problem addressed at the office encounter, the online service is separately reported (eg, **99421**). Follow payer instructions for reporting an unrelated online service within 7 days of an office E/M service (eg, append modifier **XU** [unusual nonoverlapping service]).

➤ **A 10-year-old patient is seen in the office by a pediatrician for complaint of otitis media on January 9.** On January 11, a caregiver contacts the pediatrician via secure email with concern that the patient's symptoms have worsened, and the pediatrician prescribes an antibiotic. Only the office encounter (eg, **99213**) is reported because the online digital E/M service is provided within 7 days for the same problem.

➤ **A patient receives an online digital E/M service on January 9.** The physician's total time spent providing the service is 10 minutes. On January 15, the same patient receives an online digital E/M service for an unrelated problem with total physician time of 15 minutes. The 2 services occurring within 7 days are combined (even though each service addressed different problems) and reported with code **99423**.

Do not include the time of separately reported online digital E/M services in the time attributed to other services (eg, care plan oversight [**99339, 99340, 99374, 99375, 99377–99380**] or chronic care management services [**99487, 99489, 99490, 99439, 99491**]).

Remote Interprofessional Consultations

99446   Interprofessional telephone/Internet/electronic health record assessment and management service provided by a consultative physician including a verbal and written report to the patient's treating/requesting physician/qualified health care professional; 5–10 minutes of medical consultative discussion and review

99447   11–20 minutes of medical consultative discussion and review

99448   21–30 minutes of medical consultative discussion and review

99449   31 minutes or more of medical consultative discussion and review

#99451   Interprofessional telephone/Internet/electronic health record assessment and management service provided by a consultative physician including a written report to the patient's treating/requesting physician or other qualified health care professional, 5 or more minutes of medical consultative time

#99452   Interprofessional telephone/Internet/electronic health record referral service(s) provided by a treating/requesting physician or qualified health care professional, 30 minutes

Remote interprofessional consultations include a request by a patient's attending or primary physician or other QHP soliciting opinion and/or treatment advice by telephone, internet, or EHR from a physician with specialty expertise (ie, consultant). This consultation does not require face-to-face contact with the patient by the consultant. The patient may be in the inpatient or outpatient setting.

> See Chapter 12 for information on care management services that may include online communications.

Interprofessional Consultation Reporting by an Attending/Primary Physician

The treating/requesting physician or other QHP may report code **99452** or prolonged service (**99417, 99354–99357; 99358, 99359**).

- Code **99452** may be reported when 16 to 30 minutes is spent by the requesting individual in a service day preparing for the referral and/or communicating with the consultant.
- Time spent in discussion with the consultant may also be reported with prolonged service codes (in lieu of **99452**) *if the requirements for the appropriate prolonged service codes are met.*
  - Direct prolonged service code **99417** may be reported when the requesting physician has had a face-to-face encounter with the patient in the office or other outpatient setting on the same day that extends at least 15 minutes beyond the total time of the associated E/M service (**99205, 99215**).
  - Direct prolonged service in conjunction with inpatient, observation or outpatient services, except with office or other outpatient services, may be reported with codes **99354** and **99355** or **99356** and **99357**.
  - Prolonged service of more than 30 minutes in a day without the patient present are reported with codes **99358** and **99359**.

> For more information on prolonged services, see chapters 7 and 8 for prolonged office E/M service and prolonged service in other nonhospital settings and Chapter 16 for prolonged services in an inpatient setting.

Interprofessional Consultation Reporting by a Consultant

Guidelines for the consultant reporting interprofessional telephone/internet/EHR consultations include

- Telephone/internet/EHR consultations of less than 5 minutes are not reported. For codes **99446–99449**, more than 50% of the time reported as interprofessional consultation must have been spent in medical consultative verbal or internet discussion rather than review of data (eg, medical records, test results).
- Code **99451** is reported based on the total time of review and interprofessional consultation.
- Both verbal and written reports are required for completion of the services represented by codes **99446–99449**. Only a written report is required for code **99451**.
- A single interprofessional consultation code is reported for the cumulative time spent in discussion and information review regardless of the number of contacts necessary to complete the service.
- Codes **99446–99451** are not reported more than once in a 7-day interval.
- Time spent in telephone or online consultation directly with the patient and/or family may be reported using codes **99441–99443, 99421–99423, 98966–98968**, or **98970–98972**, and the time related to these services is not included in the time attributed to interprofessional consultation services.
- When the purpose of communication is to arrange a transfer of care or face-to-face patient encounter, interprofessional consultation codes are not reported.

- Interprofessional consultation services are not reported if the consultant has provided a face-to-face service to the patient within the past 14 days or when the consultation results in scheduling of a face-to-face service within the next 14 days or at the consultant's next available appointment date.
- Time spent by the consultant reviewing pertinent medical records, studies, or other data is included in the time of the interprofessional consultation and not separately reported.
- Do not report prolonged E/M service before and/or after direct patient care (**99358**, **99359**) for any time within the service period if reporting codes **99446–99451**.
- As with all consultations, the request for advice or opinion should be documented in the patient record. For a new patient with no record, create a record to document this service.

Examples

➤ **The parents of a child with perennial allergies and chronic allergic otitis media, currently with drainage from tubes, and history of adenoidectomy contact the child's pediatrician about the number of school days she has missed due to illness and want to discuss allergy treatment.** The child's pediatrician arranges a telephone consultation with an allergist located several hours away and forwards the child's health records prior to the telephone consultation. The pediatrician and allergist spend a total of 16 minutes in discussion of treatment options.

On a second date, the pediatrician provides a face-to-face E/M service to the child and her parents to discuss recommendations based on the prior interprofessional consultation. Options of allergy testing to determine allergens that may be avoided, contraindication of allergen therapy due to the child's weight, and the importance of daily use of nasal spray and nonsedating antihistamines. The pediatrician's total time on the date of the visit is 25 minutes.

Service	International Classification of Diseases, 10th Revision, Clinical Modification (ICD-10-CM)	CPT	
First date of service (interprofessional consultation)	Both physicians report **J30.89** (other allergic rhinitis) and **H65.413** (chronic allergic otitis media, bilateral)	The consultant reports **99447** (11–20 minutes of medical discussion and review) for the service on the first date.	The pediatrician reports **99452** for the 16 minutes spent in interprofessional referral service.
Second date of service (pediatrician only)			The pediatrician reports **99213** (office E/M, 20–29 minutes total time) for services on the second date.

Teaching Point: In this vignette, the patient and parents are not present for the interprofessional consultation. The primary care physician may report code **99452** for 16 to 30 minutes of interprofessional consultation.

➤ **A physician at a rural hospital admits a child with cystic fibrosis for treatment of pneumonia.** The physician communicates with the child's pulmonologist, who is located several hours away, via a secure health information exchange for advice about treatment. The pulmonologist spends a total of 25 minutes reviewing hospital records and communicating with the attending physician. The attending physician's total time spent on the unit/floor providing and/or coordinating care for this patient is 70 minutes, with 40 minutes in preparation for and participation in the interprofessional consultation service and another 5 minutes counseling the patient and caregivers following the consultation.

ICD-10-CM	CPT	
Both physicians report **E84.0** (cystic fibrosis with pulmonary manifestations) and a code to identify the infectious agent, if known.	The consultant reports **99448** (21–30 minutes of medical consultative discussion and review).	The pediatrician reports **99223** (typical time 70 minutes) based on time spent in counseling and/or coordination of care.

Teaching Point: Interprofessional consultation services would not be reported if the consultant has provided a face-to-face service to the patient within the past 14 days or if the consultation results in scheduling of a face-to-face service within the next 14 days or at the consultant's next available appointment date.

➤ **A hospitalized 2-day-old develops poor feeding and tachypnea and is diagnosed with group B streptococcal septicemia.** The patient's primary care physician telephones an infectious disease specialist located several hours away for treatment advice. The physicians spend 8 minutes discussing the child's condition and treatment options.

ICD-10-CM	CPT
The infectious disease specialist reports this service with **P36.0** (sepsis of newborn due to streptococcus, group B).	The consultant reports **99446** (interprofessional consultation, 5–10 minutes). The pediatrician will report the appropriate E/M service.

Teaching Point: The attending physician will include this work in the per diem charge for intensive or critical care services based on the type of care rendered.

Utilization of Remote Physiologic Data

CPT describes multiple services that may include utilization of data acquired remotely by
- Patient self-collection and data submission to a physician outside of a face-to-face visit
- A single collection of data digitally stored over a specific period with interpretation and report
- By ongoing management or treatment in conjunction with continuous monitoring and response to alerts

Self-measured Blood Pressure Monitoring

#99473 Self-measured blood pressure using a device validated for clinical accuracy; patient education/training and device calibration

#99474 separate self-measurements of two readings one minute apart, twice daily over a 30-day period (minimum of 12 readings), collection of data reported by the patient and/or caregiver to the physician or other qualified health care professional, with report of average systolic and diastolic pressures and subsequent communication of a treatment plan to the patient

Self-measured blood pressure monitoring is a non–face-to-face service in which the patient or caregiver uses a home blood pressure measurement device to measure and record readings that are then provided to the ordering physician on paper or digitally (eg, email). Self-measured blood pressure monitoring is used for
- Ruling out white coat hypertension, which can avoid unnecessary treatment, adverse medication effects, and laboratory or diagnostic costs
- Identifying masked hypertension, which, if left untreated, carries a higher risk of cardiovascular disease and stroke
- Assessing control of hypertension and ensuring appropriate treatment is being ordered

Codes **99473** and **99474** are not reported for automated ambulatory blood pressure monitoring using report-generating software worn continuously for 24 hours or longer; see codes **93784–93790**. **Table 20-1** provides an overview of work included in each code.

Table 20-1. Self-measured Blood Pressure Monitoring by Patient	
#99473	Clinical staff or physician work ● Patient education/training on self-measurement and reading collection ● Home blood pressure monitoring device calibration Report once per device.
#99474	Physician work ● Review report of individual and average systolic/diastolic blood pressure readings (must include ≥12 readings; patient performs/documents 2 readings 1 minute apart at each measurement). ● Communicate treatment plan to clinical staff or patient/caregiver. Report for a 30-day period.

Do not report **99473** or **99474** when reporting collection and interpretation of physiologic data (**99091**), remote physiologic monitoring (**99453**, **99454**, **99457**, **99458**), or chronic care management (**99487**, **99489**, **99490**, **99439**, **99491**) in the same calendar month.

Example

> **A 14-year-old boy has presented with high blood pressure readings at several encounters.** The physician orders a blood pressure device validated for clinical accuracy and instructs the patient to obtain 2 readings twice daily for a 7-day period with at least 12 separate readings and provide the results to the physician's clinical staff. The clinical staff received the patient's documented readings and average the systolic and diastolic pressures. The readings and calculated averages are reviewed by the physician, who develops a treatment plan that is communicated to the patient and/or caregivers.

ICD-10-CM	CPT
R03.0 (elevated blood-pressure reading, without diagnosis of hypertension)	**99474** (collection and averaging of blood pressure readings with communication of plan of care)

Teaching Point: At least 12 blood pressure readings must be obtained and averaged to create a treatment plan for the patient. Code **99474** includes collection, analysis, and communication of treatment plan(s) within a 30-day period.

If the patient returned for an office or other outpatient E/M service to review the readings and obtain the physician's recommended care plan, an E/M service (eg, **99213**) would be reported in lieu of **99474**.

Collection and Interpretation of Digitally Stored Data

Nonspecific Physiologic Data Collection and Interpretation

#99091 Collection and interpretation of physiologic data (eg, ECG, blood pressure, glucose monitoring) digitally stored and/or transmitted by the patient and/or caregiver to the physician or other qualified health care professional, qualified by education, training, licensure/regulation (when applicable) requiring a minimum of 30 minutes of time, each 30 days

Code **99091** represents a 30-day episode of care. Time spent by a physician or other QHP in activities listed in **Table 20-2** is included in the time supporting code **99091**.

Code **99091** does not require active monitoring of physiologic data or live interactive communication with the patient during the service period as is required for remote physiologic monitoring treatment management service codes **99457** and **99458** (discussed later in this chapter).

Table 20-2. Collection and Interpretation of Physiologic Data	
99091	Physician work ● Data access, review, and interpretation. ● Modify care plan as necessary and communicate to patient/caregiver. ● Associated documentation. ● Report for minimum of 30 minutes, each 30 days.

- Do not report **99091** if other, more specific *CPT* codes exist (eg, **93227**, **93272** for electrocardiographic services; **95250** for continuous glucose monitoring).
- If the services described by code **99091** are provided on the same day the patient presents for an E/M service, these services should be considered part of the E/M service and not separately reported.
- Do not report **99091** for transfer and interpretation of data from hospital or clinical laboratory computers.
- Do not report **99091** in the same calendar month as, or within 30 days of reporting, care plan oversight services (**99374–99380**, **99339**, **99340**) or remote physiologic monitoring services (**99457**, **99458**).
- Code **99091** was assigned 1.64 relative value units (RVUs) in 2020 (facility or non-facility).

Example

➤ **A child with epilepsy is prescribed a US Food and Drug Administration (FDA)-approved wearable device that detects seizures and notifies caregivers.** The data collected by the device is transmitted to a server from which the child's physician downloads a report at the end of each 30-day period that provides the frequency of seizure detection; detailed physiologic data collected before, during, and after each seizure; and information on the patient's sleep and wake times. An additional report provides information the patient or caregiver has entered into the device diary during the reporting period. The physician spends 30 minutes or more reviewing and interpreting the data and communicating by phone with the patient or caregiver about the treatment plan. The physician reports **99091** linked to a diagnosis code for the epilepsy.

Remote Physiologic Monitoring Services

CPT includes codes for specific types of remote physiologic monitoring (eg, pediatric home apnea monitoring [**94772–94777**]). For other types of remote physiologic monitoring, for which there are no specific codes, remote physiologic monitoring service codes are reported.

See discussion of coding for continuous glucose monitoring and home apnea monitoring services later in this chapter for information on reporting these services.

- Report codes **99453**, **99454**, **99457**, and **99458** for remote physiologic monitoring services when the parameters monitored are not more specifically identified by other codes.
- A physician practice may provide all components (eg, equipment supply, initial setup, calibration, training, monitoring, treatment management services) or, perhaps more frequently, only the remote physiologic monitoring treatment management component (ie, **99457** and **99458**).

> In 2019, 22 Medicaid programs provided payment for remote patient monitoring per the Center for Connected Health Policy (www.cchpca.org; accessed June 25, 2020).

Remote Monitoring Setup and Supply

#99453 Remote monitoring of physiologic parameter(s) (eg, weight, blood pressure, pulse oximetry, respiratory flow rate), initial; set-up and patient education on use of equipment

#99454 device(s) supply with daily recording(s) or programmed alert(s) transmission, each 30 days

To report codes **99453** and **99454**, the device used must be a medical device as defined by the FDA (eg, blood glucose monitor) and the service must be ordered by a physician or QHP. Do not report when monitoring is fewer than 16 days.

- Codes **99453** and **99454** represent practice expense only; no physician work is valued in these codes. The time spent by a physician or QHP in activities listed in **Table 20-3** is included in the time supporting codes **99453** and **99454**.
- Do not report codes **99453** and **99454** in conjunction with codes for more specific physiologic parameters (eg, pulse oximetry [**94760**]).
- Do not report **99453** and **99454** when these services are included in other *CPT* codes for the duration of time of the physiologic monitoring service (eg, **95250**, ambulatory continuous glucose monitoring of interstitial tissue fluid via a subcutaneous sensor).
- Initial setup and patient education on use of equipment (**99453**) is reported for each episode of care (begins when the remote monitoring physiologic service is initiated and ends with attainment of targeted treatment goals).

Table 20-3. Remote Monitoring of Physiologic Parameters: Setup and Device Supply	
99453	Clinical staff work includes setup and patient education on use of equipment. Report once per episode of care.
99454	Supply expense. Supplies for daily recordings or programmed-alert transmissions. Report once per episode of care.

●=New code ▲=Revised code #=Re-sequenced code +=Add-on code

Remote Physiologic Monitoring Treatment Management Services

#99457   Remote physiologic monitoring treatment management services, clinical staff/physician/other qualified health care professional time in a calendar month requiring interactive communication with the patient/caregiver during the month; first 20 minutes

#+99458   each additional 20 minutes

Remote physiologic monitoring treatment management services include time spent using the results of physiologic monitoring to manage a patient under a specific treatment plan. The associated monitoring device(s) must be defined as a medical device by the FDA. These services may be rendered by physicians, QHPs, and/or clinical staff working under supervision of a physician or QHP. The time spent by a physician or QHP in activities listed in **Table 20-4** is included in the time supporting codes **99457** and **99458**.

Table 20-4. Remote Physiologic Monitoring Treatment Management Services	
#99457	Physician work ● Data access, review, and interpretation. ● Modify care plan as necessary and communication to patient/caregiver. ● Associated documentation. ● Report for minimum of 20 min, each calendar month.
#+99458	Physician work Each additional 20 min (as previous)

Documentation of remote physiologic monitoring treatment management must include
● An order by a physician or QHP
● Live interactive communication (eg, two-way conversation via telephone or email) with the patient and/or caregiver
● Time of service of 20 or more minutes in a calendar month

Reporting instructions
● Report code **99457** once with 1 unit of service for the initial 20 minutes of service regardless of the number of physiologic monitoring modalities performed in a given calendar month. When the time of service extends a full 20 minutes beyond the first 20 minutes, report code **99458** in addition to **99457**.
● Do not count any time on a day when the physician or QHP reports an E/M service (office or other outpatient services [**99202–99205, 99211–99215**]; domiciliary, rest home services [**99324–99328, 99334–99337**]; home services [**99341–99345, 99347–99350**]).
● Do not count any time related to other reported services (eg, **93290**, interrogation of implantable cardiovascular physiologic monitor system).
● Do not report **99457** or **99458** in conjunction with collection and interpretation of physiologic data (**99091**).
● Codes **99457** and **99458** may be reported during the same service period as chronic care management (**99439, 99487–99491**), transitional care management (**99495, 99496**), and behavioral health integration services (**99492–99494, 99484**). However, the time for each service must be distinct and not overlapping and must be separately documented.
● Code **99457** was assigned 0.91 RVUs in a facility setting and 1.43 in a non-facility setting in 2020. Code **99458** was assigned 0.91 RVUs in a facility setting and 1.17 in a non-facility setting.

Examples

➤ **A child with epilepsy is prescribed an FDA-approved wearable device that detects seizures and notifies caregivers in addition to transmitting data to the prescribing physician.** The patient is provided with setup and education for use of the device and the program's monitoring application. The practice directly receives and monitors daily recordings and/or programmed alerts for at least a 16-day period. Education on equipment use is provided as needed. Codes **99453** and **99454** are reported.

Teaching Point: The device must be used for monitoring for at least 16 days to report **99453** and/or **99454**. The patient and caregivers are provided separately reported treatment management services (**99457, 99458**) of at least 20 minutes in the month, as indicated.

Chapter 20. Digital Medicine Services: Technology-Enhanced Care Delivery

➤ **A child with poorly controlled asthma is enrolled in a remote monitoring program.** A Bluetooth-enabled device that promotes and monitors effective inhaler use and measures forced expiratory volume in 1 second and peak expiratory flow is provided to the patient by a durable medical equipment provider. The patient's physician and/or clinical staff provide education to the patient and caregivers on device use. The physician reports code **99453**.

Teaching Point: Because the physician practice furnishes only the initial setup and patient education, only code **99453** is reported for the initial 16 to 30 days of monitoring. Code **99454** would be reported by the provider of the equipment and monitoring service. See codes **99457** and **99458** for reporting 20 or more minutes of remote physiologic monitoring treatment management services during a calendar month.

Pediatric Home Apnea Monitoring

94772	Circadian respiratory pattern recording (pediatric pneumogram), 12-24-hour continuous recording, infant
94774	Pediatric home apnea monitoring event recording including respiratory rate, pattern and heart rate per 30-day period of time; includes monitor attachment, download of data, review, interpretation, and preparation of a report by a physician or other qualified health care professional
94775	monitor attachment only (includes hook-up, initiation of recording and disconnection)
94776	monitoring, download of information, receipt of transmission(s) and analyses by computer only
94777	review, interpretation and preparation of report only by a physician or other qualified health care professional

- Report code **94772** when circadian respiratory pattern recording (pediatric pneumogram), 12- to 24-hour continuous recording, is performed on an infant.
  - Physicians may be required to append modifier **26** to indicate only the professional component of this service was provided.
  - Report 1 unit per recording period unless otherwise instructed by a payer.
  - This code is not assigned RVUs in the Medicare Physician Fee Schedule (used by many payers). Allowable fees are determined by the payer.
- Codes **94774–94777** are reported once per 30-day period.
- Codes **94775** and **94776** are reported by the home health agency because there is no physician work involved.
- Codes **94774** and **94777** are reported by the physician.
  - Code **94774** is reported by the physician when he or she orders home monitoring, chooses the monitor limits, and arranges for a home health care provider to teach the parents. It includes reviewing and interpreting data and preparation of the report.
  - Code **94777** is reported when the physician receives the downloaded information on disc or hard copy or electronically, reviews the patterns and periods of abnormal respiratory or heart rate, and summarizes, in a written report, the findings and recommendations for continuation or discontinuation of monitoring. This information is provided to the primary care physician and/or the family.
  - Codes **94774–94777** are not reported in conjunction with codes **93224–93272** (electrocardiographic monitoring). The apnea recording device cannot be reported separately. When oxygen saturation monitoring is used in addition to heart rate and respiratory monitoring, it is not reported separately.

Example

➤ **An infant born at 23 weeks' gestation, now 2 months old, has chronic lung disease and requires prolonged low-flow oxygen.** She continues to have occasional episodes of self-stimulated apnea lasting less than 15 seconds. She goes home with heart rate and respiratory monitoring during unattended periods and sleep. The physician orders the monitor, contacts the home health agency for its provision, and instructs the home health agency to teach the parents about cardiopulmonary resuscitation, proper attachment of the monitor leads, and resetting of the monitor. The home health agency provides the physician with the downloaded recordings. The first month's data are interpreted by the physician and a written report generated. The physician counsels the parents about the need to continue monitoring.

Teaching Point: Report code **94774** and the appropriate *ICD-10-CM* code (eg, **G47.35** for congenital central alveolar hypoventilation/hypoxemia).

In subsequent months, the physician receives the downloaded recordings, interprets them, and generates reports with recommendations for continued or discontinuation of monitoring. These services are reported with code **94777**.

Ambulatory Continuous Glucose Monitoring

95250	Ambulatory continuous glucose monitoring of interstitial tissue fluid via a subcutaneous sensor for a minimum of 72 hours; physician or other qualified health care professional (office) provided equipment, sensor placement, hook-up, calibration of monitor, patient training, removal of sensor, and printout of record
#95249	patient-provided equipment, sensor placement, hook-up, calibration of monitor, patient training, and printout of recording
95251	Ambulatory continuous glucose monitoring of interstitial tissue fluid via a subcutaneous sensor for a minimum of 72 hours; analysis, interpretation and report

- When ambulatory glucose monitoring using monitoring equipment is initiated and data are captured for a minimum of 72 hours, report code **95249** or **95250** based on the supplier of the equipment (patient or physician office).
- Codes **95249** and **95250** do not include physician work (ie, valued for practice expense and liability only). **Table 20-5** lists the physician and clinical staff work components of codes **95249–95251**.
- Physicians report code **95249** only if the patient brings the data receiver into the physician's or other QHP's office with the entire initial data collection procedure conducted in the office.
- Report code **95249** only once for the entire duration that a patient has a receiver, even if the patient receives a new sensor and/or transmitter. If a patient receives a new or different model of receiver, code **95249** may be reported again when the entire initial data collection procedure is conducted in the office.
  - Report **95249** on the date the continuous glucose monitoring recording is printed in the office.
  - Removal of a sensor is not a required component of **95249**.

Table 20-5. Ambulatory Continuous Glucose Monitoring of Interstitial Tissue Fluid Via a Subcutaneous Sensor	
(A minimum of 72 hours of monitoring is required for each code.)	
95251	Physician work includes correlation of individual data points with the patient daily log; and interpretation and report. Do not report more than once per month.
95249 (patient provided equipment only)	Clinical staff work includes sensor placement; hookup; calibration of the monitor; patient training; and printout of record. Report only once during the time a patient owns a given data receiver.
95250 (physician office provided equipment only)	Clinical staff work includes sensor placement; hookup; calibration of the monitor; patient training; removal of the sensor; and printout of the record. Do not report more than once per month.

- Analysis, interpretation, and report (**95251**) may be performed without a face-to-face encounter on the same date of service. This service is reported only once per month.
- Code **95251** was assigned 1.02 RVUs in either a facility or non-facility setting in 2020.

Telemedicine

Telemedicine, as defined in *CPT*, is the use of real-time audiovisual technology to bring a physician in a distant location to a patient's bedside or to a setting right in the patient's own community without the need for either party to physically travel.

- Telemedicine may also be referred to as *telehealth*; definitions for each vary by state and payer, but telehealth is more commonly used to reference any health service provided via telecommunications. Telemedicine may be more appropriate to describe services of physicians and other QHPs and is the terminology used by *CPT*.
- Without any consideration of state law or payer policies, telemedicine services might be loosely defined as audiovisual technology–enabled, patient-specific services provided by a physician or practitioner in a distant geographic location to a patient who requires medical expertise not otherwise available at his or her location.

Synchronous Versus Asynchronous Communication

Key terms in differentiating telemedicine services from other digital services are *synchronous* and *asynchronous*. Telemedicine services (other than a special Medicare demonstration project) always include synchronous communication.

- Synchronous telemedicine services include simultaneous interaction between a physician or other qualified health care professional (QHP) and a patient who is located at a distant site.
- Asynchronous communication does not require simultaneous interaction from both parties. Examples of asynchronous communication are email and data and/or images transferred for review and subsequent response.
- *Originating sites* are those sites where the patient is located while receiving a telemedicine service.
- *Distant sites* are those sites where a physician or QHP is located while providing a telemedicine service.

Payer Coverage

In recent years, legislative changes and the need for non–face-to-face health services in public health emergencies, such as the COVID-19 pandemic, are expanding the provision of telemedicine services and may provide evidence to support expansion to all patients in the future. See the payment policies of individual health plans and other payers before initiating telemedicine services.

Medicare has published a list of codes (**Table 20-6** and online at www.aap.org/cfp [access code AAPCFP26]) that are covered when provided via telemedicine, but this list may be more restrictive than the lists used by Medicaid plans and other payers. Private payers may limit telemedicine services to those described by specific codes with benefit policy based on state telemedicine or telehealth regulations. It is important to verify the services and sites of service that are covered by each patient's health plan.

Table 20-6. 2020 Telemedicine Services			
CY 2020 Telehealth Services (Please see coding reference for code descriptors.)	**HCPCS/*CPT* Code**	**CPT Allows**[a]	**Medicare Allows**
Advanced care planning	**99497** and **99498**		√
Annual alcohol misuse screening, 15 min	**G0442**		√
Annual behavioral therapy for cardiovascular disease, 15 min	**G0446**		√
Annual depression screening, 15 min	**G0444**		√
Annual wellness visit, first visit	**G0438**		√
Annual wellness visit, subsequent visit	**G0439**		√
Behavioral counseling for alcohol misuse, 15 min	**G0443**		√
Behavioral counseling for obesity, 15 min	**G0447**		√
Comprehensive assessment and care planning for chronic care management	**G0506**		√
Diabetes self-management training services	**G0108** and **G0109**		√
Electrocardiographic rhythm derived event recording	**93268, 93270–93272**	√	
ESRD-related services[b]	**90951, 90952, 90954, 90955, 90957, 90958, 90960,** and **90961**	√	√
ESRD-related services for home dialysis[b]	**90963–90970**		√
External mobile cardiovascular telemetry with electrocardiographic recording, concurrent computerized real-time data analysis	**93228** and **93229**	√	
Genetic counseling	**96040**	√	
Health and behavior assessment/re-assessment and intervention	**96158, 96159,** and **96164–96171**		√
Health risk assessment	**96160** and **96161**		√
High-intensity behavioral counseling to prevent sexually transmitted infection; 30 min	**G0445**		√
Hospital subsequent care services (payer may limit to 1 telehealth visit every 3 days)	**99231–99233**	√	√
Inpatient consultation	**99251–99255**	√	
Kidney disease education services	**G0420** and **G0421**		√
Medical nutrition therapy	**G0270**		√
	97802–97804	√	√
Neurobehavioral status exam	**96116**	√	√

Table 20-6 (*continued*)

CY 2020 Telehealth Services (Please see coding reference for code descriptors.)	HCPCS/*CPT* Code	*CPT* Allows[a]	Medicare Allows
Nursing facility subsequent care services (payer may limit to 1 telehealth visit every 30 days)	99307–99310	√	√
Office consultation	99241–99245	√	
Office or other outpatient visits	99202–99215	√	√
Pharmacologic management, telehealth, inpatient	G0459		√
Pharmacologic management performed with psychotherapy services	90863	√	
Prolonged office or other outpatient E/M on the date of the primary service (report with **99202–99215**)	99417	√	
Prolonged preventive services	G0513 and G0514		√
Prolonged service in an outpatient setting other than an office or other outpatient visit (**99202–99215**)	99354 and 99355	√	√
Prolonged service in the inpatient or observation setting	99356 and 99357		√
Psychiatric diagnostic interview examination	90791 and 90792	√	√
Psychiatric services with interactive complexity	+90785		√
Psychoanalysis	90845	√	√
Psychotherapy, family	90846 and 90847	√	√
Psychotherapy, individual	90832–90834 and 90836–90838	√	√
Psychotherapy for crisis	90839 and 90840		√
Remote imaging for detection of retinal disease	92227	√	
Remote imaging for monitoring and management of active retinal disease	92228	√	
Self-management education and training	98960–98962	√	
Smoking cessation services	G0436 and G0437		√
	99406 and 99407	√	√
Structured assessment and intervention services for alcohol and/or substance (other than tobacco) abuse	G0396 and G0397		√
	99408 and 99409	√	
Telehealth consultation, critical care, initial, physicians typically spend 60 minutes	G0508		√
Telehealth consultation, critical care, subsequent, physicians typically spend 50 minutes	G0509		√
Telehealth consultations, emergency department or initial inpatient	G0425–G0427		√
Telehealth consultations, follow-up inpatient hospital or SNF	G0406–G0408		√
Transitional care management services	99495 and 99496	√	√

Abbreviations: *CPT, Current Procedural Terminology*; CY, calendar year; E/M, evaluation and management; ESRD, end-stage renal disease; HCPCS, Healthcare Common Procedure Coding System; SNF, skilled nursing facility.

[a] Append modifier **95** (telemedicine service rendered via a real-time interactive audio and video telecommunications system).

[b] For ESRD-related services, a physician, nurse practitioner, physician assistant, or clinical nurse specialist must furnish at least 1 hands-on visit (not telehealth) each month to examine the vascular access site.

Medicaid Payment

For purposes of Medicaid, telemedicine is a service that includes 2-way, real-time interactive communication between the patient and the practitioner including, at a minimum, audio and video technology.

Medicaid plans may pay the physician or other QHP at the distant site for each service rendered via telemedicine and pay a facility fee to the originating site (eg, hospital). States can also pay any additional costs, such as technical support, transmission charges, and equipment. These add-on costs can be incorporated into the fee-for-service rates or separately paid as an administrative cost by the state. If they are separately billed and paid, the costs must be linked to a covered Medicaid service.

State telehealth laws often include mandates for coverage of telemedicine services, and some include parity of payment (ie, equal to on-site services).

States may also choose to pay for services delivered using technology that does not meet the definition of telemedicine services (eg, telephones, facsimile machines, email systems, remote patient monitoring).

States may cover telemedicine services reported with a variety of *CPT* and Healthcare Common Procedure Coding System (HCPCS) codes. Plans may also pay **T1014** (telehealth transmission, per minute) to originating sites (other than patient's home) or **Q3014** [telehealth originating site facility fee). Modifiers **95** (telemedicine service rendered via a real-time interactive audio and video telecommunications system), **GT** (via interactive audio and video telecommunication systems), or **U1–UD** (modifiers defined by the state) may be required to identify, track, and pay for telemedicine services.

Place and Site of Service

Place of service code **02** may be used to report the location where health services and health-related services are provided or received through a telecommunications system. However, some payers continue to accept the place of service code for distant site where the physician or QHP is located (eg, **11**, office) but require modifier **95** to indicate the service was delivered via telemedicine.

See an individual payer's telemedicine policy to determine if there are reporting requirements for the specific site of service (eg, physical location from which services were rendered or received).

Field 32 of the 1500 paper claim form and its electronic equivalent is used to report the site of service (eg, hospital name, address, National Provider Identifier). This is typically the physical location of the physician or other provider of service at the time of service when payment is influenced by geographic location.

Critical access hospitals billing under Method II report modifier **GT** (via interactive audio and video telecommunication systems) because no place of service code is reported on Method II claims to identify telemedicine services. Some health plans may also require the **GT** modifier.

Reporting Telemedicine Services

From a *CPT* coding perspective, telemedicine services are face-to-face services reported using the same E/M codes that would be appropriate for in-person encounters.

Documentation of Services

Documentation of telemedicine services should be similar to that of services provided in traditional patient care settings. For E/M services, *other than* **99202–99205** and **99211–99215**, this means that documentation supports reporting of services based on the required key components (ie, history, examination, and/or MDM) or typical time of service (when >50% of the face-to-face time of the encounter is spent in counseling and/or coordination of care). The MDM or total time of service on the date of service should support telemedicine E/M services reported with **99202–99205** and **99211–99215**.

> **See Chapter 7 for more information on documentation of office and other outpatient evaluation and management services and instructions for reporting based on time.**

Telemedicine Modifier

CPT modifier **95** is appended to the appropriate procedure code to identify telemedicine services when rendered via real-time interactive audio and video telecommunications. This modifier is not applied if the communication is not real-time interactive audio and video. Telephone care is not telemedicine.

95   Telemedicine service rendered via a real-time interactive audio and video telecommunications system: Synchronous telemedicine service is defined as a real-time interaction between a physician or other qualified health care professional and a patient who is located at a distant site from the physician or other qualified health care professional. The totality of the communication of information exchanged between the provider or other qualified health care professional and the patient during the course of the synchronous telemedicine service must be of an amount and nature that would be sufficient to meet the key components and/or requirements of the same service when rendered via a face-to-face interaction. Modifier **95** may only be appended to the services listed in Appendix P. Appendix P is the list of *CPT* codes for services that are typically performed face-to-face but may be rendered via a real-time (synchronous) interactive audio and video telecommunications system.

In addition to modifier **95**, *CPT* includes Appendix P, listing all codes to which the **95** modifier is applicable, and adds a star symbol (★) to the listing of each code included in Appendix P in the main body of the manual. Appendix P codes that may be of particular interest to pediatricians include

- New and established patient office or other outpatient E/M services (**99202–99205**, **99212–99215**, **99417**)
- Subsequent hospital care (**99231–99233**)
- Inpatient (**99251–99255**) and outpatient (**99241–99245**) consultations
- Subsequent nursing facility care (**99307–99310**)
- Prolonged services in the outpatient setting (**99354**, **99355**)
- Individual behavior change interventions (**99406–99409**)
- Transitional care management services (**99495**, **99496**)

Appendix P also includes codes for services such as psychotherapy, health and behavior assessment and intervention, medical nutrition therapy, and education and training for patient self-management, allowing for telemedicine services provided by certain qualified nonphysician health care professionals in addition to subspecialty physicians.

Healthcare Common Procedure Coding System (HCPCS) Telehealth Codes and Modifiers

While *CPT* codes are accepted by most plans covering telemedicine services, payers may require HCPCS codes that are used in the Medicare program for consultations and other services with specific coverage policies (eg, telehealth critical care consultation).

- HCPCS codes are used for telemedicine consultations with Medicare beneficiaries because *CPT* consultation codes are not payable under the Medicare Physician Fee Schedule.
- Only specific services are eligible for Medicare payment when provided via telemedicine. The following codes do not apply in all potential settings where telemedicine might be provided (eg, Medicare does not cover telemedicine services to patients in observation settings).
- Exceptions apply for telemedicine services rendered as part of certain demonstration projects (eg, under telehealth waiver for patients associated with a Next Generation accountable care organization).

G0406   Follow-up inpatient consultation, limited, physicians typically spend 15 minutes communicating with the patient via telehealth

G0407   intermediate, physicians typically spend 25 minutes communicating with the patient via telehealth

G0408   complex, physicians typically spend 35 minutes communicating with the patient via telehealth

G0425   Telehealth consultation, emergency department or initial inpatient, typically 30 minutes communicating with the patient via telehealth

G0426   typically 50 minutes communicating with the patient via telehealth

G0427   typically 70 minutes or more communicating with the patient via telehealth

G0459   Inpatient telehealth pharmacologic management, including prescription, use, and review of medication with no more than minimal medical psychotherapy

G0508   Telehealth consultation, critical care, physicians typically spend 60 minutes communicating with the patient via telehealth (initial)

G0509   Telehealth consultation, critical care, physicians typically spend 50 minutes communicating with the patient via telehealth (subsequent)

When a payer uses Medicare program policies for telemedicine services, it is important to learn which services are and are not covered when delivered via telemedicine. A current listing of services covered under the Medicare program is available in Chapter 12 of the *Medicare Claims Processing Manual* (www.cms.gov/Regulations-and-Guidance/Guidance/Manuals/downloads/clm104c12.pdf).

Examples of Coding for Telemedicine Services (*Current Procedural Terminology,* HCPCS)

Examples

➤ **A consultation is requested of a cardiologist at a children's hospital for an inpatient in a rural hospital, 75 miles away.** Through real-time interactive technology, the physician performs a consultation, including a comprehensive history, comprehensive examination (assisted by clinical staff of the facility), and MDM of moderate complexity. The total time of the interactive communication is 30 minutes. A written report to the requesting physician is transmitted via secure electronic health information exchange.

MDM: Moderate *History:* Comprehensive *Physical examination:* Comprehensive	**CPT** **99254 95** (initial inpatient consultation, which requires these 3 key components: ● a comprehensive history; ● a comprehensive examination; ● MDM of moderate complexity) or, if payer requires HCPCS codes, **G0425** (telehealth consultation, emergency department [ED] or initial inpatient, typically 30 minutes communicating with the patient via telehealth)

Teaching Point: If payer policy allows payment for overhead expenses related to telemedicine services, also report **T1014**, telehealth transmission, per minute, professional services bill separately. Because this is billed per minute, 30 units are reported. The rural hospital, as the originating facility, may also report **Q3014**, telehealth originating site facility fee.

A payer that does not accept consultation codes may require that the physician report a code for initial hospital care **(99221–99223 95)** in lieu of the previous codes.

➤ **A child with end-stage renal disease is seen in an ED of a rural hospital.** The ED physician elects to consult the child's nephrologist, who is 250 miles away at a large children's hospital. The nephrologist spends 10 minutes prior to initiation of the interactive telecommunications discussing the case with the attending physician and reviewing prior medical records. The nephrologist then evaluates the patient using audiovisual technology and recommends a plan of care. The nephrologist's total time of interactive communication is 30 minutes, with more than 50% spent in counseling and/or coordination of care. The nephrologist spends another 10 minutes writing orders and documenting the encounter.

Initial outpatient consultation	**CPT** **99242 95** (outpatient consultation for a new or established patient, typical time of 30 minutes) or, if payer requires HCPCS codes, **G0425** (telehealth consultation, ED or initial inpatient, typically 30 minutes communicating with the patient via telehealth) or, if a health plan does not accept consultation codes, **99215 95** for 50 minutes of total physician time spent providing an established patient visit in an office or outpatient setting

Teaching Point: Because the physician spent 30 minutes in real-time audiovisual communication with the patient, code **99242** is reported with modifier **95** appended. The time spent on the phone with the ED physician and reviewing the patient record is not included in the time of the consultation. However, if an office or other outpatient E/M code **(99202–99205, 99211–99215)** is reported, the physician's total time devoted to the patient on the date of service may be used in code selection.

If the patient had been transferred and admitted to the nephrologist's care at the distant facility on the same date, all the nephrologist's E/M services provided on that date would be included in the initial hospital care.

Chapter 20. Digital Medicine Services: Technology-Enhanced Care Delivery

> See Chapter 7 for more information on selection of codes for office and other outpatient evaluation and management services (99202–99205, 99211–99215).

Critical Care Via Telemedicine

CPT codes for critical and intensive care services are not included in Appendix P. *CPT* instructs to report unlisted E/M service code **99499** for critical care provided via telemedicine. (Payers may instruct to append modifier **95** when reporting **99499**.) Payers may include HCPCS codes **G0508** and **G0509** as covered critical care consultation services when provided via telemedicine.

Example

➤ **A pediatric intensivist is contacted via live audiovisual telecommunications to provide remote critical care to an infant who presented with fever, lethargy, and suspected sepsis.** The intensivist views radiographs and other data from monitoring devices in addition to performing visual and audio examination of the infant. The attending physician at the hospital where the infant is an inpatient performs necessary procedures as advised by the intensivist (eg, lumbar puncture). The infant remains at the same hospital under the care of the pediatrician. A total of 65 minutes of remote critical care service is provided.

The neonatologist reports	**G0508** (telehealth consultation, critical care, physicians typically spend 60 minutes communicating with the patient via telehealth [initial])
	or, if a payer does not accept this code,
	99499 (unlisted E/M service) (Enter description of service on claim or attachment.)
The attending physician reports	*CPT* codes for services personally performed (eg, initial hospital care, intubation, lumbar puncture)

Teaching Point: Code **G0508** is reported only once per date of service per patient. Alternatively, the neonatologist may report an inpatient consultation (**99251–99255**) as allowed under the specific payer's policy for telemedicine.

Continuing Changes in Digital Medicine Services

Physicians providing digital medicine services may find that coding and payment policies for these services change from year to year. As adoption of technology increases and evidence of the value of digital medicine services is further demonstrated, codes and payment policies will likely be adapted. It is important that physician practices monitor local and regional payer policies for opportunities to use data in patient management and get paid for the physician work and practice expense of providing these services.

Resources

CPT Telemedicine Code List

CPT list of codes that may be reported with modifier **95** (See Appendix P of your *CPT* coding reference.)

Online Digital E/M Services

"*CPT*® Update: Online Digital Evaluation and Management Services," October 2019 *AAP Pediatric Coding Newsletter*™ (https://coding.solutions.aap.org/article.aspx?articleid=2751907; subscription required)

Health Insurance Portability and Accountability Act of 1996

American Academy of Pediatrics HIPAA privacy and security manual templates (www.aap.org/en-us/professional-resources/practice-transformation/managing-practice/Pages/HIPAA-Privacy-and-Security-Compliance-Manuals.aspx; member log-in required)

Medicare Telehealth Policies and Service List

Medicare telehealth service list (*Medicare Claims Processing Manual*, Chapter 12; www.cms.gov/Regulations-and-Guidance/Guidance/Manuals/downloads/clm104c12.pdf)

Telemedicine Originating Site Eligibility Analyzer

Health Resources and Services Administration Medicare Telehealth Payment Eligibility Analyzer for originating site payment (https://data.hrsa.gov/tools/medicare/telehealth)

Test Your Knowledge!

1. **Which of the following are *not* reported with online digital evaluation and management (E/M) codes 99421–99423?**
   a. An email exchange to answer questions about a medication prescribed at a face-to-face visit 2 days earlier
   b. An email exchange initiated by clinical staff for patient follow-up
   c. A digital encounter within 7 days of an initial encounter for the same problem
   d. All of the above

2. **Which describes the work reported with code 99091?**
   a. Live interactive communication with the patient during a 30-day period
   b. Collection and interpretation of physiologic data collected over a 30-day period
   c. Supply of monitoring equipment
   d. Monitoring of physiologic data over a 30-day period

3. **Which of the following is true regarding Medicaid coverage of telemedicine services?**
   a. Medicaid plans typically align with state regulations for telemedicine services.
   b. All Medicaid plans provide the same coverage of telemedicine services.
   c. Medicaid never covers telemedicine services.
   d. Only asynchronous store-and-forward technology is covered under Medicaid.

4. **Which is a *Current Procedural Terminology* instruction for reporting telemedicine services?**
   a. The service is provided using any digital technology (eg, email).
   b. Only consultations are provided via telemedicine.
   c. Modifier 95 should be appended to the code for telemedicine services.
   d. Telemedicine is limited to certain sites of service.

5. **What time is used to select a code for an office or other outpatient E/M code (99202–99205, 99211–99215) provided via telemedicine?**
   a. The physician's total time devoted to the patient on the date of service
   b. The physician's total time spent in the audiovisual communications
   c. Time cannot be used in code selection for telemedicine services.
   d. The combined time of physicians, other qualified health care professionals, and clinical staff are used in code selection.

Appendixes

More coding resources, including online forms for the documents listed herein, can be accessed at www.aap.org/cfp. Use access code AAPCFP26.

I. Quick Reference to 2021 *ICD-10-CM* Pediatric Code Changes

This quick reference list does not include all changes made to *International Classification of Diseases, 10th Revision, Clinical Modification (ICD-10-CM)*. We have made every effort to include the diagnosis code changes that are most applicable to pediatric practices. However, revisions and/or additional codes may have been published subsequent to the date of this printing. Refer to your 2021 *ICD-10-CM* coding reference (eg, manual, data files) for a complete listing of new and revised codes, complete descriptions, and instructions for reporting. Always begin in the *ICD-10-CM* alphabetic index to locate the code most specific to the condition or other reason for encounter. Codes are valid as of October 1, 2020.

Quick Reference to 2021 *ICD-10-CM* Pediatric Code Changes		
Codes followed by a dash (-) require an additional character. See an *ICD-10-CM* coding reference to complete these codes.		
Aromatic L-amino acid disorder	**E70.81** Aromatic L-amino acid decarboxylase deficiency **E70.89** Other disorders of aromatic amino-acid metabolism	
Arthritis of TMJ	**M26.643** Bilateral	**M26.642** Left	**M26.641** Right
Arthropathy of TMJ	**M26.653** Bilateral	**M26.652** Left	**M26.651** Right
Asthma, eosinophilic	**J82.83** Eosinophilic asthma	
Autoimmune hemolytic anemia	**D59.10** Unspecified **D59.11** Warm autoimmune hemolytic anemia **D59.12** Cold autoimmune hemolytic anemia **D59.13** Mixed type autoimmune hemolytic anemia **D59.19** Other	
Babesiosis	**B60.00** Unspecified **B60.01** Due to Babesia microti **B60.02** Due to Babesia duncani **B60.03** Due to Babesia divergens **B60.09** Other	
C3 Glomerulonephritis (in)	**N00.A** Acute nephritic syndrome **N01.A** Rapidly progressive nephritic syndrome **N02.A** Recurrent and persistent hematuria **N03.A** Chronic nephritic syndrome **N04.A** Nephrotic syndrome **N05.A** Unspecified nephritic syndrome **N06.A** Isolated proteinuria **N07.A** Hereditary nephropathy, NEC	
Cerebral ataxia	**G11.10** Early-onset cerebellar ataxia, unspecified **G11.11** Friedreich ataxia **G11.19** Other early-onset cerebellar ataxia	
Cerebrospinal fluid leak	**G96.00** Unspecified **G96.01** Cranial cerebrospinal fluid leak, spontaneous **G96.02** Spinal cerebrospinal fluid leak, spontaneous **G96.08** Other cranial cerebrospinal fluid leak **G96.09** Other spinal cerebrospinal fluid leak	
Chronic kidney disease, stage 3	**N18.30** Unspecified **N18.31** Stage 3a **N18.32** Stage 3b	
Congenital myopathy	**G71.20** Unspecified **G71.21** Nemaline myopathy **G71.220** X-linked myotubular myopathy **G71.228** Other centronuclear myopathy **G71.29** Other	

●=New code ▲=Revised code #=Re-sequenced code +=Add-on code

Appendixes

Quick Reference to 2021 *ICD-10-CM* Pediatric Code Changes (*continued*)

Codes followed by a dash (-) require an additional character. See an *ICD-10-CM* coding reference to complete these codes.

Contusion of back wall of thorax[a]	S20.223- Bilateral back wall of thorax S20.224- Middle back wall of thorax		
Corneal dystrophy, epithelial (juvenile)	**H18.523** Bilateral	**H18.522** Left	**H18.521** Right
Corneal dystrophies, hereditary	**H18.5-** (Refer to the *ICD-10-CM* manual for full details.)		
Cyclin-dependent kinase-like 5 deficiency disorder	**G40.42** Cyclin-dependent kinase-like 5 deficiency disorder		
Cytokine release syndrome	**D89.831** Grade 1 **D89.832** Grade 2 **D89.833** Grade 3 **D89.834** Grade 4 **D89.835** Grade 5 **D89.839** Grade unspecified		
Disorder of carbohydrate metabolism	**E74.810** Glucose transporter protein type 1 deficiency **E74.818** Other disorders of glucose transport **E74.819** Disorders of glucose transport, unspecified **E74.89** Other specified		
Disorder of central nervous system	**G96.89** Other specified		
Dravet syndrome, intractable	**G40.833** With status epilepticus **G40.834** Without status epilepticus		
Elevation of lactic acid dehydrogenase	**R74.02** Elevation of levels of lactic acid dehydrogenase (LDH)		
Elevation of liver transaminase	**R74.01** Elevation of levels of liver transaminase levels		
Eosinophilia	**D72.10** Eosinophilia, unspecified **D72.110** Idiopathic hypereosinophilic syndrome (IHES) **D72.111** Lymphocytic Variant Hypereosinophilic Syndrome (LHES) **D72.118** Other hypereosinophilic syndrome **D72.119** Hypereosinophilic syndrome (HES), unspecified **D72.12** Drug rash with eosinophilia and systemic symptoms syndrome **D72.18** Eosinophilia in diseases classified elsewhere **D72.19** Other eosinophilia		
Esophagitis	**K20.80** Other esophagitis without bleeding **K20.81** Other esophagitis with bleeding **K20.90** Esophagitis, unspecified without bleeding **K20.91** Esophagitis, unspecified with bleeding		
Foreign body suspected, ruled out after observation	**Z03.821** Suspected ingested foreign body **Z03.822** Suspected aspirated (inhaled) foreign body **Z03.823** Suspected inserted (injected) foreign body		
Gastroesophageal reflux disease with esophagitis	**K21.00** Without bleeding **K21.01** With bleeding		
Headache	**R51.0** With orthostatic component, NEC **R51.9** Unspecified		

Quick Reference to 2021 *ICD-10-CM* Pediatric Code Changes (*continued*)

Codes followed by a dash (-) require an additional character. See an *ICD-10-CM* coding reference to complete these codes.

Immunodeficiency	**D84.81**	Due to conditions classified elsewhere
	D84.821	Due to drugs
	D84.822	Due to external causes
	D84.89	Other immunodeficiencies
Injury, superficial, bilateral front wall of thorax[a]	**S20.313-**	Abrasion
	S20.323-	Blister (nonthermal)
	S20.213-	Contusion
	S20.343-	External constriction
	S20.363-	Insect bite (nonvenomous)
	S20.373-	Other superficial bite
	S20.303-	Unspecified superficial injuries
	S20.353-	Superficial foreign body
Injury, superficial, middle front wall of thoraxa	**S20.314-**	Abrasion
	S20.324-	Blister (nonthermal)
	S20.214-	Contusion
	S20.344-	External constriction
	S20.364-	Insect bite (nonvenomous)
	S20.374-	Other superficial bite
	S20.304-	Unspecified superficial injuries
	S20.354-	Superficial foreign body
Intracranial hypotension	**G96.810**	Unspecified
	G96.811	Spontaneous
	G96.819	Other intracranial hypotension
	G97.83	Following lumbar cerebrospinal fluid shunting
	G97.84	Following other procedure
Joint-related disorder, other specified joint	**M24.19**	Other articular cartilage disorders
	M24.29	Disorder of ligament, other specified site
	M24.39	Pathological dislocation, NEC
	M24.49	Recurrent dislocation
	M24.59	Contracture
	M24.69	Ankylosis
	M24.89	Other specific joint derangement, NEC
	M25.39	Other instability
	M25.59	Pain
	M25.69	Stiffness, NEC
Juvenile arthritis, unspecified	**M08.9A**	Other specified site

Juvenile osteochondrosis	Right leg	Left leg	Bilateral leg
Proximal tibia	**M92.511**	**M92.512**	**M92.513**
Tibia and fibula, other	**M92.591**	**M92.592**	**M92.593**
Tibia tubercle	**M92.521**	**M92.522**	**M92.523**
Unspecified	**M92.501**	**M92.502**	**M92.503**

Neonatal cerebral infarction	**P91.821**	Right side of brain
	P91.822	Left side of brain
	P91.823	Bilateral
	P91.829	Unspecified side
Powassan virus disease and other tick-borne viral encephalitis	**A84.81**	Powassan virus disease
	A84.89	Other tick-borne viral encephalitis

Appendixes

Quick Reference to 2021 *ICD-10-CM* Pediatric Code Changes (*continued*)

Codes followed by a dash (-) require an additional character. See an *ICD-10-CM* coding reference to complete these codes.

Rheumatoid arthritis, other specified site	M05.7A	With rheumatoid factor without organ or systems involvement
	M05.8A	Other, with rheumatoid factor
	M06.0A	Without rheumatoid factor
	M06.8A	Other specified
	M08.0A	Unspecified juvenile
	M08.2A	Juvenile with systemic onset
	M08.4A	Pauciarticular juvenile
Sickle cell disorders, other	D57.813	With cerebral vascular involvement
	D57.818	With crisis with other specified complication
Sickle cell/Hb-C disease	D57.213	With cerebral vascular involvement
	D57.218	With crisis with other specified complication
Sickle cell/Hb-SS disease	D57.03	With cerebral vascular involvement
	D57.09	With other specified complication
Sickle cell thalassemia, unspecified	D57.413	With cerebral vascular involvement
	D57.418	With crisis with other specified complication
Sickle cell thalassemia beta zero	D57.42	Without crisis
	D57.431	With acute chest syndrome
	D57.432	With splenic sequestration
	D57.433	With cerebral vascular involvement
	D57.438	With crisis with other specified complication
	D57.439	With crisis, unspecified
Sickle cell thalassemia beta plus	D57.44	Without crisis
	D57.451	With acute chest syndrome
	D57.452	With splenic sequestration
	D57.453	With cerebral vascular involvement
	D57.458	With crisis with other specified complication
	D57.459	With crisis, unspecified

Withdrawal due to	Uncomplicated	With withdrawal delirium	With perceptual disturbance	Unspecified
Abuse of other psychoactive substance	F19.130	F19.131	F19.132	F19.139
Abuse of sedative, hypnotic, or anxiolytic	F13.130	F13.131	F13.132	F13.139
Alcohol abuse	F10.130	F10.131	F10.132	F10.139
Alcohol use	F10.930	F10.931	F10.932	F10.939
Cannabis abuse	F12.13	Cannabis abuse with withdrawal		
Cocaine abuse/use	F14.13	Cocaine abuse, unspecified with withdrawal		
	F14.93	Cocaine use, unspecified with withdrawal		
Opioid abuse	F11.13	Opioid abuse with withdrawal		
Other stimulant abuse	F15.13	Other stimulant abuse with withdrawal		

External Injury Causes: Several new codes were added to indicate that an injury or other medical issue was caused by accidents involving an e-scooter or other electronic mobility device, such as a Segway or hoverboard.

Abbreviations: NEC, not elsewhere classified; TMJ, temporomandibular joint.

ª Seventh character required (**A, D,** or **S**). See *ICD-10-CM* tabular list for full codes.

II. Quick Reference to 2021 *CPT®* Pediatric Code Changes

We have made every effort to include changes to procedures and services that are applicable to pediatric practices in this appendix. However, revisions and/or additional codes may have been published subsequent to the date of this printing. This list does not include all changes made to *Current Procedural Terminology (CPT) 2021.* Also, not all codes included in the quick reference table are further discussed in this publication (typically due to limited use by most pediatricians). Codes not discussed elsewhere are shaded in gray. Always refer to *CPT 2021* for a complete listing of new codes, complete descriptions, and revisions. For questions or additional information on codes not discussed in this publication, please contact the American Academy of Pediatrics Coding Hotline (https://form.jotform.com/Subspecialty/aapcodinghotline). Any errata to *CPT 2021* will be posted to the American Medical Association website, https://www.ama-assn.org/practice-management/cpt/errata-technical-corrections. These changes take effect January 1, 2021. Do not report the changes or codes prior to that date.

Quick Reference to 2021 *CPT* Pediatric Code Changes	
2020	**2021**
Evaluation and Management	
★**99201** Office or other outpatient visit for the evaluation and management of a new patient, which requires these 3 key components: ● A problem focused history; ● A problem focused examination; ● Straightforward medical decision making. ● Counseling and/or coordination of care with other physicians, other qualified health care professionals, or agencies are provided consistent with the nature of the problem(s) and the patient's and/or family's needs. ● Usually, the presenting problem(s) are self-limited or minor. Typically, 10 minutes are spent face-to-face with the patient and/or family.	See **99202**. See **Chapter 7** for more information.
★**99202** Office or other outpatient visit for the evaluation and management of a new patient, which requires these 3 key components: ● An expanded problem focused history; ● An expanded problem focused examination; ● Straightforward medical decision making. ● Counseling and/or coordination of care with other physicians, other qualified health care professionals, or agencies are provided consistent with the nature of the problem(s) and the patient's and/or family's needs. ● Usually, the presenting problem(s) are of low to moderate severity. Typically, 20 minutes are spent face-to-face with the patient and/or family.	★▲**99202** Office or other outpatient visit for the evaluation and management of a new patient, which requires a medically appropriate history and/or examination and straightforward medical decision making. When using time for code selection, 15–29 minutes of total time is spent on the date of the encounter.
★**99203** Office or other outpatient visit for the evaluation and management of a new patient, which requires these 3 key components: ● A detailed history; ● A detailed examination; ● Medical decision making of low complexity. ● Counseling and/or coordination of care with other physicians, other qualified health care professionals, or agencies are provided consistent with the nature of the problem(s) and the patient's and/or family's needs. ● Usually, the presenting problem(s) are of moderate severity. Typically, 30 minutes are spent face-to-face with the patient and/or family.	★▲**99203** Office or other outpatient visit for the evaluation and management of a new patient, which requires a medically appropriate history and/or examination and low level of medical decision making. When using time for code selection, 30–44 minutes of total time is spent on the date of the encounter.

Appendixes

Quick Reference to 2021 *CPT* Pediatric Code Changes (*continued*)	
2020	**2021**
Evaluation and Management (*continued*)	
★99204 Office or other outpatient visit for the evaluation and management of a new patient, which requires these 3 key components: ● A comprehensive history; ● A comprehensive examination; ● Medical decision making of moderate complexity. ● Counseling and/or coordination of care with other physicians, other qualified health care professionals, or agencies are provided consistent with the nature of the problem(s) and the patient's and/or family's needs. ● Usually, the presenting problem(s) are of moderate to high severity. Typically, 45 minutes are spent face-to-face with the patient and/or family.	★▲99204 Office or other outpatient visit for the evaluation and management of a new patient, which requires a medically appropriate history and/or examination and moderate level of medical decision making. When using time for code selection, 45–59 minutes of total time is spent on the date of the encounter.
★99205 Office or other outpatient visit for the evaluation and management of a new patient, which requires these 3 key components: ● A comprehensive history; ● A comprehensive examination; ● Medical decision making of high complexity. ● Counseling and/or coordination of care with other physicians, other qualified health care professionals, or agencies are provided consistent with the nature of the problem(s) and the patient's and/or family's needs. ● Usually, the presenting problem(s) are of moderate to high severity. Typically, 60 minutes are spent face-to-face with the patient and/or family.	★▲99205 Office or other outpatient visit for the evaluation and management of a new patient, which requires a medically appropriate history and/or examination and high level of medical decision making. When using time for code selection, 60–74 minutes of total time is spent on the date of the encounter.
99211 Office or other outpatient visit for the evaluation and management of an established patient, that may not require the presence of a physician or other qualified health care professional. Usually, the presenting problem(s) are minimal. Typically, 5 minutes are spent performing or supervising these services.	▲99211 Office or other outpatient visit for the evaluation and management of an established patient, that may not require the presence of a physician or other qualified health care professional. Usually, the presenting problem(s) are minimal.
★99212 Office or other outpatient visit for the evaluation and management of an established patient, which requires at least 2 of these 3 key components: ● A problem focused history; ● A problem focused examination; ● Straightforward medical decision making. ● Counseling and/or coordination of care with other physicians, other qualified health care professionals, or agencies are provided consistent with the nature of the problem(s) and the patient's and/or family's needs. ● Usually, the presenting problem(s) are self-limited or minor. Typically, 10 minutes are spent face-to-face with the patient and/or family.	★▲99212 Office or other outpatient visit for the evaluation and management of an established patient, which requires a medically appropriate history and/or examination and straightforward medical decision making. When using time for code selection, 10–19 minutes of total time is spent on the date of the encounter.
★99213 Office or other outpatient visit for the evaluation and management of an established patient, which requires at least 2 of these 3 key components: ● An expanded problem focused history; ● An expanded problem focused examination; ● Medical decision making of low complexity. ● Counseling and coordination of care with other physicians, other qualified health care professionals, or agencies are provided consistent with the nature of the problem(s) and the patient's and/or family's needs. ● Usually, the presenting problem(s) are of low to moderate severity. Typically, 15 minutes are spent face-to-face with the patient and/or family.	★▲99213 Office or other outpatient visit for the evaluation and management of an established patient, which requires a medically appropriate history and/or examination and low level of medical decision making. When using time for code selection, 20–29 minutes of total time is spent on the date of the encounter.

Quick Reference to 2021 *CPT* Pediatric Code Changes (*continued*)

2020	2021
Evaluation and Management (*continued*)	

2020	2021
★**99214** Office or other outpatient visit for the evaluation and management of an established patient, which requires at least 2 of these 3 key components: ● A detailed history; ● A detailed examination; ● Medical decision making of moderate complexity. ● Counseling and/or coordination of care with other physicians, other qualified health care professionals, or agencies are provided consistent with the nature of the problem(s) and the patient's and/or family's needs. ● Usually, the presenting problem(s) are of moderate to highseverity. Typically, 25 minutes are spent face-to-face with the patient and/or family.	★▲**99214** Office or other outpatient visit for the evaluation and management of an established patient, which requires a medically appropriate history and/or examination and moderate level of medical decision making. When using time for code selection, 30–39 minutes of total time is spent on the date of the encounter.
★**99215** Office or other outpatient visit for the evaluation and management of an established patient, which requires at least 2 of these 3 key components: ● A comprehensive history; ● A comprehensive examination; ● Medical decision making of high complexity. ● Counseling and/or coordination of care with other physicians, other qualified health care professionals, or agencies are provided consistent with the nature of the problem(s) and the patient's and/or family's needs. ● Usually, the presenting problem(s) are of moderate to high severity. Typically, 40 minutes are spent face-to-face with the patient and/or family.	★▲**99215** Office or other outpatient visit for the evaluation and management of an established patient, which requires a medically appropriate history and/or examination and high level of medical decision making. When using time for code selection, 40–54 minutes of total time is spent on the date of the encounter.
99490 Chronic care management services, at least 20 minutes of clinical staff time directed by a physician or other qualified health care professional, per calendar month, with the following required elements: ● multiple (two or more) chronic conditions expected to last at least 12 months, or until the death of the patient; ● chronic conditions place the patient at significant risk of death, acute exacerbation/decompensation, or functional decline; ● comprehensive care plan established, implemented, revised, or monitored.	#▲**99490** Chronic care management services, with the following required elements: ● multiple (two or more) chronic conditions expected to last at least 12 months, or until the death of the patient, ● chronic conditions place the patient at significant risk of death, acute exacerbation/decompensation, or functional decline, ● comprehensive care plan established, implemented, revised, or monitored; first 20 minutes of clinical staff time directed by a physician or other qualified health care professional, per calendar month. #+●**99439** each additional 20 minutes of clinical staff time directed by a physician or other qualified health care professional, per calendar month (List separately in addition to code for primary procedure)

Appendixes

Quick Reference to 2021 *CPT* Pediatric Code Changes (*continued*)	
2020	**2021**
Evaluation and Management (*continued*)	
99487 Complex chronic care management services, with the following required elements: • multiple (two or more) chronic conditions expected to last at least 12 months, or until the death of the patient, • chronic conditions place the patient at significant risk of death, acute exacerbation/decompensation, or functional decline, • establishment or substantial revision of a comprehensive care plan, • moderate or high complexity medical decision making; • 60 minutes of clinical staff time directed by physician or other qualified health care professional, per calendar month. **+99489** each additional 30 minutes of clinical staff time directed by a physician or other qualified health care professional, per calendar month (List separately in addition to code for primary procedure)	**▲99487** Complex chronic care management services, with the following required elements: • multiple (two or more) chronic conditions expected to last at least 12 months, or until the death of the patient, • chronic conditions place the patient at significant risk of death, acute exacerbation/decompensation, or functional decline, • comprehensive care plan established, implemented, revised, or monitored, • moderate or high complexity medical decision making; first 60 minutes of clinical staff time directed by physician or other qualified health care professional, per calendar month. **+▲99489** each additional 30 minutes of clinical staff time directed by a physician or other qualified health care professional, per calendar month (List separately in addition to code for primary procedure)
★+99354 Prolonged evaluation and management or psychotherapy service(s) (beyond the typical service time of the primary procedure) in the office or other outpatient setting requiring direct patient contact beyond the usual service; first hour (List separately in addition to code for office or other outpatient Evaluation and Management or psychotherapy service) **★+99355** each additional 30 minutes	**★+▲99354** Prolonged service(s) in the outpatient setting requiring direct patient contact beyond the time of the usual service; first hour (List separately in addition to code for outpatient Evaluation and Management or psychotherapy service, except with office or other outpatient services [**99202–99215**]) **★+▲99355** each additional 30 minutes
#+99415 Prolonged clinical staff service (the service beyond the typical service time) during an evaluation and management service in the office or outpatient setting, direct patient contact with physician supervision; first hour (List separately in addition to code for outpatient Evaluation and Management service) **#+99416** each additional 30 minutes (List separately in addition to code for prolonged service)	**#+▲99415** Prolonged clinical staff service (the service beyond the highest time in the range of total time of the service) during an evaluation and management service in the office or outpatient setting, direct patient contact with physician supervision; first hour (List separately in addition to code for outpatient Evaluation and Management service) **#+▲99416** each additional 30 minutes (List separately in addition to code for prolonged service)
No code (previously reported with **99354–99355** or **99358**)	**#+●99417** Prolonged office or other outpatient evaluation and management service(s) beyond the minimum required time of the primary procedure which has been selected using total time, requiring total time with or without direct patient contact beyond the usual service, on the date of the primary service, each 15 minutes of total time (List separately in addition to codes **99205**, **99215** for office or other outpatient Evaluation and Management services)
Musculoskeletal System	
29822 Arthroscopy, shoulder, surgical; debridement, limited	**▲29822** debridement, limited, 1 or 2 discrete structures (eg, humeral bone and articular cartilage, glenoid bone and articular cartilage, biceps and biceps anchor complex, labrum, articular capsule, articular side of the rotator cuff, bursal side of the rotator cuff, subacromial bursa, foreign bodies)

●=New code   ▲=Revised code   #=Re-sequenced code   +=Add-on code

Quick Reference to 2021 *CPT* Pediatric Code Changes (*continued*)

2020	2021
Musculoskeletal System (*continued*)	
29823 Arthroscopy, shoulder, surgical; debridement, extensive	▲29823 debridement, extensive, 3 or more discrete structures (eg, humeral bone/humeral articular cartilage, glenoid bone/glenoid articular cartilage, biceps and biceps anchor complex, labrum, articular capsule, articular side of the rotator cuff, bursal side of the rotator cuff, subacromial bursa, foreign bodies)
Respiratory	
30999 Unlisted procedure, nose	●30468 Repair of nasal valve collapse with subcutaneous/submucosal lateral wall implant(s)
Cardiovascular	
92992 Atrial septectomy or septostomy; transvenous method, balloon (eg, Rashkind type) (includes cardiac catheterization) 92993 blade method (Park septostomy) (includes cardiac catheterization)	●33741 Transcatheter atrial septostomy (TAS) for congenital cardiac anomalies to create effective atrial flow, including all imaging guidance by the proceduralist, when performed, any method (eg, Rashkind, Sang-Park, balloon, cutting balloon, blade) ●33745 Transcatheter intracardiac shunt (TIS) creation by stent placement for congenital cardiac anomalies to establish effective intracardiac flow, all imaging guidance by the proceduralist, when performed, left and right heart diagnostic cardiac catheterization for congenital cardiac anomalies, and target zone angioplasty, when performed (eg, atrial septum, Fontan fenestration, right ventricular outflow tract, Mustard/Senning/Warden baffles); initial intracardiac shunt +●33746 each additional intracardiac shunt location (List separately in addition to code for primary procedure)
Immune Globulins, Serum, or Recombinant Products	
No code	●90377 Rabies immune globulin, heat- and solvent/detergent-treated (RIg-HT S/D), human, for intramuscular and/or subcutaneous use
Audiologic Function Tests	
92585 Auditory evoked potentials for evoked response audiometry and/or testing of the central nervous system; comprehensive 92586 Auditory evoked potentials for evoked response audiometry and/or testing of the central nervous system; limited	#●92650 Auditory evoked potentials; screening of auditory potential with broadband stimuli, automated analysis #●92651 for hearing status determination, broadband stimuli, with interpretation and report #●92652 for threshold estimation at multiple frequencies, with interpretation and report #●92653 neurodiagnostic, with interpretation and report
Pulmonary	
94617 Exercise test for bronchospasm, including pre- and post-spirometry, electrocardiographic recording(s), and pulse oximetry	▲94617 Exercise test for bronchospasm, including pre- and post-spirometry and pulse oximetry; with electrocardiographic recording(s) ●94619 without electrocardiographic recording(s)

Appendixes

Quick Reference to 2021 *CPT* Pediatric Code Changes (*continued*)	
2020	**2021**
Medicine: Special Services, Procedures, and Reports	
No specific code	●**99072** Additional supplies, materials, and clinical staff time over and above those usually included in an office visit or other non-facility service(s), when performed during a Public Health Emergency as defined by law, due to respiratory-transmitted infectious disease
Category III	
No specific codes	●**0604T** Optical coherence tomography (OCT) of retina, remote, patient-initiated image capture and transmission to a remote surveillance center unilateral or bilateral; initial device provision, set-up and patient education on use of equipment ●**0605T** remote surveillance center technical support, data analyses and reports, with a minimum of 8 daily recordings, each 30 days ●**0606T** review and interpretation and report by the prescribing physician or other qualified health care professional of remote surveillance center data analyses, each 30 days
No specific code	●**0615T** Eye movement analysis without spatial calibration, with interpretation and report
No specific code	●**0594T** Osteotomy, humerus, with insertion of an externally controlled intramedullary lengthening device, including intraoperative imaging, initial and subsequent alignment assessments, computations of adjustment schedules, and management of the intramedullary lengthening device
No specific code	●**0639T** Wireless skin sensor thermal anisotropy measurement(s) and assessment of flow in cerebrospinal fluid shunt, including ultrasound guidance, when performed

Appendixes

III. Vaccine Products: Commonly Administered Pediatric Vaccines

This list was current as of September 1, 2020. For updates, visit www.aap.org/cfp (access code AAPCFP26).

CPT Product Code	Separately report the administration with *CPT*® codes 90460–90461 or 90471–90474. See below.	Manufacturer	Brand	# of Vaccine Components
90702	Diphtheria and tetanus toxoids (**DT**), adsorbed when administered to <7 years, for IM use	SP	**Diphtheria and tetanus toxoids adsorbed (no trade name)**	2
90700	Diphtheria, tetanus toxoids, and acellular pertussis vaccine (**DTaP**), when administered to <7 years, for IM use	SP GSK	**DAPTACEL Infanrix**	3
90696	Diphtheria, tetanus toxoids, and acellular pertussis vaccine and inactivated poliovirus vaccine (**DTaP-IPV**), when administered to children 4–6 years of age, for IM use	GSK SP	**KINRIX Quadracel**	4
90697	Diphtheria, tetanus toxoids, acellular pertussis vaccine, inactivated poliovirus vaccine, Haemophilus influenza type b PRP-OMP conjugate vaccine, and hepatitis B vaccine (**DTaP-IPV-Hib-HepB**), for IM use	Merck/SP	**VAXELIS**	6
90723	Diphtheria, tetanus toxoids, acellular pertussis vaccine, Hepatitis B, and inactivated poliovirus vaccine (**DTaP-HepB-IPV**), for IM use	GSK	**Pediarix**	5
90698	Diphtheria, tetanus toxoids, acellular pertussis vaccine, haemophilus influenza Type B, and inactivated poliovirus vaccine (**DTaP-IPV/Hib**), for IM use	SP	**Pentacel**	5
90633	Hepatitis A vaccine (**HepA**), pediatric/adolescent dosage, 2 dose, for IM use	GSK Merck	**Havrix VAQTA**	1
90740	Hepatitis B vaccine (**HepB**), dialysis or immunosuppressed patient dosage, 3 dose, for IM use	Merck	**Recombivax HB**	1
90743	Hepatitis B vaccine (**HepB**), adolescent, 2 dose, for IM use	Merck	**Recombivax HB**	1
90744	Hepatitis B vaccine (**HepB**), pediatric/adolescent dosage, 3 dose, for IM use	Merck GSK	**Recombivax HB Engerix-B**	1
90746	Hepatitis B vaccine (**HepB**), adult dosage, for IM use	Merck GSK	**Recombivax HB Engerix-B**	1
90747	Hepatitis B vaccine (**HepB**), dialysis or immunosuppressed patient dosage, 4 dose, for IM use	GSK	**Engerix-B**	1
90647	Hemophilus influenza B vaccine (**Hib**), PRP-OMP conjugate, 3 dose, for IM use	Merck	**PedvaxHIB**	1
90648	Hemophilus influenza B vaccine (**Hib**), PRP-T conjugate, 4 dose, for IM use	SP GSK	**ActHIB Hiberix**	1
90651	Human Papillomavirus vaccine types 6, 11, 16, 18, 31, 33, 45, 52, 58, nonavalent (9v **HPV**), 2 or 3 dose schedule, for IM use	Merck	**Gardasil**	1
#90672	**Influenza** virus vaccine, quad (LAIV), live, intranasal use	AstraZeneca	**FluMist Quadrivalent**	1

Appendixes

●=New code   ▲=Revised code   #=Re-sequenced code   +=Add-on code

CPT Product Code	Separately report the administration with *CPT* codes 90460–90461 or 90471–90474. See below.	Manufacturer	Brand	# of Vaccine Components
#90674	**Influenza** virus vaccine, quad (ccIIV4), derived from cell cultures, subunit, preservative and antibiotic free, 0.5 mL dosage, IM	Seqirus	**Flucelvax Quadrivalent**	1
90685	**Influenza** virus vaccine, quad (IIV4), split virus, preservative free, 0.25mL dose, for IM use	Seqirus GSK SP	**AFLURIA Quadrivalent Fluzone Quadrivalent**	1
90686	**Influenza** virus vaccine, quad (IIV4), split virus, preservative free, 0.5mL dose, for IM use	Seqirus SP GSK GSK	**AFLURIA Quadrivalent Fluzone Quadrivalent FluLaval Quadrivalent**	1
90687	**Influenza** virus vaccine, quad (IIV4), split virus, 0.25mL dose, for IM use	Seqirus SP	**AFLURIA Quadrivalent Fluzone Quadrivalent**	1
90688	**Influenza** virus vaccine, quad (IIV4), split virus, 0.5mL dose, for IM use	Seqirus SP	**AFLURIA Quadrivalent Fluzone Quadrivalent**	1
#90756	**Influenza** virus vaccine, quad (ccIIV4), derived from cell cultures, subunit, antibiotic free, 0.5mL dose, for IM use	Seqirus	**Flucelvax Quadrivalent**	1
90707	Measles, mumps, and rubella virus vaccine (**MMR**), live, for subcutaneous use	Merck	**M-M-R II**	3
90710	Measles, mumps, rubella, and varicella vaccine (**MMRV**), live, for subcutaneous use	Merck	**ProQuad**	4
#90620	**Meningococcal** recombinant protein and outer membrane vesicle vaccine, serogroup B (MenB-4C), 2 dose schedule, for IM use	GSK	**Bexsero**	1
#90621	**Meningococcal** recombinant lipoprotein vaccine, serogroup B, 2 or 3 dose schedule, for IM use	Pfizer	**TRUMENBA**	1
90734	**Meningococcal** conjugate vaccine, serogroups A, C, W, and Y, quad, diphtheria toxoid carrier (MenACWY-D) or CRM197 carrier (MenACWY-CRM), for IM use	SP GSK	**Menactra Menveo**	1
#90619	**Meningococcal** conjugate vaccine, serogroups A, C, W, Y, quad, tetanus toxoid carrier (MenACWY-TT), for IM use	SP	**MenQuadfi**	1
90670	**Pneumococcal** conjugate vaccine, 13 valent (PCV13), for IM use	Pfizer	**Prevnar 13**	1
90732	**Pneumococcal** polysaccharide vaccine, 23 valent (PPSV23), adult or immunosuppressed patient dosage, when administered to ≥2 years, for subcutaneous or IM use	Merck	**Pneumovax 23**	1
90713	**Poliovirus** vaccine (IPV), inactivated, for subcutaneous or IM use	SP	**IPOL**	1
90680	**Rotavirus** vaccine, pentavalent (RV5), 3 dose schedule, live, for oral use	Merck	**RotaTeq**	1
90681	**Rotavirus** vaccine, human, attenuated (RV1), 2 dose schedule, live, for oral use	GSK	**ROTARIX**	1

Appendixes

CPT Product Code	Separately report the administration with *CPT*® codes 90460–90461 or 90471–90474. See below.	Manufacturer	Brand	# of Vaccine Components
90714	Tetanus and diphtheria toxoids (**Td**) adsorbed, preservative free, when administered to ≥7 years, for IM use	MBL SP	**TDVAX** **TENIVAC**	2
90715	Tetanus, diphtheria toxoids and acellular pertussis vaccine (**Tdap**), when administered to ≥7 years, for IM use	SP GSK	**Adacel** **Boostrix**	3
90716	**Varicella** virus vaccine (VAR), live, for subcutaneous use	Merck	**Varivax**	1
90749	**Unlisted vaccine or toxoid**	Please see *CPT* manual.		
Immunization Administration (IA) Codes				
IA Through Age 18 With Counseling				
90460	IA through 18 years of age via any route of administration, with counseling by physician or other qualified health care professional; first or only component of each vaccine or toxoid component administered (Do not report with **90471** or **90473**)			
+90461	IA through 18 years of age via any route of administration, with counseling by physician or other qualified health care professional; each additional vaccine or toxoid component administered			
Immunization Administration				
90471	IA, one injected vaccine (*Do not report with* **90460** *or* **90473***)*			
+90472	IA, each additional injected vaccine			
90473	IA by intranasal/oral route; one vaccine (Do not report with **90460** or **90471**)			
+90474	IA by intranasal/oral route; each additional vaccine			
# Re-sequenced code, + Add-on code				

Appendixes

●=New code   ▲=Revised code   #=Re-sequenced code   +=Add-on code

IV. Global Per Diem Critical Care Codes: Direct Supervision and Reporting Guidelines

Global Per Diem Critical Care Codes: Direct Supervision and Reporting Guidelines

The delivery of neonatal and pediatric critical care has undergone significant changes in the last 2 decades, incorporating expanded technology and services as well as new patterns of delivery of care. Neonatal intensive care units (NICUs) have grown dramatically as improvements in perinatal care have led to markedly improved survival rates of the small preterm neonate. There has also been a growing national population with major socioeconomic shifts. These changes have led to a large increase in NICU beds. Simultaneous to these demographic and epidemiologic changes, serious Accreditation Council for Graduate Medical Education and Residency Review Committee limitations in resident and fellow work hours and, more specifically, to those hours allocated to clinical care in the NICU have reduced the number of house officers providing neonatal critical care. There has been a rapid expansion of other neonatal providers working as a team in partnership with an attending physician to meet expanding bedside patient care needs. These nonphysician providers (NPPs by Centers for Medicare & Medicaid Services nomenclature) are primarily neonatal nurse practitioners (NNPs). They have assumed a critical role in assisting the attending physician in caring for this expanding population of patients.

Neither NNPs nor residents or fellows are substitutes for the attending physician, who continues to remain fully in charge of these patients and directly supervises NNPs and residents or fellow physicians as well as other ancillary providers (eg, registered nurses, respiratory therapists, nutritionists, social workers, physical therapists, occupational therapists), who all play important contributory roles in the care of these critical patients. Unlike the supervision for residents or fellows enrolled in graduate medical education programs, the attending physician's supervision and documentation of care provided by NNPs is not covered by Physicians at Teaching Hospitals (PATH) guidelines. The attending physician is not "sharing services" with the NNP or resident or fellow. The attending physician (the physician responsible for the patient's care and reporting the service for that date) remains solely responsible for the supervision of the team and development of the patient's plan of care. In developing that plan, the attending physician will use the information acquired by and discussed with other members of the care team, including that of the resident or fellow and NNP.

When supervising residents or fellows, the attending physician will use this collective information as part of his or her own documentation of care. The attending physician must demonstrate in his or her own note that he or she has reviewed this information, performed his or her own focused examination of the patient, documented any additional findings or disagreements with the resident's or fellow's findings, and discussed the plan of care with the resident or fellow to meet PATH guideline requirements. These rules allow the attending physician to use the resident or fellow note as a major component of his or her own note and in determining the level of care the attending physician will report for that patient on that date.

Physicians at Teaching Hospitals guidelines do not apply to patients cared for by NNPs because NNPs are not enrolled in postgraduate education. This is true whether the NNP is employed by the hospital, medical group, or independent contractor. Centers for Medicare & Medicaid Services rules prohibit NPPs (in this case NNPs) and the reporting physician from reporting "shared or split services" when critical care services are provided. The reporting physician may certainly review and use the important information and observation of the NNPs, but the physician also provides his or her own evaluation along with documentation of the services he or she personally provided. Documentation expectations for the reporting physician include review of the notes and observations of other members of the care team; an independent-focused, medically appropriate bedside examination of the patient; and documentation that he or she has directed the plan of care for each patient whose services the physician reports. In many critically ill but stable patients, this requirement can be met by a single daily note. In situations in which the patient is very unstable and dramatic changes and major additional interventions are required to maintain stability, more extensive or frequent documentations are likely and may be entered by any qualified member of the care team.

In some states, NNPs, through expanded state licenses, are permitted to independently report their services. If these NNPs are credentialed by the hospital and health plan to provide critical care services and procedures and possess their own National Provider Identifier (NPI), they may independently report the services they provide. In these states, they can function as independent contractors or as employees of the hospital or a medical group, reporting their services under their own NPI. It is important to emphasize again that the NNP and the physician do not report a shared critical care service. Critical care services are reported under the NNP or physician NPI, dependent on who was primarily providing the patient service and directing the care of the patient. Two providers may not report a global per diem critical care code (eg, **99468**, **99469**) on the same date of service. In most situations, the physician is serving as responsible and supervising provider and the NNP (employed by the group or hospital) is acting as a member of the team of providers the physician supervises.

Physician Supervision

Current Procedural Terminology ® states that codes **99468–99476** (initial and subsequent inpatient neonatal and pediatric critical care, per day, for the evaluation and management of a critically ill neonate or child through 5 years of age) are used to report services provided by a physician directing the inpatient care of a critically ill neonate or young child. *Current Procedural Terminology* makes clear that the reporting provider is not required to maintain a 24-hour, in-hospital physical presence. *Current Procedural Terminology* notes that the physician or other reporting provider must be physically present and at bedside at some time during the 24-hour period to examine the patient and review and direct the patient's care with the health care team. The physician must be readily available to the health care team if needed

●=New code   ▲=Revised code   #=Re-sequenced code   +=Add-on code

Global Per Diem Critical Care Codes: Direct Supervision and Reporting Guidelines

but does not have to provide 24-hour, in-house coverage. One provider reports the appropriate code only once per day, even though multiple providers may have interacted with the patient during the 24-hour global period (eg, on-call physician, NNP).

Medical Record Documentation

The medical record serves the dual purposes of communicating the medical status and progress of the patient and documenting the work of the reporting provider.

Based on the information presented previously, it is the suggestion of the American Academy of Pediatrics Committee on Coding and Nomenclature that the medical record documentation by the reporting physician or NPP supporting critical care codes should contain the following at a minimum:

- Documentation of the critical status of the infant or child (This is not to be inferred.)
- Documentation of the *bedside* direction and supervision of all aspects of care
- Review of pertinent historical information and verification of significant physical findings through a medically indicated, focused patient examination
- Documentation of all services provided by members of the care team and discussion and direction of the ongoing therapy and plan of care for the patient
- Additional documentation of any major change in patient course requiring significant hands-on intervention by the reporting provider

The following are *not* required of the reporting physician or NPP:

- Twenty-four–hour presence in the facility or bedside
- Two or more documented notes a day
- Personally ordering all tests, medications, and therapies
- Performing all or any of the bundled procedures
- Documenting a daily comprehensive physical examination
- Documenting stable or unstable status so long as the infant or child meets critical care criteria

Each patient has a different level of illness(es), grouping of diagnoses, and medical and socioeconomic problems. The following are only examples of notes and should not be interpreted as requirements in every note for each patient:

A. The following note represents a sample attestation that could be appended to a resident or fellow's progress note:

"I have reviewed the resident's progress note and the baby has been seen and examined by me. He continues to be critically ill with respiratory failure requiring mechanical ventilation. I concur with the resident's evaluation and findings, though I did not appreciate abdominal tenderness on examination. I have discussed and agreed on a plan of care with the resident."

B. The following 2 paragraphs represent a single sample documentation that a reporting physician might write when care is delivered by an NNP and physician team. This note could be appended by the reporting physician to the NNP documentation or written as separate physician documentation.

"(Name) has been seen and examined by me on bedside rounds. The interval history, laboratory findings, and physical examination of the patient have been reviewed with members of the neonatal team. The notes have been reviewed. All aspects of care have been discussed, and I have agreed on an assessment and plan for the day with the care team.

"(Name) continues to be critically ill, requiring high-frequency jet ventilation. On examination, her breath sounds are coarse but equal, there is no heart murmur, and the abdomen is soft and non-tender. Her oxygen requirements have been at 100% for the past 12 hours. She remains on antibiotics for *Proteus* sepsis. At the recommendation of infectious disease, we have changed her antibiotic coverage to cefotaxime and gentamicin. Her blood pressure is acceptable today, but her urine output is only at 1 mL/kg/h. We are watching this closely and may need to restart dopamine. She remains NPO and is on total parenteral nutrition."

Approach to Documentation

This information deals largely with neonatal care. However, the same coding and documentation principles apply for critical care services provided to all children through the age of 5 years. The guidelines provided in this statement represent clarification of documentation recommendations for this unique code set. They are intended to create clarity going forward for physicians and other parties as they incorporate this new guidance into their documentation processes. Physicians should structure their documentation such that on review of a medical record representing a physician-rendered per-day neonatal or pediatric critical care service, one should be able to discern the reporting physician's unique documentation in support of the physician's role in that patient's care. It is especially important that an electronic health record used in documenting these services be configured to uniquely identify the author of each entry and allow for timely response to requests for documentation substantiating billed services. It is equally as important to log out of the record when your documentation is complete.

Appendixes

V. Test Your Knowledge! Answer Key

Chapter 1

1. *d.* The medical record should be complete and legible.

2. *c.* The code assigned for the condition chiefly responsible for the services provided

3. *b.* Do not report codes for conditions that have been previously treated but no longer exist.

4. *d.* Extremely low birth weight newborn, unspecified weight (**P07.00**) indicates that either the birth weight was undocumented or the wrong code was selected.

5. *a.* Three categories are included in the *Current Procedural Terminology* (*CPT*®) (Healthcare Common Procedure Coding System Level I) code set. Certain codes may be updated more frequently than the annual update.

Chapter 2

1. *a.* Modifiers add context to how or when the service was provided.

2. *d.* Modifier **24** is appended to a code for an unrelated E/M service during the postoperative period of a procedure provided by the physician or other qualified health care professional.

3. *b.* **XS**, separate structure (site/organ), is a potential substitute for modifier **59**, as are modifiers **XE**, **XP**, and **XU**.

4. *a.* Modifier **66** is appended to the basic procedure code when highly complex procedures are carried out under the surgical team concept.

5. *a.* A code pair identifies services that should not normally be billed by the same physician for the same patient on the same date of service.

Chapter 3

1. *c.* When the period for which information is needed overlaps with the period for which the patient is or was enrolled in the health plan

2. *b.* The percentage of children 2 years of age who had 1 or more capillary or venous lead blood test for lead poisoning on or by their second birthday would not apply to a child who turns 3 years old during the measurement year.

3. *b.* False. Modifier **8P** allows the reporting of circumstances when an action described in a measure's numerator is not performed and the reason is not otherwise specified.

4. *c.* The Alphabetical Clinical Topics Listing does not provide a complete description of each measure. The listing directs the reader to the measure developer's website to access the complete description of the measure.

Chapter 4

1. *d.* Physician work, practice expense, and professional liability are components of the Resource-Based Relative Value Scale.

2. *c.* *International Classification of Diseases, 10th Revision, Clinical Modification* codes selected in the electronic health record for an encounter should be placed in the order of responsibility for the service(s) provided.

3. *a.* Place of service **11** designates that services were provided in a physician's office.

4. *b.* Review claim adjustment reason and remittance advice remark codes.

5. *c.* The practice shares either reward or loss depending on actual total costs versus budgeted costs.

Chapter 5

1. *a.* Coding all services at the same level is an abusive billing practice. Answers b, c, and d are examples of fraudulent practices.

2. *a.* Privacy concerns and federal and state regulatory requirements should be taken into consideration.

3. *d.* A desired attribute or qualification of a compliance officer is experience in billing and coding.

4. *d.* Contact legal counsel as soon as possible. Make sure the attorney or legal practice has experience with audits.

Chapter 6

1. *d.* Office and other outpatient E/M services **99202–99205** and **99211–99215**

2. *b.* History, examination, and medical decision-making are the key components in selecting the level of E/M services.

3. *b.* History of present illness. If the information was gathered as a description of the development of the problem, consider it as history of present illness.

4. *a.* Performance and documentation of at least 6 elements identified by a bullet (●) in 1 or more areas or systems supports a problem-focused general multisystem examination.

5. *b.* Low. Use of over-the-counter medication supports low risk. The highest level of risk in any one category (ie, presenting problem[s], diagnostic procedure[s], or management options) determines the overall risk.

Chapter 7

1. *a.* Because the allergist and primary care physician are not of the same specialty, the patient is new.

2. *d.* A schoolteacher is an example of a professional who is not a health care professional but may be involved in the management of the patient.

3. *c.* All of the physician's or QHP's time on the date of service spent on care of the patient may be included. Clinical staff time is not included.

4. *a.* The number of categories and requirements vary for each level.

5. *b.* Any 2 of 3 elements (ie, problems addressed, data, risk) must be met.

Chapter 8

1. *a.* The request for consultation must be documented.

2. *b.* False. Travel time to and from a patient's home is assumed to be in the level of care, just as travel time to and from the hospital is included in hospital care codes and is not counted in the time spent.

3. *d.* An interval history, not requiring past, family, or social history, is used in selecting the level of history.

4. *a.* Prolonged service codes **99356** and **99357** are used to report 30 minutes or more of a physician's or other qualified health care professional's prolonged unit/floor time of an evaluation and management service provided on the same date as nursing facility services.

Chapter 9

1. *d.* A new complaint is an abnormal finding. A known or chronic condition that has increased in severity is also an abnormal finding.

2. *a.* Codes **90460** and **90461** are reported for immunization administration when a physician or other qualified health care professional counsels the patient who is 18 years or younger.

3. *d.* Code **96110** is reported with either 2 units or on 2 claim lines with modifier **59** (distinct procedure) appended to **96110** on the second claim line.

4. *c.* Code **36410** is reported for venipuncture on a 4-year-old but only when a physician's skill is required. Otherwise, **36415** is reported.

5. *d.* Behavior change services may be reported when documentation supports that the time requirements of the selected code were met.

Chapter 10

1. *a.* The appropriate procedure code appended with modifier **24** (unrelated E/M service by the same physician during a postoperative period) would be reported.

2. *a.* A zero (0)-day global period applies to simple skin wound repair.

3. *c.* Layered closure of 1 or more of the deeper layers of subcutaneous tissue and superficial (non-muscle) fascia is an intermediate repair.

4. *c.* Codes **96360** and **96361** describe the initial infusion of hydration (prepackaged fluid and electrolytes) for the initial 31 minutes to 1 hour and each additional hour.

5. *b.* 1 unit of service is reported per injection (**96372**). Multiple units of service would be reported in conjunction with a Healthcare Common Procedure Coding System code describing the medication.

   ●=New code   ▲=Revised code   #=Re-sequenced code   +=Add-on code

Appendixes

Chapter 11

1. *a.* Modifier **26** indicates that only the professional component is reported.

2. *b.* Report code **36410** for venipuncture requiring a physician's skill for a child aged 3 years or older.

3. *c.* Report code **94060** for spirometry performed before and after inhalation treatment.

4. *d.* No modifier is required, as all audiological function testing services are bilateral.

5. *a.* An acute abdomen series (**74022**) includes 2 abdominal views and a single chest view.

Chapter 12

1 *d.* All are true for transitional care management (TCM) services.

2. *a.* All patients receiving CCM services must be provided a copy of their plan of care. Twenty minutes of clinical staff time is required for **99490**, and patients must have 2 chronic conditions.

3. *b.* At least moderate-complexity medical decision-making is required for patients receiving TCM.

4. *c.* Physician time integrating new information into the patient's care plan may be credited to the time of care plan oversight.

5. *b.* **99358** × 1, **99359** × 1 are correct for 75 to 104 minutes of prolonged service.

Chapter 13

1. *d.* Scope of practice is used by state licensing boards to define the procedures, actions, and processes that are permitted for a licensed individual.

2. *c.* Clinical staff may administer an injection under direct supervision of the ordering physician under incident-to policy.

3. *c.* Assessment and management are required to report **99211**.

4. *d.* In the absence of a newborn or infant feeding problem, the mother is typically the patient and claims are filed to her health benefit plan.

5. *c.* **AE** is used to indicate services by a registered dietitian. **AJ** indicates services by a clinical social worker. **RD** (not discussed in this chapter) indicates a drug was provided to a beneficiary, but not administered incident to. MN is not a valid modifier.

Chapter 14

1. *d.* Health plans often cover mental and behavioral health services under a provider network separate from other health services.

2. *c.* Report **96112** for the first 60 minutes and **96113** × 2 for the final 60 minutes.

3. *b.* False. At least 2 distinct tests must be administered and scored to report codes **96136–96139**. Do not separately count subtests in a multifaceted test (eg, Wechsler Preschool and Primary Scale of Intelligence is 1 test with 14 subtests).

4. *a.* Code **97155** is only reported when a physician or other qualified health care professional (QHP) provides face-to-face care to a single patient. For **0373T**, a physician or QHP is on-site during the service.

5. *d.* Psychiatric collaborative care management is reported by a primary care physician for supervision of a behavioral health manager working in collaboration with a psychiatric consultant.

Chapter 15

1. *b.* The neonate who is born on September 1 (day 0) is 29 days old on September 30.

2. *b.* **99460** and **99238** or **99239** are reported for the physician's initial care on February 16, 2021, and discharge services on the next calendar date, February 17, 2021.

3. *b.* **99462**. The service to an asymptomatic neonate who is monitored but not treated is subsequent normal newborn care.

4. *d.* Physician time of more than 30 minutes on unit/floor devoted to care of the individual patient is reported with code **99239**.

5. *a.* **99231–99233** (subsequent hospital care) is reported by the pediatrician who assumes management of a sick neonate transferred from intensive or critical care.

●=New code ▲=Revised code #=Re-sequenced code +=Add-on code

Chapter 16

1. *c.* Physicians select codes based on the total unit/floor time dedicated to 1 patient. Time spent off the unit/floor is not included in the total unit/floor time.

2. *c.* Comprehensive history and physical examinations are required for both **99219** and **99220**. However, medical decision-making is moderate for **99291** and high for **99220**.

3. *c.* Codes **99234–99236** are reported based on the total care provided when a patient is admitted and discharged on the same date.

4. *d.* Codes **99221–99223** include all evaluation and management (E/M) services by the same physician (or physicians of the same specialty and same group practice) on the date of the initial hospital care.

5. *b.* The E/M service extended 65 minutes beyond the typical time of 25 minutes. Code **99356** includes 30 to 74 minutes beyond the time of the related E/M service.

Chapter 17

1. *c.* The physician must designate only 1 sign, symptom, disease, or injury as the chief complaint.

2. *b.* All 3 key components must support code selection except when the ED caveat applies.

3. *d.* Certain procedures, as specified in *CPT*, are included in critical care services. Time of separately reported procedures is not included in the time of critical care.

4. *d.* All of the above, including permanent image documentation, thorough evaluation, and a written report, are required.

5. *c.* Modifier **26** (professional component) is required. The facility may report the same code with modifier **TC** (technical component).

Chapter 18

1. *a.* The time required to report code **99291** must be met by a single physician. However, cumulative time spent by physicians or other qualified health care professionals of the same specialty and same group practice later on the same date may be reported with **99292**.

2. *c.* Provision of positive-pressure ventilation in response to respiratory instability supports neonatal resuscitation code **99465**.

3. *d.* All of the answers must be true for a cardiologist to report hourly critical care when a neonatologist is reporting daily neonatal critical care.

4. *c.* **99480** (subsequent intensive care) is reported for a second initial intensive care service in 1 admission for a patient with present body weight of 2,501 to 5,000 g.

5. *b.* The same physician may report overall patient management (eg, **99468**) and/or cannula insertion in addition to initiation of extracorporeal membrane oxygenation/extracorporeal life support, when provided.

Chapter 19

1. *c.* Services during the postoperative period to manage complications *that do not require return to the operating room* are included in the global period as defined by the Centers for Medicare & Medicaid Services.

2. *a.* No modifier is required when a physician other than the surgeon (or the surgeons in the same group practice) provides unrelated services to a patient during the postoperative period.

3. *d.* The teaching physician must be present only for the critical or key portions of a surgery that is not a minor or a complex or high-risk procedure.

4. *a.* Codes **36568** and **36569** are reported for peripherally inserted central catheter insertion without a subcutaneous port *and without imaging guidance* based on the patient's age.

5. *c.* **99155**, **99157** × 1. Code **99155** represents the first 15 minutes of service. Because the intraservice time extended 9 minutes past the first 15-minute period (ie, past the midpoint between the first and second 15-minute period), code **99157** is reported for the final 9 minutes of intraservice time.

●=New code   ▲=Revised code   #=Re-sequenced code   +=Add-on code

Appendixes

Chapter 20

1. **d.** None of these would be reported as an online digital evaluation and management (E/M) service based on *Current Procedural Terminology* guidelines, which require patient initiation, no related E/M service within 7 days, and service by a physician or other qualified health care professional.

2. **b.** Collection and interpretation of physiologic data collected over a 30-day period is included in the service reported with **99091**. Code **99457** is reported for remote physiologic monitoring treatment management services requiring interactive communication.

3. **a.** Medicaid plans typically align with state regulations for telemedicine services.

4. **c.** Modifier **95** should be appended to the code for telemedicine services.

5. **a.** The physician's total time devoted to the patient on the date of service is used in code selection only for office E/M services. Time of other E/M services may be limited to time spent in communication with the patient and/or caregivers via telemedicine technology.

Appendixes

INDEXES

Subject Index
Code Index

Subject Index

Digital medicine services. *See also* Telemedicine
collection and interpretation of digitally stored
data, 500–504
continuing changes in, 510
online digital E/M, 305–306, 495–496
remote interprofessional consultations, 497–499
remote physiologic data, 306, 499–504
Dilantin, 276
Diphenhydramine hydrochloride, 276
Diphtheria, tetanus toxoids, acellular pertussis,
inactivated poliovirus, and *Haemophilus
influenzae* type b (DTaP-IPV/Hib)
combination vaccine, 206–207
Direct optical observation, 269
Direct prolonged services, 402–403
Discharge day management
hospital, 394–395
observation care, 388–389
perinatal care, 374
Discharge services
nursing facility, 191
observation or inpatient hospital care services
(including admission and discharge
services), 389–391
Discharge summary, 18
Discharge versus subsequent hospital services,
395–396
Discontinued procedure, 37–38
Distinct procedural service, 40
Documentation
advice from payers, 105
coding audits and, 90, 107, 109
compliance programs for medical record,
103–104
evaluation and management (E/M). *See*
Evaluation and management (E/M)
documentation and coding guidelines
general principles of medical record, 120
incident-to services, 316
records retention, 105
telemedicine services, 507
time, 18
*Documentation Guidelines for Evaluation and
Management Services,* 117–118
Domiciliary, rest home, or custodial care services,
188–189
Drainage
integumentary, 237–238
pericardial, 473
Drug amount discarded/not administered to any
patient, 48
Drug tests, presumptive, 272
Drug therapy requiring intensive monitoring for
toxicity, 155
DuoNeb, 276
Dyslipidemia, 218

E

Ear, nose, mouth, and throat procedures
adenoidectomy and tonsillectomy, 463, 481
control of nasal hemorrhage, 246–247
examination, 128, 131–132
foreign body removal from, 35
laryngoplasty, 480
removal of impacted cerumen, 247–248
Eating habits, 220
ECLS. *See* Extracorporeal life support (ECLS)
ECMO. *See* Extracorporeal membrane oxygenation
(ECMO)

Edits, coding
appropriate modifiers, 49–50
keeping up to date with, 51–52
Medically Unlikely, 50–51
NCCI, 49
procedure-to-procedure, 49
reviewing and using, 52
Education and training for patient self-
management, 318–319
EHR. *See* Electronic health records (EHRs)
Electrocardiogram, 266
Electronic health records (EHRs), 80
capturing encounter and billing information
in, 80–81
consultation, 306, 400
pitfalls of coding, 104
E/M. *See* Evaluation and management (E/M)
Emergency department (ED) services. *See also*
Critical care services
asthma, 427–428
code modifiers, 423–425
comanagement of ED patients, 417–418
common procedures, 421
critical care in, 418–420
diagnosis code reporting, 411–412
directing emergency medical technicians, 418
E/M codes, 412–418
head injury, 429
laceration, 430–431
point-of-care ultrasound, 421–423
reporting procedures in, 420–425
sedation, 425–426
special service codes, 426–427
Emergency medical services (EMS)
direction of, 418, 451–452
patient transport, 449–451
Emergency office services, 173–174
Emotional/behavioral assessment, 214–215, 283
Encounter dominated by counseling or
coordination of care, 142
Encounter forms, 81–84
Encounter story, telling the, 5–6
Endocrinology services, 282–283
Endoscopy, 467
End-stage renal disease, 509
Enteral feeding, 302, 304
Enterostomy, 482
EOB. *See* Explanation of benefits (EOB)
EP (modifier), 47
Epilepsy, 70, 348, 501, 502
Epinephrine, 276
auto-injector administration, 281
EpiPen kits, 281
Established patient(s). *See also* New patient(s)
domiciliary, rest home, or custodial care
services, 188
home care services, 187
initial nursing facility care, 190
office and outpatient consultation codes, 184
office visit codes, 151–152
preventive medicine E/M services, 199–200
Evaluation and management (E/M)
code categories, 118
code components, 118–119
coded from clinical perspective, 118
coding guidelines. *See* Evaluation and
management (E/M) documentation and
coding guidelines
contributory factors, 119
critical care, 194–196

documentation guidelines. *See* Evaluation and
management (E/M) documentation and
coding guidelines
domiciliary, rest home, or custodial care
services, 188–189
emergency department (ED) services codes,
412–418
hearing and vision screening, 211–213
home care services, 186–187
modifiers and, 29
neonate, 372
new versus established patients in, 151–152
noncritical hospital. *See* Noncritical hospital
E/M services
in noncritical nonhospital settings. *See*
Noncritical nonhospital E/M services
nonphysician services, 317–318
nursing facility care, 189–192
office and other outpatient. *See* Office and other
outpatient E/M services
office and other outpatient consultations,
182–186
online digital services, 305–306, 495–496
out-of-office service add-on codes, 192
preventive services. *See* Preventive services
prolonged, in the inpatient setting, 402–404
psychiatric evaluation and psychotherapy
without, 328–329
psychotherapy with, 352–353
shared/split, 142–143, 156, 172
significant, separately identifiable E/M service
by the same physician or other qualified
health care professional on the same day of
the procedure or other service, 31–32
telephone services, 193, 306
time of E/M services, 16–19
unrelated E/M service by the same physician
or other qualified health care professional
during a postoperative period, 30
in urgent care facilities, 152–153
Evaluation and management (E/M) documentation
and coding guidelines, 117–118
categories of E/M codes, 118
chief complaint (CC), 121, 122
CMS guidelines, 117–118
code components, 118–119
coding E/M services from a clinical
perspective, 118
coding tips, 143
complexity of medical decision-making, 139–142
contributory factors, 119
counseling or coordination of care, 142
CPT guidelines, 117
documentation of E/M services, 120–142
encounter dominated by counseling or
coordination of care, 142
examination, 126–139
explicit component (time), 119
general principles of medical record
documentation, 120
history, 121–125
history of present illness (HPI), 121–123
importance of documentation, 119–120
key components, 118–119
level of history performed, 125
medical student, 144–145
past, family, and social history (PFSH), 122,
123, 124–125
payers, 120
primary care exception rule, 145
review of systems (ROS), 122, 123–124

CODE INDEX

References are to pages. **Boldfaced** page numbers indicate the pages on which the primary code descriptions reside. *Current Procedural Terminology (CPT®)* codes begin on this page; *International Classification of Diseases 10th Revision, Clinical Modification (ICD-10-CM)* codes begin on page 553; and Healthcare Common Procedure Coding System (HCPCS) codes begin on page 555.

CPT Codes

HCPCS Codes